General Ophthalmology

. . . Now do you not see that the eye embraces the beauty of the whole world? It is the lord of astronomy and the maker of cosmography; it counsels and corrects all the arts of mankind; it leads men to the different parts of the world; it is the prince of mathematics, and the sciences founded on it are absolutely certain. It has measured the distances and sizes of the stars; it has found the elements and their locations; it . . . has given birth to architecture, and to perspective, and to the divine art of painting. Oh excellent thing, superior to all others created by God! . . . What peoples, what tongues will fully describe your true function? The eye is the window of the human body through which it feels its way and enjoys the beauty of the world. Owing to the eye the soul is content to stay in its bodily prison, for without it such bodily prison is torture.

–Leonardo da Vinci (1452– 1519)

ELEVENTH EDITION

General Ophthalmology

Daniel Vaughan, MD

Clinical Professor of Ophthalmology
University of California, San Francisco
Member, Francis I. Proctor Foundation
for Research in Ophthalmology

Taylor Asbury, MD

Clinical Professor of Ophthalmology
College of Medicine
University of Cincinnati

Illustrated by
Laurel V. Schaubert

LMP LANGE Medical Publications/Los Altos, California

APPLETON-CENTURY-CROFTS/Norwalk, Connecticut ACC

Copyright © 1986 by Appleton-Century-Crofts
A Publishing Division of Prentice-Hall
Copyright © 1983, 1980, 1977, 1974, 1971, 1968, 1965, 1962, 1960, 1958
by Lange Medical Publications

Italian Edition: *Piccin Nuova Libraria, S.p.A., Via Altinate, 107, 35121 Padua, Italy*
Spanish Edition: *Editorial El Manual Moderno, S.A. de C.V.,*
Av. Sonora 206, Col. Hipodromo, 06100-Mexico, D.F.
Polish Edition: *Panstwowy Zaklad Wydawnictw Lekarskich,*
P.O. Box 379, 00-950 Warsaw 1, Poland
Portuguese Edition: *Atheneu Editora São Paulo Ltda., Rua Marconi, 131-2.o andar,*
01047 São Paulo, Brazil
German Edition: *Springer-Verlag GmbH & Co. KG, Postfach 10 52 80,*
6900 Heidelberg 1, West Germany

87 88 89 90 / 10 9 8 7 6 5 4 3 2

Prentice-Hall of Australia, Pty. Ltd., Sydney
Prentice-Hall Canada, Inc.
Prentice-Hall Hispanoamericana, S.A., Mexico
Prentice-Hall of India Private Limited, New Delhi
Prentice-Hall International (UK) Limited, London
Prentice-Hall of Japan Inc., Tokyo
Prentice-Hall of Southeast Asia (Pte.) Ltd., Singapore
Whitehall Books Ltd., Wellington, New Zealand
Editora Prentice-Hall do Brasil Ltda., Rio de Janeiro

ISBN: 0-8385-3108-3

PRINTED IN THE UNITED STATES OF AMERICA

This edition of
General Ophthalmology
is dedicated to
Dr. and Mrs. Heinrich König

Table of Contents

8. Conjunctiva (cont'd)

Michael D. Sanders, FRCP, FRCS, & Elizabeth M. Graham, MRCP, DO

The Authors

Taylor Asbury, MD
Clinical Professor of Ophthalmology, University of Cincinnati School of Medicine, Cincinnati.

Roderick Biswell, MD
Assistant Clinical Professor of Ophthalmology, University of California School of Medicine, San Francisco.

J. Brooks Crawford, MD
Associate Clinical Professor of Ophthalmology, University of California School of Medicine, San Francisco.

Howard M. Eggers, MD
Assistant Professor of Ophthalmology, Columbia University School of Medicine, New York.

Philip P. Ellis, MD
Professor of Ophthalmology and Chairman of Department of Ophthalmology, University of Colorado School of Medicine, Denver.

F. T. Fraunfelder, MD
Professor of Ophthalmology and Chairman of Department of Ophthalmology, The Oregon Health Sciences University, Portland, Oregon.

Elizabeth M. Graham, MRCP, DO
Research Fellow in Medical Ophthalmology, St. Thomas' Hospital and National Hospital for Nervous Diseases, London.

S. Martha Meyer, BS
Research Associate, Department of Ophthalmology, The Oregon Health Sciences University, Portland, Oregon.

Conor O'Malley, MD
220 Meridian Avenue, San Jose, California.

Michael D. Sanders, FRCP, FRCS
Consultant Ophthalmologist, St. Thomas' Hospital and National Hospital for Nervous Diseases, London.

John P. Shock, MD
Professor of Ophthalmology and Chairman of Department of Ophthalmology, University of Arkansas School of Medicine, Little Rock.

John H. Sullivan, MD
Associate Clinical Professor of Ophthalmology, University of California School of Medicine, San Francisco.

Khalid F. Tabbara, MD
Professor of Ophthalmology and Chairman of Department of Ophthalmology, King Khaled Eye Specialist Hospital, Riyadh, Saudi Arabia.

Daniel Vaughan, MD
Clinical Professor of Ophthalmology, University of California School of Medicine, San Francisco; Member, Francis I. Proctor Foundation for Research in Ophthalmology, San Francisco.

Orson W. White, MD
Associate Clinical Professor of Ophthalmology, University of Utah School of Medicine, Salt Lake City.

Acknowledgments

Arthur K. Asbury
Crowell Beard
Diane Beeston
Laurie Vaughan Campbell
Patricia Cunnane
Chandler Dawson
J. Winston Duggan
Mitchell H. Friedlaender
Hans Beat Gassmann
Margaret Henry
Harry Hind
William F. Hoyt
Geraldine Hruby
Marianne Thalmann Huslid
Vicente Jocson
Philip Knapp

Raga Malaty
G. Richard O'Connor
Patrick O'Malley
Bruce Ostler
Patricia Pascoe
Kenneth D. Rogers
Joel G. Sacks
Robert N. Shaffer
Lionel W. Sorenson
Christopher B. Stephenson
Ralph T. Sutton
Phillips Thygeson
Ruth Lee Thygeson
Margot Vaughan
H. Ward Wick

Preface

In keeping with our goal of presenting the most current, complete, and authoritative treatment of the subject, the eleventh edition of *General Ophthalmology* represents a major revision and updating of the work. It contains the following changes from the tenth edition:

- A completely rewritten chapter on Strabismus, featuring modern concepts of surgical and nonsurgical treatment.
- A revised chapter on the Vitreous, introducing new concepts of fluid dynamics in retinal detachment. The illustrations are unique and instructive.

All references have been brought up to date, and the following additional improvements have been introduced:

- A new section on ocular and systemic side effects of drugs has been added to the chapter on Commonly Used Eye Medications.
- The chapter on Optics and Refraction is simplified and appropriately illustrated to make it more accessible to the ophthalmology resident. These improvements reflect the increasing importance of optics, especially in view of the popularity of contact lenses and intraocular lenses.
- Discussion of the ocular effects of AIDS is incorporated into appropriate chapters.
- The section on Special Ophthalmologic Examinations has been expanded to include discussions of automated perimetry, potential acuity measurement, CT scan, MRI, and ultrasonography.
- The chapter on the Cornea now has a discussion of refractive corneal surgery, including the new and controversial procedures radial keratotomy, keratomileusis, and epikeratophakia.
- The Lens chapter revision details recent developments in intraocular lenses and neodymium-YAG laser therapy for after-cataract.
- The Glaucoma chapter includes discussions of pressure dynamics, laser trabeculoplasty and iridectomy, therapeutic ultrasound, and some very new drug regimens.
- The chapter on Neuro-ophthalmology has been updated with new photos showing CT scans and MRI.
- The chapter on Systemic Diseases has been extensively revised. Immunosuppressive agents are discussed, and many new photos of retinal disorders have been added.
- The Pediatrics chapter now includes the most modern concepts of retinopathy of prematurity, ophthalmia neonatorum, and amblyopia.
- The Genetics chapter emphasizes the latest information on the mechanisms of inheritance in genetic ocular disorders.

Additionally,

- Prevention of iatrogenic ocular infections is now covered in Chapter 26.
- Chapter 27 includes coverage of blindness associated with xerophthalmia and cataracts and a discussion of low vision aid clinics.
- The Glossary of Terms has been expanded to reflect new information in the book.

As before, it remains the objective of *General Ophthalmology* to present a concise and current review of the subject for medical students, ophthalmology residents, practicing ophthalmologists, nurses, optometrists, and our colleagues in other fields of medicine and surgery, as well as allied health personnel. In achieving this objective we have relied on the assistance of many authorities in special fields, who have reviewed the manuscript of the eleventh edition with great care and given us the benefit of their advice.

We wish to express our gratitude in particular to Dr. Paul Riordan Eva, who made a monumental effort to review the entire manuscript, and to Dr. David F. Chang, who revised the retina and examination chapters.

Daniel Vaughan
Taylor Asbury

May, 1986

Anatomy

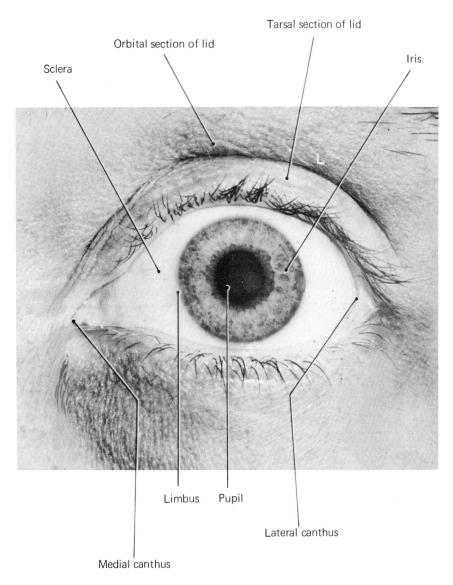

Figure 1–1. External landmarks of the eye. The sclera is covered by transparent conjunctiva. (Photo by HL Gibson, from: *Medical Radiography and Photography*. Labeling modified slightly.)

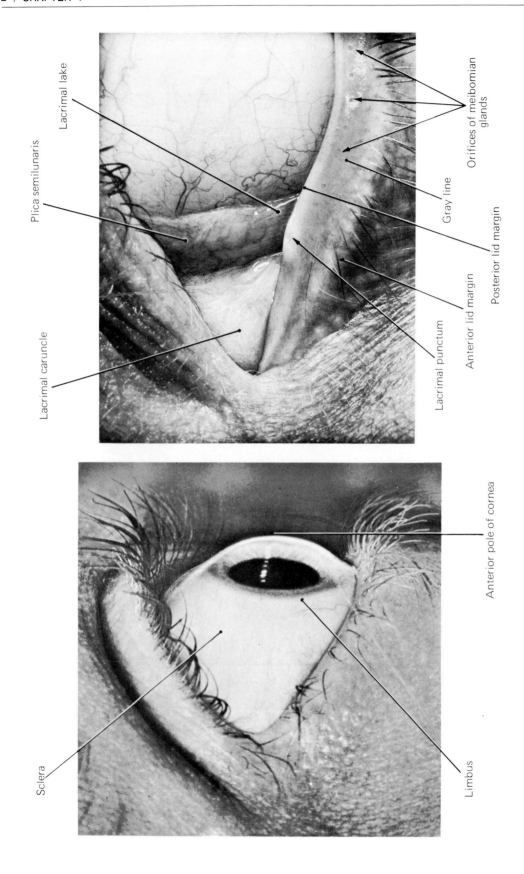

Figure 1–2. External landmarks of the eye. The sclera is covered by transparent conjunctiva. (Photos by HL Gibson, from: *Medical Radiography and Photography*. Labeling modified slightly.)

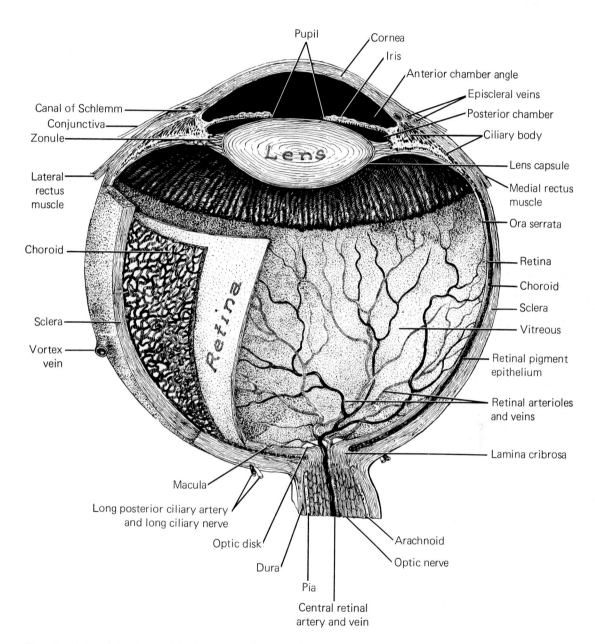

Pupil
Cornea
Iris
Anterior chamber angle
Episcleral veins
Posterior chamber
Ciliary body
Lens capsule
Medial rectus muscle
Ora serrata
Retina
Choroid
Sclera
Vitreous
Retinal pigment epithelium
Retinal arterioles and veins
Lamina cribrosa
Arachnoid
Optic nerve

Canal of Schlemm
Conjunctiva
Zonule
Lateral rectus muscle
Choroid
Sclera
Vortex vein
Macula
Long posterior ciliary artery and long ciliary nerve
Optic disk
Dura
Pia
Central retinal artery and vein

Lens
Retina

Figure 1–3. Internal structures of the human eye. (Redrawn from an original drawing by Paul Peck and reproduced, with permission, from: *The Anatomy of the Eye.* Courtesy of Lederle Laboratories.)

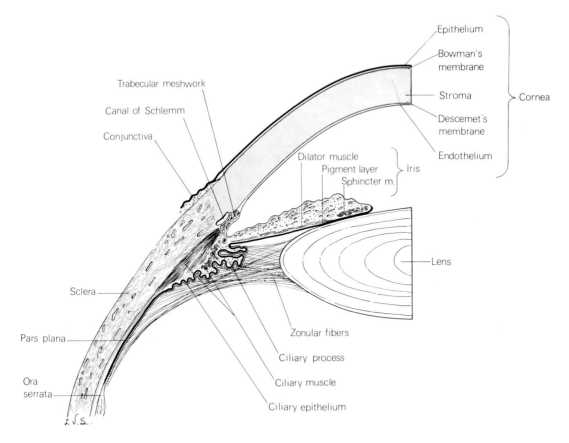

Figure 1–4. Anterior chamber angle and surrounding structures.

Figure 1–5. Photomicrograph of anterior chamber angle and related structures. (Courtesy of I Wood and L Garron).

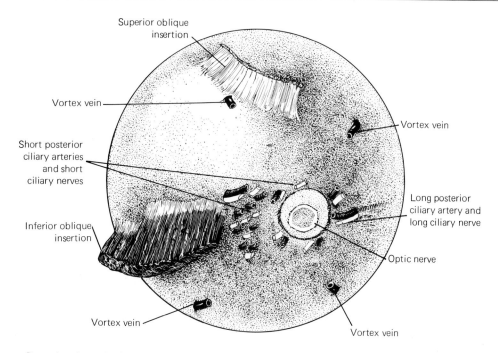

Figure 1–6. Posterior view of left eye. (Redrawn and reproduced, with permission, from Wolff E: *Anatomy of the Eye and Orbit,* 4th ed. Blakiston-McGraw, 1954.)

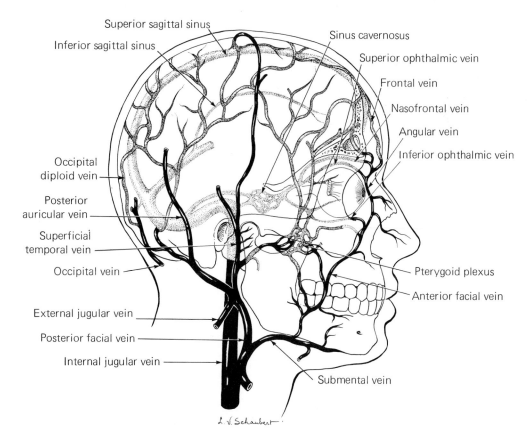

Figure 1–7. Venous drainage system of the eye. (Redrawn and reproduced, with permission, from Wolff E: *Anatomy of the Eye and Orbit,* 4th ed. Blakiston-McGraw, 1954.)

Figure 1–8. Lateral view of eye and surrounding structures.

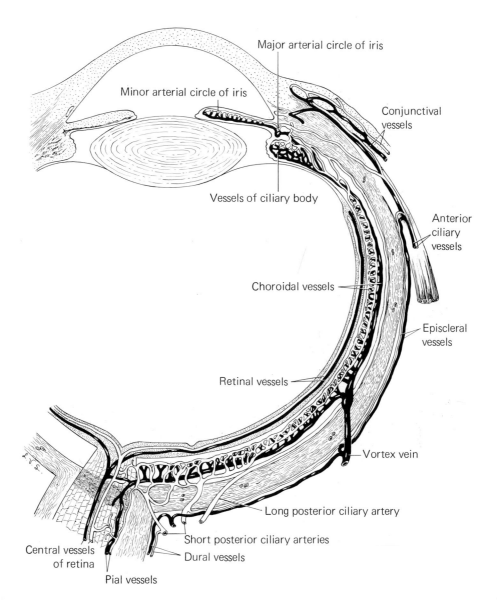

Figure 1–9. Vascular supply to the eye. All arterial branches originate with the ophthalmic artery. Venous drainage is through the cavernous sinus and the pterygoid plexus.

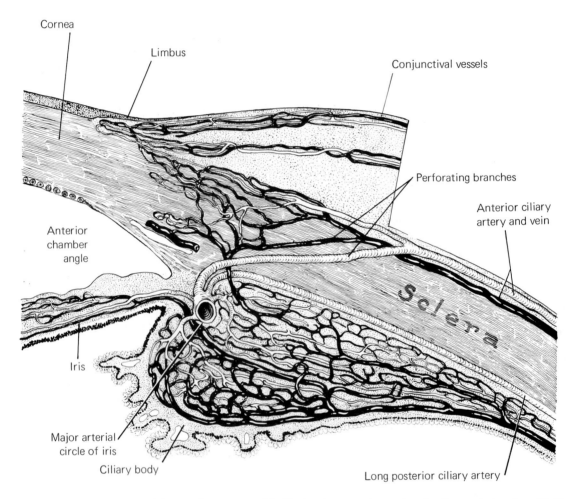

Figure 1–10. Vascular supply of the anterior segment. (Modified, redrawn, and reproduced, with permission, from Wolff E: *Anatomy of the Eye and Orbit,* 4th ed. Blakiston-McGraw, 1954.)

Growth, Development, & Senescence 2

EMBRYOLOGY OF THE EYE
(Fig 2–1)

OPTIC VESICLE STAGE

The earliest embryonic stage at which ocular structures can be differentiated from the rest of the fetus is the embryonic plate stage. The site of the eye is indicated by flattened areas on both sides of the anterior end of the neural groove. The edges of the neural groove (2.5-mm stage or 2-week stage) thicken to form the neural folds. The folds fuse to form the neural tube, which sinks into the underlying mesoderm and detaches from the surface ectoderm. Before the anterior end of the neural tube is completely closed, buds of neural ectoderm grow toward the surface ectoderm on either side to form the spherical optic vesicles (4-mm or 3-week stage). These vesicles are connected to the forebrain by the optic stalks. At the 4-mm stage, a thickening of the surface ectoderm, the lens plate, begins to form just opposite the ends of the optic vesicles.

OPTIC CUP STAGE

The optic vesicle invaginates to produce the optic cup, so that the original outer wall of the optic vesicle becomes approximated to its inner wall. Invagination of the lower surface of the optic stalk and the optic vesicle occurs simultaneously, creating a groove known as the choroidal (fetal) fissure. At the same time, the lens plate also invaginates to form first a cup and then a hollow sphere known as the lens vesicle. By the 9-mm (4-week) stage, the lens vesicle separates completely from the surface ectoderm to lie free in the rim of the optic cup.

The choroidal fissure permits entrance into the optic stalk of the vascular mesoderm that eventually forms the hyaloid system. As invagination becomes complete, the choroidal fissure narrows until it becomes completely closed (13-mm or 6-week stage), leaving one small permanent opening at the anterior end of the optic stalk through which pass the hyaloid artery until the 100-mm (4-month) stage and the central retinal artery and vein thereafter.

At this point, the ultimate general structure of the eye has been determined. Further development consists of differentiation into individual structures. In general, differentiation occurs relatively more rapidly in the posterior than in the anterior segment early in gestation and more rapidly in the anterior segment later in gestation.

EMBRYONIC ORIGINS OF INDIVIDUAL EYE STRUCTURES*

Surface Ectoderm
Lens; epithelium of cornea, conjunctiva, lacrimal gland and drainage system; vitreous (mesoderm also contributes to vitreous).

Neural Ectoderm
Vitreous, retina; epithelium of iris, ciliary body, and retina; pupillary muscle sphincter and dilator, optic nerve.

Mesoderm
Sclera; stroma of cornea, conjunctiva, iris, ciliary body, choroid; extraocular muscles, lids (except epithelium and conjunctiva), hyaloid system (gone by birth), sheaths of the optic nerve; connective tissue and blood supply of eye, bony orbit, and vitreous.

EMBRYOLOGY OF SPECIFIC STRUCTURES

Lens
Soon after the lens vesicle lies free in the rim of the optic cup (13-mm or 6-week stage), the cells of its posterior wall elongate, encroach on the empty cavity, and finally fill it in (26-mm or 7-week stage). At about this stage (13-mm or 6-week), a hyaline capsule is secreted by the lens cells. Secondary lens fibers elongate from the equatorial region and grow forward under the subcapsular epithelium, which remains as a single layer of cuboid epithelial cells, and backward under the lens capsule. These fibers meet to form the lens sutures (upright "Y" anteriorly and inverted "Y" posteriorly), which are complete by the seventh month. (This growth and proliferation of secondary lens fibers continues at a decreasing rate

*Endoderm does not contribute to the formation of the eye.

2.5-mm stage

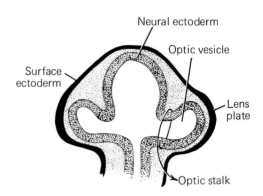

Forebrain of 4-mm embryo, optic vesicle stage

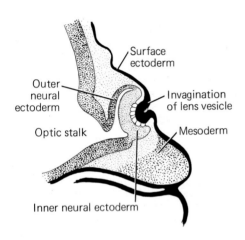

5-mm stage. Beginning formation of optic cup by invagination.

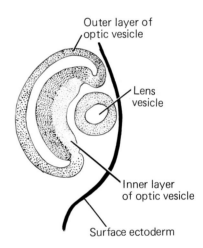

9-mm stage. Lens vesicle has separated from surface ectoderm and lies free in rim of optic cup.

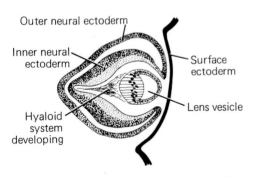

13-mm stage. Choroidal fissure closed. Posterior lens cells growing forward.

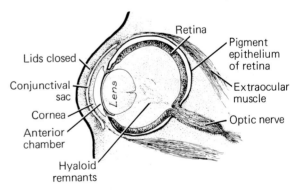

65-mm stage (3 months)

Figure 2–1. Embryologic development of ocular structures. (Redrawn and reproduced, with permission, from Mann IC: *The Development of the Human Eye,* 2nd ed. British Medical Association, 1950.)

throughout life; the lens therefore continues to enlarge slowly, causing compression of the lens fibers.)

Retina

The outer layer of the optic cup remains as a single layer and becomes the pigment epithelium of the retina. Pigmentation begins at the 10-mm (5-week) stage. The inner layer undergoes a complicated differentiation into the other 9 layers of the retina. This occurs slowly throughout gestation. By the seventh month, the outermost cell layer (consisting of the nuclei of the rods and cones) is present as well as the bipolar, amacrine, and ganglion cells and nerve fibers. The macular region is thicker than the rest of the retina until the eighth month, when macular depression begins to develop. Macular development is not complete until 6 months after birth.

Optic Nerve

The axons of the ganglion cell layer of the retina form the inner nerve fiber layer. The fibers slowly form the optic stalk and then the optic nerve (26-mm or 7-week stage). Mesodermal elements enter the surrounding tissue to form the vascular septa of the nerve. Medullation extends from the brain peripherally down the optic nerve, and at birth has reached the lamina cribrosa. Medullation is completed by age 3 months.

Iris & Ciliary Body

During the third month (50-mm stage), the rim of the optic cup grows forward in front of the lens as a double row of epithelium and lies posterior to mesoderm, which becomes the stroma of the iris. These 2 epithelial layers become pigmented in the iris, whereas only the outer layer is pigmented in the ciliary body. Folds appear in the epithelial layers of the ciliary body; mesoderm grows into this fold to form the ciliary processes. By the fifth month (150-mm stage), the sphincter muscle of the pupil is developing from a bud of nonpigmented epithelium derived from the anterior epithelial layer of the iris near the pupillary margin. Soon after the sixth month, the dilator muscle appears in the anterior epithelial layer near the ciliary body.

Choroid

At the 6-mm (3½-week) stage, a network of capillaries encircles the optic cup and develops into the choroid. By the 13-mm (6-week) stage, the outer neural epithelial layer has secreted Bruch's membrane. By the third month, the intermediate and large venous channels of the choroid are developed and drain into the vortex veins to exit from the eye.

Vitreous
(Fig 2–2)

A. First Stage: (Primary vitreous, 4.5- to 13-mm or 3- to 6-week stage.) At about the 4.5-mm stage, fibrils grow in from the inner layer of the optic vesicle to join elements from the lens vesicle that—along with some mesoderm fibrils associated with the hyaloid

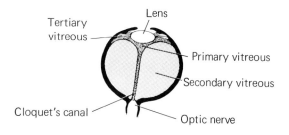

Figure 2–2. The vitreous. (Redrawn and reproduced, with permission, from Duke-Elder WS: *Textbook of Ophthalmology.* Vol 1. Mosby, 1942.)

artery—form the primary vitreous. This stage ends as the lens capsule appears, precluding any further lens participation in vitreous formation. The primary vitreous does not atrophy and ultimately lies just behind the posterior pole of the lens as the hyaloid canal.

B. Second Stage: (Secondary vitreous, 13- to 65-mm or 3- to 10-week stage.) Müller's fibers of the retina become continuous with vitreous fibrils, so that the secondary vitreous is mainly derived from retinal ectoderm. The hyaloid system develops a set of vitreous vessels as well as vessels on the lens capsule surface (tunica vasculosa lentis). The hyaloid system is at its height at 40 mm and then atrophies from posterior to anterior.

C. Third Stage: (Tertiary vitreous, 65 mm or 10 weeks on.) During the third month, the marginal bundle of Drualt is forming. This consists of vitreous fibrillar condensations extending from the future ciliary epithelium of the optic cup to the equator of the lens. Condensations then form the suspensory ligament of the lens, which is well developed by the 100-mm or 4-month stage. The hyaloid system atrophies completely during this stage.

Blood Vessels

Long ciliary arteries bud off from the hyaloid at the 16-mm (6-week) stage and anastomose around the optic cup margin with the major circle of the iris by the 30-mm (7-week) stage.

The hyaloid system (see Vitreous) atrophies completely by the eighth month. The hyaloid artery gives rise to the central retinal artery and its branches (100-mm or 4-month stage). Buds begin to grow into the retina and develop the retinal circulation, which reaches the ora serrata at 8 months. The branches of the central retinal vein develop simultaneously.

Cornea

The epithelium is derived from surface ectoderm, whereas the rest of the cornea comes from mesodermal structures. The earliest differentiation is seen at about the 12-mm (5-week) stage, when endothelial cells appear. Descemet's membrane is secreted by the flattened endothelial cells by the 75-mm (12-week) stage. The stroma slowly thickens, largely by an increase in the number of elastic fibers, and forms an anterior condensation just under the epithelium that is recognizable at 100 mm (4 months) as Bowman's membrane. A definite corneoscleral junction is present at 4 months.

Anterior Chamber

The anterior chamber of the eye first appears at 20 mm (7 weeks) and remains very shallow until birth. At 65 mm (9–10 weeks), Schlemm's canal appears as a vascular channel at the level of the recess of the angle and gradually assumes a relatively more anterior location as the angle recess develops. The iris, which in the early stages of development is quite anterior, gradually lies relatively more posteriorly as the chamber angle recess develops, most likely because of the difference in rate of growth of the anterior segment structures. The trabecular meshwork develops from the loose vascular mesodermal tissue lying originally at the margin of the optic cup. The aqueous drainage system is ready to function before birth.

Sclera & Extraocular Muscles

The sclera and extraocular muscles are formed from condensations of mesoderm encircling the optic cup and are first identifiable at the 20-mm (7-week) stage. Development of these structures is well advanced by the fourth month. Tenon's capsule appears about the insertions of the rectus muscles at the 80-mm (12-week) stage and is complete at 5 months.

Lids & Lacrimal Apparatus

The lids develop from mesoderm except for the skin and conjunctiva. The lid buds are first seen at 16 mm (6 weeks) growing in front of the eye, where they meet and fuse at the 37-mm (8-week) stage. They separate during the fifth month, and lashes and meibomian and other lid glands develop. The lacrimal gland (including the accessory glands and the conjunctiva) and drainage system develop from ectoderm. The canaliculi, lacrimal sac, and nasolacrimal duct are developed by burying a solid epithelial cord between the maxillary and nasal processes. This cord canalizes just before birth.

PATHOLOGY OF CONGENITAL OCULAR ABNORMALITIES

Congenital defects of the ocular structures have been described under 2 main headings: (1) developmental anomalies or dysplasias of embryonal origin and (2) tissue reactions to intrauterine inflammation in the latter months of gestation. Examples of the first type are the colobomas, dermoid tumors, anophthalmos, and microphthalmos. In the second category belong certain lesions of chorioretinitis similar to those seen in postnatal life and some forms of cataract.

Heredity plays a major role in many congenital deformities.

In reviewing the embryologic development of the eye, with its complex folds to form the optic vesicles, cornea, lens, and anterior chamber, it is obvious that any failure of regression of primitive vascular tissue at the proper stage, or failure of fusion of embryonic tissue, would lead to a defect of development, eg, of the iris or choroid (coloboma). These developmental defects commonly occur at any point from a segment of the optic nerve itself at the disk, along the choroidal structure and the ciliary body, or in an iris segment. These defects are often seen grossly as a missing wedge of iris tissue or may be seen with the ophthalmoscope as a large white strip extending radially along the inner surface of the eye toward the periphery.

An eye may be missing (anophthalmos) or smaller than normal (microphthalmos). A small eye is quite often deficient in function.

Congenital lens opacities may occur at any time during the formation of the lens, and the stage at which the opacity began to develop is often measurable by the depth of the opacity. The innermost fetal nucleus of the lens forms early in embryonal life and is surrounded by the embryonal nucleus. Adult addition to the lens is a peripheral subcapsular growth in postnatal life. Certain types of congenital cataracts are familial, whereas others may occur as reactions to intrauterine influences.

Congenital rests, such as dermoids, occur frequently in the ocular structures.

GROWTH & DEVELOPMENT

Eyeball

At birth, the eye is larger in relation to the rest of the body than is the case in children and adults. In relation to its ultimate size (reached at 7–8 years), it is comparatively short, averaging 17.3 mm in anteroposterior length (the only optically significant dimension). This would make the eye quite hyperopic if it were not for the refractive power of the nearly spherical lens.

Cornea

The newborn infant has a relatively large cornea that reaches adult size by the age of 2 years. It is flatter than the adult cornea, and its curvature is greater at the periphery than in the center. (The reverse is true in adults.)

Almost all astigmatic refractive errors are produced by differences in curvature in the various meridians of the cornea. In the infant, the vertical meridian usually has the greatest curvature. In adult life the cornea tends to flatten, and the flattening is more marked in the vertical than the horizontal, changing the axis of astigmatism. However, the degree of astigmatism changes very little throughout life.

Lens

At birth, the lens is more nearly spherical in shape than later in life, producing a greater refractive power that helps to compensate for the short anteroposterior diameter of the eye. The lens grows throughout life as new fibers are added to the periphery, making it flatter.

The consistency of the lens material changes throughout life. At birth, it may be compared with soft plastic; in old age, the lens is of a glasslike consistency. This accounts for the greater resistance to change of shape in accommodation as one grows older.

Refractive State

About 80% of children are born hyperopic, 5% myopic, and 15% emmetropic. Hyperopia often gradually decreases prior to puberty and may even become myopia. Myopia usually increases after age 7–8 years and develops in some children not previously affected. The increase in the myopic refractive error usually ceases or is much diminished by age 16 years. Refractive errors tend to stabilize during the 20s and 30s. The onset of presbyopia is at age 42–46 years in nearly everyone.

Iris

At birth, there is little or no pigment on the anterior surface of the iris; the posterior pigment layer showing through the translucent tissue gives the eyes of most infants a bluish color. As the pigment begins to appear on the anterior surface, the iris assumes its definitive color. If considerable pigment is deposited, the eyes become brown. Less iris stroma pigmentation results in blue, hazel, or green.

Position

During the first 3 months of age, eye movements may be so poorly coordinated (because of the normally slow development of reflexes) that doubt may exist about the straightness of the eyes. Most of the binocular reflexes should be well developed by 6 months of age. Deviation that persists beyond age 6 months should be investigated (see Chapter 16).

Nasolacrimal Apparatus

The cord of cells that hollows out to form the nasolacrimal duct between the tear sac and the nose usually becomes patent at about the time of birth. Failure to function may not be noticed for some time because of lack of tear secretion in the first few weeks of life. Failure of tear production by 3 months of age demands attention.

Optic Nerve

The completion of the medullation process around the optic nerve fibers usually occurs within a few weeks after birth.

AGING CHANGES IN THE EYE

Eyelids

Aging of the skin tissues produces gradual loss of elasticity, with wrinkling and drooping folds (dermatochalasis). There may be fatty alteration of the tissues (xanthelasma).

Conjunctiva

Senile plaques and degenerative infiltrates occasionally are found.

Cornea

The cornea may show circular infiltration of degenerative material within the limbus ("arcus senilis"). A flattening of curvature of the vertical meridian tends to produce distorted vision.

Lens

The lens continues to grow throughout life, although in senescence the rate of growth decreases. The consistency changes from the soft plastic juvenile lens to an almost "glasslike" character, with increasing difficulty in change of shape with attempted accommodation (presbyopia).

Disturbances of lens metabolism may produce tissue changes with resultant loss of transparency (cataract). Most older people have some degree of cataract.

Vitreous

Increase in "floaters" (muscae volitantes) due to fibrillar condensations, exudates, degenerative deposits, or asteroid hyalosis; detachment and liquefaction of vitreous.

Choroid & Retina

Arteriosclerosis of the vessels of the choroid and retina may be followed by degenerative changes in these tissues.

Examination*

ROUTINE EYE EXAMINATION

The routine ophthalmologic examination consists of careful elicitation of the patient's history, physical examination of the eyes, and assessment of visual function. The history should include not only the patient's ocular manifestations but general information about age, occupation, and physical health. Special examinations may be required to determine ocular pathophysiology or to establish the presence of associated systemic disease. The patient's pertinent past medical records are often helpful.

GENERAL INFORMATION

Age

The age of the patient is important not only as an etiologic factor in senile changes but also for the purpose of comparing individual abilities with established norms for the age group and in helping to determine what one might expect in the way of performance without discomfort. For example, in cases of amblyopia, occlusive treatment should improve the visual acuity of a child under age 6, whereas the same treatment in a child over 6 would be less effective. In a young child it is not too important to correct the visual acuity to 6/6 (20/20), since demands for clear distance visual acuity are much less at an early age than is the case with older schoolchildren or adults. Age also plays a role in the rate of progression of myopia, which tends to increase during the teens and levels off in the third decade.

Age is also an important factor in visual disability in the prepresbyopic or early presbyopic period, as the symptoms of presbyopia are often quite disconcerting to a person who has had good eyesight throughout life. Proper explanation of these symptoms to the patient may postpone the need for the first pair of reading glasses or facilitate the adjustment to the first pair.

Occupation

Occupational demands for visual acuity are important in determining the treatment of visual symptoms. Special requirements, such as those involved in working with small objects or at unusual working distances, must be considered in the work-fatigue balance of the visual effort. Even in the same age group, marked differences in symptoms may be noted between 2 individuals with the same refractive error whose work makes widely different demands on their eyes. Small refractive errors that produce discomfort in an accountant, for example, may be unnoticed by a laborer.

In presbyopic patients requiring occupational bifocals, special work requirements play an important role in the prescription of bifocal segments.

In industrial injuries a careful record should be made of time and circumstances of injury, previous emergency treatment, and visual acuity.

SYMPTOMS & SIGNS

Most of the presenting manifestations of eye involvement fall into one of 5 categories: (1) subnormal visual acuity; (2) pain or discomfort; (3) change of appearance of lids, orbit, or eye; (4) diplopia or dizziness; and (5) discharge or increased conjunctival secretion. Some of the important features of each complaint are discussed below.

Subnormal Visual Acuity

A. Duration: Is visual acuity the same as it has been for most of the patient's life? Was the change noted recently? Was it found by accidentally covering one eye? Has there been a gradual diminution of acuity over months or years?

B. Difference in Visual Acuity in the 2 Eyes: Is the patient certain that visual acuity was formerly the same in both eyes? Has the patient passed an eye examination as part of a driver's test or military physical examination? At that time was the visual acuity the same in both eyes?

C. Disturbances of Vision:

1. Distortion of the normal shapes of objects (metamorphopsia) is most often due to astigmatism or macular lesions.

2. Photophobia is commonly due to corneal inflammation, aphakia, iritis, and ocular albinism. Some drugs may produce increased light sensitivity (eg, chloroquine, acetazolamide).

3. Color change (chromatopsia), such as yellow, white, or red vision, may be due to chorioretinal lesions or lenticular changes, or may be associated with systemic disturbances (eg, yellow vision of jaundice)

*Ophthalmoscopic examination: See Chapter 4.

or certain medications (eg, yellow or white vision in digitalis toxicity).

4. Halos, or rings seen when viewing lights or bright objects, are typically thought of as accompanying glaucoma but are also found with other processes causing corneal edema or infiltration as well as with lens changes. Incipient cataract is the most common cause of halos.

5. "Spots" before the eyes, seen as dots or filaments that move with the eye, are usually due to benign vitreous opacities.

6. Visual field defects may be due to disorders of the lids, media, retina, optic nerve, or brain. Quivering or scintillating blind spots (scotomas) may occur transiently as a result of localized constriction of cerebral or retinal arteries.

7. Night blindness, or difficulty seeing in the dark (nyctalopia), may be congenital (retinitis pigmentosa, hereditary optic atrophy) or acquired (vitamin A deficiency, glaucoma, optic atrophy, cataract, retinal degeneration).

8. Momentary loss of vision (amaurosis fugax) may imply impending cerebrovascular accident, spasm of the central retinal artery, or partial occlusion of the internal carotid artery.

Pain or Discomfort

The usual painful symptoms mentioned are headache, "eye-ache," and burning or itching of the eyes or eyelids. Photophobia (sensitivity to light) may cause great discomfort; fatigue symptoms such as "pull," "tired eyes," and "a feeling of pressure" may be described. Acute localized pain intensified by movement of the eye or lid suggests a foreign body or corneal abrasion.

Headache is a common complaint causing a patient to go to an ophthalmologist for an eye examination. If the eye examination discloses no pathologic abnormalities that may account for the symptom, a careful description of the type of headache and a history of its onset, relationship to use of the eyes, duration, and associated symptoms may not only rule out eye disease as a probable cause but may indicate the proper diagnosis.

For example, the headache that occurs upon arising in the morning and disappears soon afterward is seldom caused by eye disorders; a general medical examination is indicated. On the other hand, mild to moderate headaches that occur toward the end of a day of exacting eye work and that are relieved by a few hours of rest or sleep are more probably due to ocular disorders. Any case of severe headache that is becoming worse should suggest an intracranial lesion; visual field tests, ophthalmoscopy, and neurologic consultation are indicated.

"Eye-ache" often accompanies extreme fatigue with or without excessive use of the eyes. It is more common in patients with muscle imbalances, but it may be present with inflammatory lesions involving the episclera, iris, or choroid. The eyes may also ache with the increased pressure of glaucoma. In severe acute congestive glaucoma, the pain may be so intense as to radiate throughout the cranium and be accompanied by nausea and vomiting. Ocular pain may also be caused by fever, neuralgia, retrobulbar neuritis, and temporal arteritis. Aching eyes constitute one of the first symptoms of severe influenza and dengue.

Burning and itching may be a symptom of eyestrain, but the most frequent cause is inflammation of the lids or conjunctiva, eg, chronic blepharitis, conjunctivitis, and allergic reactions of the hay fever type. Itching, in particular, is a symptom of ocular allergy.

A sensation of "pull" is often described in adjusting to a new lens prescription, particularly if the prescription incorporates a change in astigmatic correction. There may also be sensations of pull or actual ache in adjusting to the first pair of bifocals.

Change in Appearance

A. Discoloration: Redness or congestion of the lids, conjunctiva, or scleras may be due to an acute inflammatory reaction to infection, trauma, or allergy or to acute glaucoma. Subconjunctival hemorrhage is sudden in onset and bright red in appearance. (Gross intraocular hemorrhage gives no external ocular sign.) Change of color of the cornea may occur with corneal ulcer or intraocular infection, producing cloudiness of the anterior chamber or an actual level of purulent material in the anterior chamber (hypopyon). Change of color of the "white" of the eye may be noted. Yellow scleras are usually seen with jaundice or antimalarial drug toxicity (eg, quinacrine). Blue scleras are associated with osteogenesis imperfecta. Dark discoloration may follow prolonged local or systemic use of silver compounds (rare) or may be due to scleral thinning and degeneration.

B. Swelling: One or both lids may be swollen. Swelling of one lid suggests a local abscess; bilateral swelling indicates a more generalized reaction such as blepharitis, allergy, myxedema, or malignant exophthalmos.

C. Mass: An orbital mass may occur, causing displacement of the globe.

D. Displacement: The eyes may be displaced forward or in other directions. There may be a change of position of the lids, either drooping (ptosis) or retracted (elevated).

Diplopia & Vertigo

It is difficult to differentiate diplopia and vertigo without a careful history. Both may be described by the patient as "dizziness." If double vision is described, it is important to know the time of onset, whether it is constant or intermittent, whether it occurs in certain positions of gaze or at certain distances, and whether the 2 objects seen are horizontal or vertical. Monocular diplopia occurs in lenticular changes, macular lesions, malingering, or hysteria.

Vertigo or light-headedness is often (but seldom justifiably) ascribed to eye disorders, since the patient frequently notes that during this time it is difficult to focus on any object or that "things seem to go around."

The attacks are frequently associated with sudden changes in posture, such as arising suddenly from a lying or seated position, or sudden changes in the position of the head or neck muscles.

Discharge (Exudate or Epiphora)

It is important to know the type and amount of discharge, when it occurs, and whether chronic crusting or "granulation" of the lid margins occurs. If the discharge is watery (epiphora) and not associated with redness or pain, it is usually due to excessive formation of tears or obstruction of the lacrimal drainage system. The patency of the drainage system may be examined by irrigating the canaliculi and nasolacrimal ducts. If the discharge is watery but accompanied by photophobia or burning, viral conjunctivitis or keratoconjunctivitis may be present. A purulent discharge usually indicates a bacterial infection. A discharge seen with allergic conditions often contains a large number of eosinophils. Samples of the exudate may be stained with methylene blue, Giemsa's, Gram's, or other stains for microscopic identification of cell types and bacteria. If necessary, further identification of bacteria may be done by culture.

Decreased or Increased Lacrimation

Many systemic disorders are marked by decreased tearing. Dryness of the eyes is a frequent complaint in elderly patients and also occurs in several of the collagen disorders (eg, Sjögren's syndrome) and in patients taking tranquilizers. Excessive tearing (epiphora) may be due to chemical irritation (eg, smog), allergy, acute inflammatory disease of the eye, or tear duct obstruction.

PHYSICAL EXAMINATION OF THE EYE BY THE GENERAL PHYSICIAN

VISUAL ACUITY

Visual acuity determination should be part of the routine examination of all patients—not only those who present with eye complaints.

Technique

The usual method of testing visual acuity is with one of various types of special charts of test letters. (The Snellen chart is most commonly used.)

The patient faces the test chart at a distance of 6 meters (or 20 feet). A clean card or occluder is placed in front of the left eye without pressure on the globe, and the patient is asked to read as far down the chart as possible with the right eye. If the patient is able to read the line marked 6/6 (20/20), this is recorded and the same procedure repeated for the left eye. If

Figure 3–1. E game: Measuring visual acuity in preschool children.

the patient can read the large letters at the top of the chart but cannot read down to the 6/6 (20/20) line, the value that corresponds to the smallest line that can be read is recorded. A patient who is unable to read the large letters at the top of the chart should be moved progressively closer to the chart until they can be read; this distance is then recorded as the distance from the chart over 12 meters (40 feet) or 60 meters (200 feet), ie, x/12 (if meters are used), x/40 (if feet are used). If glasses for distance are worn, the test should be repeated with glasses on and the results recorded as "uncorrected" and "corrected." Corrected visual acuity is far more important than uncorrected visual acuity.

Preschool children or illiterates should be instructed in the "E" game and then tested with the illiterate E chart (Fig 3–1). In this test the patient is taught to point a finger in the same direction as the bars of the E. The average 4-year-old child can cooperate satisfactorily in this test. Charts with test pictures have been devised but are not as accurate.

A corrected visual acuity of less than 6/9 (20/30) is abnormal.

INSPECTION

Inspection of external ocular structures (lids, conjunctiva, corneas, scleras, and lacrimal apparatus) should include everting the upper eyelids for inspection of the conjunctival surface with the patient looking down. This can be done easily by grasping the lashes of the upper eyelid with one hand, pulling out and down slightly to put the tissue on stretch, and then pressing on the lid with a thin applicator stick at the superior border of the tarsal plate.

Fovea
Macula
Optic disk
Arteriole
Vein

Figure 3–2. The normal fundus. Diagram at left shows landmarks of photograph at right. (Photo by Diane Beeston.)

The exposed surfaces are inspected for defects, foreign bodies, inflammation, discharge, epiphora, dryness, or any other abnormality.

With a history of injury in which the coats of the eye may have been lacerated, great care should be taken in opening the lids to avoid pressure upon the eyeball. In the presence of pain and lid spasm, it may be necessary to instill a few drops of sterile anesthetic solution in order to examine the eye. In small children it may even be necessary to give a short-acting, light general anesthetic.

Pupils

The pupils should be inspected for size, color, shape, reaction to the stimulation of light, the effect of accommodation, and the presence or absence of the consensual light response. (Light directed into the pupil of one eye normally constricts the pupils of both eyes.) Examination for reaction to light is best performed in a darkened room with the examiner to the side of the patient. The pupils may be markedly constricted (miotic) due to the effects of bright illumination, central nervous system syphilis, or narcotic or parasympathomimetic drugs. They may be dilated as a result of dim illumination, myopia, or sympathomimetic drugs. Unequal pupils (anisocoria) may be normal but suggest neurologic disease if one or both pupils do not react well to light. Argyll Robertson pupil is one in which there is failure of direct and consensual light response with retention of the normal response of pupillary constriction on accommodation (focusing on a near object). The tonic pupil of Adie's syndrome (see Chapter 18) must be differentiated from Argyll Robertson pupil.

Position of the Eyes

Note the size (microphthalmos or enophthalmos), prominence (exophthalmos), and position (orbital tumor, strabismus) of the eyes. Palpation may be helpful in locating orbital tumors and determining their size, consistency, and pulsation.

The eyes should be observed for alignment as well as for movement of the eyes together in all fields of gaze. Any limitation can be further investigated as described in the section on strabismus evaluation in Chapter 16.

CONFRONTATION VISUAL FIELD TESTS

Many conditions are associated with loss of side vision. If special instruments for a careful perimetric field study are not available, the simple confrontation test should be performed as a rough test for gross defects.

Equipment & Materials

The only equipment needed is a simple wand, such as a pencil with a white eraser, a small white bead, or the examiner's finger.

Technique

The observer and patient face each other at arm's length. The patient is then told to hold one hand lightly over the left eye and look with the right eye at the examiner's left eye. The examiner then holds the target as far to the side as possible at middle distance from the patient. The target is then slowly brought into the line of sight, and the patient is instructed to respond as soon as the target can be identified. This is repeated at intervals of 30–45 degrees around the 360-degree periphery. The fullness of the reported field is compared to that of the observer's. The test is then repeated for the other eye.

Interpretation of Findings

Gross hemianopia, bitemporal defects, or large unilateral defects can be detected by confrontation.

The test should not be considered a substitute for a careful tangent screen or perimetric visual field examination but merely as a gross screening test.

SPECIAL OPHTHALMOLOGIC EXAMINATIONS

SLIT LAMP EXAMINATION (Biomicroscopy)

The slit lamp consists of a microscope and special light source. Slit lamp examination is indicated in any condition of the eyelids or eyeball that can be better diagnosed and treated by having a well illuminated and highly magnified view of the area involved (eg, dendritic keratitis, corneal foreign body, iris tumor).

Equipment & Materials
A slit lamp is shown in Fig 3–3.

Technique
Both the patient and the examiner are seated. The patient places chin on chin rest and forehead against frame while the examiner views the eyes through the microscope.

The lids, cornea, anterior chamber, and iris can be easily and quickly studied by moving the focus of both the microscope and the light back and forth. Since the strong light of the slit lamp causes the iris to contract, a mydriatic may be necessary to study lens detail.

For detailed binocular viewing of the vitreous, optic nerve, posterior and peripheral retina, and choroid, a specialized contact lens is used, following dilation of the pupil.

PERIMETRY

Perimetry is used to examine the central and peripheral visual fields. This technique, which is performed separately for each eye, measures the function of the retina, the optic nerve, and the intracranial visual pathway. It is used clinically to detect or monitor field loss due to disease at any of these locations. Because perimetry relies on subjective patient responses, the results will depend on the patient's mental, as well as visual, status.

The visual field of the eye is measured and plotted in degrees of arc (the measurement of degrees of arc remains constant regardless of the distance from the eye at which it is taken). The sensitivity of the field is greatest in the center (corresponding to the fovea) and least at the periphery.

Equipment & Materials
The **tangent screen** is the simplest apparatus for standardized perimetry. It utilizes different-sized pins on a wand presented against a black screen and is used primarily to test the central 30 degrees of the visual field. The advantages of this method are its simplicity and rapidity, the possibility of placing the subject at various distances from the screen, and the option of using any assortment of fixation and test objects (including colors).

Significantly more sophisticated, **Goldmann perimetry** (Fig 3–4) uses a hollow white spherical bowl, in front of which the patient is positioned at a set distance. A light of variable intensity and size can be manually presented by the examiner in either a static or kinetic fashion (see below). This method can test the full limits of the field and has for years been the primary method for plotting fields in glaucoma patients.

More recently, **computerized automated perimetry** has become available (Figs 3–5 and 3–6). This method also uses test lights projected into a hollow

Figure 3–3 (at left). Eye examination with Zeiss slit lamp. (Photo by Diane Beeston.)

Figure 3–4 (at right). Goldmann perimeter. (Photo by M Narahara.)

bowl but with a static threshold testing method that is more precise and comprehensive. One distinct advantage is that the test presentation is programmed and automated, eliminating any variability on the part of the examiner.

Despite the growing sophistication of these devices, perimetry is still a subjective test and must always be performed and interpreted with this in mind.

Technique

The various methods of perimetry have been standardized to enable reproducibility and subsequent comparison. The subjectiveness of patient responses prevents the test from being wholly objective, however. It requires steady fixation by the eye, a constant amount of background illumination and contrast, and a known distance from the eye to the screen or testing device. As the patient's eye fixates on a central target, test objects are presented at different locations throughout the field, and the patient responds if they are seen. By varying the target's size or brightness, the sensitivity of different areas in the field can be quantified.

There are 2 basic methods of target presentation, static and kinetic, which are often used in combination during an examination. In **static perimetry,** a test object is presented at a particular location. If it is not seen, the size or intensity of the object can be increased. The threshold level of that location is determined by that object which is just large or bright enough to be detected. In this fashion, the sensitivity of multiple points in the field can be evaluated.

In **kinetic perimetry,** a test object of fixed size and brightness is moved toward the center from a peripheral area until it is first spotted. By moving the same object inward from multiple different directions, a boundary called an **isopter** can be mapped out, which is specific for that target. The object can be

Figure 3–5 (at right). Computerized automated perimeter. (Photo by M Narahara.)

Figure 3–6. Glaucomatous visual field by computerized perimeter.

Figure 3–7. Measuring the intraocular pressure with a Schiotz tonometer. (Photo by Diane Beeston.)

seen within the isopter but not beyond it. Smaller or dimmer test objects will therefore have smaller isopters.

SCHIOTZ TONOMETRY
(Fig 3–7)

Tonometry is the determination of intraocular pressure by means of an instrument that measures the amount of corneal indentation produced by a given weight. It can be performed as part of the general physical examination by internists and general physicians as well as ophthalmologists.

Indications

Tonometer readings should be taken on all patients over the age of 20 having a routine eye examination or general physical examination and on any patient suspected of having increased intraocular pressure for any reason.

Contraindications & Precautions

Tonometry should be done with great caution on patients with corneal ulcers. It is extremely important to clean the tonometer before each use by carefully wiping the footplate with a moist sterile cotton swab and to sterilize the instrument once a day (dry heat).

Corneal abrasions are rarely caused by Schiotz tonometry. Epidemic keratoconjunctivitis can be spread by tonometry, and this can be prevented if the tonometer is cleaned before each use and the physician washes hands between patients.

Equipment & Materials

Local anesthetic solution and a Schiotz tonometer.

Technique

Anesthetic solution is instilled into each eye. The patient lies supine and is asked to stare at a spot on the ceiling with both eyes or at a finger placed directly in the line of gaze overhead. The tonometer is then placed on the corneal surface of each eye and the scale reading taken from the tonometer. The intraocular pressure is determined by referring to a chart that converts the scale reading to millimeters of mercury. If the scale reading is 4 or less, the 7.5- and 10-g weights are added separately to gain further information concerning the intraocular pressure.

Normal Findings

12–20 mm Hg.

Interpretation of Abnormalities

If the intraocular pressure is 20–30 mm Hg or more, further investigation is indicated to determine whether or not glaucoma is present—ie, tonometry is a screening device to select patients for glaucoma testing. Visual field and ophthalmoscopic examinations should be done and the tonometer readings repeated several times at different hours of the day or on different days before the diagnosis of glaucoma can be regarded as established. If the pressure remains high on successive readings and there is a characteristic visual field defect or cupping of the optic disks, the diagnosis of glaucoma may be established (see Chapter 15).

Figure 3–8. Applanation tonometer mounted on a Zeiss slit lamp. (Photo by Diane Beeston.)

Accuracy of Method & Sources of Error

Schiotz tonometry is accurate for clinical purposes. Sources of error include scleral rigidity, a poorly calibrated tonometer, improper application of the tolnometer to the cornea, or an uncooperative patient who squeezes the eyelids shut. (The abnormal pressure of the orbicularis muscles on the eye artificially elevates the intraocular pressure.)

APPLANATION TONOMETRY

Applanation tonometry (Fig 3–8) measures the force required to flatten rather than indent a small area of the central cornea and is more accurate than Schiotz tonometry. Applanation tonometry is widely used by ophthalmologists, but the equipment is impractical for the nonophthalmologist because it is fairly sophisticated and very expensive.

GONIOSCOPY

Gonioscopy consists of direct visualization of the anterior chamber angle, using a lens with a special mirror. It should be performed in all cases of suspected glaucoma. It is also useful to estimate the extent of involvement of tumors of the iris and to look for suspected foreign bodies in the anterior chamber angle.

Equipment & Materials

Local anesthetic solution, a goniolens, and a source of illumination depending on the type of goniolens (Fig 3–9).

Technique

The patient is seated at the slit lamp, and following topical anesthesia, the goniolens is placed on the eye (Fig 3–10). The anterior chamber angle and the iris are then viewed with magnification through the special mirror. The mirror can be rotated so that the full 360-degree circumference of the angle can be examined. The same lens can be used to direct laser treatment toward the angle.

The **Koeppe lens,** another goniolens, requires a special illuminator and a hand-held microscope. It is used with the patient in the supine position and can thus be used in the operating room for either examination or surgery.

Figure 3–9 (at right). Three types of goniolenses. *Left:* Goldmann-type lens. *Center:* Koeppe lens. *Right:* Posner/Zeiss-type lens. (Photo by M Narahara.)

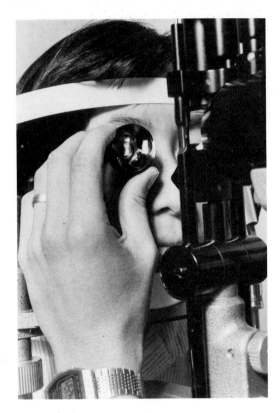

Figure 3–10. Gonioscopy with slit lamp and Goldmann-type lens. (Photo by M Narahara.)

Normal & Abnormal Findings

Normally (and in most cases of chronic glaucoma), the structures of the anterior chamber angle can be clearly visualized. If the angle is extremely narrow and the intraocular pressure normal, the patient is at risk of developing angle-closure glaucoma following spontaneous or pharmacologic pupillary dilation.

SCHIRMER TEST

The Schirmer test is a gross measurement of the quantity of tear fluid in the conjunctival sac. It is indicated in any patient who complains of dry or chronically irritated eyes. The test is performed with standardized 5- by 35-mm Schirmer strips. One end of the filter paper is bent and inserted into the conjunctival sac near the inner angle and left for 5 minutes with the eyes closed.

The tears from the conjunctival sac should wet at least 10 mm of the filter paper strip in 5 minutes. If less than 10 mm of wetting occurs on repeated examinations, this is evidence of decreased tear production (see Chapter 7).

CORNEAL STAINING

Corneal staining consists of the instillation of fluorescein or other dyes (eg, rose bengal) into the conjunctival sac to outline irregularities of the corneal surface. Staining is indicated in corneal trauma or other corneal disorders (eg, herpes simplex keratitis) when examination with a loupe or slit lamp in the absence of a stain has not been satisfactory.

Precautions

Because the corneal epithelium, the chief barrier to corneal infection, is usually interrupted when corneal staining is indicated, be certain that whatever dye is used (particularly fluorescein) is sterile.

Equipment & Materials

Fluorescein on papers or sterile individual dropper units are safest. Fluorescein solution may be used, but the physician runs the risk of introducing a new organism into the eye.

Technique

The individually wrapped fluorescein paper is wetted with sterile saline or touched to the wet conjunctiva so that a thin film of fluorescein spreads over the corneal surface. Any irregularity in the cornea is stained by the fluorescein and is thus more easily visualized, especially with blue light.

Normal & Abnormal Findings

If there is no superficial corneal irregularity, a uniform film of dye covers the cornea. If the corneal surface has been altered, the affected area absorbs more of the dye and will stain a deeper green. It is customary to sketch the staining area on the patient's record for later comparison to show the progress of healing.

MEASUREMENT OF THE REFRACTIVE POWER OF THE CORNEA

Although originally designed for measuring corneal astigmatism as part of refraction, the keratometer is now used primarily to measure the radii of anterior corneal curvature (in millimeters) for contact lens fitting and intraocular lens power determination. It is also a helpful diagnostic aid in some corneal conditions, particularly keratoconus.

THE KERATOSCOPE

The keratoscope is used to study the regularity of the corneal light reflection in the examination of suspected keratoconus. It is a round disk with alternating black and white concentric rings and a hole in the center. The cornea is examined through the keratoscope much as one would use an ophthalmoscope.

The reflections of the rings are not distorted in a

normally curved cornea but are in corneas of patients with keratoconus.

IRRIGATION OF THE LACRIMAL DRAINAGE SYSTEM

Irrigation of the lacrimal drainage system is a diagnostic or therapeutic procedure that consists of injecting fluid through the upper or lower punctum into the upper or lower canaliculus, whence it will normally flow into the lacrimal sac and down through the nasolacrimal duct into the nasopharynx. Irrigation is done in patients of all ages who complain of tearing. In infants who are not cured of dacryocystitis by massage and irrigation of the lacrimal sac and by antibacterial drops, probing of the nasolacrimal duct is indicated.

Equipment & Materials

Local anesthetic solution, a punctum dilator, a 3-mL syringe with a lacrimal irrigation cannula, and sterile water or physiologic saline solution (Fig 3–11). One must be certain that the cannula has a dull tip so that the wall of the canaliculus will not be punctured.

Technique

Adults require one instillation of anesthetic solution in the conjunctival sac.

The upper and lower puncta in the affected eye are first dilated and the lacrimal needle then passed into the canaliculus. Sterile water or saline solution injected into the canaliculus and tear sac normally passes down the nasolacrimal duct into the nasopharynx.

Normal & Abnormal Findings

If the lacrimal drainage system is patent and an individual sits with head back, the fluid will be immediately felt in the throat. If the fluid is injected into the lower punctum and comes out of the upper punctum and does not go into the nose or throat, the site of obstruction is in the nasolacrimal duct or the common canaliculus at the entrance to the tear sac. If the fluid will not enter the canaliculus under pressure and does not come out of the opposite punctum or in the throat, the site of obstruction is in the canaliculus.

PROBING OF THE LACRIMAL DRAINAGE SYSTEM

Probing the lacrimal drainage system consists of passing a metal (preferably silver) probe of uniform caliber through the upper or lower punctum and the upper or lower canaliculus into the tear sac and down the nasolacrimal duct into the nose. It is indicated in obstruction of the upper or lower canaliculus or the nasolacrimal duct (particularly in infants) that is not relieved by irrigation.

Probing of the lacrimal drainage system should not be done in patients with acute dacryocystitis. It should always be done gently in order to avoid making a false passage through the canaliculus or lacrimal sac.

Equipment & Materials

Local anesthetic solution, a punctum dilator, and a flexible silver probe about 15 cm long should be used. The probes vary in diameter (Fig 3–12) and are numbered accordingly from No. 1 (smallest) upward to No. 8.

Technique

In adults, anesthetic drops are instilled into the conjunctival sac and the area of the tear sac is infiltrated with anesthetic.

The upper and lower puncta are dilated and the probe is passed into the tear sac. Lateral pressure on the lid is maintained until the probe is obstructed by the bony nasal wall; the probe is then withdrawn slightly, turned approximately 90 degrees, and passed through the nasolacrimal duct.

Normal & Abnormal Findings

The probe should pass freely and easily through all of the lacrimal passages and should be easily visualized with a nasal speculum in the inferior meatus of the nose. The point of obstruction may be noted when the probe cannot be passed farther with undue force.

Figure 3–11. Syringe with gold cannula and punctum dilator.

Figure 3–12. Lacrimal probes of various diameters. (Photo by Diane Beeston.)

The most common site of obstruction in patients of all ages is the nasolacrimal duct.

Probing is almost always successful in relieving the obstruction in infants but is seldom successful in adults, for whom dacryocystorhinostomy is usually required.

LIGHT & COLOR PERCEPTION

When the fundus is obscured by opaque media, gross tests of retinal function may be performed by stimulating the macula with light or by merely testing light and color perception.

Technique

A. Test of Macular Function: The patient sits with eyes closed as the examiner massages the eyeball gently with the lighted end of a small flashlight. The patient is then asked to describe what is seen. If the macula is functioning properly, the patient will see a red central area surrounded by the retinal blood vessels. If macular function is impaired, the central area will be dark rather than red and no blood vessels will be seen. Two disadvantages of the test are that it is highly subjective and is difficult for some patients to comprehend.

B. Color Perception and Light Projection: A bandage is placed over one eye and the patient's hand is placed over the bandage to exclude all light. The patient is then asked to look straight ahead with the other eye. A light is held in 4 different quadrants and the patient is asked to identify the direction from which the light is approaching the eye. A red lens is then held in front of the light, and the patient is asked to differentiate the red from the white light. If all questions are answered correctly, it suggests that the retina is functioning normally.

POTENTIAL ACUITY MEASUREMENT

When opacities of the cornea or lens coexist with disease of the macula or optic nerve, the visual potential of the eye is in doubt. The benefit of corneal transplantation or cataract extraction will depend on the degree of retinal or optic nerve impairment. In addition to the methods listed above, sophisticated quantitative instruments have been developed for more direct determination of visual potential in these situations. These instruments project a narrow beam of light containing a pattern of images through a relatively clear portion of the media and onto the retina. The patient's vision is then graded according to the size of the smallest patterns that can be resolved.

Two different types of imaging patterns are used. **Laser interferometry** employs laser light to generate interference fringes or gratings, which the patient sees as a series of parallel lines. By progressively narrowing the width and spacing of the lines, an end point will be reached where the patient can no longer discern the orientation of the lines. The narrowest image width that the patient can resolve is then correlated with a Snellen acuity measurement to determine the visual potential of that eye. The **potential acuity meter** projects a standard Snellen acuity chart onto the retina (Fig 3–13). The patient is then graded in the usual fashion, according to the smallest line of letters read.

Although both methods appear to be reliable means of measuring visual acuity, false-positive and false-negative results do occur, with a frequency dependent on the type of disease present. Thus, these instruments are helpful but not completely reliable in determining visual potential in eyes with cloudy media.

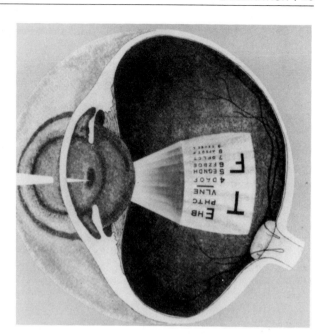

Figure 3–13 (at right). Method of potential acuity meter examination. (Courtesy of Mentor O & O, Inc.)

EXOPHTHALMOMETRY

The exophthalmometer is an instrument for determining the degree of anterior projection of the eyes. This is an accurate method of diagnosing and, more particularly, following the course of a patient with exophthalmos.

Equipment & Materials

An exophthalmometer is shown in Fig 3–14.

Technique

The patient stands with his or her back against the wall and looks into the examiner's eyes. The 2 small concave parts of the exophthalmometer are placed against the lateral orbital margins and the bar reading is noted. This reading represents the distance between the lateral orbital walls. It must be constant for successive examinations if the course is to be judged accurately.

The examiner then views the cornea of the patient's right eye in the mirror with the patient fixing the right eye on the examiner's left eye. The cornea is simultaneously lined up in the mirror with a scale that reads directly in millimeters. The left eye is then observed in the same way, with the patient fixing the left eye on the examiner's right eye. Both the bar reading and the degree of exophthalmos are recorded in millimeters. (A typical reading: with a bar reading of 96 mm, RE = 17 mm, LE = 17 mm.)

Figure 3–14 (at right). Hertel exophthalmometer. (Photo by M Narahara.)

Normal & Abnormal Findings

The normal range of bar readings is 12–20 mm. The reading is usually the same in each eye and indicates the anterior distances from the corneas to the lateral orbital margins. When exophthalmos is diagnosed (bar readings > 20 mm), one must look for some underlying cause, eg, thyroid disease or orbital tumor. Periodic exophthalmometer readings aid greatly thereafter in observing the course of the disease.

COLOR VISION TESTS

Determination of a person's ability to perceive the primary colors and shades thereof is performed as part of the physical examination of military recruits, transportation workers, and others whose occupations require the best possible color perception.

The term color blindness is something of a misnomer. Because color blindness is such a relative thing, color deficient might be a more descriptive term. No one is ever disabled by being color deficient. People are merely tested by our somewhat crude methods and are excluded from certain job categories if they fail the tests.

Equipment & Materials

The most commonly used polychromatic plates are those of Ishihara, Stilling, and Hardy-Rand-Rittler (Fig 3–15). The plates are made up of dots of the primary colors printed on a background of similar dots in a confusion of colors. The dots are set in patterns (eg, numbers) that are indiscernible by persons with color perception defects.

Technique

Under adequate illumination, the various polychromatic plates are presented to the patient, who is asked to identify the patterns.

Normal & Abnormal Findings

All of the patterns are recognizable to the person with normal color vision. A color-blind person is unable to identify the various figures and forms on the polychromatic plates. The type of color blindness is diagnosed according to the plates used. Red-green blindness is diagnosed in about 8% of the male population and 0.4% of the female population. Blue-yellow or violet blindness is extremely rare.

Accuracy of Method & Sources of Error

An experienced color-defective person may have memorized the plates. If this is suspected, some other test, such as examination with the Eldridge-Green lamp, should be used. Abnormalities of the ocular media, the retina, or the optic nerve can affect the test and should be ruled out if color blindness is discovered.

TESTS FOR MALINGERING

Utilizing the refractor, place a strong convex lens in front of the good eye and a weak convex lens in front of the "blind" eye. If the patient reads small letters on the test chart, the eye under consideration is not blind. This test can be more subtly done with the refractor than with the trial frame, since the strong convex lens is not visible to the patient when the refractor is used.

Place a 10-diopter base-out prism in front of the "blind" eye. If there is sight in the eye, diplopia will result and the eye will be seen to move inward to correct the diplopia.

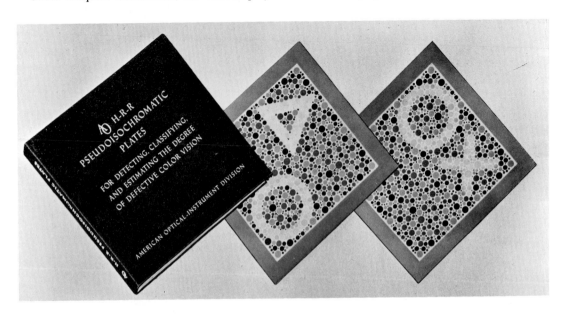

Figure 3–15. H-R-R (Hardy-Rand-Rittler) pseudoisochromatic plates.

Place a pair of red-green glasses on the patient, with the red lens in front of the right eye and the green lens in front of the left eye. If the left eye is the suspected eye and the patient can read green letters with this eye, the eye is not blind; the green letters will not be transmitted through the red lens in front of the right eye.

BINOCULAR INDIRECT OPHTHALMOSCOPY

Binocular indirect ophthalmoscopy (Fig 3–16) is a means of observing the posterior segment of the eye with a strong source of illumination and a convex lens held before the patient's eye. The observer views an inverted image of the retina that is formed between the lens and the observer's eye.

Binocular indirect ophthalmoscopy can be used to advantage whenever ophthalmoscopic examination is indicated. The advantages of this technique over direct ophthalmoscopy are that the field is larger; the view is stereoscopic; there is more illumination; and the peripheral retina can be more easily visualized, especially when combined with the technique of scleral depression. The disadvantages are the inverted image, decreased magnification, and the fact that the pupil must be dilated with a mydriatic strong enough to

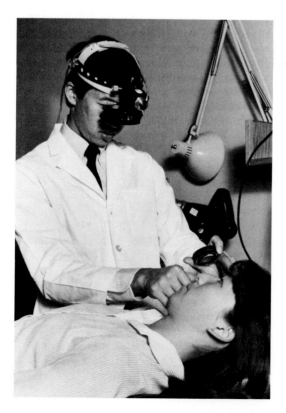

Figure 3–16. Examination with binocular indirect ophthalmoscopy. (Photo by M Narahara.)

overcome the pupillary constrictive effect of the bright light. Retinal surgeons rely heavily on indirect ophthalmoscopy both for preoperative diagnostic evaluation and during retinal detachment surgery.

OPHTHALMODYNAMOMETRY

Ophthalmodynamometry gives an approximate measurement of the relative pressures in the central retinal arteries and is an indirect means of assessing the carotid artery flow on either side. It is performed with the patient in a sitting position with the head supported. The test consists of exerting pressure on the sclera with a spring plunger while observing with an ophthalmoscope the vessels emerging from the optic disk. The pressure is gradually increased until the central retinal artery begins to pulsate at the point where it or one of its branches leaves the disk. This reading represents the diastolic pressure in the ophthalmic artery on that side, and this pressure is approximately half the brachial blood pressure. The procedure is then repeated in the other eye. The 2 readings are recorded directly from the scale in millimeters of mercury.

Ophthalmodynamometry is indicated in the neurologic evaluation of patients who complain of "blacking out" (amaurosis fugax) in one eye, spells of weakness on one side of the body, or other symptoms of impending cerebrovascular accident. No significant complications have been reported with its use.

A difference of more than 20% in the diastolic pressures between the 2 eyes suggests insufficiency of the carotid arterial system on the side with the lower reading.

FLUORESCEIN ANGIOGRAPHY

Ophthalmoscopy following the intravenous injection of fluorescein has gained great diagnostic importance in ophthalmology. This specialized technique provides sequential evaluation of the anatomic and physiologic status of the choroidal and retinal vasculature.

Equipment & Materials

The following items are needed: sterile aqueous sodium fluorescein solution, 10%; 5-mL syringe with 21-gauge needle; indirect ophthalmoscope with cobalt filter; and, if permanent photographic records are to be made, a fundus camera with appropriately paired filters, eg, Nos. 47 and 15 Kodak Wratten filters (Fig 3–17).

Technique

Following maximum mydriasis, 5 mL of 10% aqueous sodium fluorescein is rapidly injected into the antecubital vein with the patient in a sitting position. Black and white photographs are taken with a

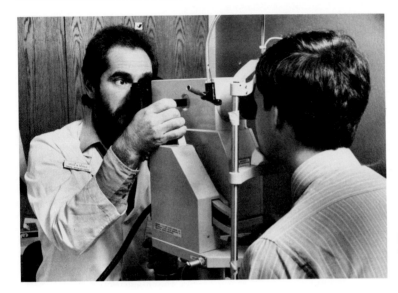

Figure 3–17 (at left). Fluorescein angiography with fundus camera. (Photo by M Narahara.)

camera equipped with a motorized film advance and a high-intensity flash generator capable of recycling at approximately 1-second intervals. Photographs are taken prior to injection and then at half-second intervals for 20 seconds. Additional exposures are made at intervals up to 5 minutes. Valuable information can be obtained by simply observing the fundus after the injection of fluorescein (fluorescein angioscopy). A cobalt or Wratten 47A filter should be placed before the light source of the indirect ophthalmoscope.

Normal Findings

The normal pattern of fluorescein angiography can be divided into 3 phases:

A. Filling Phase: (8–20 seconds.) The choroidal circulation (choroidal flush) precedes retinal arterial filling. It is first seen in the macular area and spreads toward the periphery. A cilioretinal artery is observed at this stage. The fluorescein leaks from the choroidal vessels to the extravascular space.

The retinal arterial filling phase starts 0.5 second after the choroidal flush (Fig 3–18). This is followed by capillary transition and a venous drainage phase.

The retinal pigment epithelium acts as a physical and optical barrier to fluorescein. It prevents leakage of the dye into the inner retina and, except in albino patients, masks most of the fluorescence of the underlying choroidal circulation.

B. Recirculation Phase: (3–5 minutes.) The fluorescein concentration in the choroidal intravascular and extravascular spaces is equal. In the normal retina, fluorescein is confined to the intravascular space and there is no leakage to surrounding tissue.

C. Late Phase: (30–60 minutes.) There is little or no fluorescein in the retinal vessels. There may be very faint staining in the choroid and lamina cribrosa. This stage marks the elimination of fluorescein from the body.

Abnormal Findings (Fig 3–19)

Vascular abnormalities such as arteriovenous shunts, microaneurysms, and neovascularization are detected early in the filling phase. Vascular leakage can be observed later. Window defects in the retinal pigment epithelium eliminate the optical barrier between the retina and choroid and transmit underlying fluorescence. Hyperpigmented areas and retinal hemorrhages, on the other hand, obscure the underlying fluorescence. Serous choroidal fluid accumulated under the retinal pigment epithelium shows early fluorescence. Serous fluid between the sensory and pigment epithelium fluoresces more slowly and at a later stage. Retinal edema or inflammation and fibrous tissue may show variable degrees of fluorescence. Suspected papilledema can be confirmed by vascular leakage in the area of the disk.

Figure 3–18. Normal angiogram, mid venous phase. (Photo courtesy of Roger Griffith and Terry King.)

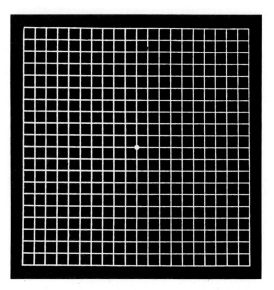

Figure 3–19. Abnormal angiogram showing prominent perifoveal detachment of the retinal pigment epithelium. (Photo courtesy of Roger Griffith and Terry King.)

Figure 3–20. Amsler grid.

AMSLER GRID

The Amsler grid is useful for detecting and following central scotomas.

Equipment & Materials
The Amsler grid is shown in Fig 3–20.

Technique
With one eye occluded, the patient holds the Amsler grid chart at the customary reading distance with glasses on. While fixating the central dot, the individual is asked to describe and outline any area of distortion or absence of the grid.

This test may be used by patients at home to detect progression of macular disease.

Normal & Abnormal Findings
Abnormal findings include all positive and negative scotomas. The patient may describe a gray area, an area where the lines are missing, or an area where the grid is distorted (metamorphopsia).

OPHTHALMIC RADIOLOGY
(X-Ray, CT Scan, MRI)

Plain x-ray, tomography, and CT scan are useful in the evaluation of any orbital or intracranial condition. CT scan in particular has become the primary method of localizing and characterizing structural disease in the extraocular visual pathway (for further discussion, see Chapters 17 and 18).

The intraocular applications for radiology are primarily the detection of foreign bodies following trauma and the demonstration of intraocular calcium in tumors such as retinoblastoma. CT scan is the most important means of foreign body localization because of its multidimensional reformatting capabilities and its ability to image the ocular walls.

Although not yet of uniform quality, magnetic resonance imaging (MRI) is a promising new diagnostic tool. Its resolving capability is better than that of CT scan and should prove to be of significant value in intracranial studies. However, the practical advan-

Figure 3–21. Intraocular metallic foreign body as seen by x-ray. (Left lateral view.)

tages of MRI for ophthalmic evaluation have yet to be convincingly demonstrated.

See Fig 3–21 and Chapters 17 and 18 for illustrations of x-ray, CT scan, and MRI.

ELECTRORETINOGRAPHY

The normal retina exhibits certain electrical changes when exposed to light. Measurement of the changes in potential under the influence of light is known as electroretinography. The recorded electroretinogram (ERG) represents the difference in potential between an electrode placed in a corneal contact lens and an electrode placed on the forehead. The ERG is a composite curve resulting from several superimposed events and consists of 4 waves:

a **wave:** The initial negative response after a latency period following the light stimulus (photoreceptor cell layer).

b **wave:** The positive deflection (bipolar cell layer).

c **wave:** A slight positive deflection.

d **wave (off effect):** A positive potential occurring when the light is turned off.

The ganglion cell layer and the nerve fiber layer do not contribute to the ERG.

Electroretinography is usually performed under both photopic (light-adapted) and scotopic (dark-adapted) conditions.

ERG has a number of clinical applications. It may be a helpful diagnostic aid in patients with *diffuse* retinal damage with or without ophthalmoscopic changes. It is also of great help in the evaluation of the retina if the optical media are opaque. Local macular diseases are not detected by electroretinography.

VISUAL EVOKED RESPONSE (VER)
(Visual Evoked Potential, VEP)

When a flash of light strikes the retina, it evokes a volley of nerve impulses that are transmitted along the visual pathways to the occipital cortex. The response to the light stimulus can be recognized only after an averaging computer eliminates asynchronous spontaneous activity and thus enhances the response to repeated (50–100) light stimulations.

Fig 3–22 shows the normal response to 100 flash stimuli recorded from over the occipital lobes. The first upward deflection at a latency of 40–50 ms gives data on the velocity and quality of conduction along the visual pathways. Later components show the response as the visual information is processed in the brain.

By stimulating each eye separately, optic nerve lesions can be recognized in the absence of hemisphere response from the affected nerve (Fig 3–23). Partial optic nerve lesions result in delayed conduction and reduced amplitude. Retrochiasmatic lesions are recognized by the different hemispheric responses (Fig 3–24).

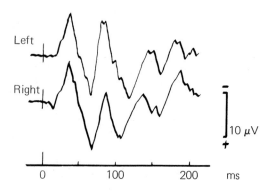

Figure 3–22. Normal VER recorded from over the left and right occipital poles. (Courtesy of M Feinsod.)

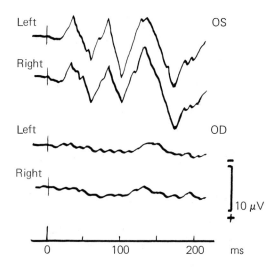

Figure 3–23. Complete right optic nerve lesion. No response is evoked by stimulating the right eye (OD). (Courtesy of M Feinsod.)

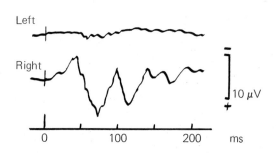

Figure 3–24. Right homonymous hemianopia. No response is recorded from over the left hemisphere. (Courtesy of M Feinsod.)

Figure 3–25. Ultrasonography using B-scan probe. (Photo by M Narahara.)

Visual evoked response is becoming an important tool in the objective investigation of the visual system in babies or nonresponsive patients. It is of recognized value in the detection of subclinical lesions in the visual pathways, eg, as may occur in multiple sclerosis. With the use of a patterned light of various gratings, the VER has become a major tool in research on amblyopia.

ULTRASONOGRAPHY

Ultrasonography utilizes the principle of sonar to allow viewing of structures that might otherwise not be directly visible. High-frequency sound waves are emitted from a transmitter toward the target organ. As the sound waves bounce back off the various tissue components, they are collected by a receiver that amplifies and displays them on an oscilloscope screen.

A single probe that contains both the transmitter and receiver is placed against the eye and used to aim the beam of sound (Fig 3–25). Various structures in its path will reflect separate echoes (which arrive at different times) back toward the probe. Those derived from the most distal structures arrive last, having traveled the farthest.

There are 2 methods of clinical ultrasonography, A scan and B scan. In **A scan,** the sound beam is aimed in a straight line. Each echo is displayed as a spike, the amplitude of which is dependent on the

Figure 3–26. A scan *(left)* and B scan *(right)* of an intraocular tumor (melanoma). C = cornea; I = iris; L = posterior lens surface; O = optic nerve; R = retina; T = tumor. (Courtesy of RD Stone.)

density of the reflecting tissue and its degree of perpendicularity to the probe (which maximizes the strength of reflection toward the probe). The spikes are arranged in temporal sequence, with the latency of each signal corresponding to that structure's distance from the probe (Fig 3–26). If the same probe is now swept across the eye, a series of individual A scans is obtained; from these scans, a 2-dimensional image, or **B scan,** can be constructed.

Although therapeutic applications are being investigated, ophthalmic ultrasonography is currently used mainly for diagnosis and measurement. Both A and B scans can be used to image and differentiate orbital disease or intraocular anatomy concealed by opaque media. In addition to defining the size and location of intraocular and orbital masses, A and B scans can provide clues to the tissue characteristics of a lesion (eg, solid, cystic, vascular, calcified).

Quantitatively, A scan is the most accurate method. The temporal separation of echoes arriving from 2 different points can be used to calculate the distance between the points, based on the speed of sound in the tissue medium. The most commonly used ocular measurement is the axial length (cornea to retina); this is important in cataract surgery in order to calculate the power for an intraocular lens implant. A scans can also be used to monitor tumor growth over time.

REFERENCES

Boyd BF (editor): *Highlights of Ophthalmology.* 2 vols. Highlights of Ophthalmology Press, 1981.

Braley AE et al: *Stereoscopic Atlas of Slit-Lamp Biomicroscopy.* 2 vols. Mosby, 1970.

Dallow RL: Reliability of orbital tests: Ultrasonography, computerized tomography, and radiography. *Ophthalmology* 1978;**85:**1218.

Feinsod M et al: Visually evoked response. *Arch Ophthalmol* 1976;**94:**237.

Green DG, Cohen MM: Laser interferometry in the evaluation of potential macular function in the presence of opacities in the ocular media. *Trans Am Acad Ophthalmol Otolaryngol* 1971;**75:**629.

Guyton DL: Instruments for measuring retinal visual acuity behind cataracts. *Ophthalmology* 1982;**89(8S):**34.

Harrington DO: *The Visual Fields: A Textbook and Atlas of Clinical Perimetry,* 5th ed. Mosby, 1981.

Heijl A et al: A clinical comparison of three computerized automatic perimeters in the detection of glaucoma defects. *Arch Ophthalmol* 1981;**99:**832.

Keeney AH: *Ocular Examination: Basis and Technique,* 2nd ed. Mosby, 1976.

Krimsky E: Simple eye tests. *Postgrad Med* (Dec) 1966;**40:**697.

Miller BW: A review of practical tests for ocular malingering and hysteria. *Surv Ophthalmol* 1973;**17:**241.

Miller NR: *Walsh & Hoyt's Clinical Neuro-Ophthalmology,* 4th ed. Vol 1. Williams & Wilkins, 1982.

Minkowski JS, Palese M, Guyton DL: Potential acuity meter using a minute aerial pinhole aperture. *Ophthalmology* 1983;**90:**1360.

Moses R (editor): *Adler's Physiology of the Eye,* 7th ed. Mosby, 1981.

Norton EWD (editor): Symposium: The value of fluorescein angiography in the study of choroidal and pigment epithelial disease. *Trans Am Acad Ophthalmol Otolaryngol* 1973;**77:**724.

Perkins ES: Tonometry. *Proc R Soc Med* 1976;**60:**63.

Pinschmidt NW: Evaluation of the Schirmer tear test. *South Med J* 1970;**63:**1256.

Richard JM (editor): *A Manual for the Beginning Ophthalmology Resident,* 3rd ed. American Academy of Ophthalmology, 1980.

Shammas HJ: *Atlas of Ophthalmic Ultrasonography and Biometry.* Mosby, 1984.

Smith SE: Mydriatic drugs for routine fundal inspection. *Ophthalmol Digest* 1972;**34:**10.

Thompson HS: Functional visual loss. *Am J Ophthalmol* 1985;**100:**209.

Walsh TJ: *The Interpretation of Visual Fields,* 4th ed. American Academy of Ophthalmology, 1979.

Ophthalmoscopic Examination

Hermann von Helmholtz, a German physicist and physiologist, invented the ophthalmoscope in 1851. In so doing, he provided the medical practitioner—ophthalmologist, internist, or neurologist—with an instrument that has become indispensable to the study of eye diseases and systemic diseases with ocular manifestations. Nowhere else in the body is it possible to examine living vascular and nerve tissue under magnification, and the information gained in this way can be of great diagnostic importance. It can also be of value in the management of a recognized disease process, providing a ready means of estimating changes in established lesions.

The principal contribution of the ophthalmoscope is of course the remarkable view of the inner eye it provides. Ophthalmoscopy, or examination of the fundus—optic disk, retina, retinal vessels, macula, and choroid—is therefore of prime ophthalmoscopic importance. However, examination of other ocular tissues—cornea, iris, lens, and vitreous—with the ophthalmoscope also yields valuable information. Although the slit lamp is a better instrument for this purpose, it is often not available, since it is used principally by the ophthalmologist. Inspection of the anterior ocular structures with the ophthalmoscope may alert the examiner to a wide variety of changes that are indicative of ocular or systemic diseases. It is possible in this way to recognize vascular changes and opacities in the cornea; hemorrhages and exudates in the anterior chamber; the location and nature of opacities in the lens; irregularities of the pupil; and opacities, detachments, and degenerative changes in the vitreous.

For all of these reasons, ophthalmoscopy should be an integral part of every general physical examination; and since both the ocular media and the fundus can be examined quickly and easily with the modern ophthalmoscope once its principles are understood, everyone doing general physical examinations—medical students, interns, general practitioners, internists, pediatricians, and others—should feel obliged to master the use of this extraordinary but essentially quite simple instrument.

The Use of Mydriatics

For the purposes of routine physical examination, it is almost always possible to visualize the ocular media and fundus adequately without dilating the pupil if the lighting in the examining room is sufficiently subdued and the light in the ophthalmoscope is strong (fresh batteries). If mydriasis is indicated, however

(eg, to investigate impaired vision of unknown cause), the mydriatic should be short-acting and should not affect accommodation.

Phenylephrine hydrochloride (2.5–10%) is an excellent mydriatic for this purpose. Others are mentioned briefly in Chapter 28. The drug acts rapidly; and dilation of the pupil can be accomplished by one or 2 instillations. A heavily pigmented iris is less responsive than a lightly pigmented one to phenylephrine alone, and such a patient may require the use of a cycloplegic, such as homatropine or cyclopentolate, along with phenylephrine.

Since any mydriatic agent can precipitate acute angle-closure glaucoma in an eye with a shallow anterior chamber, mydriatics must always be used with caution. In young patients the danger is negligible, but in adults the depth of the anterior chamber should be estimated by oblique illumination with a flashlight (Fig 15–8).

TYPES OF OPHTHALMOSCOPY

There are 2 types of ophthalmoscopy: indirect and direct. Each has special uses as well as special advantages and disadvantages (Table 4–1). Both require a darkened room and an ophthalmoscope supplied with an electrical source strong enough to produce a bright light. As a rule, the patient is sitting down and the examiner is standing—at the right side of the patient and holding the ophthalmoscope in the right hand when the right eye is examined; at the left side and using the left hand when the left eye is examined (Fig 4–5).

1. INDIRECT OPHTHALMOSCOPY (Fig 4–2)

Indirect ophthalmoscopy has been performed for many years by holding a convex lens (objective) between the ophthalmoscope and the patient's eye. The ophthalmoscope, with a +3 or +4 diopter lens in the aperture to neutralize the observer's accommodation, is held several centimeters from the patient's eye.

The disk is brought into view by having the patient look over the examiner's right shoulder at ear level when examining the right eye, and over the left shoulder at the same level when examining the left eye. Areas of interest near the disk can then be examined by having the patient move the eyes slightly in various directions.

Indirect ophthalmoscopy has 2 distinct advantages over direct ophthalmoscopy: It provides a large field of vision that gives the examiner a good view of the fundus even through an undilated pupil and in spite of opacities in the media, and it is not affected by major refractive errors in the patient's eyes. The disadvantages are the lower magnification and the inverted image. In making and recording observations, the observer must never forget that the image is inverted.

Binocular Indirect Ophthalmoscopy

The binocular indirect ophthalmoscope began to come into wide use among ophthalmologists in the 1950s. Its use is now being taught to all students of ophthalmology, and in the specialist's hands, it is being used almost to the exclusion of the standard monocular ophthalmoscope. Its advantages are a more powerful light source that can cut through cloudy media (eg, incipient cataract); its binocularity; and the fact that the entire peripheral retina can be viewed with it. It is unlikely, however, that this instrument will meet the needs of medical students and other physicians doing general physical examinations, since it is relatively cumbersome and expensive, the technique of using it is difficult to master, and the pupil must be widely dilated because of its very strong light.

This instrument is further discussed and illustrated in Chapter 3.

2. DIRECT OPHTHALMOSCOPY
(Figs 4–3, 4–4, 4–5)

The use of the direct ophthalmoscope is the principal subject matter of this chapter. Unless otherwise specified, all further references are understood to be to direct ophthalmoscopy.

The instrument has been greatly improved since Helmholtz published the first description of the ophthalmoscope, but the principle is the same. The basic unit is a strong light that can be directed into the patient's eye by reflection from a small mirror. The light is then reflected from the fundus of the patient's eye back through a small aperture in the ophthalmoscope to the examiner's eye. Various models of electric and battery-powered ophthalmoscopes are available.

In direct ophthalmoscopy, the aperture of the instrument is held as close as possible to the observer's eye and the subject's eye. The details of the inner eye will then be in focus if both eyes (examiner's and patient's) are emmetropic. If either eye is ametropic, a graduated series of convex (plus) or concave (minus) lenses can be moved into the aperture (by rotating the lens wheel with one finger) to bring the details into focus.

As the examiner directs the beam of the ophthalmoscope into the patient's eye and moves the plus lenses successively into the aperture (from +20 diopters down to about +4 diopters), the magnified details of the anterior segment of the eye (cornea, iris, and lens) will first be visualized. As the examiner gradually reduces the strength of the plus lenses, the focus of observation gradually extends posteriorly through the vitreous until the retinal and other fundus details come into view.

The fundi of aphakic eyes (eyes without lenses) are examined with a lens in the range of +8 to +12 in the aperture or with the patient's own corrective lenses in place.

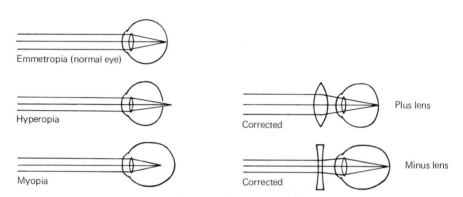

Figure 4–1. Common defects of the optical system of the eye. In hyperopia the eyeball is too short, and light rays come to a focus behind the retina. A biconvex lens corrects this by adding to the refractive power of the lens of the eye. In myopia the eyeball is too long, and light rays focus in front of the retina. Placing a biconcave lens in front of the eye causes the light rays to diverge slightly before striking the eye, so that they are brought to a focus on the retina. (Modified and reproduced, with permission, from Ganong WF: *Review of Medical Physiology*, 12th ed. Lange, 1985.)

Table 4—1. Comparison of indirect and direct ophthalmoscopy.

	Indirect	Direct
Area of field examined	Eight disk diameters	Two diameters
Area accessible to view	Up to ora serrata	Up to equator
Stereopsis	Yes	No
Image	Inverted, virtual	Erect, true
Magnification	2—4 ×	15—15 ×

Red Fundus Reflection

The first step in ophthalmoscopy is to look for the red fundus reflection, which can be seen without magnification from a comfortable distance of 25– 40 cm. The experienced examiner, when seeing the fundus reflection, can immediately rule out gross corneal lesions, dense opacities of the media, and complete detachment of the retina.

If opacities are present, they will appear as black forms against the red background.

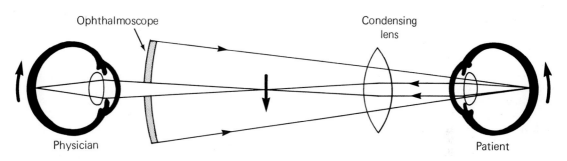

Figure 4 –2. Indirect ophthalmoscopy. Arrow at focal point represents inverted image of patient's ocular fundus.

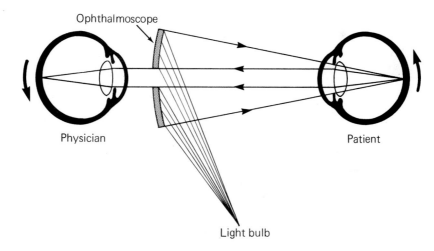

Figure 4 –3. Direct ophthalmoscopy. Arrows show spatial orientation of images in examiner's and patient's eyes. (Modified and reproduced, with permission, from Nover A: *The Ocular Fundus,* 2nd ed. Lea & Febiger, 1971.)

Figure 4–4. Ophthalmoscope. (Courtesy of Propper Manufacturing Co., Inc.)

Figure 4–5. Position of patient and examiner for direct ophthalmoscopy.

Cornea, Aqueous, Iris, & Lens

A. Cornea: In order to examine the cornea at close range, a strong plus lens is introduced into the aperture of the ophthalmoscope. For example, a dendritic lesion of the cornea is easy to see with a +20 diopter lens from a distance of approximately 2 cm, and with the same lens one can see corneal scars, ulcers, foreign bodies, pterygiums, and vascularization. (Figs 4–6 to 4–10.)

Figure 4–6 (at right). Examination of the cornea with a strong convex lens at close range.

Figure 4–7. Dendritic figures seen in herpes simplex keratitis.

Figure 4–9. Pterygium, right eye. (Photo by Diane Beeston.)

Figure 4–8. Trachomatous pannus. (Courtesy of P Thygeson.)

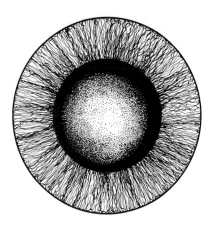

Figure 4–10. Disciform herpes simplex keratitis.

B. Aqueous: The examiner can get a magnified view of abnormalities in the aqueous with the ophthalmoscope, eg, blood (hyphema) resulting from trauma or pus (hypopyon) in association with bacterial corneal ulcer. (Figs 4– 11 and 4– 12.)

C. Iris: Since the iris is behind the cornea, a weaker lens is required in the ophthalmoscope to make it clearly visible. With a +15 diopter lens, for example, such disorders of the iris as tumors, nodules, pigmentary abnormalities, and synechiae can be seen in adequate detail. (Figs 4– 13 and 4– 14.)

D. Lens: The lens is still farther posterior and can be seen quite well with a lens in the range of +8 to +12 diopters. If there are lens opacities, their location, shapes, sizes, and degrees of density can all be clearly viewed. (Figs 4– 15 to 4– 19.)

Figure 4–13. Examination of the iris with a strong convex lens.

Figure 4–11. Hypopyon. (Courtesy of K Tabbara.)

Figure 4–14. Tumor of iris. (Courtesy of K Tabbara.)

Figure 4–12. Blood in the anterior chamber (hyphema). (Courtesy of M Hogan.)

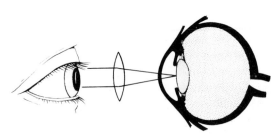

Figure 4–15 (at right). Examination of the lens with a weaker convex lens.

Figure 4–16. Senile cataract, "cuneiform" type. (Reproduced, with permission, from Cordes FC: *Cataract Types,* 3rd ed. American Academy of Ophthalmology and Otolaryngology, 1965.)

Figure 4–18. Traumatic "star-shaped" cataract in the posterior lens. (From Cordes FC: Ibid.)

Figure 4–17. Mature senile cataract. (Courtesy of A Rosenberg.)

Figure 4–19. "Vossius' ring." (From Cordes FC: Ibid.)

Vitreous (Fig 4–20)

As the examiner gradually rotates the lens wheel to bring lenses of from +8 to +4 diopters into the aperture, the focus extends posteriorly into the vitreous. Cloudiness of the vitreous may occur as a result of various inflammatory diseases of the optic disk, retina, and uvea. Vitreous hemorrhages give a very dark picture. Even a small amount of blood in the vitreous may appear almost black and can completely obstruct the view of the fundus. Fibrovascular proliferation in the vitreous can be seen in patients with advanced diabetic retinopathy. Degenerative changes—asteroid hyalosis and synchysis scintillans—can easily be seen with the ophthalmoscope.

Fundus (Figs 4–21 and 4–22)

Examination of the fundus includes inspection of the optic disk, macula, retina, retinal vessels, choroid, and sclera. These structures can be brought into clear focus with a wide range of lenses depending on the refractive error of the patient and the examiner. If the patient has high myopia, the size of the image is greatly increased; with high hyperopia, it is greatly decreased. The retina can be examined by direct ophthalmoscopy as far anteriorly as the equator of the eyeball in patients with widely dilated pupils; but the area from the equator to the ora serrata can be examined adequately only with the binocular indirect ophthalmoscope.

Examination of the fundus must proceed systematically if lesions of diagnostic importance are not to be overlooked. A sketch of the disk, macula, and major blood vessels will help to localize the lesions, and all fundus lesions should be described and sketched for the case record. If the lesion is one that should be observed periodically, fundus photographs are highly desirable.

Figure 4–20. Metallic foreign body in vitreous as seen with ophthalmoscope.

Figure 4–21. Examination of retina with a zero lens (assuming that the physician is emmetropic).

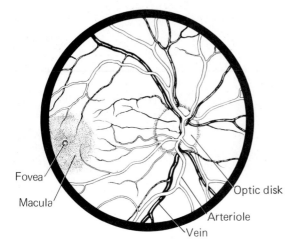

Fovea

Macula

Optic disk

Arteriole

Vein

Figure 4–22. The normal fundus. Diagram at left shows landmarks of the photograph at right. (Photo by Diane Beeston.)

A. Optic Disk: (Figs 4–23 to 4–31.) Under the strong light of an ophthalmoscope and with adequate magnification, observation of the optic disk can yield clinical information that is not available about any other nerve in the body. As a first step in the examination, the disk's size, color, and vascularity and the degree of cupping should be assessed.

Although the diameter of the normal optic disk in adults averages only about 1.5 mm, with the ophthalmoscope it appears quite large. All of the details are clearly visible, including the central artery and vein and the numerous capillaries on the disk's surface that produce the pink color.

The disk is round or oval, and the nasal edge is less distinct than the temporal edge. A white crescent may appear around the temporal edge, especially in myopic patients. This is bare sclera exposed by a normal break in the choroid.

The optic disk usually has a white central depression (cup) whose diameter averages approximately one-third of the disk diameter. This is referred to as the cup/disk ratio and should be noted on the patient's record (eg, 0.3 cup). In normal individuals the cup/disk ratio ranges from 0.0 (flat disk) to 0.9 (huge cup). In some patients, the disk is elevated, and if the elevation is significant the condition is referred to as pseudopapilledema. In patients with glaucoma, recording the cup/disk ratio is especially important, since the breadth and depth of the cup increase in uncontrolled glaucoma with the death of the nerve fibers. In this situation, the cup/disk ratio becomes a measure of the progress of the disease.

In optic neuritis the disk becomes abnormally vascular and slightly elevated. Small hemorrhages are sometimes seen.

In papilledema, the essential feature is bulging forward (elevation) of the disk due to pressure (usually intracranial) from behind. The vessels on the disk's surface are engorged, and hemorrhages may occur.

In optic atrophy, there is reduction in the vascularity of the optic nerve head. With reduction in vascularity, the normal pink color of the healthy disk turns white.

In central retinal artery occlusion, the disk immediately becomes pale. Weeks to months later, the nerve whitens.

Occlusion of the central retinal vein produces a dramatic clinical picture. Extensive hemorrhages in the region of the optic disk make the area look as if it had been "slapped with a red paintbrush."

Figure 4–23. Normal optic disk and peripapillary retina. Note rich vascular network supplying the retinal nerve fiber layer surrounding the disk. (Courtesy of WF Hoyt.)*

*(Photos on pp 351–355 are by Ron Eckelhoff.)

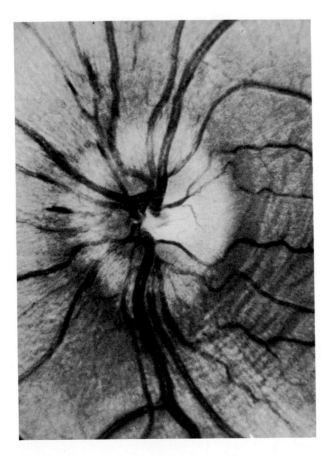

Figure 4–24. Early papilledema showing blurring of disk margins and peripapillary nerve fiber layer. Vessels are buried (blurred by surrounding edema), resulting in absence of highlights and fine detail in retina. (Courtesy of WF Hoyt.)

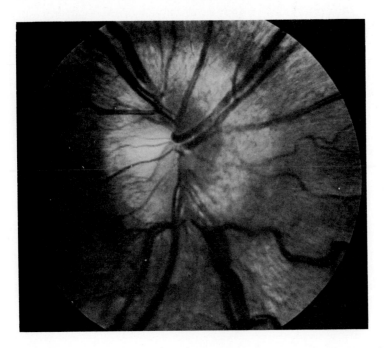

Figure 4–25. Papilledema causing moderate disk elevation without hemorrhages. (Courtesy of WF Hoyt.)

Figure 4–26. Pseudopapilledema. Note vessels on top (not buried). (Courtesy of WF Hoyt.)

Figure 4–27. Congenitally "full" optic disk. There is no edema, and the disk is not choked. (Courtesy of WF Hoyt.)

Figure 4–28. Optic neuritis (papillitis) with disk changes, including capillary hemorrhages and minimal edema. (Courtesy of WF Hoyt.)

Figure 4–29. Optic atrophy. Note avascular white disk and avascular network in surrounding retina. (Courtesy of WF Hoyt.)

Figure 4–30. Chorioretinal peripapillary scar with atrophy of overlying nerve fiber layer, perhaps due to toxoplasmosis. Central vision was defective. (Courtesy of WF Hoyt.)

Figure 4–31. Arteriovenous malformation of retina and disk (Wyburn-Mason syndrome). (Courtesy of WF Hoyt.)

B. Macula: (Figs 4–32 to 4–35.) The macula is an oval area situated about 2 disk diameters temporally to and slightly below the optic disk. It is devoid of blood vessels and appears to be darker than the surrounding retina. There is a central light reflection from the centrally located, slightly depressed fovea.

The commonest affliction of the macula is disciform macular degeneration. In its end stage this appears as a round, fairly well circumscribed, elevated white mass. Other types of macular degeneration (hereditary, cystic, circinate, etc) are described in Chapter 14.

In central retinal artery occlusion, the macula is edematous and ischemic. With the choroidal blood supply showing through, the fovea, in contrast to the ischemic retina, appears as a "cherry-red spot."

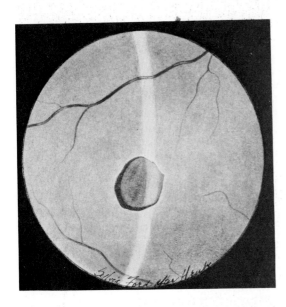

Figure 4–32. Hole in retina, macular area, posttraumatic.

Figure 4–34. Twenty-four hours after closure of central retinal artery, left eye. The macular area shows a "cherry-red spot."

Figure 4–33. Healed disciform macular degeneration (drawing). (Courtesy of F Cordes.)

Figure 4–35. Juvenile macular degeneration (hereditary). (Courtesy of WF Hoyt. Photo by Ron Eckelhoff.)

C. Retina: Retinal detachment appears ophthalmoscopically as a gray, elevated cloud affecting part or all of the retina. Detachments are associated with one or more orange-red retinal tears.

A variety of retinal disturbances (eg, those associated with retinitis pigmentosa) can be seen with the ophthalmoscope. (Figs 4–36 to 4–45.)

Figure 4–36. Retinitis pigmentosa. *Left:* Typical "bone spicule" arrangement of pigmentary changes. *Right:* Clumped, scattered pigment, attenuated arteries, and choroidal sclerosis. (Photos by L Arlinghaus.)

Figure 4–37. Thrombosis of superior temporal retinal vein. (Courtesy of K Tabbara.)

Figure 4–38. Subhyaloid hemorrhage around optic disk associated with subarachnoid hemorrhage (drawing).

Figure 4–40. Hemangiomas of the retina (drawing). (Courtesy of F Cordes.)

Figure 4–39. Tuberous sclerosis.

Figure 4–41. Retinoblastomas after x-ray radiation.

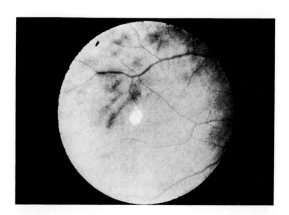

Figure 4 –42. Retinal fat embolism. (Courtesy of K Tabbara.)

Figure 4 –44. "Histo spot"—a depigmented area in peripheral retina. (Courtesy of K Tabbara.)

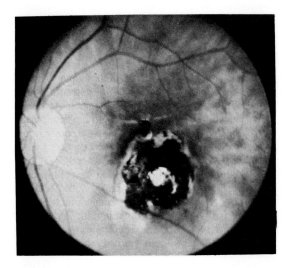

Figure 4 –43. Healed toxoplasmic chorioretinitis. Note scarring in left macular area.

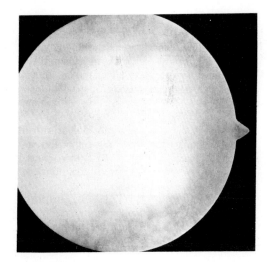

Figure 4 –45. Acute toxoplasmic chorioretinitis. (Courtesy of K Tabbara.)

D. Retinal Vessels: The retinal arteries and veins can be seen clearly with the ophthalmoscope. After the first bifurcation of the central retinal artery, the vessels are called arterioles. They should be examined for caliber, occlusion, color of the blood column, course and contour, light reflection from the blood column, pulsation, compression, and aneurysms.

In arteriosclerosis, the walls of the retinal arterioles are infiltrated with lipids and cholesterol. Sclerosis supervenes, and the sclerotic changes are easy to see ophthalmoscopically.

In hypertension, the changes in the retinal arterioles include vasospasm, narrowing, sclerosis, and eventually occlusion. If severe enough, hypertensive retinopathy can lead to retinal edema, cotton wool patches, hemorrhages, and eventually papilledema.

These changes are classified according to the Keith-Wagener system (Fig 4–46).

Retinal changes associated with diabetes mellitus are similar to the changes associated with hypertension but more devastating (Fig 4–47). They include microaneurysms, dilated veins, hemorrhages and exudates, and neovascularization. When major hemorrhages are absorbed, fibrous tissue forms along with the neovascularization. This gives the picture of proliferative diabetic retinopathy, which is usually destructive enough to cause blindness. (See also Chapter 14.)

Retinal hemorrhages and exudates can also be caused by other systemic disorders, including lupus erythematosus and blood dyscrasias (Figs 4–48 and 4–49).

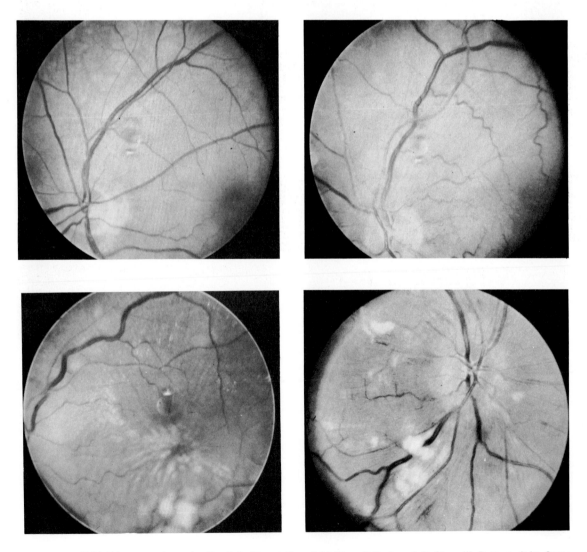

Figure 4–46. Keith-Wagener retinopathy. *Top left:* Stage I. *Top right:* Stage II. *Bottom left:* Stage III. *Bottom right:* Stage IV.

Figure 4–47. *Top left:* Background diabetic retinopathy. *Top right:* Background diabetic retinopathy with hard exudate (arrows). (Courtesy of P O'Malley.) *Lower left:* Preproliferative retinopathy with multiple cotton wool spots (incorrectly named soft exudates). (Courtesy of E Ai.) *Lower right:* Proliferative diabetic retinopathy. Fundus photograph of left eye, showing neovascularization of the disk and along the inferotemporal arcade (arrows). The latter area has bled, producing a preretinal hemorrhage (open arrow).

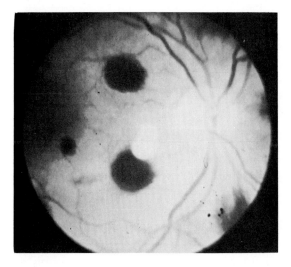

Figure 4–48. Retinal hemorrhages associated with severe pernicious anemia.

Figure 4–49. Engorged and markedly tortuous veins of polycythemia vera. (Photo by L Arlinghaus.)

E. Choroid and Sclera: (Figs 4–50 to 4–52.) If the pigment epithelium, which normally precludes visualization of the choroidal vessels and sclera, is congenitally absent or has degenerated, the vessels can be easily seen. In some myopic individuals, the sclera is visible near the temporal edge of the optic disk. In individuals who have punched-out lesions of the retina and choroid, which follow focal necrotizing retinochoroiditis (eg, toxoplasmosis, histoplasmosis), the sclera can be seen in the vicinity of the lesions surrounded by pigmentary proliferation.

Sclerosis of the choroidal vessels is seen in association with thinning and degeneration of the retina. A choroidal tear is quite likely to occur after a severe contusion of the globe.

Malignant melanoma appears ophthalmoscopically as a pigmented, elevated mass located most commonly in the posterior choroid on the temporal side.

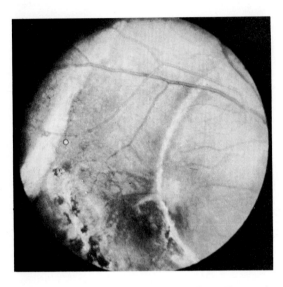

Figure 4–50. Choroidal tears. (Photo by Diane Beeston.)

Figure 4–52. Malignant melanoma of choroid, macular area, left eye (drawing). (Courtesy of F Cordes.)

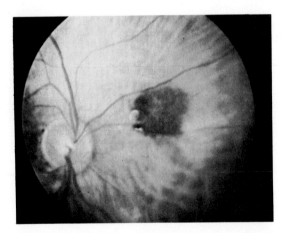

Figure 4–51. Nevus of choroid. (Photo by Diane Beeston.)

REFERENCES

Cogan DG: *Ophthalmic Manifestations of Systemic Vascular Disease*. Saunders, 1974.

Havener WH: *Synopsis of Ophthalmology: The Ophthalmoscopy Book*,6th ed. Mosby, 1984.

Jensen PE, Kalina RE: Congenital anomalies of the optic disk. *Am J Ophthalmol* 1976;**82**:27.

Jones WL, Reidy RW: *Atlas of the Peripheral Ocular Fundus*. Butterworth, 1985.

Keeney AH: *Ocular Examination: Basis and Techniques*, 2nd ed. Mosby, 1976.

Michaelson IC: *Ballantyne's Textbook of the Fundus of the Eye*, 3rd ed. Churchill Livingstone, 1980.

Nover A: *The Ocular Fundus*, 4th ed. Lea & Febiger, 1981. [Translated from the German by F Blodi.]

Orth DH: *Color and Fluorescein Angiographic Atlas of Retinal Vascular Disorders*. Williams & Wilkins, 1984.

Rucker CW: *History of the Ophthalmoscope*. Whiting Printers & Stationers, 1971.

Sauter H et al: *Atlas of the Ocular Fundus*. Urban & Schwarzenberg, 1984. [Translated from the German by F Blodi.]

5

Principles of Management of Common Ocular Disorders

It is not necessary to refer every patient with an eye disease to an ophthalmologist for treatment. In general, sties, bacterial conjunctivitis, superficial trauma to the lids, cornea, and conjunctiva, and superficial corneal foreign bodies can be treated just as effectively by the internist or general physician as by the ophthalmologist. On the other hand, more serious eye diseases or symptoms such as the following should be referred as soon as possible for specialized care: iritis, glaucoma, retinal detachment, strabismus, eye pain or blurred vision of undetermined origin, double vision, and corneal trauma or infection.

In the management of acute ocular disorders, it is most important to establish a definitive diagnosis before prescribing treatment. "All red eyes are not pinkeye," is a useful maxim, and the physician must be alert for the more serious iritis, keratitis, or glaucoma (see chart on inside front cover). The common practice of prescribing "shotgun" topical antibiotic combinations containing corticosteroids is to be discouraged, principally because of the inherent danger of incautious steroid treatment.

This chapter is an attempt to summarize the basic principles and techniques of diagnosis and management of common ocular problems. All of the disorders discussed here are dealt with in greater detail elsewhere in this book.

OFFICE EQUIPMENT & SUPPLIES

Basic Equipment

A great many specialized instruments have been devised for the investigation of eye disorders. However, most diseases of the eye can be diagnosed with the aid of a few relatively simple instruments:

(1) Hand flashlight.
(2) Binocular loupe.
(3) Ophthalmoscope.
(4) Visual acuity chart (Snellen).
(5) Tonometer. (Tonometry should be performed on all patients over 20 years of age having a physical examination.)

Basic Medications
A. Local Anesthetics:
1. Proparacaine, 0.5%.
2. Tetracaine, 0.5%.
B. Dyes: Sterile fluorescein papers, rose bengal solution.
C. Mydriatics: Phenylephrine, 2.5%, is a satis-

factory mydriatic when the examiner wishes to obtain a clearer view of the lens, vitreous, or ocular fundus.
D. Miotics: Pilocarpine, 1%.
E. Antibacterial Agents: Sulfisoxazole, 4% ophthalmic solution or ointment; and gentamicin, 0.3% solution or ointment.

HISTORY & PHYSICAL EXAMINATION

History

When taking a history from a patient who presents with an eye problem, a useful initial question is, "How do your eyes bother you?" After the patient has described the present difficulty, inquire specifically about glasses, blurred vision, pain, red eyes, double vision, trauma to the eyes or head, headaches, and "eyestrain." Information concerning the patient's general health is also relevant, particularly with regard to diabetes mellitus and hypertension. Since many eye diseases have a genetic pattern, the family history should be obtained. The patient's age and occupation are important factors in many ocular difficulties. Patients with glasses should be asked how long it has been since their prescription was changed.

Physical Examination

An adequate gross physical examination of the eye can be performed easily and quickly with a minimum of equipment (see above). By far the most important single examination is visual acuity testing in each eye. This should be done on all patients and the results noted in the clinical record. Visual acuity is tested at a distance of 6 meters (20 feet) using the Snellen chart. It is usually noted with and without glasses. However, corrected visual acuity has greater significance, since it is presumably the best possible visual acuity.

Inspection is facilitated by adequate illumination and should include a mental note of the patient's age, body build, and the structure of the head, face, and eyelids (eg, a patient with Marfan's syndrome is tall and thin and has long fingers). Bell's palsy and acromegaly may also be noted. Observe the eyes grossly for evidence of exophthalmos or enophthalmos.

Using a hand flashlight, examine the lids, conjunctivas, and corneas to rule out inflammation. Observe for icteric scleras (eg, hepatitis), pale conjunctivas (anemia), tumors, and scars. The pupillary light response should also be noted at this time. Gross disorders of ocular movements can be observed by having the patient follow the light of a moving flashlight by moving the eyes to the right, left, up, down, and inward while holding the head in fixed position.

Pressure over the tear sac will produce a mucoid or purulent discharge if significant infection is present.

With the ophthalmoscope, one can judge the clarity of the aqueous, lens, and vitreous as well as the appearance of the optic nerve, macula, retina, retinal blood vessels, and choroid. The ophthalmoscopic examination is facilitated by dim illumination in the examining room and a strong, well-focused light in the ophthalmoscope. If the ocular fundi cannot be easily inspected through the normal pupil, the pupil should be dilated. *Caution:* Before instilling the mydriatic, examine the anterior chamber by oblique illumination with a hand light (see p 193). If the anterior chamber is shallow (iris and lens quite close to the cornea), dilation of the pupils should be performed only by an ophthalmologist, since in these cases dilation may precipitate an attack of acute glaucoma.

In any patient over 20 years of age, tonometry should be performed as a screening test for glaucoma. Determining the intraocular pressure by finger palpation of the eyes (tactile tension) is not a reliable procedure.

BACTERIOLOGIC & MICROSCOPIC EXAMINATION

In the management of all serious external eye infections, the first step is to obtain a stained smear of the exudate. In conjunctivitis, for example, the scraping is taken directly from the conjunctival surface, and in corneal ulcer the scraping is taken directly from the advancing border of the lesion. The equipment necessary for the study of stained smears is as follows: sterile spatula, glass slides, stains (methylene blue, Wright's, Gram's, and Giemsa's), microscope, light, and immersion oil. Pull down on the patient's lower lid to expose the conjunctiva, make 3–4 horizontal scrapings, and smear on a clean glass slide. Allow to dry in air, fix with methanol, and stain. Prior instillation of local anesthetic drops minimizes discomfort from the scraping.

Cultures and antibiotic sensitivity studies should be done in *all* cases of corneal ulcer and in severe cases of bacterial conjunctivitis.

Study of the stained smear is far more important than culturing in the average ocular infection, since by this means one can immediately determine whether the causative agent is bacterial, viral, fungal, or allergic and because in some instances the exact cause can be determined on the spot. This information serves as a guide to treatment. For example, if pneumococci are found, almost any type of antibiotic will be effective, whereas staphylococcal infection will require more specific measures. If there is considerable inflammation of the conjunctiva, if no bacteria are found, and if monocytes are present in increased numbers in the smear, a diagnosis of viral conjunctivitis can be

made, and the physician knows that the condition will probably last 10–14 days with or without treatment. If many eosinophils are noted in the stained conjunctival smear, the conjunctivitis is probably due to allergy.

TREATMENT OF SPECIFIC EYE CONDITIONS

LIDS

Marginal Blepharitis

Marginal blepharitis is the most common disorder of the lids. The most important factor in its treatment is cleanliness, which is best maintained by rubbing the scales from the eyelid margins daily with a wet cotton applicator or clean washcloth or by scrubbing the lid margin and the base of the eyelashes with baby shampoo. Since this disorder is frequently associated with dandruff, vigorous efforts to keep the scalp clean are warranted. Specific antibiotic ointment should be applied to the lid margins once daily at bedtime when the condition is associated with microbial infection.

Internal Hordeolum

This common condition is essentially a meibomian gland abscess caused by infection with *Staphylococcus aureus.* The treatment is similar to that of a boil elsewhere on the body. Warm compresses should be applied for 15 minutes 3–4 times daily, followed by the instillation of sulfonamide or antibiotic ointment. Incision or expression is required when the hordeolum is pointing. If the hordeolum points toward the conjunctival surface, the incision should be a vertical one on the conjunctival side to avoid cutting across the meibomian glands. If the hordeolum is pointing on the lid side, a horizontal incision is made through the skin, since most of the lines of the skin in this region are horizontal.

External Hordeolum (Sty)

Infection of Zeis's or Moll's glands (sty) is smaller and more superficial than internal hordeolum (meibomian gland abscess). Pain and redness are the principal symptoms. Treatment is similar to that outlined for internal hordeolum.

Chalazion

A chalazion is a nontender lipogranulomatous inflammation of a meibomian gland. It should be excised by an ophthalmologist.

Dacryocystitis

A. In Adults: Acute dacryocystitis in adults usually implies that the nasolacrimal duct is completely blocked. Systemic administration of penicillin is effective treatment. Local treatment is generally ineffective. Operation is indicated if the infection does not respond to medical treatment. Dacryocystorhinostomy is the operation of choice for the prevention of recurrences of dacryocystitis.

B. In Infants: In infantile dacryocystitis, the tear sac should be massaged 3–4 times daily. Following the massage, instill sulfonamide or antibiotic drops into the conjunctival sac. If this is not successful, probing of the nasolacrimal duct by an ophthalmologist is indicated.

Tumors

Verrucae and papillomas are common and can usually be easily excised as well by the general physician as by the ophthalmologist as long as they are not near the lid margin. All lid tumors should be examined microscopically to rule out malignancy. Improper excision of tumors near the lid margin may result in lid abnormalities.

CONJUNCTIVA

Hyperemia of the conjunctival vessels is the most common cause of red eyes. Smog, smoke, and other irritants found in the environment may cause hyperemia of the conjunctival vessels. Local vasoconstrictors or cold compresses may be helpful in alleviating the symptoms and the redness.

Conjunctivitis caused by allergy can be helped by local vasoconstrictors and cold compresses. Topical corticosteroid drops may be used in severe cases under ophthalmologic supervision.

Conjunctivitis due to microbial agents—bacterial, viral, fungal, chlamydial, or parasitic—may be treated specifically after proper identification of the agent. Because treatment with ointments may cause blurring of vision for half an hour after instillation, eye drops are prescribed during the day; ointment can be used at bedtime to ensure prolonged effect during the sleeping hours. Patients are cautioned to wash their hands frequently and not to touch their eyes. This is to prevent spread of infection to the other eye as well as to other people. Individual washcloths and towels should be used. Systemic therapy may be indicated in certain forms of conjunctivitis (eg, chlamydial).

CORNEA*

Corneal Foreign Bodies

Note the time and place of the accident and what the patient was doing when it occurred. Visual acuity testing—if possible, before treatment is instituted—is important for legal as well as medical reasons in all cases.

If the patient complains of a foreign body sensation and gives a consistent history, there usually is one

*All corneal conditions except superficial foreign bodies should be treated by an ophthalmologist.

even though it may not be readily visible on the initial examination. However, if oblique illumination is used with the hand flashlight, almost all foreign bodies can be detected. If no corneal foreign bodies are seen and the patient continues to have a foreign body sensation, instill a local anesthetic and turn the upper lid to exclude the possibility of an upper tarsal conjunctival foreign body. If there is no conjunctival foreign body, stain the cornea with fluorescein paper. When the corneal foreign body is found, remove it with a wet cotton applicator or spud under good illumination, using an ocular loupe if one is available. Instill gentamicin ointment to prevent contamination with a gram-negative or gram-positive organism. It is not necessary to patch the eye, but it is essential that the patient be observed on the following day to exclude the possibility of secondary infection of the crater. If no infection occurs, the corneal wound will heal by epithelial regeneration. If infection occurs, the wound area may take weeks or months to heal.

Untreated infection may cause severe corneal ulceration with consequent marked visual loss. Early infection is manifested by a white necrotic area around the foreign body crater and a slight gray exudate. *Note:* These patients should be referred immediately to an ophthalmologist.

Corneal Abrasions

The history should be taken and visual acuity tested before treatment. A patient with a corneal abrasion complains of severe pain, especially with movement of the lid over the cornea. The surface of the cornea may be examined with a light and loupe. If an abrasion is suspected but cannot be seen, stain the cornea with sterile 2% fluorescein solution. The area of corneal abrasion will have a deeper green stain than the surrounding cornea.

Instill gentamicin ophthalmic ointment. Apply a tight pressure bandage to prevent movement of the lid and resultant irritation of the abraded corneal area. Bed rest may be necessary. The patient should be observed on the following day to be certain that the cornea is healing. Corneal abrasions heal in 24–72 hours if a pressure bandage is properly applied. In contrast to corneal foreign body wounds, there is little chance of infection. The main dangers are delayed healing and recurrent corneal erosion due to imperfect healing. Do not use corticosteroids or topical anesthetics in any form of physical injury of the cornea. Systemic analgesics may be necessary in certain cases.

UVEAL TRACT

Any uveal tract disorder may lead to permanent visual impairment. Therefore, the treatment should be supervised by an ophthalmologist.

Acute Anterior Uveitis (Iritis)

This is the most common disorder of the uveal tract and can easily be confused with both conjunctivitis and acute glaucoma. Treatment with local cycloplegics and steroids is usually effective within 10 days. However, recurrences are common.

Posterior Uveitis

This disorder is more difficult to diagnose than anterior uveitis, and treatment is much less effective.

Neoplasms of the Uveal Tract

Melanoma is a primary tumor of the uveal tract. Its usual location is in the posterior choroid, where it can be seen with the ophthalmoscope. The method of treatment is determined by the size, location, and growth characteristics of the melanoma. If a melanoma is situated in the iris, iridectomy is usually successful in removing the growth.

VITREOUS

One of the most common of eye complaints is "spots before the eyes." These are usually due to vitreous opacities (visible upon ophthalmoscopic examination). In the absence of significant pathologic findings in the vitreous or retina, the patient may be reassured that they are not serious, only "little spots floating in the jellylike fluid [vitreous] inside the eye."

There is no treatment. With time, the opacities tend to fall inferiorly in the vitreous and thus out of the patient's line of sight. The examiner must bear in mind that vitreous floaters are occasionally the forerunners of retinal detachment.

RETINA

Retinal Detachment

This is an extremely important condition to keep in mind, since the diagnosis is fairly simple, and surgery is often effective if undertaken soon after onset. A complaint of sudden loss of vision, a shower of floaters, "soot," "lightning flashes," or "a curtain coming up [or down] in front of my eye," is an indication for examination with the ophthalmoscope through a dilated pupil for the presence of retinal detachment. This is particularly true if the patient is myopic, has undergone cataract surgery, or has sustained recent trauma.

A patient with retinal detachment should be hospitalized without delay and prepared for surgery. During transportation, a patient with retinal detachment should keep both eyes closed to avoid undue ocular movement. The area of the detachment should be in the dependent position. For example, the patient with a superior temporal retinal detachment of the right eye should be supine with the head turned to the right; if the right inferior nasal retina is detached, the patient should be transported sitting up with the head turned to the left.

Retinoblastoma

Retinoblastoma is the most common intraocular tumor in childhood. Any child with a suspected retinoblastoma should be referred to the ophthalmologist for prompt treatment.

LENS

Cataract

There is no medical treatment for cataract. The only treatment is lens extraction, which is indicated when visual acuity decreases to the point where the patient can no longer lead a normal life. Congenital cataracts should be removed as early as possible to prevent amblyopia.

Dislocated Lens

Lens dislocation may be genetically determined (eg, as one component of Marfan's syndrome) or may be caused by trauma. Visual impairment and secondary glaucoma are the principal indications for lens removal.

OPTIC NERVE

Optic Neuritis

Optic neuritis occurs as a manifestation of several neurologic diseases. It may be the first sign of multiple sclerosis. The presenting complaint is sudden loss of central vision with pain on moving the globe. On ophthalmoscopic examination, the optic disk may appear normal or may be slightly elevated, with increased vascularity. Systemic corticosteroid treatment has not been effective.

The vision ordinarily returns to normal in a matter of weeks.

Papilledema

Papilledema is most commonly caused by increased intracranial pressure, malignant hypertension, or thrombosis of the central retinal vein. It is manifested as an elevation of the optic disk and dilatation of the veins in the optic disk area. Parapapillary hemorrhages may occur. Papilledema can be observed easily with the ophthalmoscope through an undilated pupil. Intracranial tumors in the posterior fossa characteristically produce papilledema because of their blocking effect on the cerebrospinal fluid. Conversely, frontal lobe tumors usually do not produce papilledema. The rate of onset of papilledema after increased intracranial pressure produced by trauma (eg, subdural hematoma) is extremely variable and is of course related to the magnitude of the process. Moderate degrees of papilledema will not affect visual acuity, but the blind spots will be enlarged as shown by central visual field testing.

Optic Atrophy

In this condition, the disk is pale or white. Optic

atrophy is usually an end-stage process for which no treatment is available. (See fuller discussion on p 239.)

Visual Field Loss in Intracranial Diseases

Some tumors of the central nervous system that produce gross visual defects in moderately advanced but still treatable stages can be suspected by the general physician on the basis of confrontation field tests. These include pituitary tumors, meningiomas, and posterior fossa tumors. These patients should be referred to a neurosurgeon for treatment.

STRABISMUS

There are 3 principal objectives in the treatment of strabismus: (1) to develop good visual acuity in each eye; (2) to straighten the eyes, for cosmetic purposes; and (3) to develop coordinate function of the 2 eyes (binocular vision). The best time to initiate nonsurgical treatment of a strabismus patient is by age 6 months. If treatment is delayed beyond this time, the child will favor the straight eye and suppress the image in the other eye; this results in failure of visual development (amblyopia) in the deviating eye. In such a case, patching of the good eye should be instituted without delay.

If the child is under 6 years of age and has an amblyopic eye, the amblyopia can be cured by patching the good eye. At 1 year of age, patching may be successful within 1 week; at 6 years, it may take a year to achieve the same result, ie, to equalize the visual acuity in the 2 eyes.

There is no firm rule about the proper time for surgery. Some surgeons operate as early as age 6 months; in some cases, there may be valid reasons for deferring strabismus surgery. If the visual acuity is equal and the eyes are made reasonably straight with surgery (or with glasses, as in the case of accommodative esotropia), eye exercises (orthoptics) may assist the patient in learning to use the eyes together. This is the seldom achieved ideal result in strabismus therapy. The prognosis is more favorable for strabismus with onset at age 2 or 3 than for strabismus present at birth; better for divergent (outward deviation of the eyes) than for convergent (inward deviation) strabismus; and better for intermittent than for constant strabismus.

GLAUCOMA

Ninety to 95% of glaucoma cases are of the chronic open-angle type. There are no symptoms in the early stages of open-angle glaucoma. The best means of detection is by routine tonometry and ophthalmoscopic inspection of the optic disk in all persons old enough to cooperate. Chronic glaucoma comes on insidiously and causes slowly progressive loss of peripheral vision by damaging the optic nerve. The response to antiglaucoma eye drops is usually good, and surgery is seldom necessary.

Acetazolamide and other carbonic anhydrase inhibitors (eg, dichlorphenamide) have been shown to be extremely effective in inhibiting the production of aqueous by the ciliary body. Consequently, they are helpful as preoperative adjuncts in the treatment of acute glaucoma and in the management of secondary glaucoma. Because of their side effects (particularly renal calculi), long-term therapy of open-angle glaucoma with such drugs is not always feasible.

Epinephrine, 0.5–2%, when instilled as drops into the conjunctival sac, lowers the intraocular pressure.

Timolol is a beta-adrenergic agent effective in lowering the intraocular pressure by decreasing aqueous production. It is available as drops containing 0.25% and 0.5%.

Pilocarpine continues to be a commonly used antiglaucoma drop.

Laser trabeculoplasty is indicated if topical treatment is ineffective (see Chapter 15).

It is essential to diagnose glaucoma before significant visual loss has occurred, since visual field loss is not reversible. Tonometry, ophthalmoscopy, visual field tests, and gonioscopy are the most important procedures in evaluating and treating a glaucoma patient.

Approximately 5% of cases are angle-closure glaucoma, which produces pain, injection, and blurred vision. The patient seeks treatment immediately because of the pain. Acute glaucoma is treated by laser iridectomy. The laser treatment is preceded by intensive miotic therapy and carbonic anhydrase inhibitors over a period of hours. If miotics and carbonic anhydrase inhibitors do not lower the intraocular pressure sufficiently, glycerin or isosorbide by mouth or intravenous mannitol will nearly always do so within 2 hours.

TRAUMA

Chemical Conjunctivitis & Keratitis

This is best treated with irrigation of the eyes with isotonic saline solution or water immediately after exposure. It is wise not to try to neutralize an acid or alkali by using its chemical counterpart, as the heat generated by the reaction may cause further damage. If the chemical irritant is an alkali, the irrigation should be continued for at least 1 hour; this is because alkalies are not precipitated by the proteins of the eye, as acids are, but tend to linger in the tissues, producing further damage for hours after exposure. A local anesthetic solution is instilled before the irrigation to relieve pain. The pupil should be dilated with 5% homatropine or 0.2% scopolamine solution. Collagenase inhibitors such as sodium edetate (EDTA) or acetylcysteine (Mucomyst) are now being used in the treatment of severe alkali burns. Acetylcysteine is available as 10% or 20% solution in a preparation suitable for ophthalmic use. Sodium edetate solution must be specially prepared for the purpose. The patient's own serum (full strength or diluted 2:1) may also be used for its lubricant and mild anticollagenase activity. The patient must be watched carefully for such complications as symblepharon, corneal scarring, closure of the puncta, and secondary infection. Soft contact lenses may sometimes be helpful in such patients.

Lids

Lacerations of the lids not involving the lid margins, no matter how deep, can be sutured just as any other skin laceration. If the lid margin is involved, whether the canaliculi are also involved or not, the patient should be referred for specialized care; permanent notching of the lid margin may occur if the edges are not properly sutured.

Conjunctiva

In minor lacerations of the conjunctiva, sutures are not necessary. To prevent infection, instill an antibiotic 2–3 times a day until the laceration is healed.

Cornea, Sclera; Intraocular Foreign Bodies

The best emergency treatment for a laceration of the cornea or sclera or an intraocular foreign body is to bandage the eye lightly and cover the bandage with a metal shield that rests on the orbital bones superiorly and inferiorly and is held in place with tape passing over the shield from the forehead to the cheek. Examination, manipulation, and eye movement should be kept to the absolute minimum, since any undue pressure on the eye may cause extrusion of the intraocular contents.

OCULAR EMERGENCIES

Ocular emergencies may be classified as true emergencies and urgent cases. A true emergency is defined as one in which a few hours' delay in treatment can lead to permanent ocular damage or extreme discomfort to the patient. An urgent case is one in which treatment should be started as soon as possible but in which a delay of a few days can be tolerated.

TRUE EMERGENCIES

Trauma

Corneal foreign bodies and corneal abrasions must be treated early in order to relieve the progressively more severe pain and irritation. Lacerations of the eyeball should be sutured as soon as possible in order to avoid extrusion of the internal contents of the eye. Intraocular foreign bodies should be removed without delay. It is sometimes possible to remove them through the point of entry with a magnet. Because the ocular media become cloudy if the foreign body is not re-

moved, a foreign body that is visible with the ophthalmoscope shortly after the injury might not be visible several hours or a day later. These procedures are best undertaken by an ophthalmologist.

A foreign body beneath the upper lid is suggested by blepharospasm and a history of foreign body but no foreign body that is visible. Evert the lid by grasping the lashes gently and exerting pressure in the midportion of the outer surface of the upper lid with a cotton applicator. If a foreign body is present on the tarsal conjunctiva, it can be easily seen when the lid is everted and then removed with a wet cotton applicator.

Corneal Ulcer

Corneal tissue is a good culture medium for bacteria, particularly *Pseudomonas aeruginosa*. Specific treatment of any corneal wound or infection by an ophthalmologist should be instituted as soon as possible to avoid corneal perforation and possible loss of the eye.

Severe Conjunctivitis

Most cases of conjunctivitis are not urgent. One exception to this rule is gonococcal conjunctivitis, which has the serious complication of corneal ulceration; a delay in treatment of 1–2 days may result in corneal ulceration or perforation.

Orbital Cellulitis

Orbital cellulitis may be complicated by brain abscess. Immediate treatment with systemic antibiotics is indicated. The bacteriology of orbital cellulitis is similar to that of sinusitis. For example, pneumococci, staphylococci, and *Haemophilus* species are common invaders and require intensive systemic antibiotic therapy.

Chemical Burns

Chemical burns of the external ocular tissues must be treated immediately by copious irrigation with sterile water or saline, if available, or tap water, for at least 5 minutes. Do not use chemical antidotes, since the heat generated by the reaction may increase the degree of injury. After irrigation, instill sterile local anesthetics as necessary to relieve pain, and dilate the pupil. Local corticosteroid therapy may limit the degree of corneal damage. These patients should be referred to an ophthalmologist as soon as possible after injury.

Acute Iritis

Severe acute iritis causes extreme pain and photophobia. The pupil should be dilated as soon as possible to prevent the formation of posterior synechiae, which further increase the possibility of secondary cataract and glaucoma. Slit lamp examination is necessary to confirm the diagnosis.

Acute Glaucoma

If the intraocular pressure is unusually high

(60–100 mm Hg), permanent optic nerve damage can occur within 24–48 hours. Therefore, these patients should be referred immediately for definitive care.

Occlusion of the Central Retinal Artery

This is a true emergency because the retina is completely without blood as long as the artery is occluded, and the visual receptors in the retina will degenerate within 30–60 minutes if the flow of blood is not restored. The diagnosis is based upon a history of sudden, complete, painless loss of vision in one eye in an older person and the following ophthalmoscopic findings: pallor of the optic disk, edema of the macula, cherry-red fovea, bloodless arterioles that may be difficult to detect, and "boxcar" segmentation of the blood in the veins.

The best treatment (of value only when the patient is seen within 30–60 minutes of onset) is to pass a sharp instrument such as a No. 11 Bard-Parker blade or No. 25 needle (see p 165) into the anterior chamber. The knife is inserted at the limbus and passed into the anterior chamber on a plane with the iris. The objective is to permit the extrusion of some of the anterior chamber fluid (aqueous) without striking the lens with the knife. This sudden decrease in the intraocular pressure may restore the flow of blood in the central retinal artery. No treatment is required for the wound. There are some favorable reports on the use of anticoagulants in cases of partial occlusion of the central retinal artery or its branches.

Retinal Detachment

Retinal detachment is a true emergency if the macula is threatened. If the macula is detached, permanent loss of central vision usually occurs even though the retina is eventually reattached successfully by surgical means.

URGENT CASES

Strabismus or Anisometropia in a Preschool Child With Amblyopia

The sense of sight develops from birth to about 6 years of age. If a child tends to favor one eye as a result of strabismus or anisometropia, vision may fail to develop in the other eye. These children should be treated without delay with glasses and alternate patching of the eyes. Surgery is performed if indicated after visual acuity has been equalized in the 2 eyes.

Chronic Glaucoma

Antiglaucoma therapy should be instituted without delay in order to decrease the intraocular pressure and preserve the remaining visual field.

Vitreous Hemorrhage

A patient with hemorrhage into the vitreous body should be referred, as the hemorrhage may later clear to reveal a retinal detachment.

Unilateral Exophthalmos of Recent Origin

Exophthalmos most commonly occurs in association with thyroid disease. In some cases of hyperthyroidism, it develops only after thyroidectomy. Unilateral exophthalmos may also be due to an orbital tumor, cavernous sinus thrombosis, or carotid cavernous fistula. These disorders are treatable.

Acute Dacryocystitis

Early treatment with warm compresses and systemic antibiotics is usually effective. If not, surgery is indicated.

Ocular Tumors

Many tumors of the ocular adnexa can be completely excised if they are diagnosed in an early stage. Malignant intraocular tumors (except those of the iris) may require enucleation.

Optic Nerve Disorders

Optic nerve disorders are quite serious and may indicate accompanying intracranial or systemic disease. The patient should be examined from a neurologic as well as an ophthalmologic standpoint.

Sympathetic Ophthalmia

With the availability of effective steroid treatment, sympathetic ophthalmia is now a condition that should be referred for immediate local and systemic corticosteroid or other immunosuppressive therapy. Sympathetic ophthalmia should be suspected if the patient has inflammation in both eyes and a history of penetrating injury to one eye.

PRINCIPLES OF ANTIBIOTIC & CHEMOTHERAPEUTIC TREATMENT OF OCULAR INFECTIONS

In the treatment of infectious eye disease, eg, conjunctivitis, one should always use the drug that is most effective, least likely to cause complications, least likely to be used systemically at a later date, and least expensive. Of the available antibacterial agents, the sulfonamides come closest to meeting these specifications. Two reliable sulfonamides are sulfisoxazole and sodium sulfacetamide. The sulfonamides have the added advantage of low allergenicity. They are available in ointment or solution form.

If sulfonamides are not effective, the antibiotics can be used. One of the most effective broad-spectrum antibiotics for ophthalmic use is gentamicin. It has some effect against gram-negative as well as gram-positive organisms. Other antibiotics frequently used are erythromycin, tetracycline, bacitracin, and polymyxin. Combined bacitracin-polymyxin ointment is often used prophylactically for the protection it affords against both gram-positive (bacitracin) and gram-negative (polymyxin) organisms.

The great majority of antibiotic and chemotherapeutic medications for eye infections are administered locally. Systemic administration is required for all intraocular infections, corneal ulcer, chlamydial conjunctivitis (trachoma and inclusion blennorrhea), orbital cellulitis, dacryocystitis, and any serious external infection that does not respond to local treatment.

Ointments have greater therapeutic effectiveness than solutions, since in this way contact can be maintained for at least 1 hour. However, they do have the disadvantage of causing blurred vision; where this must be avoided, solutions should be used.

Before one can determine the drug of choice, the causative organisms must be known. For example, a pneumococcal corneal ulcer will respond to treatment with a sulfonamide or any broad-spectrum antibiotic, but this is not true in the case of corneal ulcer due to *P aeruginosa*, which responds only to vigorous treatment with polymyxin, colistin, gentamicin, or tobramycin. Another example is staphylococcal dacryocystitis; staphylococci not sensitive to penicillin are most likely to be susceptible to erythromycin or methicillin.

Caution: It is well to keep in mind that the antibiotics, like the steroids, when used over a prolonged period of time in bacterial corneal ulcers, favor the development of secondary fungal infection of the cornea. This is another reason for using the sulfonamides whenever they are adequate for the purpose.

COMMON TECHNIQUES USED IN THE TREATMENT OF OCULAR DISORDERS

Liquid Medications

Place the patient in a sitting position with both eyes open and looking up. Pull down slightly on the lower lid and instill 1 drop in the lower cul-de-sac. The patient is then asked to look down while finger contact on the lower lid is maintained. Do not let the patient squeeze the eye shut.

Ointments

Ointments are instilled in the same way as liquids. While the patient is looking down, lift out the lower lid to trap the medication in the conjunctival sac. The lids should be kept closed for at least 1 minute to allow the ointment to melt.

Eye Bandages

Eye bandages should be applied firmly enough to hold the lid fairly securely against the cornea. A single patch consisting of gauze-covered cotton is usually sufficient. A wraparound head bandage is seldom necessary. Tape is passed from the cheek to the forehead. If more pressure is desired, use 2 or 3 patches.

Warm Compresses

Use a clean towel or washcloth soaked in hot tap water well below the temperature that will burn the thin skin covering the eyelids. Warm compresses are usually applied for 15 minutes 4 times a day. The therapeutic rationale is to increase blood flow to the affected area and decrease pain and inflammation.

Removal of Superficial Corneal Foreign Body

The main considerations are good illumination, magnification, anesthesia, position of the patient, and sterile technique. If possible, the patient's visual acuity is always recorded first.

The patient may be in the sitting or supine position. The examiner should use a loupe unless a slit lamp is available. An assistant should direct a strong flashlight into the eye with the rays of light striking the cornea at an oblique angle. The examiner may then see the corneal foreign body and remove it with a wet cotton applicator. If this is not successful, the foreign body may be removed with a metal spud while the lids are held apart with the other hand to prevent blinking. An antibacterial ointment is instilled after the foreign body has been removed. For more specific anti-infective measures, see Chapter 28.

Most patients are more comfortable without a patch on the eye after removal of a foreign body.

Note: It is essential to see the patient the next day to be certain that no infection has occurred and that healing is under way.

Home Medication

At home, the same techniques should be used as described above except that drops should be instilled with the patient in the supine position. Experienced patients (eg, those with glaucoma) are usually quite skillful in self-administration of eye drops.

COMMON PITFALLS TO BE AVOIDED IN THE MANAGEMENT OF OCULAR DISORDERS

Dangers in the Use of Local Anesthetics

Unsupervised self-administration of local anesthetics is dangerous because the patient may further injure an anesthetized eye without knowing it. Furthermore, most anesthetics delay healing. *Caution:* Do not give patients local anesthetics to take home with them. Eye pain should be controlled by systemic analgesics.

Errors in Diagnosis

Of these the most common is a diagnosis of conjunctivitis when the correct diagnosis is iritis (anterior uveitis), glaucoma, or corneal ulcer (especially herpes simplex). The differentiation between iritis and acute glaucoma may be difficult also.

Misuse of Atropine

Atropine must never be used in routine diagnosis or treatment. It causes cycloplegia (paralysis of the ciliary muscle) of about 14 days' duration and can precipitate an attack of glaucoma if the patient has a narrow anterior chamber angle (see p 373).

Dangers of Local Corticosteroid Therapy

Local ophthalmologic corticosteroid preparations, eg, prednisolone, are often used for their anti-inflammatory effect on the conjunctiva, cornea, and iris. Although it is true that a patient with conjunctivitis, corneal inflammation, or iritis can be made more comfortable with local corticosteroids, it must be stressed that the corticosteroids are associated with 4 very serious complications when used in the eye over a long period of time: herpes simplex keratitis, open-angle glaucoma, cataract formation, and fungal infection. The most common complications are herpes simplex keratitis and glaucoma. Corticosteroids enhance the activity of the herpes simplex virus, apparently by increasing the destructive effect of collagenase on the collagen of the cornea. This is evidenced by the fact that perforation of the cornea occasionally occurs when the corticosteroids are used during the more active stage of a herpes simplex corneal infection. Corneal perforation was a very rare complication of dendritic keratitis before the corticosteroids came into general use. In the treatment of any corneal inflammation, particularly if the corneal epithelium is not intact, the prolonged use of corticosteroids is sometimes complicated by fungal infection (eg, *Candida albicans*), and this may lead to loss of the eye. Topical corticosteroids can cause or aggravate open-angle glaucoma and, less commonly, can produce cataracts.

For these reasons, although the corticosteroids are valuable in the treatment of ocular disease, any patient on whom they are being used should be watched carefully for the development of complications. The corticosteroids should not be used unless specifically indicated, eg, in iritis, certain types of keratitis, and acute allergic disorders.

Use of Contaminated Eye Medications

The external coats of the eye, including the sclera and the corneal epithelium, are resistant to infection. However, once the corneal epithelium or sclera is broken by trauma, the tissues become markedly susceptible to bacterial infection. For this reason, ophthalmic solutions that may be used in injured eyes must be prepared with the same degree of caution as fluids intended for intravenous administration.

Sterile, single-use disposable units of the common ophthalmic solutions should be used whenever liquid medication is instilled into an injured eye. For routine use in intact eyes, nearly all eye medications are now available in small plastic containers. It is perfectly safe to use these provided they are not kept a long time after opening and are not contaminated accidentally.

Overtreatment

Some patients with chronic conjunctivitis or keratitis may be made worse by overtreatment with topical medications. If a patient is not improving as expected, make certain the preservative in the local medication is not the cause.

REFERENCES

Cogan DG: *Ophthalmic Manifestations of Systemic Vascular Disease.* Saunders, 1974.

Deutsch TA, Feller DB: *Paton and Goldberg's Management of Ocular Injuries,* 2nd ed. Saunders, 1985.

Ellis PP, Smith DL: *Ocular Therapeutics and Pharmacology,* 7th ed. Mosby, 1985.

Ernest TJ (editor): *Year Book of Ophthalmology 1985.* Year Book, 1986.

Fraunfelder FT: *Drug-Induced Ocular Side Effects and Drug Interactions,* 2nd ed. Lea & Febiger, 1982.

Gardiner PA: ABC of ophthalmology: Accidents and first aid. (ABC of Ophthalmology Series.) *Br Med J* 1978;**2:**1347.

Gombos GM: *Handbook of Ophthalmologic Emergencies,* 2nd ed. Medical Examination Publishing Co, 1977.

Harrington DO: *The Visual Fields: A Textbook and Atlas of Clinical Perimetry,* 5th ed. Mosby, 1981.

Havener WH: *Ocular Pharmacology,* 5th ed. Mosby, 1983.

Henkind P et al (editorial consultants): *Physicians' Desk Reference (PDR) for Ophthalmology,* 13th ed. Medical Economics, 1985.

Keeney AH: *Ocular Examination: Basis and Techniques,* 2nd ed. Mosby, 1976.

Kolker AE, Hetherington J: *Becker-Shaffer's Diagnosis and Therapy of the Glaucomas,* 5th ed. Mosby, 1983.

Miller NR (editor): *Walsh & Hoyt's Clinical Neuro-ophthalmology,* 4th ed. Vols 1 and 2. Williams & Wilkins, 1982, 1984.

Miller SJ: *Parson's Diseases of the Eye,* 17th ed. Churchill Livingstone, 1984.

Newell FW: *Ophthalmology: Principles and Concepts,* 5th ed. Mosby, 1982.

Thygeson P: The unfavorable role of corticosteroids in herpetic keratitis. Page 450 in: *Controversy in Ophthalmology.* Brockhurst RJ et al (editors). Saunders, 1977.

von Noorden GK: *Von Noorden-Maumenee's Atlas of Strabismus,* 4th ed. Mosby, 1983.

Lids & Lacrimal Apparatus

6

John H. Sullivan, MD

THE LIDS

Anatomy (Fig 6–1)

The eyelids are movable folds of tissue that serve to protect the eye. The skin of the lids, the thinnest in the body, is loose and elastic, permitting extreme swelling and subsequent return to normal shape and size. The tarsal plates consist of dense fibrous tissue with some elastic tissue. They are lined posteriorly by conjunctiva. The **orbital septum** is the fascia lying posterior to the portion of the orbicularis muscle between the orbital rim and the tarsi and serves as a barrier between the lid and the orbit.

The **orbicularis oculi** muscle, which receives its innervation from the seventh cranial nerve, is roughly circular. Its function is to close the lids. The muscle is divided into **orbital, preseptal,** and **pretarsal** por-

tions. The preseptal and pretarsal muscles have deep points of origin over the fascia of the lacrimal sac. Contraction causes lacrimal secretions to be pumped into the nasolacrimal duct.

The **levator palpebrae** muscle is supplied by the third nerve; its aponeurosis inserts into the anterior surface of the tarsal plate and the skin and serves to elevate the lid. The superior tarsal muscle (of Müller), supplied by sympathetic nerves, originates at the levator muscle and inserts at the superior edge of the tarsus, coursing deep to the levator aponeurosis.

The 4 types of glands in the lid are the meibomian glands, the glands of Moll and Zeis, and the accessory lacrimal glands (of Krause and Wolfring). The meibomian glands are long sebaceous glands in the tarsal plate. They do not communicate with the hair follicles. There are about 25 in the upper lid and 20 in the lower lid, and they appear as yellow vertical streaks deep to the conjunctiva. The meibomian glands produce a sebaceous substance that creates an oily layer on the

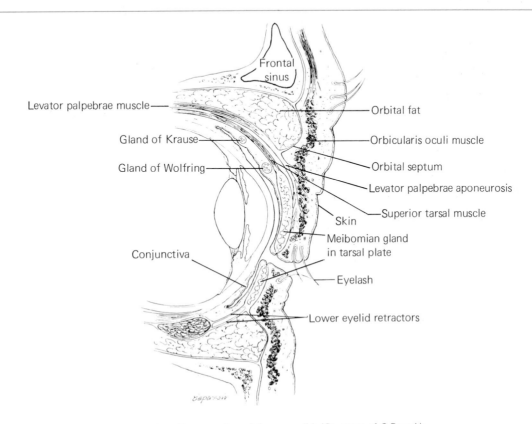

Figure 6–1. Cross section of the upper lid. (Courtesy of C Beard.)

surface of the tear film. This helps to prevent rapid evaporation of the normal tear layer. The glands of Zeis are smaller, modified sebaceous glands that are connected with the follicles of the eyelashes. The sweat glands of Moll are unbranched sinuous tubules that begin in a simple spiral and not in a glomerulus, as do ordinary sweat glands. Accessory lacrimal glands (Krause and Wolfring) are formed beneath the palpebral conjunctiva. They supply most of the needed moisture to the conjunctival sac and cornea.

There is a **gray line** (mucocutaneous border) on the margins of both the upper and lower eyelids. If an incision is made along this line, the lid can be cleanly split into a posterior portion, containing the tarsal plate and conjunctiva, and an anterior portion, containing the orbicularis oculi muscle, skin, and hair follicles.

The blood supply to the lids is derived mainly from the ophthalmic, zygomatic, and angular arteries. The lymphatics drain into the preauricular, parotid, and submaxillary lymph glands.

Physiology of Symptoms

Lid disorders are among the most common of all ocular problems. The patient with disorders of the eyelids will have varied complaints. There are many pain fibers in the tissues near the lid margins. Consequently, if there is inflammation with stretching of tissues, as in hordeolum, the patient complains of moderately severe pain. In marginal blepharitis there is no pain, but the patient complains of red-rimmed eyes; because of the proximity of the lid margins to the conjunctiva, frequent attacks of conjunctivitis are a common complaint.

If the patient has a foreign body sensation, entropion, with eyelashes rubbing on the cornea, should be ruled out. If the diagnosis is not immediately apparent, entropion will be produced by asking the patient to close the eyelids tightly. If the lid falls away from the eyeball, as in ectropion, tearing will be the chief complaint, since the tears do not have access to the lower punctum. Exposure keratitis may also occur with ectropion.

Technique of Upper Lid Eversion

Have the patient look down. Grasp the lashes gently and exert pressure posteriorly and medially on the upper lid at the upper tarsal border with a cotton applicator.

INFECTIONS & INFLAMMATIONS OF THE LIDS

1. HORDEOLUM

Hordeolum is a common staphylococcal infection of the lid glands that is characterized by a localized red, swollen, and acutely tender area. It is essentially an abscess, as there is pus formation within the lumen

Figure 6–2. Internal hordeolum, left upper eyelid, pointing on skin side. This should be opened by a horizontal skin incision. (Courtesy of A Rosenberg.)

of the affected gland. When it affects the meibomian glands it is relatively large and is known as an **internal hordeolum** (Fig 6–2). The smaller and more superficial **external hordeolum** (sty) is an infection of Zeis's or Moll's glands. Pain is the primary symptom, and the intensity of the pain is in direct proportion to the amount of lid swelling. An internal hordeolum may point to the skin or to the conjunctival side of the lid; external hordeolum always points to the skin side of the lid margin.

Treatment of both internal and external hordeolum is with warm compresses for 10–15 minutes 3–4 times a day, and incision and drainage of the purulent material if the process does not begin to resolve within 48 hours. An antibacterial ophthalmic ointment instilled into the conjunctival sac every 3 hours is beneficial. A large internal hordeolum can be complicated by cellulitis of the entire lid.

2. CHALAZION

Chalazion (Fig 6–3) is a sterile granulomatous inflammation of a meibomian gland, of unknown cause, characterized by localized swelling in the upper or lower eyelid. It may begin with inflammation and tenderness similar to a hordeolum and develop over a period of weeks. The majority point toward the conjunctival side of the lid. When the lid is everted, the conjunctiva over the chalazion is seen to be reddened and elevated.

If sufficiently large, a chalazion may press upon the eyeball and cause astigmatism.

In general, a fully developed chalazion is differentiated from hordeolum by the absence of acute inflammatory signs.

Chalazion seldom subsides spontaneously; if it is large enough to distort vision or to be a cosmetic

Figure 6–3. Chalazion, right lower eyelid. (Courtesy of K Tabbara.)

blemish, excision is indicated. Pathologically, there is proliferation of the endothelium of the acinus and a granulomatous inflammatory response, including some Langhans type giant cells.

If chalazions are recurrent in the same area, biopsy should be performed to rule out malignant disease.

3. MARGINAL BLEPHARITIS (Granulated Eyelids)

Blepharitis is a common chronic bilateral inflammation of the lid margins. There are 2 main types: staphylococcal and seborrheic. Staphylococcal blepharitis is usually ulcerative. Seborrheic blepharitis (nonulcerative) is usually associated with the presence of *Pityrosporon ovale*, although this organism has not been shown to be the etiologic factor. Often, both types are present (mixed infection). Seborrhea of the scalp, brows, and ears is frequently associated with seborrheic blepharitis.

The chief symptoms are irritation, burning, and itching of the lid margins. The eyes are "red-rimmed." Many scales or "granulations" can be seen clinging to the lashes of both the upper and lower lids. In the staphylococcal type, the scales are dry, the lids are red, tiny ulcerated areas are found along the lid margins, and the lashes tend to fall out. In the seborrheic type, the scales are greasy, ulceration does not occur, and the lid margins are less red. In the more common mixed type, both dry and greasy scales are present and the lid margins are red and may be ulcerated. *Staphylococcus aureus* and *P ovale* can be seen together or singly in stained material scraped from the lid margins.

Conjunctivitis, superficial keratitis of the lower third of the cornea, and chronic meibomianitis are the main complaints in the early morning hours. Seborrheic blepharitis is occasionally complicated by a mild keratitis. Persons with staphylococcal blepharitis are prone to develop chalazions and hordeola.

The scalp, eyebrows, and lid margins must be kept clean, particularly in the seborrheic type of blepharitis, by means of soap and water shampoo. Scales must be removed from the lid margins daily with a damp cotton applicator.

Staphylococcal blepharitis is treated with antistaphylococcal antibiotic or sulfonamide eye ointment applied on a cotton applicator once daily to the lid margins.

Meibomianitis is very resistant to treatment and requires repeated expression of the glands. It may be complicated by secondary infection with one of the prominent gram-negative organisms (eg, *Pseudomonas aeruginosa*).

The seborrheic and staphylococcal types usually become mixed and may run a chronic course over a period of months or years if not treated adequately; associated staphylococcal conjunctivitis or keratitis usually disappears promptly following local antistaphylococcal medication.

4. MEIBOMIANITIS

Bilateral, chronic inflammation of the meibomian glands is an uncommon disease of unknown cause that occurs during or after the middle years of life. It is generally preceded by or associated with blepharitis.

The patient complains of chronically red and irritated eyes and a slight but continuous discharge. The meibomian glands are prominent, the lid margins are red, and there is a frothy conjunctival discharge. A soft, cheesy, yellow material that contains no organisms can be expressed from the glands. An irritative conjunctivitis due to contact with meibomian secretion is a frequent complication, especially in the morning upon awakening.

The only treatment is repeated expression of the meibomian glands. However, because this treatment never produces dramatic results, the patient usually neglects to do it or have it done, and the disease process continues indefinitely with a slight tendency to become worse.

POSITIONAL DEFECTS OF THE LIDS

1. ENTROPION

Entropion (turning inward of the lid) (Fig 6–4) usually affects the lower lid but may affect the upper lid. It seldom occurs in persons under 40 years of age. Entropion is categorized as senile (spastic) or cicatricial. Senile entropion is due to a degeneration of fascial attachments in the lower eyelid, including a dehiscence of the lower eyelid aponeurosis (retractors) from the lower eyelid tarsus. This allows preseptal orbicularis to override pretarsal orbicularis and rotate the lid margin inward. Cicatricial entropion is due to

Figure 6–4. Entropion. (Courtesy of M Quickert.)

scarring of the palpebral conjunctiva and the tarsus and is therefore common in trachoma. Trichiasis (turning inward of the lashes so that they rub on the cornea) results from entropion, but it may also be the result of misdirected eyelashes without entropion. It causes corneal irritation and may encourage corneal ulceration.

Surgery to evert the lid is effective in the treatment of both types of entropion. A useful temporary measure is to tape the lower lid to the cheek with tension temporally and inferiorly. Trichiasis without entropion can be relieved temporarily by plucking the offending eyelashes. Permanent relief may be obtained with electrolysis or, in more extensive cases, with cryosurgery.

2. ECTROPION

Ectropion (sagging and eversion of the lower lid) (Fig 6–5), is usually bilateral and is a frequent finding in older persons. Ectropion may be caused by relaxation of the orbicularis oculi muscle, either as part of the aging process or following seventh nerve palsy. The symptoms are tearing and irritation. Exposure keratitis may occur.

Marked ectropion is treated by surgical shortening of the lower lid in a horizontal direction. Cicatricial ectropion is caused by contracture of the anterior lamella of the lid. It requires surgical revision of the scar and often skin grafting for relief. Minor degrees of ectropion can be treated by several fairly deep electrocautery penetrations through the conjunctiva 4–5 mm from the lid margins at the inferior aspect of the tarsal plate. The fibrotic reaction that follows will often draw the lid up to its normal position.

ANATOMIC DEFORMITIES OF THE LIDS

1. DERMATOCHALASIS & BLEPHAROCHALASIS

Dermatochalasis (Fig 6–6) is redundancy and loss of elasticity of skin such that a skin fold covers the tarsal portion of the eyelid. It is a common condition that is most often a function of aging, although occasionally it may be the result of repeated episodes of lid edema. When severe, pseudoptosis may result. Excision of a portion of the skin is required if vision is affected or for cosmetic reasons.

Blepharochalasis (Fig 6–7) is a rare condition caused by recurrent episodes of edema, resulting in thin, wrinkled, and redundant eyelid skin sometimes described as resembling cigarette paper. Atrophic changes of all eyelid tissues frequently produce ptosis and a sunken appearance in the location of the medial fat pads. Symptoms of edema begin around puberty and diminish with age. Surgery consists of removal of the redundant skin and repair of the levator aponeurosis.

Figure 6–5. Ectropion. (Courtesy of M Quickert.)

Figure 6–6. Dermatochalasis of upper lids and herniation of orbital fat of lower lids. (Courtesy of M Quickert.)

2. EPICANTHUS

Epicanthus (Fig 6–8) is characterized by vertical folds of skin over the medial canthi. It is characteristic of Asians and is present to some degree in most children of all races. The skin fold is often large enough to cover part of the nasal sclera and cause "pseudoesotropia," as the eyes appear to be crossed when a normal amount of medial sclera is not visible. Prominent epicanthal folds in children gradually decrease as the child grows older and are seldom apparent by school age.

BLEPHAROSPASM
(Tic)

Blepharospasm is persistent or repetitive involuntary contraction of the orbicularis oculi muscle. It is usually bilateral and is more common in older persons. The cause is not known. It may be due to irritative lesions of the cornea and conjunctiva or of the seventh cranial nerve. Emotional stress and fatigue make it worse. The eyes should be examined carefully to rule out irritative lesions such as corneal foreign body, meibomianitis, and trichiasis.

Treatment consists of removal of the causative factor if possible. If the specific cause is not known, explanation and reassurance are in order. Intractable cases may require alcohol injection of the orbicularis oculi muscle to produce temporary paralysis. Seventh nerve block with a long-acting local anesthetic should be tried before alcohol injection is resorted to. Plastic surgery designed to weaken orbicularis function and selective removal of seventh nerve branches have been successful in some cases.

Intramuscular botulinum toxin injections have recently been used successfully for temporary relief of blepharospasm.

BLEPHAROPTOSIS

Ptosis (drooping of the upper lid) is an uncommon disorder that may be unilateral or bilateral. Congenital cases are usually seen in children and acquired cases in adults. Most cases can be corrected with surgery.

Classification

It is important to identify the type of ptosis, as a guide to appropriate treatment. The following scheme has been found to be useful.

A. True Congenital Ptosis: True congenital ptosis is caused by isolated dystrophy of the levator muscle, affecting both contraction and relaxation of the fibers. This results in ptosis in the primary position of gaze, reduced movement of the lid in upgaze, and impaired closure on downgaze. This relative lagophthalmos is an important clue to differentiation of congenital from acquired ptosis. The different forms of congenital ptosis may be classified as follows:

1. Ptosis with normal superior rectus function.

2. Ptosis with weakness of the superior rectus (25% of cases).

3. Marcus Gunn syndrome (jaw-winking syndrome)–Marcus Gunn syndrome occurs in 5% of cases and is a manifestation of a neurologic misconnection. Contraction of the levator muscle occurs when the jaw is open or deviated to the opposite side. Such cases present a difficult surgical challenge.

4. Blepharophimosis–Another unusual form of congenital ptosis is blepharophimosis. In addition to severe ptosis with poor levator function, the patient displays epicanthal folds, telecanthus, and lower lid ectropion.

B. Acquired Ptosis: Acquired ptosis may be present at birth and may be confused with true congenital ptosis.

1. Neurogenic ptosis–Horner's syndrome, caused by paralysis of the cervical sympathetic nerves, is a neurogenic ptosis that is usually acquired but may be present at birth. In **myasthenia gravis,** diplopia almost always develops. Intravenous edrophonium

Figure 6–7. Blepharochalasis.

Figure 6–8. Epicanthus.

Figure 6–9. Surgical correction of ptosis. *Left:* Before operation, ptosis of the upper lid was present. *Right:* After the operation (levator resection), the ptosis was well corrected and a natural-appearing upper lid fold produced. (Courtesy of C Beard.)

chloride (Tensilon) temporarily reverses the ptosis and is used for diagnostic testing in that way. In oculomotor nerve paralysis, ptosis is severe and there is no levator function. There is also pupillary mydriasis and paralysis of the superior, inferior, and medial rectus muscles.

2. Myogenic ptosis–Myogenic ptosis is the most common form of acquired ptosis and usually presents in geriatric patients as disinsertion or dehiscence of the levator aponeurosis.

3. Traumatic ptosis–Traumatic ptosis may be a combination of neurogenic, myogenic, and mechanical ptosis and is therefore often the most difficult to treat.

4. Mechanical ptosis–Tumors of the upper lid, if sufficiently large, may restrict the lid from opening, as may conjunctival adhesions.

C. Pseudoptosis: In pseudoptosis, the lid appears to be ptotic, but surgical correction usually involves structures other than the levator complex.

1. Microphthalmos–With a small or sunken eye, the lid may droop because of poor support from the globe.

2. Hypotropia–In hypotropia, the lid follows the globe down unless the eye is moved back to fixation.

3. Dermatochalasis–In dermatochalasis, an additional fold of skin hangs over the lid margin like a curtain (see discussion above).

Clinical Findings

The upper lid normally lies about 2 mm below the limbus. The degree of ptosis can be reasonably estimated by noting the position of the lid in relation to the limbus and pupillary margin. The most important measurement is the degree of levator function, since in most instances this determines the magnitude of surgery to be performed. With the brow immobilized, the full vertical excursion of the lid is noted. Poor levator function is suggested by absence of the lid crease. Severe ptosis may be associated with ipsilateral astigmatism but is seldom the cause of amblyopia ex anopsia.

Treatment

With the exception of cases associated with myasthenia gravis, treatment of ptosis requires surgery (Fig 6–9). The technique and extent of surgery differ according to the type of ptosis. Perfect correction is usually possible only when excellent (> 8 mm) levator function is present. The surgeon (and the patient) should understand that the object of surgery is to balance the lids in primary position. With unilateral ptosis, the degree of symmetry in other positions of gaze is inversely proportionate to levator function.

Most operations involve resection of the levator or superior tarsal muscle (or both). Patients with no levator function require an alternative elevating force and are usually treated by brow suspension; autogenous fascia lata is used to suspend the lid to the frontalis muscle.

In recent years, it has been demonstrated that some cases of acquired ptosis are the result of disinsertion of the levator aponeurosis. The condition is suspected when excellent levator function is associated with moderate or severe ptosis. A high lid fold and very thin lid may be features.

COSMETIC MICROPIGMENTATION OF THE LIDS

Tattooing of the lids in women is a controversial new procedure. Its purpose is to reduce the necessity for applying cosmetic eyeliner. It is performed in the office under local anesthesia. The long-term consequences of dye impregnation at the lid margin are unknown.

THE LACRIMAL APPARATUS*

Anatomy (Fig 6–10)

The lacrimal apparatus consists of the lacrimal gland, accessory glands, puncta, canaliculi, tear sac, and nasolacrimal duct. The lacrimal gland is a tear-secreting gland located in the anterior superior temporal portion of the orbit. Several secretory ducts connect the gland to the superior conjunctival fornix. The tears pass down over the cornea and the bulbar and palpebral conjunctiva, moistening the surfaces of these structures. They drain into the lacrimal canaliculi through the lacrimal puncta, round apertures about 0.5 mm in diameter on the medial aspect of both the upper and lower lid margins. The canaliculi are about 1 mm in diameter and 8 mm long and join to form a common canaliculus just before opening into the lacrimal sac. Diverticula may be a part of the normal structure and are susceptible to higher bacteria (*Actinomyces*) or fungal infection.

The lacrimal sac is the dilated portion of the lacrimal drainage system that lies in the bony lacrimal fossa.

The nasolacrimal duct is the downward continuation of the lacrimal sac. It opens into the inferior meatus lateral to the inferior turbinate.

All of the passages of the lacrimal drainage system are lined with epithelium. The tears pass into the puncta by capillary attraction. The combined forces

*See also Chapter 7.

of the capillary attraction in the canaliculi, gravity, and the pumping action of the orbicularis oculi muscle on the lacrimal sac tend to continue the flow of tears down the nasolacrimal duct into the nose and nasopharynx.

Physiology of Symptoms

Disorders of the lacrimal system are manifested either by excess tearing (**epiphora**) or dryness of the eyes (**keratitis sicca**). There are many causes of epiphora, eg, conjunctivitis, keratitis, iritis, corneal or conjunctival foreign body, and (rarely) primary hypersecretion. If epiphora is the only symptom, the cause in the great majority of cases is in the lacrimal drainage apparatus. **Paradoxic lacrimation (crocodile tears)** may be congenital or acquired and is the result of neurologic misconnection between the seventh cranial nerve (salivation) and the nervus intermedius (lacrimation).

Examination for epiphora involves inspection of the puncta for atresia or malposition. Irrigation and probing of the canaliculi and fluorescein dye are used to test the functional patency of the system. In difficult cases, dacryocystography and scintigraphy can sometimes be helpful.

Inadequate tear production is a common complaint of old people and is often associated with Sjögren's syndrome. Drying of the corneal epithelium (keratitis sicca) is painful and can lead to loss of vision. Secretions from the accessory glands of the conjunctiva and the lids are more important than those of the lacrimal gland. The Schirmer test can be used to measure the function of the lacrimal gland and accessory lacrimal glands (see Chapter 7 for detailed discussion).

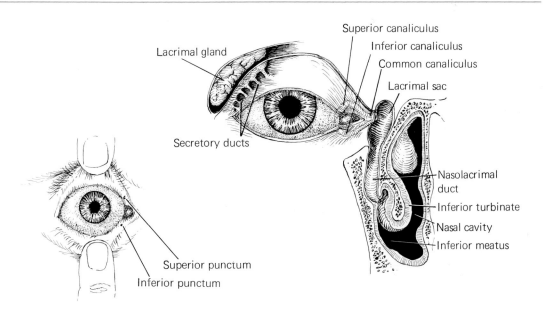

Figure 6–10. The lacrimal drainage system. (Redrawn with modifications and reproduced, with permission, from Thompson J, Elstrom ER: Radiography of the nasolacrimal passageways. *Med Radiogr Photogr* 1949;25(3):66.)

INFECTIONS OF THE LACRIMAL APPARATUS

1. DACRYOCYSTITIS (Fig 6–11)

Infection of the lacrimal sac is a common acute or chronic disease that usually occurs in infants or in persons over 40 (about 9 out of 10 chronic adult cases occur in menopausal women); it is uncommon in the intermediate age groups unless it follows trauma or is caused by a fungal infection. It is most often unilateral and is always secondary to obstruction of the nasolacrimal duct. In most adult cases, the cause of the obstruction remains unknown. Acute cases are often preceded by chronic dacryocystitis; some cases are preceded by chronic conjunctivitis (eg, trachoma). In acute dacryocystitis the usual infectious agent is *S aureus* or, occasionally, beta-hemolytic *Streptococcus*. In chronic dacryocystitis, *Streptococcus pneumoniae* is the predominant organism (rarely, *Candida albicans*).

In fungal dacryocystitis, obstruction of the nasolacrimal duct by a dacryolith sometimes occurs. Spontaneous improvement follows passage of the stone, but recurrence is the rule.

It is curious that dacryocystitis is seldom complicated by conjunctivitis even though the conjunctival sac is constantly being bathed with pus exuding through the lacrimal puncta.

Clinical Findings

The chief symptoms are tearing and discharge. In the acute form, inflammation, pain, swelling, and tenderness are present in the tear sac area; purulent material can be expressed from the tear sac. In the chronic form, tearing is usually the only sign; mucoid material can usually be expressed from the tear sac.

The infectious agent can be identified microscopically by staining a conjunctival smear taken after expression of the tear sac.

Corneal ulcer occasionally occurs following minor corneal trauma in the presence of pneumococcal dacryocystitis. Perforation of the skin and fistula formation may also occur. If a corneal ulcer occurs, vigorous local and systemic treatment is indicated and a dacryocystectomy or dacryocystorhinostomy should be done without delay.

Figure 6–11. Acute dacryocystitis.

Treatment

A. Adult Dacryocystitis: Warm compresses to the affected eye at frequent intervals during the acute stage.

1. Acute–Specific treatment for acute staphylococcal or pneumococcal dacryocystitis consists of systemic antibiotics until the inflammation subsides.

2. Chronic–Since an obstruction of the nasolacrimal duct is the basic cause of dacryocystitis, the disease is usually persistent until the obstruction is relieved. However, probing is notably unsuccessful in adults, and dacryocystorhinostomy is usually necessary if symptoms are severe. If chronic tearing is the only symptom, many patients prefer the tearing to surgery.

B. Infantile Dacryocystitis: Normally, the nasolacrimal ducts open spontaneously before birth or during the first month of life. Occasionally, one of the ducts fails to canalize and a secondary *Haemophilus influenzae* dacryocystitis develops. When this happens, forceful massage of the tear sac is indicated, and antibiotic or sulfonamide drops should be instilled in the conjunctival sac 4–5 times daily. If this is not successful after a few weeks, probing of the nasolacrimal duct is indicated regardless of the infant's age. One probing is effective in about 75% of cases; in the remainder, cure can almost always be achieved by repeated probings in fracture of the inferior turbinate or by a temporary silicone lacrimal drainage splint.

Course & Prognosis

Acute adult dacryocystitis responds well to systemic antibiotic therapy. Recurrences are common if the nasolacrimal duct obstruction is not removed. The chronic form can be kept latent by using antibiotic eye drops, but relief of the obstruction is the only cure.

2. CANALICULITIS

Canaliculitis is an uncommon chronic unilateral condition caused by infection with *Actinomyces israelii, C albicans,* or *Aspergillus* species (Fig 6–12). It affects the lower canaliculus more often than the upper, occurs exclusively in adults, and causes a secondary purulent unilateral conjunctivitis that frequently escapes etiologic diagnosis. Canalicular stenosis can also result from viral infections, notably varicella and herpes.

The patient complains of a mildly red and irritated eye with a slight discharge. The punctum usually pouts; material can be readily expressed from the canaliculus. The organism can be seen microscopically on a direct smear taken from the canaliculus.

Curettage of the necrotic material in the involved canaliculus, followed by forceful irrigation, is usually effective. Canaliculotomy is sometimes necessary. Tincture of iodine should be applied to the lining of the canaliculus after canaliculotomy.

Figure 6–12. *Actinomyces israelii* canaliculitis, left eye. (Courtesy of P Thygeson.)

3. DACRYOADENITIS

Acute inflammation of the lacrimal gland is a rare unilateral condition that may be seen in children as a complication of mumps, measles, or influenza, and in adults in association with gonorrhea. It may also develop following a perforating injury to the lacrimal gland or as a retrograde infection from a bacterial conjunctivitis.

In the acute type, considerable swelling, pain, and infection occur over the upper temporal aspect of the eye. The lid has an S-shaped curve.

If bacterial infection is present, antibiotics are given systemically. Incision may be necessary if pus collects in the gland under tension.

Chronic dacryoadenitis is occasionally seen bilaterally as one manifestation of sarcoidosis. This condition (which, with lacrimal gland swelling, is called Mikulicz's syndrome) usually occurs in blacks and is self-limited. The prognosis is good. Chronic dacryoadenitis may also occur in tuberculosis, lymphatic leukemia, and lymphosarcoma.

REFERENCES

Beard C: Malignancy of the eyelids. *Am J Ophthalmol* 1981;**92:**1.

Beard C: *Ptosis*, 3rd ed. Mosby, 1981.

Callahan A et al: Lid cancer: Operate or radiate? Pages 381–398 in: *Controversy in Ophthalmology*. Brockhurst RJ et al (editors). Saunders, 1977.

Callahan MA: Surgically mismanaged ptosis associated with double elevator palsy. *Arch Ophthalmol* 1981;**99:**108.

Char D: Therapeutic review: The management of lid and conjunctival malignancies. *Surv Ophthalmol* 1980;**24:**679.

Collin JRO, Rathbun JE: Involutional entropion. *Arch Ophthalmol* 1978;**96:**1058.

Custer PL, Tenzel RR, Kowalczyk AP: Blepharochalasis syndrome. *Am J Ophthalmol* 1985;**99:**424.

Frueh BR et al: Treatment of blepharospasm with botulinum toxin. *Arch Ophthalmol* 1984;**102:**1464.

Jones LT: The lacrimal secretory system and its treatment. *Am J Ophthalmol* 1966;**62:**47.

Jones LT, Wobig JL: *Surgery of the Eyelids and Lacrimal Apparatus*. Aesculapius, 1976.

Quickert MH: The eyelids. Pages 937–954 in: *Modern Ophthalmology*. Vols 3 and 4. Sorsby A (editor). Butterworth, 1972.

Richards WW: Actinomycotic lacrimal canaliculitis. *Am J Ophthalmol* 1973;**75:**155.

Salvaggio JE (editor): Primer on allergic and immunologic diseases. *JAMA* 1982;**248:**2579. [Special issue.]

Sevel D: Ptosis and underaction of the superior rectus muscle. *Ophthalmology* 1984;**91:**1080.

Stewart WB (editor): *Ophthalmic Plastic and Reconstructive Surgery*. American Academy of Ophthalmology, Manuals Program, 1984.

Sullivan JH, Beard C, Bullock JD: Cryosurgery for treatment of trichiasis. *Am J Ophthalmol* 1976;**82:**117.

Thygeson P: Complications of staphylococcic blepharitis. *Am J Ophthalmol* 1969;**68:**446.

Tears

7

Khalid F. Tabbara, MD

SOURCE & FUNCTION OF THE TEARS

The tears are a mixture of secretions from the major and minor (accessory) lacrimal glands, the goblet cells, and the meibomian glands. Under normal circumstances, the tear fluid forms a thin layer approximately 7–10 μm thick that covers the corneal and conjunctival epithelium. The functions of this ultrathin layer are (1) to make the cornea a smooth optical surface by abolishing minute surface irregularities of its epithelium; (2) to wet the surface of the corneal and conjunctival epithelium, preventing damage to the epithelial cells; and (3) to inhibit the growth of microorganisms on the conjunctiva and cornea by mechanical flushing and the antimicrobial action of the tear fluid.

The total mass of the accessory lacrimal glands has been estimated to be approximately one-tenth that of the lacrimal gland mass.

COMPOSITION OF THE TEARS

The normal tear volume is estimated to be about 6 μL in each eye, and the average rate of turnover about 1.2 μL/min. When collected with minimal trauma, tear fluid contains a high concentration of proteins. Three fractions are demonstrable by paper electrophoresis: albumin, globulins, and lysozyme. The antimicrobial activity of the tears is in the gamma globulin and lysozyme fractions.

The gamma globulins found in the normal tear fluid are IgA, IgG, and IgE. The IgA predominates and is similar to the IgA found in other body secretions bathing mucous membrane surfaces such as saliva and the bronchial, nasal, and gastrointestinal secretions. The IgA found in tears differs from serum IgA, however, and is more concentrated. In certain allergic conditions such as vernal conjunctivitis, the IgE concentration of tear fluid increases. Lysozyme may act synergistically with IgA in causing lysis of bacteria.

Although lysozyme is known to have a lytic effect on certain bacteria, its absence does not necessarily increase the risk of infection. Reduction in tear lysozyme concentration usually occurs early in the course of Sjögren's syndrome and is considered helpful in the diagnosis of that disorder. Lysozyme in tears can be measured by turbidimetric assays utilizing the microorganism *Micrococcus lysodeikticus* (heat-killed) as the substrate. This can be performed on tear samples collected on regular Schirmer strips. More recently, an antibacterial factor that is closely related to betalysin was identified and measured in human tears. It appears that betalysin is a normal constituent of human tears and complements the antibacterial action of lysozyme.

The average glucose concentration of the tears is 5 mg/dL. Unstable glucose levels have been demonstrated in tears of normal adults. Glucose levels were found to be less in tears in closed eyes than in open eyes.

The average tear urea level is 0.04 mg/dL.

Changes in the blood concentrations of both glucose and urea parallel changes in the tear glucose and tear urea levels.

K^+, Na^+, and Cl^- occur in higher concentrations in tears than in plasma. The average pH of tears is 7.35. Under normal conditions, tear fluid is isotonic. Tear film osmolarity ranges from 295 to 309 mosm/L. In keratoconjunctivitis sicca, there is hyperosmolarity of the tear film.

If collection of the tear fluid is traumatic, the normal constituents of the tears may be altered and there may be transudation of substances from the conjunctival blood vessels. In certain inflammatory conditions of the conjunctiva, there is marked transudation of immunoglobulins directly from the blood to the tear fluid.

LAYERS OF THE PREOCULAR TEAR FILM

The tear film covering the corneal and conjunctival epithelium (preocular tear film) is composed of 3 layers (Fig 7–1): (1) The superficial lipid layer is a monomolecular layer derived from the secretions of the meibomian glands and thought to retard evaporation of the aqueous layer. (2) The middle aqueous layer is elaborated by the major and minor lacrimal glands and contains water-soluble substances (salts and proteins). (3) The deep mucinous layer is composed of glycoprotein mucin and overlies the corneal and conjunctival epithelial cells. The epithelial cell membranes are composed of lipoproteins and are therefore relatively hydrophobic. Such a surface cannot be wetted with an aqueous solution alone. Mucin (glycoprotein) plays an important role in wetting this surface. It is partly adsorbed onto the corneal epithelial cell membranes and is anchored by the microvilli of the surface epithelial cells. This provides a new hy-

Lipid layer
Aqueous layer
Mucus layer
Micro-villus
Epithelial cells

Figure 7–1. The 3 layers of the tear film covering the superficial epithelial layer of the cornea.

drophilic surface for the aqueous tears to spread on, and the surface is wetted by a lowering of the tears' surface tension. Mucin is elaborated by the goblet cells of the conjunctiva, and recent studies have shown that the lacrimal gland contributes to its production.

Periodic resurfacing of the tear film is important to prevent dry spots and is accomplished by blinking. In the normal eye, blinking maintains a continuous tear film over the ocular surface.

DRY EYE SYNDROME
(Keratoconjunctivitis Sicca)

Deficiency in any of the tear film components may lead to loss of the film's stability. This will cause rapid break-up of the tear film, and dry spots will appear on the corneal and conjunctival epithelium. Dryness of the eye may therefore result from any disease associated with deficiency of the tear film components (aqueous, mucin, or lipid). Although there are many forms of keratoconjunctivitis sicca, those connected with rheumatoid arthritis or other connective tissue diseases are commonly referred to as **Sjögren's syndrome.** The etiology and diagnosis of keratoconjunctivitis sicca are summarized in Table 7–1.

Clinical Findings

A. Symptoms and Signs: Patients with dry eyes complain most frequently of a scratchy or sandy (foreign body) sensation. Other common symptoms are itching, excessive mucus secretion, inability to produce tears, a burning sensation, photosensitivity, redness, pain, and difficulty in moving the lids. In most patients, the most remarkable feature of the eye examination is the grossly normal appearance of the eye.

The most characteristic feature on slit lamp examination is the interrupted or absent tear meniscus

Table 7–1. Etiology and diagnosis of dry eye syndrome.

I. **Etiology:**
  A. Conditions Characterized by Hypofunction of the Lacrimal Gland:
    1. Congenital—
      a. Familial dysautonomia (Riley-Day syndrome).
      b. Aplasia of the lacrimal gland (congenital alacrima).
      c. Trigeminal nerve aplasia.
      d. Ectodermal dysplasia.
    2. Acquired—
      a. Systemic diseases—
        (1) Sjögren's syndrome.
        (2) Progressive systemic sclerosis.
        (3) Sarcoidosis.
        (4) Leukemia, lymphoma.
        (5) Amyloidosis.
        (6) Hemochromatosis.
      b. Infection—
        (1) Trachoma.
        (2) Mumps.
      c. Injury—
        (1) Surgical removal of lacrimal gland.
        (2) Irradiation.
        (3) Chemical burn.
      d. Medications—
        (1) Antihistamines.
        (2) Antimuscarinics: atropine, scopolamine.
        (3) General anesthetics: halothane, nitrous oxide.
        (4) Beta-adrenergic blockers: timolol, practolol.
      e. Neurogenic—Neuroparalytic (facial nerve palsy).
  B. Conditions Characterized by Mucin Deficiency:
    1. Avitaminosis A.
    2. Stevens-Johnson syndrome.
    3. Ocular pemphigoid.
    4. Chronic conjunctivitis, eg, trachoma.
    5. Chemical burns.
    6. Medications—Antihistamines, antimuscarinic agents, beta-adrenergic blocking agents (eg, practolol).
  C. Defective Spreading of Tear Film Caused by the Following:
    1. Eyelid abnormalities—
      a. Defects, coloboma.
      b. Ectropion or entropion.
      c. Keratinization of lid margin.
      d. Decreased or absent blinking.
        (1) Neurologic disorders.
        (2) Hyperthyroidism.
        (3) Contact lens.
        (4) Drugs.
      e. Lagophthalmos—
        (1) Nocturnal lagophthalmos.
        (2) Hyperthyroidism.
    2. Conjunctival abnormalities—
      a. Pterygium.
      b. Symblepharon.
    3. Proptosis.
II. **Diagnostic Tests:**
  A. Biomicroscopy.
  B. Rose Bengal Staining.
  C. Fluorescein Staining.
  D. Tear Break-Up Time.
  E. Tear Film Osmolarity.
  F. Tear Lysozyme.
  G. Schirmer Test Without Anesthesia.

Figure 7–2. Rose bengal staining of corneal and conjunctival cells in a 54-year-old woman with keratoconjunctivitis sicca.

at the lower lid margin. Tenacious yellowish mucous strands are sometimes seen in the lower conjunctival fornix. The bulbar conjunctiva loses its normal luster and may be thickened, edematous, and hyperemic.

The damaged corneal and conjunctival epithelial cells stain with 1% rose bengal (Fig 7–2), and defects in the corneal epithelium stain with fluorescein. The corneal epithelium shows varying degrees of fine punctate stippling in the interpalpebral fissure.

In the late stages of keratoconjunctivitis sicca, filaments may be seen—one end of each filament attached to the corneal epithelium and the other end moving freely (Figs 7–3 and 7–4). Three types of corneal filaments have been recognized: (1) filaments consisting entirely of mucus, (2) filaments consisting entirely of epithelial cells, and (3) filaments consisting of epithelial cells and mucus.

In patients with Sjögren's syndrome, conjunctival scrapings may show increased numbers of goblet cells (Fig 7–5). Lacrimal gland enlargement occurs uncommonly in patients with Sjögren's syndrome.

B. Schirmer Test: The use of wettable filter paper strips as a device for measuring tear secretion was first described by Köster in 1900 in connection with a study of facial nerve paralysis. Köster placed one end of a filter paper strip 1 cm wide and 20 cm long in the conjunctival sac in each eye and noted the extent of wetting by the tear fluid. In 1903, Otto Schirmer modified Köster's method by reducing the width of the strips to 0.5 cm and their length to 3.5 cm.

The accessory lacrimal glands of Wolfring and Krause secrete enough tears to keep the cornea adequately wetted under most circumstances, and the major lacrimal glands secrete enough to help cover stressful circumstances such as drying from exposure to hot air, irritation from corneal injury, foreign bodies, emotional upsets, and various noxious stimuli. Schirmer tests performed without topical anesthesia measure the function of the lacrimal gland, whose secretory activity is stimulated by the irritating nature of the filter paper. Schirmer tests performed after topical anesthesia (instillation of 0.5% tetracaine) measure the function of the accessory lacrimal glands (the basic secretors).

The Schirmer test is a good screening test—and definitely the simplest test—for the assessment of tear production. However, false-positive and false-negative results occur in 15% of eyes tested; a positive result (decreased wetting of the filter paper strip) should be confirmed and a negative result should by no means rule out dryness of the eyes, particularly if it is secondary to mucin deficiency.

A Schirmer test showing less than 10 mm of wetting in 5 minutes is considered abnormal.

C. Tear Film Break-Up Time: At present there is no practical method of measuring the mucin content of the tear fluid, but measurement of the tear film break-up time may sometimes be very useful. Defi-

Figure 7–3. Corneal filaments in a 56-year-old patient with keratoconjunctivitis sicca.

Figure 7–4. Slit lamp picture of a 48-year-old patient with keratoconjunctivitis sicca and corneal filaments.

Figure 7–5. Goblet cells in conjunctival scrapings from a patient with Sjögren's syndrome. (Stained with Giemsa's stain.)

ciency in mucin may not affect the Schirmer test but may lead to instability of the tear film. This causes the film's rapid break-up. "Dry holes" (Fig 7–6) are formed in the tear film, and a baring of the corneal or conjunctival epithelium follows. This process ultimately damages the epithelial cells, which can then be stained with rose bengal. Damaged epithelial cells may be shed from the cornea, leaving areas susceptible to punctate staining when the corneal surface is flooded with fluorescein.

The tear film break-up time can be measured by applying a slightly moistened fluorescein strip to the bulbar conjunctiva and asking the patient to blink. The tear film is then scanned with the aid of a slit lamp while the patient refrains from blinking. A cobalt blue filter and a broad light beam are used for this purpose. The time that elapses before the first hole (dry spot) appears in the corneal fluorescein layer is the tear film break-up time. Normally, the break-up time is over 15 seconds, but it can be reduced appreciably by the use of local anesthetics, by manipulating the eye, or by holding the lids open. The break-up time is shorter in eyes with aqueous tear deficiency and is always shorter than normal in eyes with mucin deficiency.

D. Ocular Ferning Test: A simple and inexpensive qualitative test for the study of conjunctival mucus has been described. The test is performed by spreading conjunctival scrapings on a clean glass slide and letting them dry. Microscopic arborization (ferning) is observed in normal eyes. In patients with cicatrizing conjunctivitis (ocular pemphigoid, Stevens-Johnson syndrome, diffuse conjunctival cicatrization), ferning of the mucus is either reduced or absent.

Complications

Early in the course of keratoconjunctivitis sicca, vision is slightly impaired and a few patients develop corneal ulceration, corneal thinning, and perforation. Secondary bacterial infection occasionally occurs, and corneal scarring and vascularization may result in marked reduction in vision. Early treatment may prevent these complications.

Treatment

Treatment depends upon the cause. In most early cases, the corneal and conjunctival epithelial changes are reversible.

Aqueous deficiency can be treated by replacement of the aqueous with various types of artificial tears (Table 7–2). Mucin deficiency can be partially compensated for by the use of ophthalmic vehicles of high molecular weight—eg, water-soluble polymers—or by the use of the patient's own serum as local eye drops. Serum used for this purpose must be kept refrigerated at all times. It acts by lowering the surface tension of the tears, assisting in the spreading of the tears, and wetting the epithelium. If the mucus is tenacious, as in Sjögren's syndrome, mucolytic agents (eg, acetylcysteine, 10%) may give some relief.

A slow-release artificial tear insert (Lacrisert) has been developed and made commercially available for clinical use. The insert is a solid 5-mg rod made of hydroxypropylcellulose. When inserted into the inferior cul-de-sac, the rod swells up to 10 times its original size by imbibition of fluid from the capillary bed, and the hydroxypropylcellulose is slowly released over a period of 12 hours. About half of patients with keratoconjunctivitis sicca have good relief with one insert in each eye once in the morning. Some patients complain of irritation or blurring of vision. Topical artificial tears may be used simultaneously with these preservative-free inserts.

Treatment with all-*trans*-retinoic acid, 0.1%, relieved symptoms and improved visual acuity in pa-

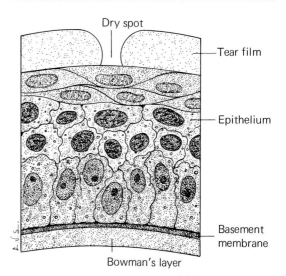

Figure 7–6. Baring of the corneal epithelium following formation of a dry spot in the tear film. (Modified and redrawn from Dohlman CH: The function of the corneal epithelium in health and disease. *Invest Ophthalmol* 1971;10:383.)

Table 7—2. Local therapy of dry eye syndrome.

Mild syndrome
(1) Artificial tears 4—5 times daily.
(2) Lubricating ointment at bedtime.

Moderate syndrome
(1) Artificial tears every 2 hours.
(2) Lubricating ointment at bedtime.
(3) Consider sustained-release tear insert (Lacrisert), one insert in each eye once daily.
(4) Mucolytic agent (acetylcysteine, 10%, 4 times daily).

Severe syndrome
(1) Artificial tears (or gum cellulose, 0.625%) every hour. Avoid benzalkonium chloride.
(2) Tight goggles.
(3) Punctal occlusion.
(4) Lubricating ointment at bedtime.
(5) Change environment; use humidifier.

tients with Sjögren's syndrome, Stevens-Johnson syndrome, ocular pemphigoid, and postoperative or postradiation dry eye syndrome. Fewer abnormalities were also seen with rose bengal staining or the Schirmer test in these patients. Topical vitamin A treatment causes reversal of squamous metaplasia.

OTHER DISORDERS OF THE LACRIMAL SYSTEM

Lacrimal Hypersecretion

The causes of excessive tearing are varied but are due to stimulation of the lacrimal gland.

Psychic lacrimation is normally associated with pain or emotional upsets. The fact that this type of lacrimation appears after the first few months of life explains why newborns do not produce tears when they cry.

Neurogenic lacrimation is brought about by reflex stimulation. Eyestrain, corneal injury, a blast of hot air, dry wind, or foreign body in the cornea or conjunctiva may cause reflex trigeminal irritation that excites lacrimation. Strong light causes reflex visual irritation and copious lacrimation. Irritation of the facial nerve, yawning, vomiting, and laughing are also associated with reflex lacrimation.

Epiphora may follow obstruction of the lacrimal drainage system. This can be caused by punctal eversion or occlusion or by canalicular or nasolacrimal duct obstruction. Most cases of nasolacrimal duct obstruction can be corrected surgically.

Paradoxic Lacrimation ("Crocodile Tears")

This is an acquired unilateral (very rarely bilateral) condition characterized by excessive tearing while eating. It occurs as a sequel to Bell's palsy (facial nerve palsy) and is the result of aberrant regeneration of the facial nerve fibers.

Bloody Tears

This is a rare clinical entity attributed to a variety of causes. It has been associated with menstruation ("vicarious menses"). Blood-tinged tears may be secondary to conjunctival hemorrhage due to any cause (trauma, blood dyscrasia, etc) or to tumors of the lacrimal sac. They have also recently been reported in a hypertensive patient suffering from epistaxis with extension through the nasolacrimal duct.

REFERENCES

Allansmith MR et al: Plasma cell content of main and accessory lacrimal glands and conjunctiva. *Am J Ophthalmol* 1976; **82**:70.

Allen M, Wright P, Reid L: The human lacrimal gland: A histochemical and organ culture study of the secretory cells. *Arch Ophthalmol* 1972;**88**:493.

Brauninger GE, Centifanto YM: Immunoglobulin E in human tears. *Am J Ophthalmol* 1971;**72**:558.

Crandall DC, Leopold IH: The influence of systemic drugs on tear constituents. *Ophthalmology* 1979;**86**:115.

Daum KM, Hill RM: Human tears: Glucose instabilities. *Acta Ophthalmol (Copenh)* 1984;**62**:472.

deLuise VP, Tabbara KF: Quantitation of tear lysozyme levels in dry-eye disorders. *Arch Ophthalmol* 1983;**101**:634.

Dohlman CH: Punctal occlusion in keratoconjunctivitis sicca. *Ophthalmology* 1978;**85**:1277.

Ford LC, DeLange RJ, Petty RW: Identification of a nonlysozymal bactericidal factor (beta lysin) in human tears and aqueous humor. *Am J Ophthalmol* 1976;**81**:30.

Frayha RA, Tabbara KF, Geha RS: Familial CRST syndrome with sicca complex. *J Rheumatol* 1977;**4**:53.

Gilbard JP, Farris RL, Santamaria J II: Osmolarity of tear microvolumes in keratoconjunctivitis sicca. *Arch Ophthalmol* 1978;**96**:677.

Gillette TE, Greiner JV, Allansmith MR: Immunohistochemical localization of human tear lysozyme. *Arch Ophthalmol* 1981;**99**:298.

Holly FJ, Lemp MA: Tear physiology and dry eyes. *Surv Ophthalmol* 1977;**22**:69.

Huth SW, Miller MJ, Leopold HI: Calcium and proteins in tears. *Arch Ophthalmol* 1981;**99**:1628.

Hypher TJ: Uptake and loss of tears from filter paper discs employed in lysozyme tests. *Br J Ophthalmol* 1979;**63**:251.

Jones DB: Prospects in the management of tear-deficiency states. *Trans Am Acad Ophthalmol Otolaryngol* 1977;**83**:693.

Katz JI, Blackman WM: A soluble sustained-release ophthalmic delivery unit. *Am J Ophthalmol* 1977;**83**:728.

Lamberts DW, Langston DP, Chu W: A clinical study of slow-releasing artificial tears. *Ophthalmology* 1978;**85**:794.

Mackie IA, Seal DV, Pescod JM: Beta-adrenergic receptor blocking drugs: Tear lysozyme and immunological screening for adverse reaction. *Br J Ophthalmol* 1977;**61**:354.

McClellan BH et al: Immunoglobulins in tears. *Am J Ophthalmol* 1973;**76**:89.

Nielsen NV, Eriksen JS: Timolol transitory manifestations of dry eyes in long-term treatment. *Acta Ophthalmol* 1979;**57**:418.

Norn MS: The conjunctival fluid, its height, volume, density of cells, and flow. *Acta Ophthalmol* 1966;**44**:212.

Ohashi Y et al: The presence of cytotoxic autoantibody to lacrimal gland cells in NZB/W mice. *Invest Ophthalmol Vis Sci* 1985;**26**:214.

Spiers ASD: Syndrome of "crocodile tears": Pharmacologic study of a bilateral case. *Br J Ophthalmol* 1970;**54**:330.

Tabbara KF: Sjögren's syndrome. Pages 309–314 in: *The Cornea: Scientific Foundation and Clinical Practice.* Smolin G, Thoft RA (editors). Little, Brown, 1983.

Tabbara KF, Okumoto M: Ocular ferning test: A qualitative test for mucus deficiency. *Ophthalmology* 1982;**89**:712.

Tabbara KF et al: Sjögren's syndrome: A correlation between ocular findings and labial salivary gland histology. *Trans Am Acad Ophthalmol Otolaryngol* 1974;**78**:467.

Terry JE, Hill RM: Human tear osmotic pressure. *Arch Ophthalmol* 1978;**96**:120.

Tseng SCG et al: Topical retinoid treatment for various dry-eye disorders. *Ophthalmology* 1985;**92**:717.

Warwick R: *Eugene Wolff's Anatomy of the Eye and Orbit,* 7th ed. Saunders, 1976.

Werblin TP, Rheinstrom SD, Kaufman HE: The use of slow-release artificial tears in the long-term management of keratitis sicca. *Ophthalmology* 1981;**88**:78.

8

Conjunctiva

ANATOMY & PHYSIOLOGY

The conjunctiva is the thin, transparent mucous membrane that covers the posterior surface of the lids (the palpebral conjunctiva) and the anterior surface of the sclera (the bulbar conjunctiva). It is continuous with the skin at the lid margin (a mucocutaneous junction) and with the corneal epithelium at the limbus.

The **palpebral conjunctiva** lines the posterior surface of the lids and is firmly adherent to the tarsus. At the superior and inferior margins of the tarsus, the conjunctiva is reflected posteriorly (at the superior and inferior fornices) and covers the episcleral tissue to become the bulbar conjunctiva.

The **bulbar conjunctiva** is loosely attached to the orbital septum in the fornices and is folded many times. This allows the eye to move and enlarges the secretory conjunctival surface. (The ducts of the lacrimal gland open into the superior temporal fornix.) Except at the limbus (where Tenon's capsule and the conjunctiva are fused for about 3 mm), the bulbar conjunctiva is loosely attached to Tenon's capsule and the underlying sclera.

A soft, movable, thickened fold of bulbar conjunctiva (the **semilunar fold**) is located at the inner canthus and corresponds to the nictitating membrane of some lower animals. A small, fleshy, epidermoid structure (the **caruncle**) is attached superficially to the inner portion of the semilunar fold and is a transition zone containing both cutaneous and mucous membrane elements.

Histology

The **conjunctival epithelium** consists of 2–5 layers of stratified columnar epithelial cells, superficial and basal. Conjunctival epithelium near the limbus, over the caruncle, and near the mucocutaneous junctions at the lid margins consists of stratified squamous epithelial cells. The **superficial epithelial cells** contain round or oval mucus-secreting goblet cells. The mucus, as it forms, pushes aside the goblet cell nucleus and is necessary for proper dispersion of the precorneal tear film. The **basal epithelial cells** stain more deeply than the superficial cells and near the limbus may contain pigment.

The **conjunctival stroma** is divided into an adenoid (superficial) layer and a fibrous (deep) layer. The **adenoid layer** contains lymphoid tissue and in some areas may contain ''folliclelike'' structures without germinal centers. The adenoid layer does not develop until after the first 2 or 3 months of life. This explains why inclusion conjunctivitis of the newborn is papillary in nature rather than follicular and why it later becomes follicular. The **fibrous layer** is composed of connective tissue that attaches to the tarsal plate in a hexagonal manner. This explains the appearance of the papillary reaction in inflammations of the conjunctiva. The fibrous layer is loosely arranged over the globe.

The **accessory lacrimal glands** (glands of Krause and Wolfring), which resemble the lacrimal gland in structure and function, are located in the stroma. Most of the glands of Krause are in the upper fornix, the remaining few in the lower fornix. The glands of Wolfring lie at the superior margin of the upper tarsus.

The conjunctival blood vessels are derived from the anterior ciliary and palpebral arteries. The nerves arise from the ophthalmic division of the fifth cranial nerve. There are only a few pain fibers. The conjunctiva is rich in lymphatics.

CONJUNCTIVITIS

Inflammation of the conjunctiva (conjunctivitis) is the most common eye disease in the western hemisphere. It varies in severity from a mild hyperemia with tearing (hay fever conjunctivitis) to a severe necrotic process (membranous conjunctivitis). The source is usually exogenous, sometimes endogenous.

The types of conjunctivitis and their commonest causes are set forth in Tables 8–1 and 8–2.

GENERAL CONSIDERATIONS

Because of its location, the conjunctiva is exposed to many microorganisms and other noxious substances. Resisting this bombardment are the tears. By diluting the infectious material and sluicing the conjunctival debris and organisms into the nasal passages for excretion, they greatly reduce the conjunctiva's vulnerability. They also contain lysozyme, betalysin, IgA, and IgG, all of which can inhibit bacterial growth.

The following factors make established conjunctivitis a self-limiting disease: tears, abundant lymphoid elements, constant epithelial exfoliation, a cool conjunctival sac due to tear evaporation, the pumping

Table 8—1. Causes of conjunctivitis.

Bacterial
Purulent
Neisseria gonorrhoeae
Neisseria meningitidis
Acute catarrhal (pinkeye)
Pneumococcus *(Streptococcus pneumoniae)* (temperate climates)
Haemophilus aegyptius (Koch-Weeks bacillus) (tropical climates)
Subacute catarrhal
Haemophilus influenzae (temperate climates)
Chronic, including blepharoconjunctivitis
Staphylococcus aureus
Moraxella lacunata (diplobacillus of Morax-Axenfeld)
Rare types (acute, subacute, chronic)
Streptococci
Branhamella (Neisseria) catarrhalis
Coliforms
Proteus
Corynebacterium diphtheriae
Mycobacterium tuberculosis
Treponema pallidum
Chlamydial*
Trachoma *(Chlamydia trachomatis)*
Inclusion conjunctivitis *(Chlamydia oculogenitalis)*
Lymphogranuloma venereum (LGV) *(Chlamydia lymphogranulomatis)*
Psittacosis *(Chlamydia psittaci)*
Rare types: Agents of feline pneumonitis and ovine abortion
Viral
Acute viral follicular conjunctivitis
Pharyngoconjunctival fever due to adenoviruses types 3 and 7
Epidemic keratoconjunctivitis due to adenovirus types 8 and 19
Herpes simplex virus
Newcastle disease
Acute hemorrhagic conjunctivitis due to enterovirus type 70; rarely, coxsackievirus type A28
Chronic viral follicular conjunctivitis
Molluscum contagiosum virus
Viral blepharoconjunctivitis
Vaccinia due to vaccinia-variola viruses
Varicella, zoster due to varicella-zoster virus
Measles virus
Rickettsial
Nonpurulent conjunctivitis with hyperemia and minimal infiltration, often a feature of rickettsial diseases
Typhus
Murine typhus
Scrub typhus
Rocky Mountain spotted fever
Mediterranean fever
Q fever
Fungal (Rare.)
Catarrhal, complicating blepharitis
Candida
Granulomatous
Rhinosporidium seeberi
Coccidioides immitis (San Joaquin Valley fever)
Sporothrix schenckii
Parasitic (Rare but important.)
Chronic conjunctivitis and blepharoconjunctivitis
Onchocerca volvulus (Central America, Africa)
Thelazia californiensis

Parasitic (Rare but important.) (cont'd)
Chronic conjunctivitis and blepharoconjunctivitis (cont'd)
Loa loa
Ascaris lumbricoides
Trichinella spiralis
Schistosoma haematobium (bladder fluke)
Taenia solium (cysticercus)
Pthirus pubis (Pediculus pubis, pubic louse)
Fly larvae (*Oestrus ovis,* etc) (ocular myiasis)
Immunologic (Allergic)
Immediate (humoral) hypersensitivity reactions
Hay fever conjunctivitis (pollens, grasses, animal dander, etc)
Vernal keratoconjunctivitis
Atopic keratoconjunctivitis
Giant papillary conjunctivitis
Delayed (cellular) hypersensitivity reactions
Phlyctenulosis
Mild conjunctivitis secondary to contact blepharitis
Autoimmune disease
Keratoconjunctivitis sicca associated with Sjögren's syndrome
Cicatricial pemphigoid
Midline lethal granuloma and Wegener's granulomatosis
Chemical or Irritative
Iatrogenic
Miotics
Idoxuridine
Other topically applied drugs
Contact lens solutions
Occupational
Acids
Alkalies
Smoke
Wind
Ultraviolet light
Caterpillar hair
Etiology Unknown
Folliculosis
Chronic follicular conjunctivitis (orphan's conjunctivitis, Axenfeld's conjunctivitis)
Ocular rosacea
Psoriasis
Erythema multiforme major (Stevens-Johnson syndrome) and minor
Dermatitis herpetiformis
Epidermolysis bullosa
Superior limbic keratoconjunctivitis
Ligneous conjunctivitis
Reiter's syndrome
Mucocutaneous lymph node syndrome (Kawasaki disease)
Associated With Systemic Disease
Conjunctivitis in thyroid disease
Gouty conjunctivitis
Carcinoid conjunctivitis
Sarcoidosis
Tuberculosis
Syphilis
Secondary to Dacryocystitis or Canaliculitis
Conjunctivitis secondary to dacryocystitis
Pneumococci or beta-hemolytic streptococci
Conjunctivitis secondary to canaliculitis
Actinomyces israelii, Candida sp, *Aspergillus* sp (rarely)
Conjunctivitis secondary to tumors of conjunctiva or lid margins

*See box on p 84 for a note on the taxonomic status of these organisms.

action of the tear drainage system (unimpeded when the lids are open), and the fact that bacteria are caught in the conjunctival mucus and then excreted.

Although organisms pathogenic for the genitourinary tract are also pathogenic for the conjunctiva, those that grow abundantly on the nasal mucosa tend to grow less well in the conjunctival sac, and vice versa. For example, whereas the conjunctiva is usually resistant to the viruses of the common cold, it is highly susceptible to the gonococcus and inclusion conjunctivitis agents, both of which are infectious for the genitourinary tract. Moreover, when these organisms are established on the conjunctiva, they are constantly washed down the nasolacrimal duct into the nose by the tears, yet they grow in the nose only rarely and with difficulty.

In the differential diagnosis of conjunctivitis as the cause of a red, painful, or irritated eye, it is important to rule out keratitis, iritis, and acute glaucoma. The causal organisms can then be identified by the microscopic examination of stained conjunctival material. Before treatment is started, culture studies should be made and antibiotic sensitivity tests performed.

Cytology of Conjunctivitis

Damage to the conjunctival epithelium by a noxious agent may be followed by epithelial edema, cellular death and exfoliation, epithelial hypertrophy, or granulomas. There may also be edema of the conjunctival stroma (chemosis) and hypertrophy of the adenoid layer of the stroma (follicle formation). Inflammatory cells, including neutrophils, eosinophils, basophils, lymphocytes, and plasma cells, may be seen and often indicate the nature of the damaging agent. The inflammatory cells migrate from the conjunctival stroma through the epithelium to the surface. They then combine with fibrin and with the mucus produced by the conjunctival goblet cells to form the conjunctival exudate, which accounts for the gumming of the eyelids noted on waking.

The inflammatory cells appear in the exudate or in scrapings taken with a sterile platinum spatula from the anesthetized conjunctival surface. The material is stained with Gram's stain (to identify the bacterial organisms) and with Giemsa's stain (to identify the cell types). A predominance of polymorphonuclear leukocytes is characteristic of both bacterial and chlamydial conjunctivitis. (Infections with *B catarrhalis* and *M lacunata* are exceptions; in a conjunctivitis arising from either of these bacteria, the inflammatory response is minimal, and mononuclear cells predominate.) As a rule, a predominance of mononuclear cells, especially lymphocytes, is characteristic of viral conjunctivitis except when a pseudomembrane forms, as it may in epidemic keratoconjunctivitis or herpes simplex virus conjunctivitis. Polymorphonuclear cells then predominate because of necrosis.

Eosinophils and basophils are found in allergic conjunctivitis, and scattered eosinophil granules and eosinophils are found in vernal keratoconjunctivitis. In all types of conjunctivitis there are plasma cells in the conjunctival stroma. They do not migrate through the epithelium, however, and are therefore not seen in smears of exudate or of scrapings from the conjunctival surface unless the epithelium has become necrosed, as it may in trachoma; in this event, the rupturing of a follicle allows the plasma cells to reach the epithelial surface. Since the mature follicles of trachoma rupture easily, the finding of large, palely staining, lymphoblastic (germinal center) cells in scrapings strongly suggests trachoma.

Symptoms of Conjunctivitis

The important symptoms of conjunctivitis are a foreign body sensation, a scratching or burning sensation, a sensation of fullness around the eyes, itching, and (when the cornea is also affected) photophobia.

Foreign body sensation and a scratching or burning sensation are often associated with the swelling and papillary hypertrophy that normally accompany conjunctival hyperemia. If there is pain, the cornea is probably also affected. Pain that is more severe on waking and improves during the day suggests staphylococcal infection, and pain that is severe during the day and better on waking suggests keratoconjunctivitis sicca. Itching, if complained of spontaneously rather than in response to questioning, usually indicates that the patient has an allergic conjunctivitis of the immediate hypersensitivity type.

Signs of Conjunctivitis
(Table 8–2)

The important signs of conjunctivitis are hyperemia, tearing, exudation, pseudoptosis, papillary hypertrophy, chemosis, follicles, pseudomembranes and membranes, granulomas, and preauricular adenopathy.

Hyperemia is the most conspicuous clinical sign of acute conjunctivitis. The redness is most marked in the fornix and diminishes toward the limbus by virtue of the dilatation of the posterior conjunctival vessels. (A perilimbal dilatation suggests inflammation of the cornea or deeper structures.) A brilliant red suggests bacterial conjunctivitis, and a milky appearance suggests allergic conjunctivitis. Hyperemia without cellular infiltration suggests irritation from physical causes such as wind, sun, smoke, etc, and also occurs occasionally as part of a general vascular dilatation, eg, acne rosacea or carcinoid.

Tearing is often prominent in conjunctivitis, the tears resulting from the foreign body sensation, the burning or scratching sensation, or the itching. Mild transudation also arises from the hyperemic vessels and adds to the tearing. An abnormally scant secretion of tears suggests granulomatous conjunctivitis or keratoconjunctivitis sicca.

Exudation is a feature of all types of acute conjunctivitis. The exudate is flaky and amorphous in bacterial conjunctivitis and stringy in allergic conjunctivitis. A mild gumming of the lids on waking occurs in almost all types of conjunctivitis, and if the exudate is copious and the lids are firmly stuck to-

Table 8–2. Differentiation of the common types of conjunctivitis.

Clinical Findings and Cytology	Viral	Bacterial	Chlamydial	Allergic
Itching	Minimal	Minimal	Minimal	Severe
Hyperemia	Generalized	Generalized	Generalized	Generalized
Tearing	Profuse	Moderate	Moderate	Moderate
Exudation	Minimal	Profuse	Profuse	Minimal
Preauricular adenopathy	Common	Uncommon	Common only in inclusion conjunctivitis	None
In stained scrapings and exudates	Monocytes	Bacteria, PMNs*	PMNs,* plasma cells, inclusion bodies	Eosinophils
Associated sore throat and fever	Occasionally	Occasionally	Never	Never

*Polymorphonuclear cells.

gether the conjunctivitis is probably bacterial or chlamydial.

Pseudoptosis is a drooping of the upper lid due to its increased weight from cellular infiltration. This sign is typical of several types of conjunctivitis (trachoma, epidemic keratoconjunctivitis, etc).

Papillary hypertrophy is a nonspecific conjunctival reaction that occurs because the conjunctiva is bound down to the underlying tarsus or limbus by fine fibrils. When the tuft of vessels that forms the substance of the papilla (along with cellular elements and exudates) reaches the basement membrane of the epithelium, it branches over the papilla like the spokes in the frame of an umbrella. An inflammatory exudate accumulates between the fibrils, heaping the conjunctiva into mounds. In necrotizing disease (eg, trachoma), the exudate may be replaced by granulation tissue or connective tissue.

When the papillae are small, the conjunctiva usually has a smooth, velvety appearance. A red papillary conjunctiva suggests bacterial or chlamydial disease (eg, a velvety red tarsal conjunctiva is characteristic of stage IIb trachoma). When the papillae are large they are flat-topped, polygonal, and milky in color. On the upper tarsus they suggest vernal keratoconjunctivitis, and on the lower tarsus they suggest atopic keratoconjunctivitis. Giant papillae may also occur at the limbus, especially in the area that is normally exposed when the eyes are open (between 2 and 4 o'clock and between 8 and 10 o'clock). Here they appear as gelatinous infiltrates that may encroach on the cornea. Limbal papillae are characteristic of vernal keratoconjunctivitis, rare in atopic keratoconjunctivitis.

Chemosis of the conjunctiva strongly suggests acute hay fever conjunctivitis but may also occur in acute gonococcal or meningococcal conjunctivitis and in epidemic keratoconjunctivitis. Chemosis of the bulbar conjunctiva is a conspicuous sign in trichinosis. Occasionally, chemosis may appear before there is any gross cellular infiltration or exudation.

Follicles are seen in most cases of viral conjunctivitis, in all cases of chlamydial conjunctivitis except neonatal inclusion conjunctivitis, and in all cases of

toxic conjunctivitis induced by topical medications such as idoxuridine and miotics. Follicles in the fornix and at the tarsal margins have limited diagnostic value, but when they are located on the tarsi (especially the upper tarsus), a chlamydial, viral, or toxic conjunctivitis following topical medication should be suspected.

The follicle is a focal lymphoid hyperplasia within the adenoid layer of the conjunctiva and usually contains a germinal center. Clinically, it can be recognized as an avascular white or gray, round structure. On slit lamp examination, small vessels can be seen arising at the border of the follicle and encircling it.

Pseudomembranes and **membranes**—the result of a coagulating process and differing only in degree—are produced by infectious or toxic agents. A pseudomembrane is a coagulum on the *surface* of the epithelium, and when it is removed the epithelium remains intact. A membrane is a coagulum involving the *entire* epithelium, and when it is removed a raw, bleeding surface remains. Pseudomembranes or membranes may accompany epidemic keratoconjunctivitis, primary herpes simplex virus conjunctivitis, streptococcal conjunctivitis, diphtheria, and erythema multiforme major. They may also be an aftermath of chemical burns, especially alkali burns.

In a peculiar form of chronic conjunctivitis (ligneous), bilateral membranes or pseudomembranes form repeatedly on the upper and lower tarsal conjunctivas and often spread out from a granulomatous area. Sometimes simulating pseudomembranes are conjunctival mucous patches—minimally elevated, whitish, and surrounded by a narrow border of erythema—seen in secondary syphilis.

Granulomas of the conjunctiva always affect the stroma. Although they usually arise endogenously (eg, from tuberculosis, syphilis, coccidioidomycosis), there are also many exogenous causes (eg, cat-scratch disease, lymphogranuloma venereum conjunctivitis, tularemia). Both chalazions (lipogranulomas) and the lesions of Parinaud's oculoglandular syndrome are granulomas, and biopsies are often necessary to determine their causes.

Phlyctenules are localized manifestations of microbial allergy (like tuberculids of the skin).

Preauricular adenopathy is an important sign. A grossly visible preauricular node is seen in Parinaud's oculoglandular syndrome and, rarely, in epidemic keratoconjunctivitis. A large or small preauricular node, sometimes slightly tender, occurs in primary herpes simplex conjunctivitis, epidemic keratoconjunctivitis, inclusion conjunctivitis, and trachoma. Small but nontender preauricular nodes occur in pharyngoconjunctival fever, Newcastle disease conjunctivitis, and acute hemorrhagic conjunctivitis. There is no preauricular adenopathy in bacterial conjunctivitis.

BACTERIAL CONJUNCTIVITIS

The acute and chronic bacterial conjunctivitides are the commonest types of conjunctivitis. The acute types occasionally become chronic but are usually self-limited, lasting a maximum of 2 weeks if untreated. Treatment with one of the many available antibacterial agents usually cures them in a few days.

Clinical Findings

A. Symptoms and Signs: The organisms listed in Table 8– 1 account for most cases of bacterial conjunctivitis. They produce bilateral irritation and injection, a purulent exudate with agglutination of the lids on waking, and occasionally lid edema. The infection usually starts in one eye and is spread to the other by the hands. It may spread from one person to another by fomites.

Purulent conjunctivitis (caused by *N gonorrhoeae* and *N meningitidis*) is marked by a profuse purulent exudate (Fig 8– 1). Meningococcal conjunctivitis is usually milder than gonococcal conjunctivitis and has fewer sequelae, but any severe, profusely exudative conjunctivitis demands immediate laboratory investigation and immediate treatment. If there is any delay, there may be severe corneal damage and the conjunctiva may become the portal of entry of the meningococcus to the bloodstream and meninges.

Acute catarrhal conjunctivitis often occurs in epidemic form and is called "pinkeye" by most laymen (Fig 8– 2). It is characterized by an acute onset of conjunctival hyperemia and a moderate amount of mucopurulent discharge. The commonest causes are the pneumococcus in temperate climates and *H aegyptius* in warm climates. Rare causes are staphylococci and streptococci. The types caused by the pneumococcus (Fig 8– 3) and *H aegyptius* may be accompanied by subconjunctival hemorrhages.

Subacute catarrhal conjunctivitis is caused most often by *H influenzae* and occasionally by *Escherichia coli* and *Proteus* sp. *H influenzae* infection is characterized by a thin, watery, or flocculent exudate.

Chronic catarrhal conjunctivitis is usually caused by *S aureus*, but *M lacunata* is also a frequent cause in warm climates. *M lacunata*—and occasionally the staphylococcus—produce a localized angular conjunctivitis that is commonly associated with dermatitis, fissuring of the external or internal canthi, and a scant conjunctival discharge.

Rare bacterial conjunctivitides may be caused by *C diphtheriae* and *Streptococcus pyogenes*. Pseudomembranes or membranes caused by these organisms may form on the palpebral conjunctiva. The rare cases of chronic conjunctivitis produced by *B catarrhalis*, the coliform bacilli, *Proteus* sp, etc, are as a rule indistinguishable clinically. Both *Mycobacterium tuberculosis* and *Treponema pallidum* produce granulomatous conjunctival disease associated with large, grossly visible preauricular nodes.

B. Laboratory Findings: In most cases of bacterial conjunctivitis, the organisms can be identified by the microscopic examination of conjunctival scrap-

Figure 8 –1. Gonorrheal conjunctivitis. Profuse purulent exudate. (Courtesy of P Thygeson.)

Figure 8 –2. Acute catarrhal conjunctivitis caused by Koch-Weeks bacillus *(Haemophilus aegyptius)*. (Courtesy of HB Ostler.)

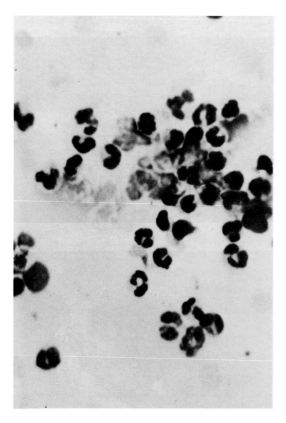

Figure 8–3. Polymorphonuclear reaction in Giemsa-stained scrapings from a patient with bacterial conjunctivitis. (Courtesy of M Okumoto.)

ings stained with Gram's stain or Giemsa's stain; this reveals numerous polymorphonuclear neutrophils (Fig 8–3). Direct examination and culture study are recommended for all cases and are mandatory if the disease is purulent, membranous, or pseudomembranous. Antibiotic sensitivity studies are also highly desirable, so that an appropriate drug can be started at once.

Complications & Sequelae

A chronic marginal blepharitis may complicate an untreated staphylococcal conjunctivitis except in very young patients who are not subject to blepharitis. Conjunctival scarring follows both pseudomembranous and membranous conjunctivitis, and in some cases the corneal nutrition may be so compromised that corneal ulceration and perforation supervene.

Marginal corneal ulceration may follow infection with *N gonorrhoeae*, *H aegyptius*, or *S aureus*, and if the toxic products of *N gonorrhoeae* diffuse through the cornea into the anterior chamber, they may cause toxic iritis.

Treatment

Specific therapy of bacterial conjunctivitis depends on the identification of the etiologic agent. While waiting for the laboratory results, the physician can start topical therapy with a sulfonamide or an antibiotic. In any purulent conjunctivitis, an antibiotic suitable for treating *N gonorrhoeae* and *N meningitidis* infection should be selected, and both systemic and topical therapy should be started immediately after material for laboratory study has been collected.

In both purulent and acute catarrhal conjunctivitis, the conjunctival sac should be irrigated with saline solution as necessary to remove the conjunctival secretions. To prevent spread of the disease, the patient and family should be instructed to give special attention to their personal hygiene.

Course & Prognosis

Acute bacterial conjunctivitis is almost always self-limited. Untreated, it usually lasts 10–14 days; if properly treated, 1–3 days. The exceptions are staphylococcal conjunctivitis (which may progress to blepharoconjunctivitis and enter a chronic phase) and gonococcal conjunctivitis (which when untreated can lead to corneal perforation and endophthalmitis). Since the conjunctiva may be the portal of entry for the meningococcus to the bloodstream and meninges, septicemia and meningitis may be the end results of meningococcal conjunctivitis.

Chronic bacterial conjunctivitis may not be self-limited and may become a troublesome therapeutic problem.

CHLAMYDIAL CONJUNCTIVITIS

1. TRACHOMA

Trachoma is one of the most ancient of known diseases. It was recognized as a cause of trichiasis as early as the 27th century BC and affects all races. With over 400 million of the world's population afflicted, it is one of the most common of all chronic human diseases. Its regional variations in prevalence and severity can be explained on the basis of variations in the personal hygiene and standards of living of the world's peoples, the climatic conditions under which they live, the prevailing age at onset, and the frequency and type of the prevailing concomitant bacterial eye infections. Although sporadic cases occur in the white population of the USA, trachoma is rare here except among the American Indians of the southwestern states, where it is now mild and relatively uncomplicated.

Trachoma has a special affinity for the eye and is usually bilateral. Spread is by direct contact or fomites, usually from mother to child or grandmother to grandchild. Family members in contact with a child with trachoma should always be investigated and should be treated when found to harbor the disease. Insect vectors, especially flies and gnats, may play a role in transmission. The acute forms of the disease are more infectious than the cicatricial forms, and the larger the inoculum the more severe the onset. Spread is often associated with epidemics of bacterial conjunctivitis and with the dry seasons in tropical and semitropical countries.

Clinical Findings

A. Symptoms and Signs: The incubation period of trachoma averages 7 days but varies from 5 to 14 days. In an infant or child the onset is usually insidious, and the disease may resolve with minimal or no complications. In the adult the onset is often subacute or acute, and complications may develop early. At onset, trachoma often resembles bacterial conjunctivitis, the signs and symptoms usually consisting of tearing, photophobia, pain, exudation, edema of the eyelids, chemosis of the bulbar conjunctiva, hyperemia, papillary hypertrophy, tarsal and limbal follicles, superior keratitis, pannus formation, and a small, tender preauricular node.

According to **MacCallan's classification,** the disease passes through the following 4 clinical stages:

Figure 8–4. Trachoma, stage IIb. Papillae and follicles in upper tarsal conjunctiva. (Courtesy of P Thygeson.)

> **Stage I** (early lymphoid hyperplasia): Papillary hypertrophy and immature (small) follicles on the upper tarsus.
> **Stage IIa** (established trachoma): Papillary hypertrophy and mature (large) follicles on the upper tarsus.
> **Stage IIb** (established trachoma): Papillary hypertrophy predominating and masking the follicles on the upper tarsus (Fig 8–4).
> **Stage III** (cicatricial trachoma): Early conjunctival scarring, shown by fine white lines in the subepithelial conjunctiva and associated with persistent follicles and papillary hypertrophy of the upper tarsal conjunctiva. (Since the agent of trachoma is epitheliotropic, the subepithelial scarring of the tarsal conjunctiva and the cornea may be due to a diffusible toxin.)

> **Stage IV** (healed trachoma): Conjunctival stellate and linear cicatrization without inflammation of the upper tarsus.

In established trachoma there may also be superior epithelial keratitis, subepithelial keratitis, pannus, superior limbal follicles, and ultimately the cicatricial remains of these follicles, known as **Herbert's peripheral pits.** Both the limbal follicles and Herbert's pits are pathognomonic of trachoma; the follicles are gelatinous, semiopaque, dome-shaped elevations surrounded by the pannus, and the pits are small depressions in the connective tissue of the limbocorneal junction. They are filled with epithelium and look like small, lucid circles or semicircles in a fibrovascular membrane arising at the limbus, from which vascular loops encroach on the cornea from above (Fig 8– 5).

Note on the Taxonomic Status of the Chlamydiae

The classification of the chlamydiae (formerly the bedsoniae) is currently the subject of a dispute reminiscent of one that arose over the classification of another group of small intracellular microorganisms: the rickettsiae. Officially, there are at present only 2 species: *C trachomatis* (also known as "subgroup A") and *C psittaci* (also known as "subgroup B"). This grouping is based on the sulfonamide susceptibility of *C trachomatis* and the iodine-staining properties of its inclusions—2 important properties not shared by *C psittaci*. But the lack of official speciation of the agents of trachoma, inclusion disease (conjunctivitis, urethritis, and cervicitis), and lymphogranuloma venereum has led to serious confusion and some startling misconceptions. For example, headlines in a recent issue of *Sight-Saving Review* stated that trachoma was the commonest cause of sexually transmitted disease in the USA!

An excellent speciation was made by Rake in 1957, who designated the agent of trachoma as *C trachomatis;* the agent of inclusion conjunctivitis, urethritis, and cervicitis as *C oculogenitalis;* and the agent of lymphogranuloma venereum as *C lymphogranulomatis.** Speciation based on biologic properties is difficult with the chlamydiae because of the many shared properties; but speciation based on immunologic typing, pathogenicity patterns in primates, tissue tropism, and disease manifestations in humans is both reasonable and inevitable. Most ophthalmic microbiologists still use the Rake classification, and we can only hope that with some slight modification it will soon become the official one.

*Breed RS et al: *Bergey's Manual of Systematic Bacteriology.* Vol 1. Williams & Wilkins, 1984.

All of the signs of trachoma are more severe in the upper than in the lower conjunctiva and cornea.

MacCallan's classification has no prognostic value. For prognostic purposes, a classification of the intensity of the inflammatory response has been developed, based on the scoring of papillae and follicles in the upper tarsal conjunctiva. The slightly simplified system presented here consists of 4 categories: severe, moderate, mild, and trivial or inactive (Table 8–3).

Other systems of classification have been devised for distortion of the eyelids due to conjunctival scarring, for trichiasis and entropion, and for corneal scarring, all of which represent potentially blinding lesions of trachoma.

B. Laboratory Findings: Giemsa-stained conjunctival scrapings show a predominantly polymorphonuclear reaction, but plasma cells, Leber cells (large macrophages containing phagocytosed debris), and follicle cells (lymphoblasts) may also be seen. Plasma cells and Leber cells suggest trachoma, but follicle cells are diagnostic. Unfortunately, they are not always present. When inclusion bodies, which cannot always be found in chronic active trachoma, appear in the Giemsa-stained preparations, they are dark purple, purplish-blue, or blue inclusions that cap the nucleus of the epithelial cell (Fig 8–6). Fluorescent antibody stains increase the likelihood of detecting inclusion bodies, but the technique is expensive and difficult.

The agent of trachoma resembles the agent of inclusion conjunctivitis morphologically, but the 2 can be differentiated serologically by microimmunofluorescence and by their pathogenicity patterns in mon-

Table 8–3. Prognostic classification of trachoma according to intensity of inflammatory response.

Intensity	Papillae (P)*	Follicles (F)†
Severe	P3	F3 or F2 or F1
Moderate	P2	F3
Mild	P1 or P2	F1 or F2
Trivial or inactive	P1	F4

*Papillae and diffuse infiltration in the upper tarsal conjunctiva are scored as follows:

P0 Absent: normal appearance.

P1 Mild: individual papillae prominent but deep subconjunctival vessels not obscured.

P2 Moderate: more prominent papillae, and normal vessels appear hazy, even to the naked eye.

P3 Severe: pronounced papillae, conjunctiva thickened and opaque, normal tarsal vessels hidden over more than half the surface.

†For the purpose of scoring follicles, the upper tarsal conjunctival surface is divided into 3 approximately equal zones by 2 imaginary lines. The lines run approximately parallel with the upper tarsal border. Zone 1, nearest to the upper tarsal border, includes the entire upper tarsal border and adjacent tarsal surface. Zone 3 includes the tarsal conjunctiva adjacent to the central half of the lid margin. Upper tarsal follicles are scored as follows:

F0 Absent: no follicles.

F1 Mild: follicles present but not more than 5 altogether in zones 2 and 3.

F2 Moderate: more follicles in zones 1 and 2 but not more than 5 in zone 3.

F3 Severe: follicles present in all 3 zones but more than 5 in zone 3.

F4 Old follicles: yellowish, angular, and depressed follicles.

Figure 8–5. Trachomatous pannus. (Courtesy of P Thygeson.)

Figure 8–6. Cytoplasmic inclusion body in conjunctival epithelial cells in trachoma. Ruptured inclusion at right. Polymorphonuclear neutrophil (typical in conjunctival scrapings of trachoma) below. (Courtesy of P Thygeson and C Dawson.)

keys and apes. Trachoma is caused by serotypes A, B, Ba, or C. Both agents can be isolated in tissue cultures, commonly using McCoy cells treated with cycloheximide, idoxuridine, or irradiation to favor the growth of chlamydiae or using the yolk sac of embryonated hen eggs. Identification of the organisms in tissue cultures is achieved by staining for inclusions with iodine, Giemsa's stain, or fluorescent antibody. Recently, specific DNA probes have also become available.

Measurement of antibody levels in the patient's serum plays no significant role in the diagnosis of ocular chlamydial infections. The prevalence of positive serology among unaffected members of most populations is much too high. Serologic testing is, however, a useful epidemiologic tool.

Differential Diagnosis

In the differentiation of trachoma from viral infections, 2 differences are important: (1) With one exception (the follicular conjunctivitis associated with a molluscum contagiosum nodule on the lid margin), all viral conjunctivitides are of less than 3 weeks' duration; and (2) unless there is a pseudomembrane, all viral infections are associated with a predominantly mononuclear inflammatory reaction. Follicular conjunctivitis following treatment with idoxuridine or miotics may simulate trachoma, but the drug-induced follicular reaction subsides when the drug is withdrawn, and a conjunctival scraping contains a limited and approximately equal number of polymorphonuclear and mononuclear cells. Long-standing dacryocystitis or chronic canaliculitis in children may occasionally be complicated by chronic follicular conjunctivitis, but there are no corneal changes in these conditions, and as soon as the underlying infections are eradicated the conjunctivitis clears and leaves no scars. In children, folliculosis of the adenoid type may simulate trachoma grossly, but there are no associated corneal changes and no papillary hypertrophy, and the conjunctiva between follicles is normal.

The agents of inclusion conjunctivitis, feline pneumonitis, and psittacosis (all chlamydial infections) may produce follicular conjunctivitis, but except for the flat scars associated with the pseudomembranes that occasionally form in neonatal inclusion conjunctivitis, there is no scarring.

Parinaud's oculoglandular syndrome in children may have an associated follicular conjunctivitis, but a prominent feature of Parinaud's syndrome, never seen in trachoma, is a grossly visible preauricular node.

Vernal keratoconjunctivitis is occasionally mistaken for trachoma because of its upper tarsal lesions, but the conjunctiva in vernal keratoconjunctivitis has a milky appearance, polygonal, flat-topped giant papillae, and numerous eosinophils and eosinophil granules in conjunctival scrapings.

Complications & Sequelae

Conjunctival scarring is a frequent complication of trachoma and can shut off the ductules of the accessory lacrimal glands and obliterate the orifices of the lacrimal gland. These effects may drastically reduce the aqueous component of the precorneal tear film, and the film's mucous components may be reduced by loss of goblet cells. The scars may also cause entropion of the upper lid, and if there is an associated trichiasis the aberrant lashes may abrade the cornea. This often leads to corneal ulceration, bacterial corneal infections, and corneal scarring (Fig 8–7).

Ptosis (Fig 8–8), nasolacrimal duct obstruction, and dacryocystitis are other common complications of trachoma.

Treatment

Tetracycline, 1– 1.5 g/d orally in 4 divided doses for 3– 4 weeks; doxycycline, 100 mg orally twice daily for 3 weeks; or erythromycin, 1 g/d orally in 4 divided doses for 3– 4 weeks, will usually result in striking clinical improvement. Several courses are sometimes necessary for actual cure. Systemic tetracyclines should

Figure 8 –7. Advanced trachoma following corneal ulceration and scarring. (Courtesy of P Thygeson.)

Figure 8 –8. Ptosis with an "S"-shaped curve of lids associated with chronic trachoma. (Courtesy of P Thygeson.)

not be given to a child under 7 years of age or to a pregnant woman since they may cause staining of the developing child's incisors and may produce epiphyseal problems in the fetus.

Topical ointments or drops, including preparations of sulfonamides, tetracyclines, erythromycin, and rifampin, used 4 times daily for 6 weeks, have had some success.

From the time therapy is begun, its maximum effect is usually not achieved for 10–12 weeks. The persistence of follicles on the upper tarsus for some weeks after a course of therapy should therefore not be construed as evidence of therapeutic failure.

Course & Prognosis

Characteristically, trachoma is a chronic disease of long duration. In an ideal environment, however, about 20% of cases detected in any one year heal spontaneously; and when treatment is given early the prognosis is excellent. Unfortunately, however, because of unfavorable conditions and lack of treatment, about 20 million people in the world today have major visual loss from trachoma.

2. INCLUSION CONJUNCTIVITIS (Inclusion Blennorrhea)

Inclusion conjunctivitis, usually bilateral, is a common disease, especially in sexually active young people. Characteristically, the chlamydial agent infects the urethra of the male and the cervix of the female. Transmission to the eyes of adults is usually from the genitourinary tract to the eye. Indirect transmission in inadequately chlorinated swimming pools can also occur, and in the newborn the agent is transmitted during birth by direct contamination of the conjunctiva with cervical secretions. The Credé prophylaxis does not protect against inclusion conjunctivitis.

Clinical Findings

A. Symptoms and Signs: Inclusion conjunctivitis may have an acute or a subacute onset. The patient frequently complains of redness of the eyes, pseudoptosis, and discharge, especially in the mornings. The newborn has a papillary conjunctivitis and a moderate amount of exudate, and in hyperacute cases pseudomembranes occasionally form and can lead to scarring. Since the newborn has no adenoid tissue in the stroma of the conjunctiva (see p 78), there is no follicle formation; but if the conjunctivitis persists for 2–3 months, follicles appear and the conjunctival picture is like that in older children and adults. In the newborn, chlamydial infection may cause pharyngitis, otitis media, and, occasionally, interstitial pneumonia.

In adults the conjunctivas of both tarsi, and especially of the lower tarsus, are loaded with both papillae and follicles (Fig 8–9). Since pseudomembranes never form in the adult, scarring does not occur. A superficial keratitis may be noted superiorly and,

Figure 8–9. Acute follicular conjunctivitis caused by inclusion conjunctivitis in a 22-year-old male with urethritis. (Courtesy of K Tabbara.)

less often, a small superior micropannus (< 1–2 mm). Rarely, subepithelial opacities, usually marginal, may develop. A complicating otitis media may arise from infection of the eustachian tube.

B. Laboratory Findings: The examination of conjunctival scrapings shows (1) a predominantly polymorphonuclear neutrophil reaction; (2) no bacteria; (3) basophilic cytoplasmic inclusion bodies in epithelial cells, identical to those seen in trachoma; and (4) free elementary bodies, the extracellular form of chlamydial organisms. Bacterial cultures are negative.

In neonatal inclusion conjunctivitis, epithelial inclusions and free elementary bodies are plentiful. Giemsa staining is usually sufficient to establish the diagnosis and is useful in excluding other causes of acute conjunctivitis. In adult inclusion conjunctivitis, epithelial inclusions and free elementary bodies are less frequently seen; fluorescent antibody techniques may be used to aid in their identification. The best method of diagnosis in these cases is isolation of the organism in tissue culture.

Inclusion conjunctivitis may be caused by serotypes D–K. Serologic determinations are not useful in the diagnosis of ocular infections, but measurement of IgM antibody levels is extremely valuable in the diagnosis of chlamydial pneumonia in infants.

Differential Diagnosis

Inclusion conjunctivitis can be clinically differentiated from trachoma on the following grounds: (1) Inclusion conjunctivitis is transmitted sexually; trachoma from eye to eye. (2) Conjunctival scarring, which is common in trachoma, occurs in inclusion conjunctivitis only in the newborn and only after the formation of a pseudomembrane. If scars develop under these circumstances, they are flat and diffuse rather than linear or stellate, as in trachoma. (3) Inclusion conjunctivitis sometimes causes a micropannus but never the gross pannus seen regularly in trachoma.

(4) The corneal scarring and Herbert's pits (limbal scars) that occur in trachoma are never seen in inclusion conjunctivitis.

Treatment

In infants, 1% tetracycline in oil or ointment, erythromycin ophthalmic ointment, or a sulfonamide drop (instilled 5– 6 times daily for 14 days) is very effective. In adults, a 3-week course of oral tetracycline, 1– 1.5 g/d; doxycycline, 100 mg orally twice daily; or erythromycin, 1 g/d, is curative. (Systemic tetracyclines should not be given to a pregnant woman or a child under 7 years of age since they cause epiphyseal problems in the fetus or staining of the young child's incisors.) The patient's sexual partners should be examined and treated.

When one of the standard therapeutic regimens is followed, recurrences are rare. If untreated, inclusion conjunctivitis runs a course of 3– 9 months or longer. The average duration is 5 months.

3. LYMPHOGRANULOMA VENEREUM CONJUNCTIVITIS

Lymphogranuloma venereum infections of the conjunctiva, which can result from accidental laboratory accidents or sexual transmission, are rare. The conjunctival reaction is nonfollicular and largely granulomatous, and there is a grossly visible preauricular node (bubo). Elephantiasis of the eyelids may occur because of lymph blockage and has been compared to the esthiomene of the female genitalia. The conjunctiva and cornea become diffusely scarred. In endogenous disease secondary to a genitourinary focus, optic neuritis, uveitis, episcleritis, and phlyctenulosis have all been reported.

The causal organism, *C lymphogranulomatis,** may be recovered by inoculating mouse brains or tissue cultures with scrapings from an infected conjunctiva. Examination of the scrapings may show typical inclusions within monocytes and macrophages but not in epithelial cells. In more than 50% of patients, the Frei test is positive, and a high titer of complement-fixing antibodies is the rule. Lymphogranuloma venereum conjunctivitis is caused by chlamydia of serotypes L1, L2, and L3.

A sulfonamide or broad-spectrum antibiotic, given systemically for 3– 4 weeks, is curative.

4. PSITTACOSIS

One reported case of conjunctivitis due to an accidental laboratory infection with *C psittaci** of parakeet origin was characterized by chronic conjunctival infiltration and papillary hypertrophy of the upper tarsus and by epithelial keratitis. No inclusions were seen in epithelial cells, but cultures were positive for chlamydia. The conjunctivitis and keratitis responded only after long-term systemic tetracycline.

*See box on p 84.

5. FELINE PNEUMONITIS

Two cases have been reported of follicular conjunctivitis associated with intimate exposure to domestic cats with feline pneumonitis (a chlamydial infection caused by *C psittaci*). In both cases the conjunctivitis was associated with central epithelial keratitis and cleared after 4 weeks of therapy with systemic tetracycline. There were no sequelae. Cytoplasmic epithelial cell inclusions were seen in Giemsa-stained scrapings from the conjunctiva. This was in sharp contrast to the absence of inclusions in the parakeet-derived disease.

VIRAL CONJUNCTIVITIS

Viral conjunctivitis, a common affliction, can be caused by a wide variety of viruses. Some of these produce severe, disabling disease; others only mild, rapidly self-limited disease.

I. ACUTE VIRAL FOLLICULAR CONJUNCTIVITIS

1. PHARYNGOCONJUNCTIVAL FEVER

Pharyngoconjunctival fever is characterized by fever of 38.3– 40 °C (101– 104 °F), sore throat, and a follicular conjunctivitis in one or both eyes. The follicles are often very prominent on both the conjunctiva (Fig 8– 10) and the pharyngeal mucosa. Bilateral and, less commonly, unilateral injection and tearing occur, and there may be transient superficial epithelial keratitis and occasionally some subepithelial opacities. Preauricular lymphadenopathy (nontender) is characteristic. The syndrome may be incomplete, consisting of only one or 2 of the cardinal signs (fever, pharyngitis, and conjunctivitis).

Figure 8–10. Acute follicular conjunctivitis due to adenovirus type 3. (Courtesy of P Thygeson.)

Pharyngoconjunctival fever is caused regularly by adenovirus type 3 and occasionally by types 4 and 7. The virus can be grown on HeLa cells and identified by neutralization tests. As the disease progresses, it can also be diagnosed serologically by a rising titer of neutralizing antibody to the virus. Clinical diagnosis is a simple matter, however, and clearly more practical.

Conjunctival scrapings contain predominantly mononuclear cells, and no bacteria grow in cultures. The condition is more common in children than in adults and can be transmitted in chlorinated swimming pools. There is no specific treatment, but the conjunctivitis is self-limited, usually lasting about 10 days.

2. EPIDEMIC KERATOCONJUNCTIVITIS

Epidemic keratoconjunctivitis is usually bilateral. The onset is often in one eye only, however, and as a rule the first eye is more severely affected. At onset the patient notes injection, moderate pain, and tearing, followed in 5– 14 days by photophobia, epithelial keratitis, and round subepithelial opacities. Corneal sensation is normal. A large, tender preauricular node, rarely grossly visible, is characteristic. Edema of the eyelids, chemosis, and conjunctival hyperemia mark the acute phase, with follicles and subconjunctival hemorrhages often appearing within 48 hours. Pseudomembranes (and occasionally true membranes) may occur and may be followed by flat scars or symblepharons (Fig 8– 11).

The conjunctivitis lasts for 3– 4 weeks at most. The subepithelial opacities are concentrated in the central cornea, sparing the periphery, and may persist for months but heal without scars.

Epidemic keratoconjunctivitis is caused by adenovirus types 8 and 19, which can be cultivated on HeLa cells and identified by neutralization tests. Rising neutralizing antibody titers during the course of the disease are diagnostic. Scrapings from the conjunctiva show a primarily mononuclear inflammatory reaction (Fig 8– 12); when pseudomembranes occur, neutrophils may also be prominent.

Epidemic keratoconjunctivitis in adults is confined to the external eye, but in children there may be such systemic symptoms of viral infection as fever, sore throat, and diarrhea. Spread takes place all too often by way of the physician's fingers or use of improperly sterilized ophthalmic instruments or contaminated solutions. Eye solutions, particularly topical anesthetics, can be contaminated when a dropper tip rubs the conjunctiva or cilia. There the virus may persist, and the solution becomes a source of spread.

The danger of contaminated solution bottles can be averted by the use of individual sterile droppers for each patient. Hand washing between examinations and meticulous sterilization, especially of tonometers, are also mandatory. The tonometer footplate should be cleansed carefully with a sterile solution after each use, and the instrument should be sterilized by flame or in a hot air tonometer sterilizer after use on an inflamed eye. Applanation tonometers should be cleaned by rinsing with a sterile nonirritating solution and careful wiping several times with a facial tissue. (Epidemic keratoconjunctivitis is the only serious eye disease known to be transmissible by tonometry.)

Figure 8 –12. Mononuclear cell reaction in conjunctival scrapings of a patient with viral conjunctivitis caused by adenovirus type 8. (Courtesy of M Okumoto.)

Figure 8 –11. Epidemic keratoconjunctivitis. Thick white membrane in lower palpebral conjunctiva. (Courtesy of P Thygeson.)

Figure 8–13. Primary ocular herpes. (Courtesy of HB Ostler.)

3. HERPES SIMPLEX VIRUS CONJUNCTIVITIS

Herpes simplex virus conjunctivitis, a disease of young children, is an uncommon entity characterized by unilateral injection, irritation, mucoid discharge, pain, and mild photophobia. It occurs only in first attacks of herpes simplex virus infection, ie, in primary infections (Fig 8– 13), and is often associated with herpes simplex virus keratitis, in which the cornea shows discrete epithelial lesions that usually coalesce to form single or multiple dendrites. The conjunctivitis is follicular or, less often, pseudomembranous. (Patients receiving idoxuridine may develop follicular conjunctivitis that is not to be confused with primary herpes simplex virus conjunctivitis.) Herpetic vesicles often appear on the eyelids and lid margins, usually associated with severe edema of the eyelids. Typically, there is a large or small tender preauricular node.

No bacteria are found in scrapings or recovered in cultures. If the conjunctivitis is follicular, the predominant inflammatory reaction is mononuclear, but if it is pseudomembranous the predominant reaction is polymorphonuclear due to the chemotaxis of necrosis. Intranuclear inclusions cannot be seen in Giemsa-stained preparations (because of the margination of the chromatin), but they appear if Bouin fixation and the Papanicolaou stain are used. The finding of multinucleated giant epithelial cells has diagnostic value.

The virus can be isolated readily by gently rubbing a dry cotton-tipped applicator over an infected conjunctiva and then transferring the infected cells on the applicator directly to either an abraded rabbit cornea or a susceptible tissue culture.

Herpes simplex virus conjunctivitis may persist for 2– 3 weeks, and if it is pseudomembranous it may leave fine linear or flat scars. Complications include corneal dendrites and vesicles on the skin. Although type 1 herpesvirus causes the overwhelming majority of cases, type 2 can be a rare cause in both the newborn and adult. In the newborn there may be generalized disease with encephalitis, chorioretinitis, hepatitis, etc.

Since the conjunctivitis is self-limited, therapy is usually not necessary. Corneal debridement may be performed, or idoxuridine ointment may be applied 4 times daily for 7– 10 days. Herpetic keratitis may be treated with 3% acyclovir ointment 5 times daily for 10 days. The use of steroids is contraindicated, since they aggravate herpes simplex infections and convert the disease from a short, self-limited process to a severe, greatly prolonged process.

4. NEWCASTLE DISEASE CONJUNCTIVITIS

Newcastle disease conjunctivitis is a rare disorder characterized by burning, itching, pain, redness, tearing, and (rarely) blurring of vision. It often occurs in small epidemics among poultry workers handling infected birds, or among veterinarians or laboratory helpers working with live vaccines or virus.

The disease often presents as chemosis and mild lid edema, and, although usually unilateral, it may sometimes affect both eyes at onset or within the first few days. There is a small nontender preauricular node, minimal discharge, and follicles that are more prominent on the lower tarsus than elsewhere. Rarely, there is corneal involvement in the form of fine epithelial keratitis or round, central subepithelial opacities. An influenzalike syndrome with mild fever, headaches, and mild arthralgia may develop. The disease subsides in less than a week, and there is no specific treatment.

No bacteria appear in scrapings or grow in cultures, and the inflammatory reaction is predominantly mononuclear. The virus can be isolated readily in embryonated hen eggs or tissue cultures, and complement-fixing, neutralizing, and hemagglutination-inhibiting antibodies can be found in the patient's serum.

5. ACUTE HEMORRHAGIC CONJUNCTIVITIS

Except for North and South America, all of the continents and most of the islands of the world have had major epidemics of acute hemorrhagic conjunctivitis. Because it was first recognized in Ghana in 1969 at the time of the Apollo XI moon trip, the disease has often been called Apollo XI conjunctivitis. It is caused by enterovirus type 70. Coxsackievirus type A24 has been found in some cases.

Characteristically, the disease has a short incubation period (8– 48 hours) and course (5– 7 days). The usual signs and symptoms are pain, photophobia, foreign body sensation, copious tearing, redness, lid edema, and subconjunctival hemorrhages (Fig 8– 14). Chemosis sometimes also occurs. The subconjunctival hemorrhages are usually diffuse but may be punctate at onset, beginning in the upper bulbar conjunctiva and spreading to the lower. Most patients have preauricular lymphadenopathy, conjunctival follicles, and

Figure 8–14. Acute hemorrhagic conjunctivitis. (Courtesy of K Tabbara.)

Figure 8–15. Molluscum contagiosum of lid margin with follicular conjunctivitis. (Courtesy of HB Ostler.)

epithelial keratitis. Anterior uveitis has been reported; fever, malaise, and generalized myalgia have been observed in 25% of cases; and motor paralysis of the lower extremities has occurred in rare cases in India and Japan.

The virus is transmitted by close person-to-person contact and by such fomites as common linens, contaminated optical instruments, and water. Recovery occurs within 5–7 days, and there is no known treatment.

6. COXSACKIEVIRUS CONJUNCTIVITIS

Various coxsackieviruses have caused acute conjunctivitis accidentally in laboratory workers and in children with hand-foot-and-mouth disease.

II. CHRONIC VIRAL CONJUNCTIVITIS

1. MOLLUSCUM CONTAGIOSUM BLEPHAROCONJUNCTIVITIS

A molluscum nodule on the lid margin, especially if it is on the upper lid, may produce unilateral chronic conjunctivitis, superior keratitis, and superior pannus, all of which are also typical of trachoma. The inflammatory reaction is predominantly mononuclear (unlike the reaction in trachoma), and the round, waxy, pearl-white, noninflammatory lesion with an umbilicated center is typical of molluscum contagiosum (Fig 8–15). Prolonged (24-hour) Giemsa staining of scrapings from the lid nodule shows small red elementary bodies, and biopsy shows eosinophilic cytoplasmic inclusions that fill the entire cytoplasm of the enlarged cell, pushing its nucleus to one side.

Excision or simple incision of the nodule to allow peripheral blood to permeate it cures the conjunctivitis. On very rare occasions (reports of only 2 cases have appeared in the literature), molluscum nodules have occurred on the conjunctiva. In these cases, excision of the nodule has also relieved the conjunctivitis.

2. VACCINIAL BLEPHAROCONJUNCTIVITIS

This was an important complication of smallpox vaccination at one time but is now of historical interest only.

3. VARICELLA-ZOSTER BLEPHAROCONJUNCTIVITIS

Hyperemia and an infiltrative conjunctivitis, associated with the typical vesicular eruption along the dermatomal distribution of the ophthalmic branch of the trigeminal nerve, are characteristic of herpes zoster (preferably called simply zoster). The conjunctivitis is usually papillary, but follicles, pseudomembranes, and transitory vesicles that later ulcerate have all been noted. A tender preauricular lymph node occurs early in the disease. Scarring of the lid, entropion, and the misdirection of individual lashes are rare sequelae.

The lid lesions of varicella, which are like the skin lesions (pox) elsewhere, may appear on both the lid margins and the lids and may leave scars on the lid margins. A mild catarrhal type of conjunctivitis often occurs, but discrete conjunctival lesions (except at the limbus) are very rare. Limbal lesions resemble phlyctenules and may go through all the stages of vesicle, papule, and ulcer. The adjacent cornea becomes infiltrated and may vascularize.

In both zoster and varicella, scrapings from lid vesicles contain giant cells and a predominance of polymorphonuclear neutrophil cells; scrapings from the conjunctiva in varicella and from conjunctival vesicles in zoster contain giant cells and monocytes. The virus can be recovered in tissue cultures of human embryo cells.

There is no satisfactory treatment, but studies with interferon and acyclovir are promising.

4. MEASLES KERATOCONJUNCTIVITIS

The characteristic enanthem of measles frequently precedes the skin eruption. At this early stage the conjunctiva may have a peculiar glassy appearance, followed within a few days by swelling of the semilunar fold (Meyer's sign). Several days before the skin eruption, a catarrhal conjunctivitis with a mucopurulent discharge develops, and at the time of the skin eruption Koplik's spots appear on the conjunctiva and occasionally on the caruncle. At some time (early in children, late in adults), epithelial keratitis supervenes.

In the immunocompetent patient, measles keratoconjunctivitis has few or no sequelae, but in malnourished or otherwise immunoincompetent patients the ocular disease is frequently associated with a secondary bacterial infection due to the pneumococcus, *H influenzae*, and other organisms. In this event there is often a severe purulent or even pseudomembranous conjunctivitis with associated corneal ulceration and perforation. In many developing countries, measles and the folk remedies used to treat measles-associated eye disease are major causes of blindness.

Conjunctival scrapings show a mononuclear cell reaction unless there are pseudomembranes or secondary infection. Giemsa-stained preparations contain giant cells. Since there is no specific therapy, only supportive measures are indicated unless there is secondary infection.

RICKETTSIAL CONJUNCTIVITIS

All rickettsiae recognized as pathogenic for humans are likely to attack the conjunctiva. The conjunctiva is in fact often their portal of entry, eg, in Q fever, Marseilles fever (boutonneuse fever), endemic (murine) typhus, scrub typhus, Rocky Mountain spotted fever, and epidemic typhus.

1. Q FEVER

In Q fever there is usually severe conjunctival hyperemia. Rarely there may also be severe inflammation followed by gangrene of the lids.

Conjunctival scrapings, in which neither bacteria nor inclusions are seen, show a predominantly polymorphonuclear cell response. Diagnosis can be verified serologically by complement fixation and the Weil-Felix reaction.

Treatment with systemic tetracyclines or chloramphenicol is curative.

2. MARSEILLES FEVER (Boutonneuse Fever)

The conjunctivitis associated with Marseilles fever is ulcerative or granulomatous and associated with a grossly visible preauricular lymph node (Parinaud's oculoglandular syndrome). The conjunctivitis usually precedes the systemic signs and symptoms by 5 or 6 days.

3. ENDEMIC (MURINE) TYPHUS, SCRUB TYPHUS, ROCKY MOUNTAIN SPOTTED FEVER

The conjunctivitis associated with these rickettsial diseases is usually mild, varying from a conjunctival hyperemia with photophobia to a mild catarrhal conjunctivitis.

4. EPIDEMIC TYPHUS

The signs of conjunctivitis in epidemic typhus vary from hyperemia alone to subconjunctival hemorrhages and a low-grade conjunctival inflammation. Small, purplish oval spots appear on the conjunctiva concurrently with the cutaneous manifestations of the disease.

FUNGAL CONJUNCTIVITIS

1. CANDIDAL CONJUNCTIVITIS

Candidal conjunctivitis of the newborn, a rare phenomenon, appears as a white conjunctival plaque that can be mistaken for a pseudomembrane. There is often some exudate. In adults, candidal blepharitis may be accompanied by ulcerative or granulomatous conjunctivitis, which in rare cases may be followed by conjunctival scarring.

Scrapings show a polymorphonuclear cell inflammatory reaction. The organism grows readily on blood agar or Sabouraud's medium and can be readily identified as a budding yeast or, rarely, as pseudohyphae.

The fungus responds to amphotericin B (3–8 mg/mL) in aqueous (not saline) solution, or to applications of nystatin dermatologic cream (100,000 units/g) 4–6 times daily. The ointment must be applied carefully to be sure that it reaches the conjunctival sac and does not just build up on the lid margins.

2. *SPOROTHRIX SCHENCKII* CONJUNCTIVITIS

Occasionally, *S schenckii* invades the conjunctiva alone or in conjunction with granulomatous lesions on the lids. The conjunctival lesion is typically a small, yellow granuloma that may ulcerate. It is associated with a grossly visible preauricular node (Parinaud's oculoglandular syndrome). The lid lesions proceed along the lymphatic chain and gradually ulcerate. The infection usually follows injury or an abrasion with thorns, often barberry bush thorns.

Microscopic examination of a biopsy of the granuloma reveals gram-positive, cigar-shaped conidia (spores). The lesions respond readily to systemic iodides, although in vitro the organism is not iodide-sensitive.

3. *RHINOSPORIDIUM SEEBERI* CONJUNCTIVITIS

R seeberi has many of the characteristics of a fungus but never has been cultivated. The ocular disease it causes may affect the conjunctiva, lacrimal sac, lids, canaliculi, and sclera.

The typical lesion is a polypoid granuloma arising from the upper or lower palpebral or bulbar conjunctiva. It is a painless, soft, pink lesion that sometimes has white spots on its surface. The patient often complains of a small mass that bleeds after minimal trauma. The rest of the conjunctiva appears to be normal, and there is no regional lymphadenopathy.

Histologic examination discloses a granuloma in which there are large spherules that contain myriads of endospores. Treatment is by simple excision of the lesion with cauterization of its base.

4. COCCIDIOIDOMYCOSIS (San Joaquin Valley Fever)

C immitis may on rare occasions cause a granulomatous conjunctivitis associated with a grossly visible preauricular node (Parinaud's oculoglandular syndrome). There is often a mucopurulent discharge and occasionally a thin, transparent pseudomembrane. The granulomas are raised, indolent, discrete or diffuse, reddish lesions showing tiny areas of focal necrosis. Primary ocular disease has not been recognized; the conjunctivitis is usually only a metastasis from the primary pulmonary infection. In disseminated coccidioidomycosis, the skin (including the skin of the lids) is more frequently affected than the conjunctiva.

The primary disease is an influenzalike illness with fever, malaise, cough, aches and pains, and night sweats. It is more common among dark-skinned than among light-skinned races, with Filipinos especially susceptible. Dissemination follows the rare failure of the body to limit the organism to its primary site.

Low titers of complement-fixing antibodies (< 1:16) indicate the usually limited spread of the disease; titers over 1:16 suggest widespread dissemination and a poor prognosis.

Histologic examination shows granulomatous lesions with spherules that are thick, doubly refractile, and filled with endospores. A fluffy, cotton-white colony grows on Sabouraud's medium.

Treatment with systemically administered amphotericin B yields the best results in disseminated cases, but transfer factor is now offering promise. In mild cases, only supportive therapy is needed.

PARASITIC CONJUNCTIVITIS

1. ONCHOCERCIASIS

Onchocerciasis is a common cause of blindness in the world today, only less common than such scourges as trachoma and vitamin A deficiency. The disease is a chronic infection with the parasite *O volvulus*. It is endemic in most of tropical Africa and in several countries of Central and South America (Mexico, Guatemala, Venezuela, Colombia). The parasites are transmitted by the bites of infected blackflies of the genus *Simulium*, which breed only in rapidly flowing streams (hence the term "river blindness").

The microfilariae present in the dermis of a human host are ingested by the female *Simulium* when she bites the host in the feeding process. The larvae develop in the fly for 6–12 days. Infective by then, they migrate to the labium and, again in the feeding process, are injected into another human host. In humans, the larvae mature for 12–18 months to form filarial adults that collect in subcutaneous nodules and may live as long as 15 years.

The adult female filaria discharges large numbers of microfilariae, which may migrate to the eye and cause a variety of anterior segment ocular lesions. Live microfilariae have been seen in the anterior chamber, and the eye lesions include conjunctivitis, keratitis, chronic uveitis, cataract, and, rarely, chorioretinitis and optic neuritis. The ocular changes are caused by local invasion of the microfilariae and by the tissue reactions that follow their death.

The disease can be diagnosed by teasing a snip of skin or conjunctiva in saline solution, or by aspirating a nodule and then examining the material for microfilariae.

Treatment with diethylcarbamazine citrate (Hetrazan)* can eradicate the filaria, but allergic reactions to the drug and allergic and febrile reactions to the disintegration of the worms often occur and may require use of corticosteroids. Nodulectomy may be of some prophylactic value.

2. *THELAZIA CALIFORNIENSIS* INFECTION

The natural habitat of this roundworm is the eye of the dog, but it can also infest the eyes of cats, sheep, black bears, horses, and deer. Accidental infection of the human conjunctival sac has occurred.

In the dog, the worms usually remain on the surface of the conjunctiva, causing irritation or tearing, but occasionally the corneal epithelium may be abraded. The eggs are laid in the lacrimal duct, conjunctival sac, or nictitating membrane, and the full life cycle may take place in the conjunctival sac and lacrimal apparatus. Transmission to other animals probably requires an intermediate arthropod host such as a fly (eg, *Fannia canicularis* or *Fannia benjamini*).

---

*Available in the USA only from Lederle Laboratories.

The disease can be treated effectively by removing the worms from the conjunctival sac with forceps or a cotton-tipped applicator.

3. *LOA LOA* INFECTION

L loa is the eye worm of Africa. It lives in the connective tissue of humans and monkeys, and the monkey may be its reservoir. The adult worm measures up to 55 mm in length. The female deposits the sheathed embryo (microfilaria) in its host's connective tissue, whence it migrates to the bloodstream and is taken up by the horse fly or mango fly as the fly bites its host. After 10 days the filariform larvae have developed, are infective, and are transferred to humans by the bite of the fly. (The fly feeds during the daylight hours only and especially in the middle of the day.)

The worm wanders in the connective tissue of humans for a year while it matures. During this time it may wander into the orbit or under the conjunctiva, sometimes giving pain or a feeling of vermiculation. Subcutaneous migration to the lid has also been seen, and the worm has been found in the anterior chamber, the vitreous, and (rarely) the retina.

Infestation with *L loa* is accompanied by a 60–80% eosinophilia, but diagnosis is made by identifying the worm on removal or by finding microfilariae in blood examined at midday.

Systemic diethylcarbamazine citrate (Hetrazan)* is the treatment of choice.

4. *ASCARIS LUMBRICOIDES* INFECTION (Butcher's Conjunctivitis)

Ascaris may cause a rare type of violent conjunctivitis. When butchers or persons performing postmortem examinations cut tissue containing *Ascaris*, the tissue juice of some of the organisms may hit them in the eye. This can be followed by a violent, toxic, painful conjunctivitis marked by extreme chemosis and lid edema. Treatment consists of rapid and thorough irrigation of the conjunctival sac.

5. *TRICHINELLA SPIRALIS* INFECTION

This parasite does not cause a true conjunctivitis, but in the course of its general dissemination there is often a doughy edema of the upper and lower eyelids, and over 50% of patients have chemosis—a pale, lemon-yellow swelling most marked over the lateral and medial rectus muscles and fading toward the limbus. The chemosis may last a week or more, and there is often pain on movement of the eyes.

The diagnosis is verified by a positive serologic test, a positive skin test, or a positive muscle biopsy. There is always eosinophilia of 10–50%.

The conjunctival aspect of the infection does not require therapy, but thiabendazole may be of value in allaying symptoms and reducing the eosinophilia.

*Available in the USA only from Lederle Laboratories.

Whether or not systemic corticosteroids should be used is controversial.

6. *SCHISTOSOMA HAEMATOBIUM* INFECTION

This parasitic disease (schistosomiasis, bilharziasis) is endemic in Egypt, especially in the region irrigated by the Nile. Granulomatous conjunctival lesions appearing as small, soft, smooth, pinkish-yellow tumors occur, especially in males. The symptoms are minimal. Diagnosis depends on the microscopic examination of biopsy material, which shows a granuloma containing lymphocytes, plasma cells, giant cells, and eosinophils surrounding the bilharzial ova in various stages of disintegration.

Treatment consists of excision of the conjunctival granuloma and systemic therapy with antimonials such as niridazole.

7. *TAENIA SOLIUM* INFECTION

This parasite occasionally causes conjunctivitis but more often invades the retina, choroid, or vitreous to produce ocular cysticercosis. As a rule, the affected conjunctiva shows a subconjunctival cyst in the form of a localized hemispherical swelling, usually at the inner angle of the lower fornix, which is adherent to the underlying sclera and painful on pressure. The conjunctiva and lid may be inflamed and edematous.

Diagnosis is based on a positive complement fixation or precipitin test or on the demonstration of the organism in the gastrointestinal tract. Eosinophilia is a constant feature.

The best treatment is to excise the lesion. The intestinal condition can be treated by niclosamide.

8. *PTHIRUS PUBIS* INFECTION (Pubic Louse Infection)

P pubis may infest the cilia and margins of the eyelids. Because of its size, the pubic louse seems to require widely spaced hair. For this reason it has a predilection for the widely spaced cilia as well as for pubic hair. The parasites apparently release an irritating substance (probably feces) that produces a toxic follicular conjunctivitis in children and an irritating papillary conjunctivitis in adults. The lid margin is usually red, and the patient may complain of intense itching.

Finding the adult organism or the ova-shaped nits cemented to the eyelashes is diagnostic.

Lindane (hexachlorocyclohexane [Kwell]) 1%, or RID (pyrethrins), applied to the pubic area and lash margins after removal of the nits, is usually curative. Application of lindane or RID to the lid margins must be undertaken with great care to avoid contact with the eye. Any ointment applied to the lid margin tends to smother the adult organisms. The patient's family and close contacts should be examined and treated. All clothes and fomites should be washed.

9. FLY LARVA CONJUNCTIVITIS (Ocular Myiasis)

Conjunctival infestation with the larvae of flies (*O ovis*, etc) occurs frequently in the tropics but rarely in the USA. Several species of flies have been incriminated. There is a mild type of larval conjunctivitis (ocular myiasis) in which the larvae are deposited in the conjunctival sac, the fly depositing them by alighting or while in flight. The symptoms are extreme itching, irritation, burning, and lacrimation. The conjunctiva is red and is infested with numerous elongated white larvae, especially in the fornices. The larvae tend to become buried in the depths of the conjunctiva and may escape detection.

Myiasis can also be destructive if the larvae are present in large numbers in compromised patients. If the larvae are numerous enough to convert the orbital tissues into a destructive mass, death may ensue as a result of meningeal involvement, often within 24– 48 hours.

Treatment consists of paralyzing the larvae with instillations of 10% cocaine and then removing them mechanically.

IMMUNOLOGIC (ALLERGIC) CONJUNCTIVITIS

I. IMMEDIATE (HUMORAL) HYPERSENSITIVITY REACTIONS

1. HAY FEVER CONJUNCTIVITIS

A mild, nonspecific conjunctival inflammation is commonly associated with hay fever (allergic rhinitis). There is usually a history of allergy to pollens, grasses, animal dander, etc. The patient complains of itching, tearing, and redness of the eyes and often states that his or her eyes seem to be sinking into the surrounding tissue. There is mild injection of the palpebral and bulbar conjunctiva, and during acute attacks there is often severe chemosis (which no doubt explains the concept that the eyes are ''sinking into the surrounding tissue''). There may be a small amount of ropy discharge, especially if the patient has been rubbing the eyes. A few eosinophils are found in conjunctival scrapings. There are no conjunctival papillae or follicles.

Treatment consists of the instillation of local vasoconstrictors during the acute phase (epinephrine, 1:1000 solution applied topically, will relieve the chemosis and symptoms within 30 minutes). Cold compresses are helpful to relieve itching, and antihistamines by mouth are of some value. The immediate response to treatment is satisfactory, but recurrences are common unless the antigen is eliminated. Fortunately, the frequency of the attacks and the severity of the symptoms tend to moderate as the patient ages.

2. VERNAL KERATOCONJUNCTIVITIS

This disease, also known as seasonal or warm weather conjunctivitis, is an uncommon bilateral allergic disease that usually begins in the prepubertal years and lasts for 5– 10 years. It occurs much oftener in boys than in girls. The identity of the specific allergen or allergens is still a mystery, but patients with vernal keratoconjunctivitis sometimes show other manifestations of allergy known to be related to grass pollen sensitivity. The disease is less common in temperate than in warm climates and is almost nonexistent in cold climates. It is almost always more severe during the spring, summer, and fall than in the winter.

The patient usually complains of extreme itching and a ropy discharge. There is often a family history of allergy (hay fever, eczema, etc) and sometimes in the young patient as well. The conjunctiva has a milky appearance, and there are many fine papillae in the lower tarsal conjunctiva. The upper palpebral conjunctiva often has giant papillae that give the conjunctiva a cobblestone appearance (Fig 8– 16). Each giant papilla is polygonal, has a flat top, and contains tufts of capillaries.

A stringy conjunctival discharge and a fine, fibrinous pseudomembrane (Maxwell-Lyons sign) may be noted. In some cases, especially in the black race, the most prominent lesions are located at the limbus, where gelatinous swellings (papillae) are noted. A pseudogerontoxon (arcus) is often noted in the cornea adjacent to the limbal papillae. Tranta's dots are whitish dots seen at the limbus in some patients with vernal keratoconjunctivitis during the active phase of the disease. Many eosinophils and free eosinophil granules are found in Giemsa-stained smears of the conjunctival exudate.

Micropannus is often seen in both palpebral and limbal vernal keratoconjunctivitis, but total pannus is extremely rare. Conjunctival scarring does not occur unless the patient has been treated with cryotherapy, surgical removal of the papillae, irradiation, or other damaging procedure. Superficial corneal ulcers (oval and located superiorly) may form and may be followed by mild corneal scarring. A characteristic diffuse epithelial keratitis frequently occurs. None of the corneal lesions responds well to standard treatment.

The disease may be associated with keratoconus.

Treatment

Since vernal keratoconjunctivitis is a self-limited disease, it must be recognized that the medication used to treat the symptoms may provide short-term benefit but do long-term harm. Topical and systemic steroids, which relieve the itching, affect the corneal disease only minimally, and their side effects (glaucoma, cataract, and other complications) can be severely damaging. Topical disodium cromoglycate (cromolyn) is a useful prophylactic agent in moderate to severe cases. Vasoconstrictors, cold compresses, and ice packs are helpful, and sleeping (if possible, also working) in cool, air-conditioned rooms can keep the patient rea-

Figure 8–16. Vernal conjunctivitis. "Cobblestone" papillae in superior tarsal conjunctiva. (Courtesy of P Thygeson.)

sonably comfortable. Probably the best remedy of all is to move to a cool, moist climate. Patients able to do so are benefited if not completely cured.

The severe symptoms of an extremely photophobic patient who is unable to function can often be relieved by a short course of topical or systemic steroids followed by vasoconstrictors and cold packs. As has already been indicated, the prolonged use of steroids must be avoided since it is all too often followed by herpes simplex keratitis, cataract, glaucoma, and fungal and other opportunistic corneal ulcers.

Desensitization to grass pollens and other antigens has not been rewarding. Staphylococcal blepharitis and conjunctivitis are frequent complications and should be treated. Recurrences are the rule, particularly in the spring and summer; but after a number of recurrences the papillae disappear completely, leaving no scars.

3. ATOPIC KERATOCONJUNCTIVITIS

Patients with atopic dermatitis (eczema) often also have atopic keratoconjunctivitis. The symptoms and signs are a burning sensation, mucoid discharge, redness, and photophobia. The lid margins are erythematous, and the conjunctiva has a milky appearance. There are fine papillae, but giant papillae are rare; when they occur they are on the lower tarsus (unlike the giant papillae of vernal keratoconjunctivitis, which are on the upper tarsus). Severe corneal signs appear late in the disease after repeated exacerbations of the conjunctivitis. Superficial peripheral keratitis develops and is followed by vascularization. In severe cases, the entire cornea becomes hazy and vascularized, and visual acuity is reduced. The disease is associated with keratoconus.

There is usually a history of allergy (hay fever, asthma, or eczema) in the patient or the patient's family. Most patients have had atopic dermatitis since 1 or 2 years of age. Scarring of the flexure creases of the antecubital folds and of the wrists and knees

is common. Like the dermatitis with which it is associated, atopic keratoconjunctivitis has a protracted course and is subject to exacerbations and remissions. Like vernal keratoconjunctivitis, it tends to become inactive when the patient reaches the fifth decade.

Scrapings of the conjunctiva show eosinophils, although not nearly so many as are seen in vernal keratoconjunctivitis. Scarring of both the conjunctiva and cornea is often seen, and an atopic cataract, a posterior subcapsular plaque, or an anterior shieldlike cataract may develop. Keratoconus, retinal detachment, and herpes simplex keratitis are all more than usually frequent in patients with atopic keratoconjunctivitis, and there are many cases of secondary bacterial blepharitis and conjunctivitis, usually staphylococcal.

The management of atopic keratoconjunctivitis is often discouraging. Any secondary infection must of course be treated. A short course of topical steroids may relieve symptoms. In advanced cases with severe corneal complications, corneal transplantation may be needed to improve the visual acuity.

4. GIANT PAPILLARY CONJUNCTIVITIS (Pseudovernal)

A type of giant papillary conjunctivitis with signs and symptoms closely resembling those of vernal conjunctivitis may develop rarely in patients wearing plastic artificial eyes or contact lenses. It is a sensitivity reaction, possibly to components of the plastic leached out by the action of the tears. Use of glass instead of plastic for prostheses and spectacle lenses instead of contact lenses is curative.

II. DELAYED (CELLULAR) HYPERSENSITIVITY REACTIONS

1. PHLYCTENULOSIS

Phlyctenular keratoconjunctivitis is a delayed hypersensitivity response to microbial proteins, including the proteins of the tubercle bacillus, staphylococcus, *Candida albicans, C immitis,* and *C lymphogranulomatis.* Until recently, by far the most frequent cause of phlyctenulosis in the USA was delayed hypersensitivity to the protein of the human tubercle bacillus. This is still the commonest cause in developing countries where tuberculosis is still prevalent. In the USA, however, most cases are now associated with delayed hypersensitivity to *S aureus.*

The conjunctival phlyctenule begins as a small lesion (usually 1–3 mm in diameter) that is hard, red, elevated, and surrounded by a zone of hyperemia. At the limbus it is often triangular in shape, with its apex toward the cornea. In this location it develops a grayish-white center that soon ulcerates and then subsides within 10–12 days. The patient's first phlyctenule and most of the recurrences develop at the limbus, but there may also be bulbar and very rarely even tarsal phlyctenules.

Unlike the conjunctival phlyctenule, which leaves no scar, the corneal phlyctenule develops as an amorphous gray infiltrate and always leaves a scar. Consistent with this difference is the fact that scars form on the corneal side of the limbal lesion and not on the conjunctival side. The result is a triangular scar with its base at the limbus—a valuable sign of old phlyctenulosis when the limbus has been involved.

Conjunctival phlyctenules usually produce only irritation and tearing; it is the typical corneal phlyctenule that is accompanied also by photophobia—severe when the disease is tuberculoprotein-induced and mild when staphylococcus protein–induced. Phlyctenulosis is often triggered by active blepharitis, acute bacterial conjunctivitis, and dietary deficiencies. Acute bacterial conjunctivitis causes hyperemia, which

facilitates transfer of the tuberculoprotein to the limbus in large amounts. Phlyctenular scarring (Fig 8–17), which may be minimal or extensive, is often followed by Salzmann's nodular degeneration.

Histologically, the phlyctenule is a focal subepithelial infiltration of small round cells, followed by a preponderance of polymorphonuclear cells when the overlying epithelium necrotizes and sloughs—a sequence of events characteristic of the delayed tuberculin type hypersensitivity reaction.

Phlyctenulosis induced by tuberculoprotein and the proteins of other systemic infections responds dramatically to topical corticosteroids. There is a major reduction of symptoms within 24 hours and disappearance of the lesion in another 24 hours. In contrast, phlyctenulosis induced by the proteins of staphylococcus (from staphylococcal blepharitis) is relatively unresponsive to the corticosteroids. Treatment should be aimed at the underlying disease, and the steroids, when effective, should be used only to control acute symptoms. A well-balanced diet is most important, and any bacterial conjunctivitis must be controlled. Severe corneal scarring may call for corneal transplantation.

2. MILD CONJUNCTIVITIS SECONDARY TO CONTACT BLEPHARITIS

Contact blepharitis caused by atropine, neomycin, broad-spectrum antibiotics, and other topically applied medications is often followed by a mild infiltrative conjunctivitis that produces hyperemia, mild papillary hypertrophy, a mild mucoid discharge, and some irritation. The examination of Giemsa-stained scrapings often shows only a few degenerated epithelial cells, a few polymorphonuclear and mononuclear cells, and no eosinophils.

Treatment should be directed toward finding the offending agent and eliminating it. The contact blepharitis may clear rapidly with topical corticosteroids, but their use should be limited. Long-term use of steroids on the lids may lead to steroid glaucoma and to skin atrophy with disfiguring telangiectasis.

III. AUTOIMMUNE DISEASE CONJUNCTIVITIS

1. KERATOCONJUNCTIVITIS SICCA (Associated With Sjögren's Syndrome)

Sjögren's syndrome is a systemic disease characterized by a triad of disorders: keratoconjunctivitis sicca, xerostomia, and connective tissue dysfunction (arthritis). To establish the diagnosis of Sjögren's syndrome, at least 2 of the 3 disorders must be present. The disease is overwhelmingly more common in women at or beyond the menopause than in others, although men and younger women can also be affected. The lacrimal gland is infiltrated with lymphocytes and occasionally with plasma cells, and this

Figure 8–17. Postphlyctenulosis. Vascularized scar in temporal portion of left cornea.

Figure 8–18. Keratoconjunctivitis sicca. (Courtesy of HB Ostler.)

leads to atrophy and destruction of the glandular structures.

Keratoconjunctivitis sicca is characterized by bulbar conjunctival hyperemia and symptoms of irritation that are out of proportion to the mild inflammatory signs. It often begins as a catarrhal conjunctivitis. Blotchy epithelial lesions appear on the cornea, more prominently in its lower half, and filaments may be seen. Pain builds up in the afternoon and evening but is absent or only slight in the morning. The tear film is diminished and often contains shreds of mucus (Fig 8– 18). Results of the Schirmer test are abnormal (see Chapter 7). Rose bengal staining is a helpful diagnostic test.

The diagnosis is confirmed by demonstrating lymphocytic and plasma cell infiltration of the accessory salivary glands in a labial biopsy obtained by means of a simple surgical procedure (Fig 8– 19).

Treatment should be directed toward preserving and replacing the tear film with artificial tears, with obliteration of the puncta, and with moisture chambers and Buller shields. As a rule, the simpler things should be tried first. Clinical trials have suggested that topical vitamin A in conjunction with artificial tears may be helpful in certain cases.

2. CICATRICIAL PEMPHIGOID

This disease usually begins as a nonspecific chronic conjunctivitis that is resistant to therapy. The conjunctiva may be affected alone or in combination with the mouth, nose, esophagus, vulva, and skin. The conjunctivitis leads to progressive scarring and obliteration of the fornices, especially the lower fornix (Fig 8– 20). The patient complains of pain, irritation, and blurring of vision. The cornea is affected only secondarily as a result of obliteration of the fornix and lack of the precorneal tear film. The disease is more severe in women than in men. It is typically a disease of middle life, occurring only very rarely before age 45. In women it may progress to blindness in a year or less; in men, progress is slower and spontaneous remission sometimes takes place.

Conjunctival scrapings usually contain a few eosinophils. Oral dapsone and immunosuppressive therapy have been effective in some cases. Treatment must always be instituted at an early stage, prior to the onset of significant scarring. Generally, the course is long and the prognosis poor, with blindness due to complete symblepharon and corneal desiccation the usual outcome.

Figure 8–19. Mononuclear infiltration of the accessory salivary glands of a patient with Sjögren's syndrome. (Courtesy of K Tabbara.)

Figure 8–20. Cicatricial pemphigoid. (Courtesy of M Quickert.)

3. MIDLINE LETHAL GRANULOMA & WEGENER'S GRANULOMATOSIS

Wegener's granulomatosis is a syndrome (assumed to be autoimmune in origin) that is characterized by necrotizing granulomatous lesions, generalized arteritis, and glomerulitis. The glomerulitis differentiates it from midline lethal granuloma. In both diseases there is progressive destruction of the soft tissues and bony structures of the ethmoid region. In Wegener's granulomatosis, the lower part of the respiratory tract may also be affected, and terminally there may be uremia.

In both of these diseases there may be one or more of the following ocular manifestations: exophthalmos, chemosis, exposure keratitis, papillitis by extension of the process into the orbit, episcleritis, scleritis, marginal corneal infiltration and ulceration, uveitis, and retinitis with hemorrhages and cytoid bodies. The typical conjunctival lesions are multiple small granulomas at the limbus.

Steroids and other immunosuppressives appear to reduce the severity of the lesions.

CHEMICAL OR IRRITATIVE CONJUNCTIVITIS

1. IATROGENIC CONJUNCTIVITIS FROM TOPICALLY APPLIED DRUGS

A toxic follicular conjunctivitis or an infiltrative, nonspecific conjunctivitis, followed by scarring, is often produced by the prolonged administration of miotics, idoxuridine, neomycin, and other drugs prepared in toxic or irritating preservatives or vehicles. Silver nitrate instilled into the conjunctival sac at birth (Credé prophylaxis) is a frequent cause of mild chemical conjunctivitis. If tear production is reduced by continual irritation, the conjunctiva can be further damaged by the lack of dilution of the noxious agent as it is instilled into the conjunctival sac.

Conjunctival scrapings often contain keratinized epithelial cells, a few polymorphonuclear neutrophils, and an occasional oddly shaped cell. The treatment is to stop the offending agent and to use bland drops or none at all. Often the conjunctival reaction persists for weeks or months after its source has been eliminated.

2. OCCUPATIONAL CONJUNCTIVITIS FROM CHEMICALS & IRRITANTS

Acids, alkalies, smoke, wind, and almost any irritating substance that enters the conjunctival sac may cause conjunctivitis. Some common irritants are fertilizers, soap, deodorants, hair sprays, tobacco, makeup preparations (mascara, etc), and various acids and alkalies. In certain areas, smog has become the commonest cause of mild chemical conjunctivitis. The specific irritant in smog has not been positively iden-

tified, and treatment is nonspecific. There are no permanent ocular effects, but affected eyes are frequently chronically red and irritated.

In acid burns, the acids denature the tissue proteins and the effect is immediate. Alkalies do not denature the proteins but tend to penetrate the tissues deeply and rapidly and to linger in the conjunctival tissue. Here they continue to inflict damage for hours or days, depending on the molar concentration of the alkali and the amount of it introduced. Adhesion between the bulbar and palpebral conjunctivas (symblepharon) and corneal leukoma are more likely to occur if the offending agent is an alkali. In either event, pain, injection, photophobia, and blepharospasm are the principal symptoms of caustic burns. A history of the precipitating event can usually be elicited.

Immediate and profuse irrigation of the conjunctival sac with water or saline solution is of first importance, and any solid material should be removed mechanically. Do not use chemical antidotes. General symptomatic measures include cold compresses for 20 minutes every hour, atropine 1% drops twice daily, and systemic analgesics as necessary. Corneal scarring may require corneal transplantation, and symblepharon may require a plastic operation on the conjunctiva. Severe conjunctival and corneal burns have a poor prognosis even with surgery, but if proper treatment is started immediately, scarring may be minimized and the prognosis improved.

3. CATERPILLAR HAIR CONJUNCTIVITIS (Ophthalmia Nodosum)

On rare occasions, caterpillar hairs are introduced into the conjunctival sac, where they produce one or many granulomas (ophthalmia nodosum). Under magnification, each granuloma is seen to contain a small foreign body.

Treatment by removal of each hair individually is effective. If a hair is retained, invasion of the sclera and uveal tract usually occurs.

CONJUNCTIVITIS OF UNKNOWN CAUSE

1. FOLLICULOSIS

Folliculosis is a widespread benign, bilateral noninflammatory conjunctival disorder characterized by follicular hypertrophy. It is more common in children than in adults, and the symptoms are minimal. The follicles are more numerous in the lower than in the upper cul-de-sac and tarsal conjunctiva. There is no associated inflammation or papillary hypertrophy, and complications do not occur.

There is no treatment for folliculosis, which disappears spontaneously after a course of 2–3 years. The cause is unknown, but folliculosis may be only a manifestation of a generalized adenoidal hypertrophy.

2. CHRONIC FOLLICULAR CONJUNCTIVITIS (Orphan's Conjunctivitis, Axenfeld's Conjunctivitis)

This is a bilateral transmissible disease of children characterized by numerous follicles in the upper and lower tarsal conjunctivas. There are minimal conjunctival exudates and minimal inflammation but no complications. Treatment is ineffective, but the disease is self-limited within 2 years.

3. OCULAR ROSACEA

Ocular rosacea is an uncommon complication of acne rosacea and occurs more often in light-skinned people, especially of Irish descent, than in dark-skinned people. It is usually a blepharoconjunctivitis, but the cornea is sometimes also affected. The patient complains of mild injection and irritation. There is frequently an accompanying staphylococcal blepharitis. The blood vessels of the lid margins are dilated and the conjunctiva is hyperemic, especially in the exposed interpalpebral region. Less often, there may be a nodular conjunctivitis with small gray nodules on the bulbar conjunctiva, especially near the limbus, which may ulcerate superficially. The lesions can be differentiated from phlyctenules by the fact that even after they subside, the large dilated vessels persist.

Microscopic examination of the nodules shows lymphocytes and epithelial cells. The peripheral cornea may ulcerate and vascularize, and the keratitis may have a narrow base at the limbus and a wider infiltrate centrally. The corneal pannus is often segmented or wedge-shaped inferiorly (Figs 8– 21 and 8– 22).

Treatment of ocular rosacea consists of the elimination of alcohol and hot, spicy food and drink that cause dilatation of the facial vessels. Any secondary staphylococcal infection should be treated. A course of oral tetracycline is often helpful and a small maintenance dose may be indicated.

The disease is chronic, recurrences are common, and the response to treatment is usually poor. If the cornea is not affected, the visual prognosis is good; but corneal lesions tend to recur and progress, and the vision grows steadily worse over a period of years.

4. PSORIASIS

Psoriasis vulgaris usually affects the areas of the skin not exposed to the sun, but in about 10% of cases lesions appear on the skin of the eyelids, and the plaques may extend to the conjunctiva, where they cause irritation, a foreign body sensation, and tearing. Psoriasis can also cause nonspecific chronic conjunctivitis with considerable mucoid discharge. Rarely, the cornea may show marginal ulceration or a deep, vascularized opacity.

The conjunctival and corneal lesions wax and wane with the skin lesions and are not affected by specific treatment. In rare cases, conjunctival scarring (symblepharon, trichiasis), corneal scarring, and occlusion of the nasolacrimal duct have occurred.

5. ERYTHEMA MULTIFORME (Major & Minor)

Erythema multiforme major (Stevens-Johnson syndrome) is a disease of the mucous membranes and skin. The skin lesion is an erythematous, urticarial bullous eruption that appears suddenly and is often distributed symmetrically. Bilateral conjunctivitis, often pseudomembranous, is a common manifestation. The patient complains of pain, irritation, discharge, and photophobia. The cornea is affected secondarily, and vascularization and scarring may seriously reduce vision. Stevens-Johnson syndrome is typically a disease of young people, occurring only rarely after age 35.

Figure 8 –21. Conjunctivitis and corneal infiltrate in a patient with acne rosacea. (Courtesy of HB Ostler.)

Figure 8 –22. Skin lesions in acne rosacea. (Courtesy of HB Ostler.)

Figure 8–23. Late sequelae of Stevens-Johnson syndrome: conjunctival and corneal cicatrization and epidermalization. (Courtesy of P Thygeson.)

Cultures are negative for bacteria; conjunctival scrapings show a preponderance of polymorphonuclear cells. Systemic steroids are thought to shorten the systemic disease but have little or no effect on the eye lesions. Careful cleansing of the conjunctiva to remove the accumulated secretion is helpful, however, and tear replacement may be indicated. If trichiasis and entropion supervene, they should be corrected. Topical steroids probably have no beneficial effect, and their protracted use can cause corneal melting and perforation.

The acute episode of Stevens-Johnson syndrome usually lasts about 6 weeks, but the conjunctival scarring, loss of tears, and complications from entropion and trichiasis may result in prolonged morbidity and progressive corneal cicatrization (Fig 8– 23). Recurrences are rare.

Erythema multiforme minor sometimes complicates a catarrhal conjunctivitis associated with tearing and mucoid discharge. The patient complains of irritation, redness, and discharge. The conjunctivitis is self-limited but may recur when the skin eruption recurs (usually in the spring and fall). Conjunctival scrapings show a polymorphonuclear cell reaction. Bacterial cultures are negative.

The cause is not definitely known, but there is growing evidence that the disease is a hypersensitivity disorder mediated by the deposition of circulating immune complexes in the superficial microvasculature of the skin and mucous membranes. The disease can be triggered by herpes simplex, by antibiotics, and especially by sulfonamides.

Erythema multiforme minor is self-limited, the conjunctiva clearing as the skin lesions clear. Steroids are often used systemically for the skin eruption. In contrast to ocular erythema multiforme major, this minor conjunctivitis does not leave scars and the cornea remains clear.

6. DERMATITIS HERPETIFORMIS

This is an uncommon skin disorder characterized by grouped erythematous, papulovesicular, vesicular, or bullous lesions arranged symmetrically. The disease has a predilection for the posterior axillary fold, the sacral region, the buttocks, and the forearms. Itching is often severe. Rarely, a pseudomembranous conjunctivitis occurs and may result in cicatrization resembling that seen in benign mucous membrane pemphigoid. The skin eruption and conjunctivitis usually respond readily to systemic sulfones or sulfapyridine.

7. EPIDERMOLYSIS BULLOSA

This is a rare hereditary disease characterized by vesicles, bullae, and epidermal cysts. The lesions occur chiefly on the extensor surfaces of the joints and other areas exposed to trauma. The severe dystrophic type that leads to scarring may also produce conjunctival scars similar to those seen in dermatitis herpetiformis and benign mucous membrane pemphigoid. No known treatment is satisfactory.

8. SUPERIOR LIMBIC KERATOCONJUNCTIVITIS

Superior limbic keratoconjunctivitis is usually bilateral and limited to the upper tarsus and upper limbus. The principal complaints are irritation and hyperemia. The signs are papillary hypertrophy of the upper tarsus, redness of the superior bulbar conjunctiva, thickening and keratinization of the superior limbus, epithelial keratitis, recurrent superior filaments, and superior micropannus. Rose bengal staining is a helpful diagnostic test. The keratinized epithelial cells and mucous debris pick up the stain. Scrapings from the upper limbus show keratinizing epithelial cells.

In about 50% of cases, the condition has been associated with abnormal function of the thyroid gland. Applying 0.5% or 1% silver nitrate to the upper tarsus and allowing the tarsus to drop back onto the upper limbus usually result in shedding of the keratinizing cells and relief of symptoms for 4– 6 weeks. This treatment can be repeated. There are no complications, and the disease usually runs a course of 2– 4 years.

9. LIGNEOUS CONJUNCTIVITIS

This is a rare bilateral, chronic or recurrent, pseudomembranous or membranous conjunctivitis that arises early in life, most commonly in young girls, and often persists for many years. Granulomas are often associated with it, and the lids may feel very hard. There is no satisfactory treatment.

10. REITER'S SYNDROME

A triad of disease manifestations—nonspecific urethritis, arthritis, and conjunctivitis or iritis—constitutes Reiter's syndrome. The disease occurs much more often in men than in women. The conjunctivitis is papillary in type and usually bilateral. Conjunctival scrapings contain polymorphonuclear cells. No bacteria grow in cultures. The arthritis usually affects the large weight-bearing joints. There is no satisfactory treatment. The disease has been found in association with HLA-B27.

11. MUCOCUTANEOUS LYMPH NODE SYNDROME (Kawasaki Disease)

This disease of unknown cause was first described in Japan in 1967. Conjunctivitis is one of its 6 diagnostic features. The others are (1) fever that fails to respond to antibiotics; (2) changes in the lips and oral cavity; (3) such changes in the extremities as erythema of the palms and soles, indurative edema, and membranous desquamation of the fingertips; (4) polymorphous exanthem of the trunk; and (5) acute nonpurulent swelling of the cervical lymph nodes.

The disease occurs almost exclusively in prepubertal children and carries a 1–2% mortality rate from cardiac failure. The conjunctivitis has not been severe, and no corneal lesions have been reported.

Treatment is supportive only.

CONJUNCTIVITIS ASSOCIATED WITH SYSTEMIC DISEASE

1. CONJUNCTIVITIS IN THYROID DISEASE

In orbital Graves' disease, the conjunctiva may be red and chemotic and the patient may complain of copious tearing. As the disease progresses the chemosis increases, and in advanced cases the chemotic conjunctiva may extrude between the lids.

Treatment is directed toward control of the thyroid disease, and every effort is made to protect the conjunctiva and cornea by bland ointment, lid adhesions if necessary, or even orbital decompression if the lids do not close enough to cover the cornea and conjunctiva.

2. GOUTY CONJUNCTIVITIS

Patients with gout often complain of a "hot eye" during their attacks. On examination, a mild conjunctivitis is found but is less severe than suggested by the symptoms. Gout may also be associated with episcleritis or scleritis, iridocyclitis, keratitis urica, vitreous opacities, and retinopathy. Treatment is aimed at controlling the gouty attack with colchicine and allopurinol.

3. CARCINOID CONJUNCTIVITIS

In carcinoid, the conjunctiva is sometimes congested and cyanotic as a result of the secretion of serotonin by the chromaffin cells of the gastrointestinal tract. The patient may complain of a "hot eye" during such attacks.

CONJUNCTIVITIS SECONDARY TO DACRYOCYSTITIS OR CANALICULITIS

1. CONJUNCTIVITIS SECONDARY TO DACRYOCYSTITIS

Both pneumococcal conjunctivitis (often unilateral and unresponsive to treatment) and beta-hemolytic streptococcal conjunctivitis (often hyperacute and purulent) may be secondary to chronic dacryocystitis. The nature and source of the conjunctivitis in both instances are often missed until the lacrimal system is investigated.

2. CONJUNCTIVITIS SECONDARY TO CANALICULITIS

Canaliculitis due to *A israelii* or *Candida* sp (or, very rarely, *Aspergillus* sp) may cause unilateral mucopurulent conjunctivitis, often chronic. The source of the condition is often missed unless the characteristic hyperemic, pouting punctum is noted. Expression of the canaliculus (upper or lower, whichever is involved) is curative provided the entire concretion is removed.

Conjunctival scrapings show a predominance of polymorphonuclear cells. Cultures (unless anaerobic) are usually negative. *Candida* grows readily on ordinary culture media, but almost all of the infections are caused by *A israelii*, which requires an anaerobic medium.

DEGENERATIVE DISEASES OF THE CONJUNCTIVA

PINGUECULA

Pinguecula is extremely common in adults. It appears as a yellow nodule on both sides of the cornea (more commonly on the nasal side) in the area of the lid fissure. The nodules, consisting of hyaline and yellow elastic tissue, rarely increase in size, but inflammation is common. In general, no treatment is required, but in certain cases of pingueculitis, weak topical steroids (eg, prednisolone 0.12%) may be given (Fig 8–24).

Figure 8–24. Pinguecula. (Courtesy of A Rosenberg.)

Figure 8–25. Pterygium encroaching on the cornea. (Courtesy of G Mintsioulis.)

PTERYGIUM

Pterygium is a fleshy, bilateral, triangular encroachment of a pinguecula onto the cornea, usually on the nasal side (Fig 8–25). (Pterygiums are often referred to erroneously by patients as cataracts.) It is thought to be an irritative phenomenon due to ultraviolet light since it is common in farmers and sheepherders who spend much of their lives out of doors in sunny, dusty, or sandy, windblown areas. The pathologic findings in the conjunctiva are the same as those of pinguecula. In the cornea there is replacement of Bowman's layer by the hyaline and elastic tissue.

If the pterygium is enlarging and encroaches on the pupillary area, it should be removed surgically, along with a small portion of superficial clear cornea beyond the area of corneal encroachment. To prevent recurrences, particularly in people who work out of doors, protective glasses should be prescribed.

MISCELLANEOUS DISORDERS OF THE CONJUNCTIVA

LYMPHANGIECTASIS

Lymphangiectasis is characterized by small, clear, tortuous, localized dilatations in the conjunctiva. They are merely dilated lymph vessels, and no treatment is indicated unless they are irritating or cosmetically objectionable. They can then be cauterized or excised.

CONGENITAL CONJUNCTIVAL LYMPHEDEMA

This is a rare entity, unilateral or bilateral, and characterized by pinkish, fleshy edema of the bulbar conjunctiva. Usually observed as an isolated entity at birth, the condition is thought to be due to a congenital defect in the lymphatic drainage of the conjunctiva. It has been observed in chronic hereditary lymphedema of the lower extremities (Milroy's disease) and is considered an ocular manifestation of this disease rather than an associated anomaly.

CYSTINOSIS

Cystinosis is a rare congenital disorder of amino acid metabolism characterized by a widespread intracellular deposition of cystine crystals in various body tissues, including the conjunctiva and cornea. Three types are recognized: childhood, adolescent, and adult. Life expectancy is reduced in the first 2 types.

SUBCONJUNCTIVAL HEMORRHAGE

This common disorder may occur spontaneously, usually in only one eye, in any age group. Its sudden onset and bright red appearance usually alarm the patient. The hemorrhage is caused by the rupture of a small conjunctival vessel, sometimes preceded by a bout of severe coughing or sneezing.

There is no treatment, and the hemorrhage usually absorbs in 2–3 weeks. The best treatment is reassurance.

In rare instances the hemorrhages are bilateral or recurrent; the possibility of blood dyscrasias should then be ruled out.

OPHTHALMIA NEONATORUM

Ophthalmia neonatorum in its broad sense refers to any infection of the newborn conjunctiva. In its narrow and commonly used sense, however, it refers to a conjunctival infection, chiefly gonococcal, that follows contamination of the baby's eyes during its passage through the mother's cervix and vagina. Since the newborn is a "compromised host," many opportunistic bacteria (and one virus: herpes simplex virus type 2) that are found in the female genital tract are capable of producing disease. For medicolegal reasons, the causes of all cases of ophthalmia neonatorum should be identified in smears of exudate, epithelial scrapings, and cultures.

The time of onset is important in clinical diagnosis since the 2 principal types, gonorrheal ophthalmia and inclusion blennorrhea, have widely differing incubation periods: gonococcal disease 2– 3 days and chlamydial disease 5– 12 days. The third important birth canal infection (herpes simplex virus type 2 keratoconjunctivitis) has a 2- to 3-day incubation period and is potentially extremely serious because of the possibility of systemic dissemination.

The Credé 1% silver nitrate prophylaxis is effective for the prevention of gonorrheal ophthalmia. (Regrettably, it is not protective against inclusion blennorrhea or herpetic infection.) The slight chemical conjunctivitis induced by silver nitrate is minor and of short duration. Accidents with concentrated solutions can be avoided by using wax ampules specially prepared for Credé prophylaxis. Silver nitrate substitutes, including penicillin and other antibiotics, are under study, and erythromycin ointment appears to be especially promising.

OCULOGLANDULAR DISEASE
(Parinaud's Oculoglandular Syndrome)

This is a group of conjunctival diseases, usually unilateral, characterized by low-grade fever, grossly visible preauricular adenopathy, and one or more conjunctival granulomas (Fig 8– 26). The commonest cause is cat-scratch disease, but there are many other causes, including *M tuberculosis, T pallidum, Francisella tularensis, Pasteurella (Yersinia) pseudotuberculosis, C lymphogranulomatis,* * and *C immitis.*

Conjunctival Cat-Scratch Disease

This protracted but benign granulomatous conjunctivitis is found most commonly in children who have been in intimate contact with cats. The child often runs a low-grade fever and develops a reasonably enlarged preauricular node and one or more conjunctival granulomas. These may show focal necrosis and may sometimes ulcerate. The regional adenopathy does

*See box on p 84.

Figure 8–26. Conjunctival granuloma. (Courtesy of P Thygeson.)

not suppurate. The clinical diagnosis is supported by a positive cat-scratch disease skin test.

The disease appears to be caused by a slender pleomorphic gram-negative bacillus, which grows in the walls of blood vessels. With special stains, this organism can be seen in biopsies of conjunctival tissue. Morphologically identical organisms have also been identified in lymph nodes from cases of nonocular cat-scratch disease, but isolation of the organism in culture has not yet been achieved. The organism closely resembles *Leptotrichia buccalis,* and the disease was previously known as leptotrichosis conjunctivae (Parinaud's conjunctivitis). *L buccalis* is commonly found in the mouth in humans and always in the mouth in cats. The eye may be contaminated by saliva on the child's fingers or by cat drool on the child's pillow.

The disease is self-limited (without corneal or other complications) and resolves in 2– 3 months. The conjunctival nodule can be excised; in the case of a solitary granuloma, this may be curative. Systemic tetracyclines may shorten the course of the disease but should not be given to children under the age of 7.

Conjunctivitis Secondary to Neoplasms
(Masquerade Syndrome)

When examined superficially, a neoplasm of the conjunctiva or lid margin is often misdiagnosed as a chronic infectious conjunctivitis or keratoconjunctivitis. Since the underlying lesion is often not recognized, the condition has been referred to as masquerade syndrome. The masquerading neoplasms on record are conjunctival capillary carcinoma, conjunctival carcinoma in situ, molluscum contagiosum, infectious papilloma of the conjunctiva, and verruca. Verruca and molluscum tumors of the lid margin may desquamate toxic tumor material that produces a chronic conjunctivitis, keratoconjunctivitis, or (rarely) keratitis alone.

REFERENCES

Allansmith MR et al: Giant papillary conjunctivitis in contact lens wearers. *Am J Ophthalmol* 1977;**83**:697.

Bullen CL et al: Ocular complications of Wegener's granulomatosis. *Ophthalmology* 1983;**90**:279.

Coad CT, Osato MS, Wilhelmus KR: Bacterial contamination of eye drop dispensers. *Am J Ophthalmol* 1984;**98**:548.

Darougar S (editor): Chlamydial disease. *Br Med Bull* (April) 1983;**39**. [Entire issue.]

Darougar S, Wishart MS, Viswalingam ND: Epidemiological and clinical features of primary herpes simplex virus ocular infection. *Br J Ophthalmol* 1985;**69**:2.

Darougar S et al: Adenovirus serotypes isolated from ocular infections in London. *Br J Ophthalmol* 1983;**67**:111.

Dawson CR: Epidemic Koch-Weeks conjunctivitis and trachoma in the Coachella Valley of California. *Am J Ophthalmol* 1960;**49**:801.

Dawson CR, Jones BR, Tarizzo ML: *Guide to Trachoma Control in Programmes for the Prevention of Blindness.* World Health Organization, 1981.

Dawson CR et al: Severe endemic trachoma in Tunisia. *Br J Ophthalmol* 1976;**60**:245.

Hadfield TL et al: Electron microscopy of the bacillus causing cat-scratch disease. *J Infect Dis* 1985;**152**:643.

Kiernan JP et al: Stevens-Johnson syndrome. *Am J Ophthalmol* 1981;**92**:543.

Lemp MA, Mahmood MA, Weiler HH: Association of rosacea and keratoconjunctivitis sicca. *Arch Ophthalmol* 1984;**102**:556.

Mondino BJ, Brown SI: Immunosuppressive therapy in ocular cicatricial pemphigoid. *Am J Ophthalmol* 1983;**96**:453.

Ostler HB: Acute chemotic reaction to cromolyn. *Arch Ophthalmol* 1982;**100**:412.

Pfister RR: Chemical injuries of the eye. *Ophthalmology* 1983;**90**:1246.

Salvaggio JE (editor): Primer on allergic and immunologic diseases. *JAMA* 1982;**248**:2579. [Special issue.]

Savino DF, Margo CE: Conjunctival rhinosporidiosis: Light and electron microscopic study. *Ophthalmology* 1983;**90**:1482.

Schachter J: Chlamydiae (psittacosis-lymphogranuloma venereum-trachoma group). Chap 85, pp 856–862, in: *Manual of Clinical Microbiology*, 4th ed. Lennette EH (editor). American Society for Microbiology, 1985.

Schwartz LK, Gelender H, Forster RK: Chronic conjunctivitis associated with "floppy eyelids." *Arch Ophthalmol* 1983;**101**:1884.

Sjögren H: Keratoconjunctivitis sicca and the Sjögren syndrome. *Surv Ophthalmol* 1971;**16**:145.

Sklar VEF et al: Clinical findings and results of treatment in an outbreak of acute hemorrhagic conjunctivitis in southern Florida. *Am J Ophthalmol* 1983;**95**:45.

Sommer A: Effects of vitamin A deficiency on the ocular surface. *Ophthalmology* 1983;**90**:592.

Stenson S, Newman R, Fedukowicz H: Conjunctivitis in the newborn: Observations on incidence, cause, and prophylaxis. *Ann Ophthalmol* 1981;**13**:329.

Tabbara KF, Ghosheh R, O'Connor GR: Ocular tissue absorption of minocycline in the rabbit. *Arch Ophthalmol* 1983;**101**:1426.

Tabbara KF et al: Effects of conjunctival resection on the corneal immune response. *Am J Ophthalmol* 1982;**94**:388.

Thygeson P: Historical review of oculogenital disease. *Am J Ophthalmol* 1971;**71**:975.

Thygeson P: Observations on conjunctival neoplasms masquerading as chronic conjunctivitis or keratitis. *Trans Am Acad Ophthalmol Otolaryngol* 1969;**73**:969.

Thygeson P, Dawson CR: Pseudotrachoma caused by molluscum contagiosum virus and various chemical irritants. Page 1894 in: *Proceedings of the 21st International Congress of Ophthalmology, 1970.* Excerpta Medica International Series, No. 222. Elsevier, 1971.

Wear DJ et al: Cat scratch disease bacilli in the conjunctiva of patients with Parinaud's oculoglandular syndrome. *Ophthalmology* 1985;**92**:1282.

Werblin TP, Rheinstrom SD, Kaufman HE: The use of slow-release artificial tears in the long-term management of keratitis sicca. *Ophthalmology* 1981;**88**:78.

Wishart PK et al: Prevalence of acute conjunctivitis caused by chlamydia, adenovirus, and herpes simplex virus in an ophthalmic casualty department. *Br J Ophthalmol* 1984;**68**:653.

Zaidman GW et al: Phlyctenular keratoconjunctivitis. *Am J Ophthalmol* 1981;**92**:178.

Cornea

ANATOMY

The cornea is a transparent avascular tissue comparable in size and structure to the crystal of a small wristwatch. It is inserted into the sclera at the limbus. At the scleral junction there is a circumferential depression called the scleral sulcus. The cornea functions as a protective membrane and a "window" through which light rays pass en route to the retina.

The average adult cornea is 0.65 mm thick at the periphery and 0.54 mm thick in the center. From anterior to posterior, it has 5 distinct layers (Fig 9–1): the epithelium (which is continuous with the epithelium of the bulbar conjunctiva), Bowman's layer, the stroma, Descemet's membrane, and the endothelium. The epithelium has 5 or 6 layers of cells, the endothelium only one. Bowman's layer is a clear acellular layer, a modified portion of the stroma. Descemet's membrane is a clear elastic membrane that can be seen on electron microscopy to comprise many fine fibrils. The corneal stroma accounts for about 90% of the corneal thickness. It is composed of intertwining lamellar fibers about 1 μm wide that run almost the full diameter of the cornea. They run parallel to the surface of the cornea and by virtue of their size and periodicity are optically clear. Each lamella possesses a flattened nucleus.

Sources of nutrition for the cornea are the vessels of the limbus, the aqueous, and tears. The superficial cornea also gets most of its oxygen from the atmosphere. The sensory nerves of the cornea are supplied by the first division of the fifth (trigeminal) cranial nerve. In the corneal epithelium there is a rich network of nerve fibers with bare ends. Whenever they are exposed, they produce a sensation of pain. The large number of nerves and the location of their endings account for the severe pain that results from even minor abrasions of the corneal epithelium.

The transparency of the cornea is due to its uniform structure, avascularity, and deturgescence. Deturgescence, or the state of relative dehydration of the corneal tissue, is maintained by the active bicarbonate "pump" of the endothelium and the anatomic integrity of the endothelium and epithelium. The endothelium is more important than the epithelium in the mechanism of dehydration, and chemical or physical damage to the endothelium is far more serious than damage to the epithelium. Destruction of the endothelial cells may cause marked swelling of the cornea and some loss of transparency. On the other hand, damage to the epithelium causes only slight transient, localized swelling of the corneal stroma that clears when the epithelial cells regenerate. Evaporation of water from the precorneal tear film produces slight hypertonicity of the film, which may be another factor in drawing water from the superficial corneal stroma, and helps to maintain the state of dehydration.

The penetration of the intact cornea by drugs is biphasic. Fat-soluble substances can pass through intact epithelium, and water-soluble substances can pass through intact stroma. To pass through the cornea, drugs must therefore have both a lipid-soluble and a water-soluble phase.

CORNEAL RESISTANCE TO INFECTION

The epithelium is a reliable barrier to the entrance of microorganisms into the cornea. Once the epithelium is traumatized, however, the avascular stroma and Bowman's layer become excellent culture media for a variety of organisms, particularly *Pseudomonas aeruginosa*. Descemet's membrane resists most bacteria but is not a barrier to fungi. *Streptococcus pneu-*

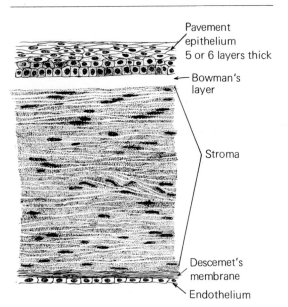

Pavement
epithelium
5 or 6 layers thick

Bowman's
layer

Stroma

Descemet's
membrane

Endothelium

Figure 9–1. Transverse section of cornea. (Reproduced, with permission, from Wolff E: *Anatomy of the Eye and Orbit,* 4th ed. Blakiston-McGraw, 1954.)

moniae (the pneumococcus) is the only true bacterial corneal pathogen; all others are opportunistic pathogens that require a heavy inoculum or a compromised host (eg, traumatized epithelium) to produce infection.

In the early days of ophthalmology, almost all bacterial ulcers were due to pneumococci and all fungal ulcers occurred in an agricultural setting. Since the advent of the corticosteroids in 1952, many opportunistic bacteria and fungi have become major causes of corneal ulcers. Local corticosteroid drops modify the immune reaction (the second line of defense against infection) and may allow opportunistic organisms to invade and flourish.

Moraxella liquefaciens, which occurs mainly in alcoholics (as a result of pyridoxine depletion), is a classic example of the bacterial opportunist, and in recent years a number of new bacterial corneal opportunists have been identified. Among them are *Serratia marcescens, Mycobacterium fortuitum, Streptococcus viridans, Staphylococcus epidermidis,* and various coliform and *Proteus* organisms.

PHYSIOLOGY OF SYMPTOMS

Since the cornea has many pain fibers, most corneal lesions, superficial or deep (corneal foreign body, corneal abrasion, phlyctenule, interstitial keratitis), cause pain and photophobia. The pain is worsened by movement of the lids (particularly the upper lid) over the cornea and usually persists until healing occurs. Since the cornea serves as the window of the eye and refracts light rays, corneal lesions usually blur vision somewhat, especially if centrally located.

Photophobia in corneal disease is the result of painful contraction of a hyperemic iris. Dilatation of iris vessels is a reflex phenomenon caused by irritation of the corneal nerve endings. Photophobia, severe in most corneal disease, is minimal in herpetic keratitis because of the hypesthesia associated with the disease, which is also a valuable diagnostic sign.

Although tearing and photophobia commonly accompany corneal disease, there is usually no discharge except in purulent bacterial ulcers.

INVESTIGATION OF CORNEAL DISEASE

Symptoms & Signs

The physician examines the cornea by inspecting it under adequate illumination. Examination is often facilitated by instillation of a local anesthetic. Fluorescein staining can outline a superficial epithelial lesion that might otherwise be impossible to see. The loupe and slit lamp are helpful but not absolutely essential aids; adequate illumination can be achieved with a hand flashlight. One should follow the course of the light reflex while moving the light carefully over the entire cornea. Rough areas indicative of epithelial defects are demonstrated in this way.

The patient's history is important in corneal disease. A history of trauma can often be elicited—in fact, foreign bodies and abrasions are the 2 most common corneal lesions. A history of corneal disease may also be of value. The keratitis of herpes simplex infection is often recurrent, but since recurrent erosion is extremely painful and herpetic keratitis is not, these disorders can be differentiated by their symptoms. The patient's use of local medications should be investigated, since corticosteroids may have been used and may have predisposed to bacterial, fungal, or viral disease, especially herpes simplex keratitis. Immunosuppression also occurs with systemic diseases, such as diabetes and malignant disease, as well as with specific immunosuppressive therapy.

Laboratory Studies

To select the proper therapy for corneal infections, especially hypopyon ulceration, laboratory aid is essential. Bacterial and fungal ulcers, for example, require completely different medications. Since a few hours' delay in determining the cause may severely prejudice the ultimate visual result, scrapings from the ulcer should be stained by both Gram's and Giemsa's stains and the infecting organism identified presumptively while the patient waits. Appropriate therapy can then be instituted immediately. Cultures for bacteria and fungi should be started at the same time, but therapy should not be withheld while awaiting confirmation of the presumptive diagnosis.

Morphologic Diagnosis of Corneal Lesions

A. Subepithelial Keratitis: Table 9–1 lists a number of important types of subepithelial lesions. These are often secondary to epithelial keratitis (eg, the nummular lesions of epidemic keratoconjunctivitis, caused by adenoviruses 8 and 19). They can usually be observed grossly but may also be recognized in the course of biomicroscopic examination of epithelial keratitis.

B. Epithelial Keratitis: The corneal epithelium is involved in most types of conjunctivitis and keratitis and in rare cases may be the only tissue involved (eg, in superficial punctate keratitis). The epithelial changes vary widely from simple edema and vacuolation to minute erosions, filament formation, partial keratinization, etc. The lesions vary also in their location on the cornea. All of these variations have incalculable diagnostic significance (Table 9–2), and biomicroscopic examination with and without fluorescein staining should be a part of every external eye examination.

Table 9–1. Subepithelial keratitis.

Types of keratitis with round, discrete, subepithelial opacities:
1. Nummular keratitis (Padi keratitis of the Orient).
2. Epidemic keratoconjunctivitis.
3. Nummular opacities in wearers of soft contact lenses.
4. Nummular opacities in zoster keratitis.
5. Nummular opacities in congenital syphilitic keratitis.

Table 9–2. Principal types of epithelial keratitis
(in order of frequency of occurrence).

Minute fluorescein-staining erosions; lower third of cornea affected predominantly. 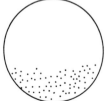 1. Staphylococcal keratitis	Typically dendritic (occasionally round or oval) with edema and degeneration. 2. Herpetic keratitis (HSK)	More diffuse than lesions of HSK; occasionally linear (pseudodendrites). 3. Varicella-zoster keratitis
Minute fluorescein-staining erosions; diffuse but most conspicuous in pupillary area. 4. Adenovirus keratitis	Minute pleomorphic, fluorescein-staining, damaged epithelium and erosions; epithelial and mucous filaments are typical; lower half of cornea affected predominantly. 5. Keratitis of Sjögren's syndrome	Minute fluorescein-staining, irregular erosions; lower half of cornea affected predominantly. 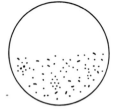 6. Exposure keratitis—due to lagophthalmos or exophthalmos
Blotchy gray, opaque, syncytiumlike lesions, most conspicuous in upper pupillary area. Sometimes a plaque of opaque epithelium forms. 7. Vernal keratoconjunctivitis	Blotchy epithelial edema; diffuse but predominant in palpebral fissure, 9–3 o'clock. 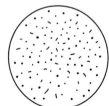 8. Trophic keratitis—sequela of herpes simplex, herpes zoster, and gasserian ganglion destruction	Minute fluorescein-staining erosions with spotty cellular edema; highly characteristic picture. 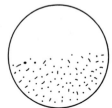 9. Drug-induced keratitis—especially by broad-spectrum antibiotics
Foci of edematous epithelial cells, round or oval; elevated when disease is active. 10. Superficial punctate keratitis (SPK)	Minute fluorescein-staining erosions of upper third of cornea; filaments during exacerbations; bulbar hyperemia, thickened limbus, micropannus. 11. Superior limbic keratoconjunctivitis	Virus-type lesions like those of SPK; in pupillary area. 12. Rubeola, rubella, and mumps keratitis

Table 9–2 (cont'd). Principal types of epithelial keratitis (in order of frequency of occurrence).

Minute fluorescein-staining epithelial erosions affecting upper third of cornea.	Spotty gray opacification of individual epithelial cells due to partial keratinization; associated with Bitot's spots.
13. Trachoma	14. Vitamin A deficiency keratitis

CORNEAL ULCERATION

Cicatrization due to corneal ulceration is a major cause of blindness and impaired vision throughout the world. Most of this visual loss is preventable, but only if an etiologic diagnosis is made early and appropriate therapy instituted. Hypopyon ulcer, the most important type, was once caused almost exclusively by the pneumococcus *(S pneumoniae)*, the only true bacterial pathogen that attacks the cornea. In recent years, however, as a result of the widespread use of compromising systemic and local medications (at least in the developed countries), opportunistic bacteria, fungi, and viruses have tended to cause more cases of corneal ulcer than the pneumococcus.

CENTRAL CORNEAL ULCERS
(Hypopyon Ulcer)

Central ulcers are infectious ulcers that follow epithelial damage. The break in the epithelium may be peripheral, but the ulcer always migrates toward the center of the cornea, away from the vascularized limbus. Hypopyon usually (not always) accompanies the ulcer. It is almost always sterile in bacterial ulcers and often contains fungal elements in fungal ulcers. The pneumococcus, historically the chief cause of hypopyon ulcer, is pathogenic, even in small numbers, for an exposed corneal stroma. If the opportunists are to cause disease, one of 2 conditions must be met: The host must have been topically immunosuppressed by anesthetics, cytotoxic drugs, or a corticosteroid preparation, or must have received an overwhelming inoculum. (This would be the case, for example, if a fluorescein solution heavily contaminated with *P aeruginosa* were instilled into an eye.)

BACTERIAL KERATITIS

Many types of bacterial corneal ulcer look alike and vary only in severity. This is especially true of ulcers caused by opportunistic bacteria (eg, alpha-hemolytic streptococci, *Staphylococcus aureus*, *Nocardia*, and *M fortuitum*), which cause indolent corneal ulcers that tend to spread slowly and superficially.

Pneumococcal Corneal Ulcer
(Acute Serpiginous Ulcer)

The pneumococcus should still be regarded as the only microorganism that is a true corneal pathogen. In some populations (eg, the Indians of the Southwestern USA), it is almost the only bacterial cause of corneal ulcer. Before the popularization of dacryocystorhinostomy, pneumococcal ulcers often occurred in coal miners or others subjected to frequent corneal abrasions that became secondarily infected from an already infected tear sac.

Pneumococcal corneal ulcer usually occurs 24–48 hours after inoculation of an abraded cornea. It typically produces a gray, fairly well circumscribed ulcer that tends to spread erratically from the original site of infection toward the center of the cornea (Fig 9–2). The advancing border shows active ulceration and

Figure 9–2. Pneumococcal corneal ulcer with hypopyon.

Table 9–3. Treatment of corneal ulceration.

Organisms	Drug Route	First Choice	Recommended Drugs Second Choice	Third Choice
Gram-positive cocci: lancet-shaped with capsule = pneumococcus	Topical	Erythromycin	Bacitracin	Vancomycin
	Subconjunctival	Cefazolin	Penicillin G	Erythromycin or methicillin
	Systemic[1]	Cefazolin	Penicillin G	Oral: Erythromycin
Other gram-positive organisms: cocci and rods	Topical	Bacitracin	Cefazolin	Gentamicin or vancomycin
	Subconjunctival	Cefazolin and gentamicin	Methicillin and gentamicin	Vancomycin and methicillin
	Systemic			
Gram-negative cocci[2]	Topical	Erythromycin	Bacitracin	Gentamicin or vancomycin
	Subconjunctival	Methicillin and gentamicin	Gentamicin and cefazolin	Erythromycin and methicillin
	Systemic	Penicillin G	Cefazolin	Oral: Erythromycin
Gram-negative rods (thin = Pseudomonas)	Topical	Tobramycin	Polymyxin B	Gentamicin and carbenicillin
	Subconjunctival	Tobramycin and carbenicillin	Gentamicin and carbenicillin	Polymyxin B
	Systemic	⋯	⋯	⋯
Gram-negative rods: large, square-ended diplobacilli = Moraxella	Topical	Rarely necessary	Sodium sulfacetamide	Zinc sulfate or chloramphenicol
	Subconjunctival	⋯	⋯	⋯
	Systemic			
Other gram-negative rods	Topical	Gentamicin	Carbenicillin	Chloramphenicol
	Subconjunctival	Gentamicin and carbenicillin	Gentamicin and cephaloridine	Carbenicillin and cephaloridine
	Systemic	Ampicillin	Cefazolin	Carbenicillin
Gram-positive rods: slender and varying in length = Mycobacterium fortuitum, Nocardia sp, Actinomyces sp	Topical	Amikacin	Amikacin	Tetracycline
	Subconjunctival	Amikacin	Rifampin	⋯
	Systemic	Oral: Sulfonamides[3]	Oral: Tetracycline[3]	⋯
Yeastlike organisms = Candida sp[4]	Topical	Amphotericin B and flucytosine	Natamycin and flucytosine	Nystatin or miconazole
	Subconjunctival	Amphotericin B	Miconazole	⋯
	Systemic	Oral: Flucytosine	Ketoconazole	⋯
Hyphaelike organisms = fungal ulcer	Topical	Natamycin	Amphotericin B	Miconazole
	Subconjunctival	Amphotericin B	Miconazole	⋯
	Systemic		Ketoconazole	⋯
No organisms identified; ulcer suggestive of bacterial type	Topical	Gentamicin and cefazolin	Gentamicin and bacitracin	Vancomycin
	Subconjunctival	Gentamicin and cefazolin	Gentamicin and methicillin	Cephaloridine and polymyxin B
	Systemic	Penicillin G	Nafcillin	Cefazolin
No organisms identified; ulcer suggestive of fungal type	Topical	Natamycin	Amphotericin B	Miconazole
	Subconjunctival	Rarely necessary: Amphotericin B	Miconazole	⋯
	Systemic	⋯	⋯	

[1] Intravenous unless otherwise stated; only when ulcer is severe.

[2] Ulcer associated with hyperacute conjunctivitis (eg, gonococcal conjunctivitis) should be treated with same drug used to treat the conjunctivitis.

[3] These 2 drugs often act synergistically.

[4] Rarely, Pityrosporum ovale or Pityrosporum orbiculare may be confused with Candida sp.

infiltration as the trailing border begins to heal. (This creeping effect suggested the term "acute serpiginous ulcer.") The superficial corneal layers become involved first and then the deep parenchyma. The cornea surrounding the ulcer is often clear.

A hypopyon of moderate size usually forms. Hypopyon is a collection of inflammatory cells, predominantly polymorphonuclear neutrophilic leukocytes with some mononuclear cells and macrophages, and is characteristic of both bacterial and fungal central corneal ulcers. Although hypopyon is sterile in bacterial corneal ulcers unless there has been a rupture of Descemet's membrane, in fungal ulcers it often contains fungal elements; this is because fungi can penetrate an intact Descemet membrane.

Scrapings from the leading edge of a pneumococcal corneal ulcer contain gram-positive lancet-shaped diplococci. Drugs recommended for use in treatment are listed in Tables 9–3 and 9–4. Concurrent dacryocystitis should also be treated.

Pseudomonas Corneal Ulcer

Pseudomonas corneal ulcer begins as a gray or yellow infiltrate at the site of break in the corneal epithelium (Fig 9–3). Severe pain usually accompanies it. The lesion tends to spread rapidly in all directions because of the proteolytic enzymes produced by the organisms. Although usually superficial at first, the ulcer may affect the entire cornea. There is often a large hypopyon that tends to increase in size as the ulcer progresses. The infiltrate and exudate may have a bluish-green color. This is due to a pigment produced by the organism and is pathognomonic of *P aeruginosa* infection.

Pseudomonas ulcer often arises from the use of a contaminated fluorescein solution or from contaminated medications used either to examine or to treat a corneal abrasion or injury. Such infections must be considered iatrogenic and are to be deplored. It is mandatory that the clinician use sterile medications

Figure 9–3. *Pseudomonas* corneal ulcer of right eye. Evisceration was done.

and a sterile technique when caring for patients with corneal injuries.

Scrapings from the ulcer contain long, thin gram-negative rods that are often few in number. Drugs recommended for use in treatment are listed in Tables 9–3 and 9–4.

Moraxella liquefaciens Corneal Ulcer

M liquefaciens (diplobacillus of Petit) causes an indolent oval ulcer that usually affects the inferior cornea and progresses into the deep stroma over a period of days. There is usually no hypopyon or only a small one, and the surrounding cornea is usually clear. *M liquefaciens* ulcer almost always occurs in a patient with alcoholism, diabetes, or other immunosuppressing disease. Scrapings contain large, square-ended gram-negative diplobacilli. Drugs recommended for use in treatment are listed in Tables 9–3 and 9–4.

Streptococcus pyogenes Corneal Ulcer

Central corneal ulcers caused by beta-hemolytic streptococci have no identifying features. The surrounding corneal stroma is often infiltrated and edematous, and there is usually a moderately large hypopyon. Scrapings contain gram-positive cocci in chains. Drugs recommended for use in treatment are listed in Tables 9–3 and 9–4.

Klebsiella pneumoniae Corneal Ulcer

The corneal ulcer caused by *K pneumoniae* is usually indolent and often without a hypopyon. There may be edema of the surrounding stroma, and scrapings contain gram-negative rods with capsules. Drugs recommended for use in treatment are listed in Tables 9–3 and 9–4.

Staphylococcus aureus, Staphylococcus epidermidis, & Streptococcus viridans Corneal Ulcers

Central corneal ulcers caused by these organisms are now being seen more often than formerly, most of them in corneas compromised by topical corticosteroids. The ulcers are often indolent but may be associated with hypopyon and some surrounding corneal infiltration. They are often superficial, and the ulcer bed feels firm when scraped. Scrapings contain gram-positive cocci—singly, in pairs, or in chains. Tables 9–3 and 9–4 show recommended drug regimens.

Mycobacterium fortuitum & Nocardia Corneal Ulcers

Ulcers due to *M fortuitum* and *Nocardia* are rare. They often follow trauma and are often associated with contact with soil. The ulcers are indolent, and the bed of the ulcer often has radiating lines that make it look like a cracked windshield. Hypopyon may or may not be present. Scrapings may contain acid-fast slender rods *(M fortuitum)* or gram-positive filamentous, often branching organisms *(Nocardia)*. See Tables 9–3 and 9–4 for recommended drug regimens.

Table 9–4. Drug concentrations and dosages for treatment of corneal ulceration.

Drug	Topical*	Subconjunctival*	Systemic* (intravenous unless otherwise indicated)
Amikacin	10 mg/mL	25 mg/0.5 mL/dose	. . .
Amphotericin B	1.5–3 mg/mL	750 μg/0.5 mL/dose every other day	. . .
Ampicillin	. . .	. . .	150–200 mg/kg body wt/d in 4 doses
Bacitracin	10,000 units/mL	. . .	. . .
Carbenicillin	4 mg/mL	125 mg/0.5 mL/dose	100–200 mg/kg body wt/d in 4 doses
Cefazolin	50 mg/mL	100 mg/0.5 mL/dose	15 mg/kg body wt/d in 4 doses
Cephaloridine	. . .	100 mg/0.5 mL/dose	. . .
Chloramphenicol	5 mg/mL	. . .	. . .
Erythromycin	5 mg/g (ointment)	100 mg/0.5 mL/dose	Oral: first dose 1 g; then 0.5 g every 6 h
Flucytosine	1% solution	. . .	Oral: 50–150 mg/kg body wt/d in 4 doses
Gentamicin	3–10 mg/mL	20 mg/0.5 mL/dose	. . .
Methicillin	. . .	100 mg/mL; dose: 0.5–1 mL	. . .
Miconazole	1% solution or 2% ointment	5 mg/0.5 mL/dose	. . .
Nafcillin	. . .	. . .	1 g every 4–6 h
Natamycin (pimaricin)	5% suspension	. . .	. . .
Nystatin	100,000 units/g (ointment)	. . .	. . .
Penicillin G	10,000–20,000 units/mL	1 million units/mL/dose	40,000–50,000 units/kg body wt/d in 4 doses or continuously
Polymyxin B	10,000–25,000 units/mL	10,000 units/mL/dose	. . .
Rifampin	1% ointment	. . .	Oral: 600 mg/d
Sodium sulfacetamide	10–15% solution	. . .	. . .
Sulfonamides	. . .	. . .	Oral: 70 mg/kg body wt/d in 4 doses, or 4 g, whichever is less
Tetracycline	5 mg/mL	. . .	Oral: 1.5 g/d in 4 doses for patients under 70 kg; 2 g/d if over 70 kg
Tobramycin	3–15 mg/mL	20 mg/0.5 mL/dose	. . .
Vancomycin	50 mg/mL	100 mg/mL; dose: 0.25 mL	. . .
Zinc sulfate	0.5 mg/mL	. . .	. . .

*Treatment schedule: Topical: Every hour during day, every 2 hours during night, for 5 days. Subconjunctival: One injection daily for 4 days unless otherwise stated; in exceptionally severe cases, initial dose sometimes repeated after 12 hours. Systemic, intravenous, or oral: One dose daily for 5 days.

FUNGAL KERATITIS

Fungal corneal ulcers, once seen only in agricultural workers, have become relatively common in the urban population since the introduction of the corticosteroid drugs for use in ophthalmology in 1952. Before the corticosteroid era, fungal corneal ulcers occurred only if an overwhelming inoculum of organisms was introduced into the corneal stroma—an event that can still take place in an agricultural setting. The uncompromised cornea seems to be able to handle the small inocula to which urban residents are ordinarily subjected.

Fungal ulcers are indolent and have a gray infiltrate, often a hypopyon, marked inflammation of the globe, superficial ulceration, and satellite lesions (usually infiltrates at sites distant from the main area of ulceration) (Fig 9–4). The principal lesion—and often the satellite lesions as well—is an endothelial plaque with irregular edges underlying the principal corneal lesions, associated with a severe anterior chamber reaction and a corneal abscess.

Most fungal ulcers are caused by opportunists such as *Candida*, *Fusarium*, *Aspergillus*, *Penicillium*, *Cephalosporium*, and others. There are no identifying features that help to differentiate one type of fungal ulcer from another.

Scrapings from fungal corneal ulcers, except those caused by *Candida*, contain hyphal elements; scrapings from *Candida* ulcers usually contain pseudohyphae or yeast forms that show characteristic budding. Tables 9–3 and 9–4 list the drugs recommended for the treatment of fungal ulcers.

VIRAL KERATITIS

Herpes Simplex Keratitis

Herpes simplex virus (HSV) keratitis is the commonest cause of corneal ulceration in the USA. It occurs in 2 forms: primary and recurrent. The primary disease is a rare keratoconjunctivitis in young children, and the recurrent disease a common ulcerative keratitis, usually but not always dendritic. Most HSV infections of the cornea are still caused by HSV type 1 (the cause of labial herpes), but in both infants and

Figure 9–4. Corneal ulcer caused by *Candida albicans*. (Courtesy of P Thygeson.)

Figure 9–5. Corneal scar caused by recurrent herpes simplex keratitis. (Courtesy of A Rosenberg.)

adults a few cases caused by HSV type 2 (the cause of genital herpes) have been reported. The corneal lesions caused by the 2 types are indistinguishable.

Herpetic keratitis is the ocular counterpart of labial herpes, and the dendritic lesion resembles the fever blister immunologically, pathologically, and in clinical course. The only difference is that the clinical course of the keratitis may be slightly prolonged because of the avascularity of the corneal stroma, which retards the migration of lymphocytes and macrophages to the lesion. HSV ocular infection is self-limited and benign in the immunocompetent host, but in the immunologically compromised host its course can be chronic and damaging.

Scrapings of the epithelial lesions of HSV keratitis contain multinucleated giant cells. The virus can be cultivated on the chorioallantoic membrane of embryonated hens' eggs and in many tissue cell lines—eg, HeLa cells, on which it produces characteristic plaques. In the majority of cases, however, diagnosis can be made clinically on the basis of typical dendritic or geographic ulcers and greatly reduced or absent corneal sensation.

Clinical Findings. Attacks of the common recurrent type of herpetic keratitis (Fig 9– 5) are triggered by fever, overexposure to ultraviolet light, trauma, psychic stress (especially anger), the onset of menstruation, or some other local or systemic source of immunosuppression. Unilaterality is the rule, but bilateral lesions develop in 4– 6% of cases and are seen most often in atopic patients.

The first symptoms are usually irritation, photophobia, and tearing. When the central cornea is affected, there is also some reduction in vision. Since corneal anesthesia usually occurs early in the course of the infection, the symptoms may be minimal and the patient may not seek medical advice. There is often a history of fever blisters or other herpetic in-

fection, but corneal ulceration can occasionally be the only sign of a recurrent herpetic infection.

Lesions. The most characteristic lesion is the **dendritic** ulcer. It occurs in the corneal epithelium, has a typical linear pattern with a tendency to branch, and has terminal bulbs at its ends (Fig 9– 6). Fluorescein staining makes the dendrite very easy to identify, but unfortunately herpetic keratitis can also simulate almost any corneal infection and must be considered in the differential diagnosis of many corneal lesions.

Other corneal epithelial lesions that may be caused by HSV are a blotchy epithelial keratitis, stellate epithelial keratitis, and filamentary keratitis. All of these are usually transitory, however, and often become typical dentrites within a day or two.

Subepithelial opacities can be caused by HSV infection. A ghostlike image, corresponding in shape to the original epithelial defect but slightly larger, can be seen in the area immediately underlying the epithelial lesion. The "ghost" remains superficial but is often enlarged by the use of antiviral drugs, especially

Figure 9–6. Dendritic figures seen in herpes simplex keratitis.

idoxuridine. As a rule, these subepithelial lesions do not persist for more than a year.

Disciform keratitis is the commonest complication of HSV infection. This round lesion is associated with moderate or severe edema of the affected stroma. Small or medium-sized white keratic precipitates sometimes lie directly under the lesions, and there may be folds in Descemet's membrane. Disciform keratitis is usually associated with local or systemic immunosuppression. Local immunosuppression is commonly produced by cauterization with strong iodine, by topical corticosteroids, or by prolonged use of idoxuridine.

Like all herpetic lesions in immunocompetent individuals, disciform keratitis is normally self-limited, lasting from several weeks to several months. Edema is the prominent sign, and healing occurs with minimal scarring and vascularization. But when immunosuppression, local or systemic, is severe, the lesion becomes chronic and may persist for years. In that event, the stroma often becomes necrotic, and an accompanying iridocyclitis may be severe. Hypopyon is rare and usually indicates secondary bacterial or fungal infection. In exceptional cases, however, it may be due to the pyogenic properties of necrotic tissue. Corneal perforation in disciform keratitis was virtually unknown prior to 1952, when the topical corticosteroids were first introduced; unfortunately, perforation has become less rare since that time.

If perforation has occurred or is imminent, immediate corneal transplantation should be considered. Alternative procedures are the application of a thin conjunctival flap, sealing the perforation with tissue glues, or protecting the eye with soft corneal contact lenses while healing takes place.

Focal avascular interstitial keratitis can also occur in HSV infection and—like stromal necrosis—is almost always associated with the use of corticosteroids. Small areas of focal infiltration and edema are surrounded by clear areas. There is no sign of vascularization, and the lesions may affect any level of the cornea. If they are examined by retroillumination at the slit lamp, their pattern often suggests a previous disciform lesion.

Peripheral lesions of the cornea can also be caused by HSV. They are usually linear and show a loss of epithelium before the underlying corneal stroma becomes infiltrated. (This is in sharp contrast to the marginal ulcer associated with bacterial hypersensitivity—eg, to S aureus in staphylococcal blepharitis, in which the infiltration precedes the loss of the overlying epithelium.) Corneal sensation is usually absent or so diminished that the patient is far less photophobic than patients with nonherpetic corneal infiltrates and ulceration usually are.

Treatment. The treatment of HSV keratitis should be directed toward elimination of the virus from the cornea. In the immunocompetent patient, the infection is self-limited and scarring minimal. Regrettably, the clinician often immunosuppresses the patient by using corticosteroids in eagerness to reduce local inflammation. This is of course based on a misconception that reducing inflammation reduces disease.

Debridement. Virus in the epithelium can be readily eliminated by debridement of the affected epithelium, which is best accomplished by removing it carefully from the anesthetized cornea with a tightly wound cotton-tipped applicator. A sterile platinum spatula or a sterile chalazion curet can also be used. The topical application of iodine or ether has no value and can produce chemical keratitis. (Unlike healthy uninfected epithelium, which adheres tightly to the cornea and is hard to remove, infected epithelium is only loosely attached to the cornea and is easy to remove.) A cycloplegic such as atropine 1% or homatropine 5% is then instilled into the conjunctival sac, and a pressure dressing is applied to promote healing. The patient should be examined daily and the dressing changed until the corneal defect has healed (usually 72 hours).

Drug Therapy. Although mechanical removal of affected epithelium is the best treatment for dendritic keratitis, topical chemotherapy with trifluridine (Viroptic), idoxuridine (IDU, Dendrid, Herplex, Stoxil) or vidarabine (Ara-A, Vira-A) is widely used. Antiviral therapy with these agents has been disappointing, and extensive research is currently under way to find more effective and less toxic preparations. The most promising of those now being tested (but not yet released in the USA) is acyclovir (acycloguanosine). Idoxuridine and vidarabine are now useful only in epithelial disease. They are ineffective in both the stromal and uveal tract forms that are now so common because of the improper use of corticosteroids. The major toxic complications of the antivirals, particularly idoxuridine, can be avoided if treatment time is limited to less than 10 days or if the drugs are discontinued promptly when found to be ineffective after a trial of 2 or 3 days. It should be borne in mind that idoxuridine is a cytotoxic drug and can be locally immunosuppressive.

Corticosteroid therapy is contraindicated at all stages of HSV disease for the following reasons: (1) The corticosteroids increase the destructive action of collagenase (produced by the damaged corneal epithelial cells or polymorphonuclear cells) on the corneal stroma; and (2) their immunosuppressive activity increases (a) the activity of the virus and (b) the susceptibility of the HSV-infected host to secondary infections with opportunistic organisms, especially fungi and such bacteria as S viridans and S epidermidis. Unfortunately, steroids are still widely used because of their anti-inflammatory effect and their temporary but dramatically beneficial effect on symptoms.

Control of trigger mechanisms that reactivate HSV infection. Recurrent HSV infections of the eye are common, occurring in about one-third of cases within 2 years of the first attack. A trigger mechanism can often be discovered by careful questioning of the patient. Once identified, the trigger can often be avoided. Aspirin can be used to avoid fever, excessive exposure to the sun or ultraviolet light can be avoided, situations that might cause psychic stress can be minimized, and aspirin can be taken just prior to the onset of menstruation.

Varicella-Zoster Viral Keratitis

Varicella-zoster virus (VZV) infection occurs in 2 forms: primary (varicella) and recurrent (zoster). Ocular manifestations are uncommon in varicella but common in ophthalmic zoster. In varicella (chickenpox), the usual eye lesions are pocks on the lids and lid margins. Rarely, keratitis occurs (typically a phlyctenulelike lesion at the limbus), and still more rarely epithelial keratitis with or without pseudodendrites. Disciform keratitis, with uveitis of short duration, has been reported.

In contrast to the rare and benign corneal lesions of varicella, the relatively frequent ophthalmic zoster is often accompanied by keratouveitis that varies in severity according to the immune status of the patient. Thus, although children with zoster keratouveitis usually have benign disease, the aged have severe and sometimes blinding disease. Corneal complications in ophthalmic zoster can be anticipated if there is a skin eruption along the branches of the nasociliary nerve.

Unlike recurrent HSV keratitis that affects only the epithelium, VZV keratitis affects the stroma and anterior uvea at onset. The epithelial lesions are blotchy and amorphous except for an occasional linear pseudodendrite that only vaguely resembles the true dendrites of HSV keratitis. Stromal opacities are prominent, characteristically nummular in shape, and largely but not exclusively subepithelial. A disciform keratitis sometimes develops and resembles HSV disciform keratitis. Loss of corneal sensation is always a prominent feature and often persists for months after the corneal lesion appears to have healed. The associated uveitis tends to persist for weeks or months, but unless corticosteroid preparations have been used it eventually heals.

In clinical trials and outside the USA, intravenous and oral forms of acyclovir have been used successfully for the treatment of herpes zoster ophthalmicus. Acyclovir is given intravenously to immunocompromised patients who develop herpes zoster infections. Corticosteroid preparations, although they do provide temporary relief, have prolonged the course of the disease and worsened its prognosis. Opportunistic superinfection, which did not occur prior to 1952, is now a common complication. Of the various complications, postherpetic neuralgia, which is particularly severe in elderly patients, is the most troublesome. Fortunately it is self-limited, and reassurance can be helpful as a supplement to analgesics.

Since zoster is a disease of immunosuppression, the restoration of immunocompetence by immunopotentiators is logical and can be looked upon as the hope of the future. The early results of the study of a number of immunopotentiating procedures are definitely encouraging.

Variola Virus Keratitis

Variola virus corneal ulcers were once a common cause of corneal scarring and blindness in developing countries. The lesions usually involved the pupillary area, and perforations with resultant adherent leukomas were common. This is one ocular disease that will be seen no more, however, for according to the World Health Organization, smallpox is now extinct.

Vaccinial Keratitis

On rare occasions vaccinial keratitis used to occur as a complication of vaccination for the prevention of smallpox. It was either a blotchy epithelial keratitis or a true corneal ulcer and was usually associated with lesions on the lid margin. Atypically, disciform keratitis sometimes occurred. Topical rifampin was apparently sometimes beneficial. Of academic interest (since vaccinial keratitis, like variolar keratitis, is no longer a problem) is the fact that intramuscular vaccinia immune globulin sometimes increased the severity of the disciform lesion.

Adenovirus Keratitis

Keratitis usually accompanies all types of adenoviral conjunctivitis, reaching its peak 5–7 days after onset of the conjunctivitis. It is a fine epithelial keratitis best seen with the slit lamp after instillation of fluorescein. The minute lesions may group together to make up larger ones.

The epithelial keratitis is often followed by subepithelial opacities. In epidemic keratoconjunctivitis (EKC), which is due to adenovirus types 8 and 19, the subepithelial lesions are round and grossly visible. They appear 8–15 days after onset of the conjunctivitis and may persist for months or even (rarely) for several years. Similar lesions occur very exceptionally in other adenoviral infections, eg, those caused by types 3, 4, and 7, but tend to be transitory and mild, lasting a few weeks at most.

Although the corneal opacities of adenoviral keratoconjunctivitis tend to fade temporarily with the use of topical corticosteroids, and although the patient is often made temporarily more comfortable thereby, corticosteroid therapy prolongs the disease and is therefore not recommended. No medication is needed.

Other Viral Keratitides

A fine epithelial keratitis may be seen in other viral infections such as measles (in which the central cornea is affected predominantly), rubella, mumps, infectious mononucleosis, acute hemorrhagic conjunctivitis, Newcastle disease conjunctivitis, and verruca of the lid margin. A superior epithelial keratitis and pannus often accompany molluscum contagiosum nodules on the lid margin. Rare cases of orf virus keratitis have been seen in sheepherders in California and Nevada. The corneal lesions resembled those of the now extinct vaccinial keratitis.

CHLAMYDIAL KERATITIS

All 5 principal types of chlamydial conjunctivitis (trachoma, inclusion conjunctivitis, primary ocular lymphogranuloma venereum, parakeet or psittacosis conjunctivitis, and feline pneumonitis conjunctivitis) are accompanied by corneal lesions. Only in trachoma and lymphogranuloma venereum, however, have they been blinding or visually damaging. The corneal lesions of trachoma have been the most studied and are of great diagnostic importance. In order of appearance they consist of (1) epithelial microerosions affecting the upper third of the cornea; (2) micropannus; (3) subepithelial round opacities, commonly called trachoma pustules; (4) limbal follicles and their cicatricial remains, known as Herbert's peripheral pits; (5) gross pannus; and (6) extensive, diffuse, subepithelial cicatrization. Mild cases of trachoma may show only epithelial keratitis and micropannus and may heal without impairing vision.

The rare cases of lymphogranuloma venereum have shown fewer characteristic changes but are known to have caused blindness by diffuse corneal scarring and total pannus. The remaining types of chlamydial infection cause only micropannus, epithelial keratitis, and rare subepithelial opacities not visually significant.

Chlamydial keratoconjunctivitis responds to treatment with the sulfonamides (except for the rare *C psittaci* infections, which are sulfonamide-resistant), and to tetracyclines and erythromycin.

DRUG-INDUCED EPITHELIAL KERATITIS

An epithelial keratitis is not uncommonly seen in patients using antiviral medications (idoxuridine and vidarabine) and the broad-spectrum and medium-spectrum antibiotics. It is usually a blotchy keratitis affecting predominantly the lower half of the cornea and interpalpebral fissure.

KERATOCONJUNCTIVITIS SICCA (Sjögren's Syndrome)

Epithelial filaments in the lower quadrants of the cornea are the cardinal signs of this autoimmune disease in which secretion of the lacrimal and accessory lacrimal glands is diminished or eliminated. There is also a blotchy epithelial keratitis that affects mainly the lower quadrants. Severe cases show mucous pseudofilaments that stick to the dry corneal epithelium.

This keratitis of Sjögren's syndrome must be distinguished from the keratitis sicca of such cicatrizing diseases as trachoma and pemphigoid, in which the goblet cells of the conjunctiva have been destroyed. Such cases sometimes still produce tears, but without mucus the corneal epithelium sheds the tears and continues to be dry.

Treatment of keratoconjunctivitis sicca calls for the frequent use of tear substitutes, of which there are many commercial preparations. When goblet cells have been destroyed, as in the cicatricial conjunctivitides, mucus substitutes must be used in addition to artificial tears. Topical vitamin A may help to reverse the epithelial keratinization.

PERIPHERAL CORNEAL ULCERS

Marginal Infiltrates & Ulcers

The majority of marginal corneal ulcers are benign but extremely painful. They are secondary to acute or chronic bacterial conjunctivitis, particularly staphylococcal blepharoconjunctivitis and less often Koch-Weeks *(Haemophilus aegyptius)* conjunctivitis. They are not an infectious process, however, and scrapings do not contain the causal bacteria. They are the result of sensitization to bacterial products, antibody from the limbus vessels reacting with antigen that has diffused through the corneal epithelium.

Marginal infiltrates and ulcers (Fig 9– 7) start as oval or linear infiltrates, separated from the limbus by a lucid interval, and only later may ulcerate and vascularize. They are self-limited, usually lasting from 7– 10 days, but those associated with staphylococcal blepharoconjunctivitis usually recur. Topical corticosteroid preparations shorten their course and relieve symptoms, which are often severe, but treatment of the underlying conjunctivitis is essential if recurrences are to be prevented. Before starting corticosteroid therapy, great care must be taken to distinguish this entity, formerly known as ''catarrhal corneal ulceration,'' from marginal herpetic keratitis. Since marginal herpetic keratitis is usually almost symptomless because of corneal anesthesia, differentiating it from the painful, hypersensitivity-type marginal ulcer is not difficult.

Figure 9–7. Marginal ulcer of temporal cornea, right eye. (Courtesy of P Thygeson.)

Ring Ulcers
(Fig 9–8)

Ring ulcers are rare but more destructive than marginal ulcers. They occasionally result from the confluence of multiple marginal ulcers secondary to conjunctivitis but are more often associated with systemic disease. They have been seen in the convalescent period of such infectious diseases as influenza and bacillary dysentery but can also be a complication of autoimmune disease. A few ring ulcers have been seen in ocular diphtheria, in severe beta-hemolytic streptococcal conjunctival infection, and (more often) in gonococcal conjunctivitis. They may also occur as a secondary manifestation of infectious endophthalmitis; in this event, the ulceration is preceded by a massive infiltration of neutrophils.

Treatment—often unsatisfactory—depends on identification of the underlying cause. Infectious ring ulcer may respond to appropriate systemic and topical antibiotics and the hypersensitivity types to topical corticosteroid therapy.

Mooren's Ulcer
(Fig 9–9)

The cause of Mooren's ulcer is still unknown, but an autoimmune origin is suspected. It is a marginal ulcer, unilateral in 60– 80% of cases and characterized by painful, progressive excavation of the limbus and peripheral cornea that often leads to loss of the eye. It occurs most commonly in old age but does not seem to be related to any of the systemic diseases that most often afflict the aged. It is unresponsive to both antibiotics and corticosteroids. Surgical excision of the limbal conjunctiva in an effort to remove sensitizing substances has recently been advocated. Past generations of ophthalmologists used repeated paracentesis with some success.

Phlyctenular Keratoconjunctivitis

This hypersensitivity disease (due to delayed hypersensitivity to bacterial products, mainly of the human tubercle bacillus) was formerly a major cause of visual loss in the USA, particularly among the Eskimos and Native Americans. Phlyctenules are localized accumulations of lymphocytes, monocytes, macrophages, and finally neutrophils. They appear first at the limbus, but in recurrent attacks they may involve the bulbar conjunctiva and cornea. Corneal phlyctenules, usually bilateral, cicatrize and vascularize, but conjunctival phlyctenules leave no trace.

Most cases of phlyctenular keratoconjunctivitis in the USA today are caused by delayed hypersensitivity to *S aureus*. The antigen is released locally from staphylococci that proliferate on the lid margin in staphylococcal blepharitis. Rare phlyctenules have occurred in San Joaquin Valley fever, a result of hypersensitivity to a primary infection with *Coccidioides immitis*. In this disease they are not visually important, however.

In the tuberculous type, the attack may be triggered by an acute bacterial conjunctivitis but is associated typically with a transient increase in the activity of a childhood tuberculosis. Untreated phlyctenules run a course to healing in 10– 14 days, but topical therapy with corticosteroid preparations dramatically shortens the course to a day or two. The corticosteroid response in the staphylococcal type is poor, however, and treatment consists essentially of eliminating the causal bacterial infection. In resistant staphylococcal cases, desensitization with *Staphylococcus* toxoid or Staphage Lysate has been useful.

Marginal Keratitis in Autoimmune Disease

The corneal periphery receives its nourishment from the aqueous humor, the limbal capillaries, and the tear film. It is contiguous with the subconjunctival lymphoid tissue and the lymphatic arcades at the limbus. The perilimbal conjunctiva appears to play an important role in the pathogenesis of corneal lesions that arise both from local ocular disease and from systemic disorders, particularly those of autoimmune origin. There is a striking similarity between the limbal capillary network and the renal glomerular capillary network: On the endothelial basement membranes of the capillaries of both networks, immune complexes

Figure 9–8. Ring ulcer of the cornea. (Courtesy of M Hogan.)

Figure 9–9. Mooren's ulcer. (Courtesy of M Hogan.)

are deposited and immunologic disease results. Thus, the peripheral cornea often participates in such autoimmune diseases as rheumatoid arthritis, polyarteritis nodosa, systemic lupus erythematosus, scleroderma, midline lethal and Wegener's granulomatosis, ulcerative colitis, Crohn's disease, relapsing polychondritis, and Reiter's syndrome. These diseases are characteristically associated with infiltration, ulceration, thinning, and (rarely) perforation of the peripheral cornea. The corneal lesions range in severity from benign and even self-limited changes to perforation and loss of the eye. Treatment is directed toward control of the underlying disease but is for the most part unsatisfactory.

CORNEAL ULCER DUE TO VITAMIN A DEFICIENCY

The typical corneal ulcer associated with avitaminosis A is centrally located and bilateral, gray and indolent, with a definite lack of corneal luster in the surrounding area (Fig 9–10). The cornea becomes soft and necrotic (hence the term, "keratomalacia"), and perforation is common. The epithelium of the conjunctiva is keratinized, as evidenced by the presence of a Bitot spot. This is a foamy, wedge-shaped area in the conjunctiva, usually on the temporal side, with the base of the wedge at the limbus and the apex extending toward the lateral canthus. Within the triangle the conjunctiva is furrowed concentrically with the limbus, and dry flaky material can be seen falling from the area into the inferior cul-de-sac. A stained conjunctival scraping from a Bitot spot will show many saprophytic xerosis bacilli (*Corynebacterium xerosis*; small curved rods) and keratinized epithelial cells.

Avitaminosis A corneal ulceration results from dietary lack of vitamin A or impaired absorption from the gastrointestinal tract and impaired utilization by the body. It may develop in an infant who has a feeding problem; in an adult who is on a restricted or generally inadequate diet; or in any person with a biliary obstruction since bile in the gastrointestinal tract is necessary for the absorption of vitamin A. Lack of vitamin A causes a generalized keratinization of the epithelium throughout the body. The conjunctival and corneal changes together are known as **xerophthalmia.** Since the epithelium of the air passages is affected, many patients, if not treated, will die of pneumonia. Avitaminosis A also causes a generalized retardation of osseous growth. This is extremely important in infants; for example, if the skull bones do not grow and the brain continues to grow, increased intracranial pressure and papilledema can result.

Vitamin A should be administered in a dosage of at least 20,000 IU/d intramuscularly. Sulfonamide or antibiotic ointment can be used locally in the eye to prevent secondary bacterial infection. The average daily requirement of vitamin A is 1500– 5000 IU for children, according to age, and 5000 IU for adults.

NEUROTROPHIC CORNEAL ULCERS

If the trigeminal nerve, which supplies the cornea, is interrupted by trauma, surgery, tumor, inflammation, or in any other way, the cornea loses its sensitivity and one of its best defenses against degeneration, ulceration, and infection. In the early stages of a typical neurotrophic ulcer, fluorescein solution will produce punctate staining of the superficial epithelium. As this process progresses, patchy areas of denudation appear. Occasionally the epithelium may be absent from a large area of the cornea.

The progress of the condition depends on the treatment. Without treatment, the denuded areas become infected. The integrity of the cornea can be maintained as long as the corneal surface is kept moist by wearing a Buller shield,* by suturing the lids together, by using a conjunctival flap, or by using a therapeutic soft contact lens. Artificial tears may be of benefit. Under the best conditions, however, the prognosis is poor, and repeated epithelial breakdown often occurs.

EXPOSURE KERATITIS

Exposure keratitis may develop in any situation in which the cornea is not properly moistened and covered by the eyelids. Examples include exophthalmos from any cause, ectropion, the absence of part of an eyelid as a result of trauma, and inability to close the lids properly, as in Bell's palsy. The 2 factors at work are the drying of the cornea and its exposure to minor trauma. The uncovered cornea is particularly subject to drying during sleeping hours. If an ulcer

Figure 9–10. Keratomalacia with ulceration associated with xerophthalmia (dietary) in an infant. (Photo by Diane Beeston.)

*The Buller shield is a watertight cone of exposed x-ray film secured to the surrounding skin with adhesive tape.

develops it usually follows minor trauma and occurs in the inferior third of the cornea.

This type of keratitis will be sterile unless it is secondarily infected, and the therapeutic objective is to provide protection and moisture for the entire corneal surface. The method depends upon the underlying condition: a plastic procedure on the eyelids, a Buller shield,* soft lens, or surgical relief of exophthalmos.

DEGENERATIVE CORNEAL CONDITIONS

KERATOCONUS

Keratoconus is an uncommon degenerative bilateral disease that may be inherited as an autosomal recessive or autosomal dominant trait. Unilateral cases of unknown cause occur rarely. Symptoms appear in the second decade of life. The disease affects all races. Keratoconus has been associated with a number of diseases, including Down's syndrome, atopic dermatitis, retinitis pigmentosa, aniridia, vernal catarrh, Marfan's syndrome, Apert's syndrome, and Ehlers-Danlos syndrome. Pathologically, there are generalized thinning and anterior protrusion of the central cornea, ruptures in Descemet's membrane, and irregular, superficial linear scars at the apex of the cone that is formed.

Acute hydrops of the cornea may occur, in which there is sudden diminution of vision associated with central corneal edema. This usually arises as a consequence of rupture of Descemet's membrane and may

*The Buller shield is a watertight cone of exposed x-ray film secured to the surrounding skin with adhesive tape.

be triggered by the patient rubbing the eye. Acute hydrops usually clears gradually without treatment.

Blurred vision is the only symptom. Signs include cone-shaped cornea (Fig 9–11), indentation of the lower lid by the cornea when the patient looks down (Munson's sign), an irregular shadow on retinoscopy, and a distorted corneal reflection with Placido's disk or the keratoscope. The fundi cannot be clearly seen because of corneal distortion.

Corneal perforation may occur in advanced cases. When this happens, the eye should be bandaged and the dressing changed daily until a corneal scar seals the wound. Corneal transplantation may be necessary. Keratoconus is one of the most common indications for keratoplasty.

Contact lenses improve visual acuity in the early stages. A corneal transplant is indicated when the corrected visual acuity decreases to the point where it interferes with the patient's normal activities.

Keratoconus is often slowly progressive between the ages of 20 and 60, although an arrest in progression of the keratoconus may occur at any time. If a corneal transplant is done before extreme corneal thinning occurs, the prognosis is excellent; about 80–95% obtain reading vision.

CORNEAL DEGENERATION

The corneal degenerations are a rare group of slowly progressive, bilateral, degenerative disorders that usually appear in the second or third decades of life. Some are hereditary. Other cases follow ocular inflammatory disease, and some are of unknown cause.

Fatty or Lipoid Degeneration
This disorder may begin in infancy or adulthood.

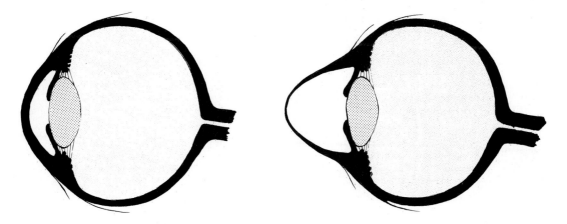

Figure 9–11. *Left:* Side view of normal cornea. *Right:* Keratoconus.

The cause is not known. There is a generalized deposition of lipid material within the corneal stroma, replacement of Bowman's layer by macrophages, and thickening of the epithelium with some infiltration of lipid material. Clinical findings include blurred vision and haziness and thickening of the cornea, particularly in the central zone.

Symptoms and signs are slowly progressive until useful vision is lost. Corneal transplant improves vision significantly in most cases.

Marginal Degeneration of the Cornea (Terrien's Disease)

This is a rare bilateral symmetric degeneration characterized by marginal thinning of the upper nasal quadrants of the cornea. Males are more commonly affected than females, and the condition occurs more frequently in the third and fourth decades. There are no symptoms except for mild irritation, and the condition is slowly progressive. The clinical picture consists of marginal thinning, arcuate opacity distal to the thinned area simulating arcus senilis, and vascularization. Perforation is a known complication of this condition and may lead to iris prolapse. Histopathologic studies of affected corneas have revealed vascularized connective tissue with fibrillary degeneration and fatty infiltration of collagen fibers.

Because the course of progression is slow and the central cornea is spared, the prognosis is good.

Calcific Band Keratopathy (Fig 9–12)

This disorder is characterized by the deposition of calcium salts in the anterior layers of the cornea. The keratopathy is usually limited to the interpalpebral area and appears as a band. The calcium deposits are noted in the basement membrane, Bowman's layer, and anterior stromal lamellas. A clear margin separates the calcific band from the limbus, and clear holes may be seen in the band, giving the Swiss cheese appearance. Symptoms include irritation, injection, and blurring of vision.

Calcific band keratopathy has been described in a number of inflammatory, metabolic, and degenerative conditions. It is characteristically associated with juvenile rheumatoid arthritis. It has been described in long-standing inflammatory conditions of the eye, glaucoma, and chronic cyclitis. Band keratopathy may also be associated with hyperparathyroidism, vitamin D intoxication, sarcoidosis, and leprosy. Treatment consists of ablation of the corneal epithelium by curettage under topical anesthesia followed by irrigation of the cornea with a sterile 0.01 M solution of ethylenediaminetetraacetic acid (EDTA) or application of EDTA with a cotton applicator.

Climatic Droplet Keratopathy (Pearl Diver's Keratopathy, Bietti's Keratopathy, Labrador Keratopathy, Spheroid Degeneration of the Cornea) (Fig 9–13)

Climatic droplet keratopathy is a relatively new clinical entity—an acquired keratopathy affecting mainly male adults who spend most of their working hours out of doors. The corneal degeneration is thought to be caused by exposure to ultraviolet light and is characterized in the early stages by fine subepithelial yellow droplets in the peripheral cornea. As the disease advances, the droplets become central, with subsequent corneal clouding causing blurred vision. Treatment in advanced cases is by corneal transplantation.

Figure 9–12. Calcific band keratopathy. (Courtesy of M Hogan.)

Figure 9–13. Climatic droplet keratopathy. Inset shows slit lamp view. (Courtesy of A Ahmad.)

Salzmann's Nodular Degeneration

This disorder is always preceded by corneal inflammation, particularly phlyctenular keratoconjunctivitis or trachoma. Symptoms include redness, irritation, and blurring of vision. There is degeneration of the superficial cornea that involves the stroma, Bowman's layer, and epithelium with superficial whitish-gray elevated nodules sometimes occurring in chains.

Corneal transplantation will significantly improve visual acuity in most cases.

ARCUS SENILIS
(Corneal Annulus, Anterior Embryotoxon)

Arcus senilis is an extremely common, bilateral, benign peripheral corneal degeneration that may occur at any age but is far more common in elderly people as part of the aging process. Arcus senilis in people under age 50 is usually associated with hypercholesterolemia.

Pathologically, lipid droplets involve the entire corneal thickness but are more concentrated in the superficial and deep layers, being relatively sparse in the corneal stroma.

There are no symptoms. Clinically, arcus senilis appears as a hazy gray ring about 2 mm in width and with a clear space between it and the limbus (Fig 9–14). No treatment is necessary, and there are no complications. Since arcus senilis causes no visual defect, it is not always classified with the corneal dystrophies.

HEREDITARY CORNEAL DYSTROPHIES

This is a group of rare hereditary disorders of the cornea of unknown cause characterized by bilateral

Figure 9–14. Arcus senilis. (Photo by Diane Beeston.)

abnormal deposition of substances and associated with alteration in the normal corneal architecture that may or may not interfere with vision. These corneal dystrophies usually manifest themselves during the first or second decade but sometimes later. They may be stationary or slowly progressive throughout life. Corneal transplantation improves vision in most patients with hereditary corneal dystrophy.

Anatomically, corneal dystrophies may be classified as anterior limiting membrane, stromal, and posterior limiting membrane dystrophies.

Anterior Limiting Membrane Corneal Dystrophies

A. Meesman's Dystrophy: This slowly progressive disorder is characterized by microcystic areas in the epithelium. The onset is in early childhood (first 1–2 years of life). The main symptom is slight irritation, and vision is slightly affected. The inheritance is autosomal dominant.

B. Cogan's Dystrophy: This condition is characterized by discrete comma-shaped or rounded, gray-white intraepithelial opacities located in the pupillary area. Fingerprint or maplike fine opacities may be seen at the level of the basement membrane. The disease is more common in females. Patients may develop recurrent erosion. Visual acuity is affected very slightly.

C. Fingerprint Dystrophy: This entity refers to fine wavy concentric lines located anterior to Bowman's layer that can be seen best by retroillumination with the slit lamp. These lines may be associated with a map- or dotlike pattern. The condition is asymptomatic but may be associated with recurrent erosion. The findings are noted during routine examination.

D. Recurrent Corneal Erosion: See p 123.

E. Others: Reis-Bücklers dystrophy is a dominantly inherited dystrophy affecting primarily Bowman's layer. The disease begins within the first decade of life with symptoms of recurrent erosion. Opacification of Bowman's layer gradually occurs and the epithelium is irregular. No vascularization is usually noted. Vision may be markedly reduced.

Vortex dystrophy, or cornea verticillata, is characterized by pigmented lines occurring in Bowman's layer or the underlying stroma and spreading over the entire corneal surface. Visual acuity is not markedly affected. Such a pattern of radiating pigmented lines may also be seen in patients suffering from chlorpromazine, chloroquine, or indomethacin toxicity as well as Fabry's disease.

Stromal Corneal Dystrophies

There are 3 types of stromal corneal dystrophies:

A. Granular Dystrophy: This usually asymptomatic, slowly progressive corneal dystrophy most often begins in early childhood. The lesions consist of central, fine, whitish "granular" lesions in the stroma of the cornea. The epithelium and Bowman's layer may be affected late in the disease. Visual acuity is slightly reduced. Histologically, the cornea shows uniform deposition of hyaline material. Corneal transplant is not needed except in very severe and late cases. The inheritance is autosomal dominant.

B. Macular Dystrophy: This type of stromal corneal dystrophy is manifested by a dense gray central opacity that starts in Bowman's layer. The opacity tends to spread toward the periphery and later involves the deeper stromal layers. Recurrent corneal erosion may occur, and vision is severely impaired. Histologic examination shows deposition of acid mucopolysaccharide in the stroma and degeneration of Bowman's layer.

The inheritance is autosomal recessive.

C. Lattice Dystrophy: Lattice dystrophy starts as fine, branching linear opacities in Bowman's layer in the central area and spreads to the periphery. The deep stroma may become involved, but the process does not reach Descemet's membrane. Recurrent erosion may occur. Histologic examination reveals amyloid deposits in the collagen fibers.

Posterior Limiting Membrane Corneal Dystrophies

A. Fuchs's Dystrophy: This disorder begins in the third or fourth decade and is slowly progressive throughout life. Women are more commonly affected than men. There are central wartlike deposits on Descemet's membrane, thickening of Descemet's membrane, and defects in the endothelium. Decompensation of the endothelium occurs and leads to edema of the corneal stroma and epithelium, causing blurring of vision. The cornea becomes progressively more opaque. Glaucoma or iris atrophy may be associated with this disorder. Histologic examination of the cornea reveals the wartlike excrescences over Descemet's membrane that are secreted by the endothelial cells. Thinning and pigmentation of the endothelium and thickening of Descemet's membrane are characteristic.

B. Posterior Polymorphous Dystrophy: This is a common disorder with onset in early childhood. Polymorphous plaques of calcium crystals are observed in the deep stromal layers. Vesicular lesions may be seen in the endothelium. Edema occurs in the deep stroma. The condition is asymptomatic in most cases, but in severe cases epithelial and total stromal edema may occur. The inheritance is autosomal dominant.

MISCELLANEOUS CORNEAL DISORDERS

SCLEROKERATITIS (Sclerosing Keratitis)

Sclerokeratitis is an uncommon, unilateral, localized inflammation of the sclera and cornea. The

Figure 9–15. Sclerokeratitis. Note fibrovascular scar in upper nasal quadrant of cornea.

cause is not known, but tuberculosis was formerly implicated. However, antituberculosis therapy is not effective. Pathologically, there are many chronic inflammatory cells (small round cells) in the involved portion of both structures. Fibrosis occurs in the later stages (Fig 9– 15). The patient complains of pain, photophobia, and irritation, but there is no discharge. A moderately severe iritis (anterior nongranulomatous uveitis) is usually associated.

No specific treatment is available. The pupil should be kept dilated with atropine, 2%, 2 drops once daily. Warm compresses and local corticosteroid drops are used to relieve the discomfort. Although the process starts as a small area of infiltration, it may progress to total corneal opacification. It may, however, subside after months or years.

SUPERFICIAL PUNCTATE KERATITIS

Superficial punctate keratitis is an uncommon chronic and recurrent bilateral disorder without regard to sex or age. It is characterized by discrete and elevated oval epithelial opacities that show punctate staining with fluorescein, mainly in the pupillary area. The opacities are not visible grossly but can be easily seen with the slit lamp or loupe. Subepithelial opacities underlying the epithelial lesions (ghosts) are often observed in patients who have been misdiagnosed as having herpes simplex keratitis and treated with topical idoxuridine.

No causative organism has been identified, but a virus is suspected. A varicella-zoster virus has been isolated from the corneal scrapings of one case.

Mild irritation, slight blurring of vision, and photophobia are the only symptoms. The conjunctiva is not involved.

Epithelial keratitis secondary to staphylococcal blepharoconjunctivitis is differentiated from superficial punctate keratitis by its involvement of the lower third of the cornea. Epithelial keratitis in trachoma is ruled out by its location in the upper third of the cornea and the presence of pannus. Many other forms of keratitis involving the superficial cornea are unilateral or are eliminated by their histories.

Short-term instillation of corticosteroid drops will often cause disappearance of the opacities and subjective improvement, but recurrences are the rule. The ultimate prognosis is good since there is no scarring or vascularization of the cornea. Untreated, the disease runs a protracted course of 1– 3 years. Long-term treatment with topical corticosteroids may prolong the course of the disease for many years and lead to steroid-induced cataract and glaucoma.

RECURRENT CORNEAL EROSION

This is a fairly common and serious mechanical corneal disorder that presents some classic signs and symptoms but may be easily missed if the physician does not look for it specifically. The patient is usually awakened during the early morning hours by a pain in the affected eye. The pain is continuous, and the eye becomes red, irritated, and photophobic. When the patient attempts to open the eyes in the morning, the lid pulls off the loose epithelium, resulting in pain and redness.

Three types of recurrent corneal erosions can be recognized:

(1) Acquired recurrent erosion (traumatic): The patient usually gives a history of previous corneal injury. It is unilateral, occurs with equal frequency in males and females, and the family history is negative. The recurrent erosion occurs most frequently in the center below the pupil no matter where the site of the previous corneal injury was.

(2) Familial recurrent erosion: This condition is bilateral and occurs more frequently in women. Patients give a family history of similar cases. There is usually no history of trauma.

(3) Recurrent erosion associated with corneal dystrophies: (See above.) Recurrent erosions of the cornea may be observed in patients with Cogan's microcystic corneal dystrophy, fingerprint dystrophy, and Reis-Bücklers corneal dystrophy.

Recurrent corneal erosion is due to a defect in the basement membrane of the corneal epithelium. The hemidesmosomes of the basal layer of the corneal epithelium fail to adhere to the basement membrane, and the corneal epithelium remains loose over the basement membrane with very slight subepithelial edema. The loose epithelial layers are vulnerable to separation and erosion.

Instillation of a local anesthetic relieves the symptoms immediately, and fluorescein staining will show the eroded area. This is typically a small area in the lower central cornea.

Treatment consists of a pressure bandage on the eye to promote healing. Mechanical denuding of the corneal epithelium may be necessary. The other eye should be kept closed most of the time to minimize movement of the lid over·the affected eye. Bed rest is desirable for 24 hours. The cornea usually heals in 2– 3 days. To prevent recurrence and to promote continued healing, it is important for these patients to use a bland ointment (eg, boric acid or other ocular lubricant) at bedtime for several months. In more severe cases, artificial tears are instilled during the day. The use of hypertonic ointment (glucose 40%) or 5% saline drops (Adsorbonac 5%) is often of value.

Rare instances of bilateral atraumatic dystrophic recurrent corneal erosion with a poor prognosis have also been reported.

INTERSTITIAL KERATITIS DUE TO CONGENITAL SYPHILIS

This self-limited inflammatory disease of the cornea is a late manifestation of congenital syphilis. There has been a sharp decrease in the incidence of the disease in recent years—almost to the point of extinction in some parts of the USA. It occasionally starts unilaterally but almost always becomes bilateral weeks to months later. It affects all races and is more common in females than males. Symptoms appear between the ages of 5 and 20. Pathologic findings include edema, lymphocytic infiltration, and vascularization of the corneal stroma.

Interstitial keratitis may be allergic in nature since *Treponema pallidum* is not found in the cornea during the acute phase. It has been postulated that these organisms enter the cornea at birth and that later in life there is a violent allergic reaction in the cornea to the organisms circulating in the bloodstream.

Clinical Findings

A. Symptoms and Signs: Other signs of congenital syphilis may be present, such as saddle nose and Hutchinson's triad (interstitial keratitis, deafness, and notched upper central incisors). The patient complains of pain, photophobia, and blurring of vision. Physical signs include conjunctival injection, corneal edema, vascularization of the deeper corneal layers, and miosis. There is an associated severe anterior granulomatous uveitis and blepharospasm due to photophobia. The grayish-pink appearance of the cornea (due to edema and vascularization) that occurs in the acute phase is sometimes referred to as a "salmon patch."

B. Laboratory Findings: Serologic tests for syphilis are positive.

Complications & Sequelae

Corneal scarring occurs if the process has been particularly severe and prolonged. Secondary glaucoma may result from the uveitis.

Treatment

There are no specific measures. Treatment is aimed at preventing the development of posterior synechiae, which will occur if the pupil is not dilated.

Both eyes should be dilated with frequent instillation of 2% atropine solution. Corticosteroid drops often relieve the symptoms dramatically but must be continued for long periods to prevent recurrence of symptoms. Dark glasses and a darkened room may be necessary if photophobia is severe. Treatment should be given for systemic syphilis, even though this usually has little effect on the ocular condition.

Corneal scarring may necessitate corneal transplant, and glaucoma, if present, may be difficult to control.

Course & Prognosis

The corneal disease process itself is not affected by treatment, which is aimed at prevention of complications. The inflammatory phase lasts 3 or 4 weeks. The corneas then gradually clear, leaving ghost vessels and scars in the corneal stroma.

INTERSTITIAL KERATITIS DUE TO OTHER CAUSES

Although congenital syphilis is no longer a common cause of interstitial keratitis, the disease still occurs as a complication of other granulomatous diseases, eg, tuberculosis and leprosy. Treatment is usually symptomatic, but it is important to establish the cause.

Cogan's syndrome is a rare disorder generally believed to be a vascular hypersensitivity reaction of unknown origin. It is a disease of young adults and is characterized by nonsyphilitic interstitial keratitis and a vestibuloauditory difficulty. Corticosteroids are reputed to be of value, but some degree of visual impairment and complete nerve deafness, with unresponsive labyrinths, usually supervene.

CORNEAL PIGMENTATION

Pigmentation of the cornea may occur with or without ocular or systemic disease. There are several distinct varieties.

Krukenberg's Spindle

In this disorder, brown uveal pigment is deposited bilaterally upon the central endothelial surface in a vertical spindle-shaped fashion. It occurs in a small percentage of people over age 20, usually in myopic women. It can be seen grossly but is best observed with the loupe or slit lamp. The visual acuity is only slightly affected, and the progression is extremely slow. Pigmentary glaucoma should be ruled out.

Blood Staining

This disorder occurs occasionally as a complication of traumatic hyphema and is due to hemosiderin in the corneal stroma. The cornea is golden brown, and vision is blurred. In most cases the cornea gradually clears in 1–2 years.

Kayser-Fleischer Ring

This is a pigmented ring whose color varies widely from ruby red to bright green, blue, yellow, or brown. The ring is 1–3 mm in diameter and located just inside the limbus posteriorly. In exceptional cases there is a second ring. The pigment is composed of fine granules immediately below the endothelium. It involves Descemet's membrane, rarely the stroma. Electron microscopic studies suggest that the pigment is a copper compound. The intensity of the pigmentation can be reduced markedly by the use of chelating agents.

These rings, which were long considered to be pathognomonic of hepatolenticular degeneration (Wilson's disease), have recently been described in 3 nonwilsonian patients with chronic hepatobiliary disease and in one patient with chronic cholestatic jaundice. Recognition of the Kayser-Fleischer rings, however, remains important, since they call attention to the possibility that the patient has Wilson's disease. Specific medical treatment with the copper chelating agent penicillamine may dramatically improve a disease that would otherwise inevitably be fatal.

Iron Lines (Hudson-Stähli Line, Fleischer's Ring, Stocker's Line, Ferry's Line)

Localized deposits of iron within the corneal epithelium may occur in sufficient quantity to become visible clinically. The Hudson-Stähli line is a horizontal line at the junction of the middle and lower thirds of the cornea, corresponding to the line of lid closure, in otherwise normal elderly patients. Fleischer's ring surrounds the base of the cone in keratoconus. Stocker's line is a vertical line associated with pterygia, and Ferry's line develops adjacent to limbal filtering blebs. Similar iron deposits are seen at the site of corneal scars.

CORNEAL TRANSPLANTATION

Corneal transplantation (keratoplasty) is indicated for a number of serious corneal conditions, eg, scarring, edema, thinning, and distortion. The term penetrating keratoplasty denotes full-thickness corneal replacement; lamellar keratoplasty denotes a partial-thickness procedure.

Young donors are preferred for penetrating keratoplasties; there is a direct relationship between age and the health of the endothelial cells. Because of the rapid endothelial cell death rate, the eyes should be enucleated soon after death and should be used within 48 hours, preferably within 24 hours.

For lamellar keratoplasty, corneas can be frozen,

Figure 9–16. Eight-millimeter Castroviejo disposable trephine. (Courtesy of R Biswell and T King.)

Figure 9–17. Penetrating keratoplasty with 10-0 nylon running suture, 3 months after operation. (Courtesy of R Biswell and T King.)

dehydrated, or refrigerated for several weeks; the endothelial cells are not important in this partial-thickness procedure.

Technique

The recipient eye is prepared by a partial-thickness cutting of a circle of diseased cornea with a trephine (cookie cutter action) (Fig 9– 16) and full-thickness removal with scissors or partial-thickness removal with dissection.

The donor eye is prepared in 2 ways. For penetrating keratoplasty, the entire cornea is placed endothelium up on a Teflon block; the trephine is pressed down into the cornea, and a full-thickness button is punched out. In lamellar keratoplasty, a partial-thickness trephine incision is made in the cornea and the lamellar button is dissected free. Certain refinements in technique, such as free hand grafts, may be necessary.

In recent years, refined sutures (Fig 9– 17) and instruments and sophisticated operating microscopes and illuminating systems have significantly improved the prognosis in all patients requiring corneal transplants.

REFRACTIVE CORNEAL SURGERY

Roderick Biswell, MD

Spectacles are considered inconvenient or unattractive by many wearers. Corneal contact lenses, invented by Kalt and improved by Tuohy, have solved many optical and cosmetic problems but have introduced other complications, and the search for an alternative solution to the correction of refractive errors continues. Refractive surgery is controversial and still regarded in most instances as only investigational.

Complications may produce visual loss, and these procedures should not be undertaken without strong justification.

Radial Keratotomy

In the late 1940s, Sato of Japan created anterior and posterior corneal incisions to alter the curvature of the cornea. Results were poor, and endothelial decompensation with corneal edema occurred frequently. In 1972, Fyodorov of the USSR began to use anterior corneal cuts only. Currently, the operation consists of radial incisions involving 90% of the corneal thickness and extending from a clear optical zone (usually the central 3 mm or more of the cornea) toward but not up to the limbus. The amount of correction achieved is modified by the size of the optical zone and the number and depth of the incisions. Various formulas and computer programs are used to determine the value of these parameters in each case.

There is general agreement that radial keratotomy does reduce the degree of myopia and is most effective for myopia in the lower range (-2 to -4 diopters). But there is a significant degree of unpredictability in the final result, with under- or overcorrection or even progressive hyperopia. Glare, fluctuations of vision during the day, and a return of increased myopia are commonly reported side effects. Delayed healing of corneal incisions, with corneal infections occurring up to 2 years after the procedure; endophthalmitis; traumatic cataract; and endothelial cell loss may all lead to permanent loss of vision. Agreement on whether the procedure should be done at all has not been reached.

Keratomileusis

In 1961, Barraquer of Colombia reported on the technique of myopic keratomileusis for the correction of high degrees of myopia. The procedure has been performed in other countries but by relatively few surgeons. A deep lamellar corneal autograft is cut;

the tissue is frozen and then reshaped with a cryolathe to obtain a flatter curvature after thawing; and the autograft is then sutured back into position. Expensive cryolathe and microkeratome equipment is required. The procedure has also been used for hyperopia.

Complications of keratomileusis include improper depth of the lamellar bed, delayed epithelialization over the resutured tissue, interface epithelial growth and opacity, and irregular astigmatism.

Keratophakia

In keratophakia, a cryolathe is used to shape a donor cornea into a lens, which is then inserted into a lamellar bed. The outer disk of the recipient cornea, which was removed prior to placement of the donor lenticule, is sutured back into position, thus thickening and steepening the cornea. Up to +15 diopters can be corrected. The procedure has been recommended for young aphakic patients who cannot tolerate contact lenses and are poor candidates for secondary lens implantation. The operation has also been performed at the time of cataract extraction. Complications have included interface opacities and astigmatism, both of which may take many months to stabilize or may never do so.

Epikeratophakia

In epikeratophakia (a rarely used procedure), an epigraft of homologous tissue is sutured to a peripheral circular groove or wedge of tissue formed in the surface corneal stroma, following removal of the host corneal epithelium. The donor lens is precut on a cryolathe and lyophilized. The procedure has been described by Kaufman and others as useful for myopia, hypermetropia, keratoconus, and even astigmatism (toric epigraft). Childhood aphakia has been mentioned prominently as an indication, since contact lenses are difficult for children to use and intraocular lens implants difficult to perform in these patients.

The procedure can be combined with congenital cataract surgery. Epikeratophakia has also been used on scarred corneas and on corneas affected with endothelial dystrophy. It has been described as having few complications because the graft can be removed at any time.

Operation to Correct Astigmatism

Various patterns of keratotomy have been described to correct corneal astigmatism. These cuts can be used alone or with radial keratotomy. Irregular astigmatism continues to be a serious problem following most corneal operations, including radial keratotomy and penetrating keratoplasty, and after cataract surgery. Troutman and others have described relaxing incisions and wedge resections for postkeratoplasty astigmatism, utilizing a surgical keratometer. Various techniques for cataract incision, such as scleral "pocket" incisions, have been reported as useful in preventing postoperative astigmatism after cataract surgery.

Alloplastic Corneal Implants

Disks of many different materials have been inserted into corneal stromal pockets, initially to control corneal edema but more recently to correct refractive errors. In most cases, the corneal tissue anterior to the implant undergoes necrosis. Hydrogel and polysulfone lenses have been more successful than other types of lenses tried so far. Use of alloplastic corneal implants would remove the need to rely on autologous or homologous material in refractive surgery.

Clear Lens Removal

A few surgeons around the world have advocated the removal of clear lenses in high degrees of myopia, suggesting that the risk of doing so is minimal owing to the safety of extracapsular lens extraction. The procedure is controversial.

REFERENCES

Adams CP Jr et al: Corneal ulcers in patients with cosmetic extended-wear contact lenses. *Am J Ophthalmol* 1983;**96:**705.

Angell LK et al: Visual prognosis in patients with ruptures in Descemet's membrane due to forceps injuries. *Arch Ophthalmol* 1981;**99:**2137.

Barraquer JI: Keratomileusis for myopia and aphakia. *Ophthalmology* 1981;**88:**701.

Baum J, Barza M: Topical vs subconjunctival treatment of bacterial corneal ulcers. *Ophthalmology* 1983;**90:**162.

Belmont SC, Troutman RC: Compensating compression sutures in wedge resection. *J Refract Surg* (July-Aug) 1985;**1:**104.

Bloomfield SE, Jakobiec FA, Theodore FH: Contact lens induced keratopathy: A severe complication extending the spectrum of keratoconjunctivitis in contact lens wearers. *Ophthalmology* 1984;**91:**290.

Boger WP III et al: Keratoconus and acute hydrops. *Am J Ophthalmol* 1981;**91:**231.

Boisjoly HM et al: Superinfections in herpes simplex keratitis. *Am J Ophthalmol* 1983;**96:**354.

Boyd BF: Does refractive surgery have a significant future? *Highlights of Ophthalmology* 1985;**13(12):**1. [Entire issue.]

Brown N, Bron A: Recurrent erosion of the cornea. *Br J Ophthalmol* 1976;**60:**84.

Brown SI, Mondino BJ: Therapy of Mooren's ulcer. *Am J Ophthalmol* 1984;**98:**1.

Cole EL et al: Herpes zoster ophthalmicus and acquired immune deficiency syndrome. *Arch Ophthalmol* 1984;**102:**1027.

Forster RK, Rebell G: The diagnosis and management of keratomycoses. *Arch Ophthalmol* 1975;**93:**975.

Friedlaender MH et al: Update on keratophakia. *Ophthalmology* 1983;**90:**365.

Goldsmith MF: Caveat emptor tops the eye chart for radial keratotomy candidates. *JAMA* 1985;**254:**3401.

Kaufman HE, Centifanto-Fitzgerald YM, Varnell ED: Herpes simplex keratitis. *Ophthalmology* 1983;**90:**700.

Kenyon KR: Decision-making in the therapy of external eye disease: Noninfected corneal ulcers. *Ophthalmology* 1982;**89:**44.

Kim HB, Ostler HB: Marginal corneal ulcer due to β-streptococcus. *Arch Ophthalmol* 1977;**95:**454.

Klintworth GK et al: Recurrence of lattice corneal dystrophy type 1 in the corneal grafts of two siblings. *Am J Ophthalmol* 1982;**94:**540.

Lemp MA et al: Gram-negative corneal ulcers in elderly aphakic eyes with extended-wear lenses. *Ophthalmology* 1984;**91:**60.

Leopold IH: Update on antibiotics in ocular infections. *Am J Ophthalmol* 1985;**100:**134.

Malbran ES: Corneal dystrophies: A clinical, pathological, and surgical approach: The 28th Edward Jackson Memorial Lecture. *Am J Ophthalmol* 1972;**74:**771.

McDonald MB et al: Alloplastic epikeratophakia for the correction of aphakia. *Ophthalmic Surg* 1983;**14:**65.

Meisler DM, Friedlander MH, Okumoto M: *Mycobacterium chelonei* keratitis. *Am J Ophthalmol* 1982;**94:**398.

Murray PI, Rahi AHS: Pathogenesis of Mooren's ulcer: Some new concepts. *Br J Ophthalmol* 1984;**68:**182.

Nassif KF et al: Factors that influence the efficacy of topical gentamicin prophylaxis for experimental *Pseudomonas* keratitis. *Am J Ophthalmol* 1982;**94:**216.

Olson R (editor): Common corneal problems. *Int Ophthalmol Clin* (Summer) 1984;**24.** [Entire issue.]

Ostler HB, Thygeson P, Okumoto M: Infectious diseases of the eye. 3. Infections of the cornea. *J Cont Educ Ophthalmol* (Sept) 1978;**40:**13.

Perry LD, Brinser JH, Kolodner H: Anaerobic corneal ulcers. *Ophthalmology* 1982;**89:**636.

Sanford-Smith JH, Whittle HC: Corneal ulceration following measles in Nigerian children. *Br J Ophthalmol* 1979;**63:**720.

Sanitato JJ et al: Acyclovir in the treatment of herpetic stromal disease. *Am J Ophthalmol* 1984;**98:**537.

Sen DK: Surgery of pterygium. *Br J Ophthalmol* 1970;**54:**606.

Shimeld C: Isolation of herpes simplex virus from the cornea in chronic stromal keratitis. *Br J Ophthalmol* 1982;**66:**643.

Sommer A: Effects of vitamin A deficiency on the ocular surface. *Ophthalmology* 1983;**90:**592.

Sommer A: Treatment of corneal xerophthalmia with topical retinoic acid. *Am J Ophthalmol* 1983;**95:**349.

Tabbara KF, Shammas HF: Bilateral corneal perforations in Stevens-Johnson syndrome. *Can J Ophthalmol* 1975;**10:**514.

Tabbara KF et al: Thygeson's superficial punctate keratitis. *Ophthalmology* 1981;**88:**75.

Thygeson P: Clinical and laboratory observations on superficial punctate keratitis. *Am J Ophthalmol* 1960;**61:**1344.

Thygeson P, Okumoto M: Keratomycosis: A preventable disease. *Trans Am Acad Ophthalmol Otolaryngol* 1974;**78:**433.

Torres MA et al: Topical ketoconazole for fungal keratitis. *Am J Ophthalmol* 1985;**100:**293.

Waring GO III et al: The corneal endothelium: Normal and pathologic structure and function. *Ophthalmology* 1982; **89:**531.

Waring GO III et al; Prospective evaluation of radial keratotomy (PERK): Clinical aspects. *Ophthalmic Forum* 1982;**1:**30.

Weiss JL et al: The use of tissue adhesive in corneal perforations. *Ophthalmology* 1983;**90:**610.

Werblin TP: Epikeratophakia: Techniques, complications, and clinical results. *Int Ophthalmol Clin* (Fall) 1983;**23:**45.

Wilson LA, Schlitzer RL, Ahearn DG: *Pseudomonas* corneal ulcers associated with soft contact-lens wear. *Am J Ophthalmol* 1981;**92:**546.

Sclera

ANATOMY & FUNCTION

The sclera is the fibrous outer protective coating of the eye. It is dense and white and continuous with the cornea anteriorly and with the dural sheath of the optic nerve posteriorly. At the insertion of the rectus muscles, it is about 0.3 mm thick; elsewhere, about 1 mm thick. A few strands of scleral tissue pass over the optic disk. This sievelike structure is known as the lamina cribrosa. Around the optic nerve, the sclera is penetrated by the long and short posterior ciliary arteries and the long and short ciliary nerves. Slightly posterior to the equator, the 4 vortex veins exit through the sclera, usually one in each quadrant. About 4 mm posterior to the limbus, the 4 anterior ciliary arteries and veins penetrate the sclera. Each set penetrates slightly anterior to the insertion of a rectus muscle.

The outer surface of the sclera is covered by a thin layer of fine elastic tissue, the episclera, containing numerous blood vessels that nourish the sclera. The brown pigment layer on the inner surface is the lamina fusca, which is continuous with the sclera and the choroid. On the inner surface at 180 degrees (in a horizontal plane through 9 and 3 o'clock), there is a shallow groove from the optic nerve to the ciliary body in which are embedded the long posterior ciliary artery and the long ciliary nerve. The nerve supply to the sclera is from the ciliary nerves.

Histologically, the sclera consists of many dense bands of parallel and interlacing fibrous tissue bundles each of which is 10–16 μm thick and 100–140 μm wide. The histologic structure of the sclera is remarkably similar to that of the cornea; this raises the question why the cornea is transparent and the sclera opaque. The apparent physiologic reason is the relative deturgescence of the cornea and the less uniform structure of the sclera. The cornea has the ability to absorb a great deal of water, whereupon it becomes opaque; the sclera is almost completely hydrated in its normal state.

DISEASES & DISORDERS OF THE SCLERA

BLUE SCLERAS

The normal sclera is white and opaque, so that the underlying uveal structures are not visible. Structural changes of the scleral collagen fibers and thinning of the sclera may allow the underlying uveal pigment to be seen, giving the sclera a bluish discoloration. Blue sclera occurs in several disorders that lead to disturbances in the connective tissues, particularly the collagen fibers. Blue scleras are part of the clinical picture in osteogenesis imperfecta, Ehlers-Danlos syndrome, pseudoxanthoma elasticum, Marfan's syndrome, and pseudohypoparathyroidism and may occur with prolonged use of corticosteroids. Blue scleras are sometimes noted in normal newborn infants, in keratoconus, and in keratoglobus.

SCLERAL ECTASIA

Prolonged elevation of intraocular pressure early in infancy, such as occurs in cases of congenital glaucoma, may lead to stretching and ectasia of the sclera. Scleral ectasia may occur as a congenital anomaly surrounding the disk or occasionally in the macular area. It may also follow inflammation or injury of the sclera.

STAPHYLOMA

Staphyloma results from bulging of the uvea into a thinned and stretched sclera. Staphylomas can be characterized as ectatic dark blue, bulging areas involving a localized segment of the eyeball. The staphyloma may be anterior, equatorial, or posterior. Anterior staphylomas are generally located over the ciliary body (ciliary staphyloma) (Fig 10–1) or between the ciliary body and the limbus (intercalary staphyloma). Equatorial staphylomas are located at the equator and posterior staphylomas posterior to the equator. Posterior staphylomas are most commonly seen at the optic nerve head. They affect the lamina cribrosa and

Figure 10–1. Ciliary staphyloma. (Courtesy of P Thygeson.)

Figure 10–2. Nodular episcleritis, right eye. (Photo by Diane Beeston.)

may follow extreme myopia. Large congenital posterior staphylomas associated with poor vision have been observed. Patients having such conditions are generally extremely myopic. Cases of congenital peripapillary staphylomas in patients with normal or nearly normal vision have been reported. Posterior staphyloma is usually associated with areas of pronounced choroidal atrophy.

Staphyloma must be differentiated from extreme myopia and scleral ectasia in a coloboma of the optic nerve head.

INTRASCLERAL NERVE LOOPS OF AXENFELD

The intrascleral nerve loops are sites of branches of the long ciliary nerves. They enter the sclera close to the ciliary body and about 3.5 mm from the limbus. They are more commonly seen nasally. They may be pigmented and are usually accompanied by the small anterior ciliary artery in its inward course.

INFLAMMATION OF THE SCLERA & EPISCLERA

Inflammation involving the episclera, the thin layer of vascular elastic tissue overlying the sclera, is referred to as **episcleritis. Scleritis** is inflammation of the sclera itself, with or without inflammation of the episclera. The 2 diseases are considered distinct clinical entities and will be considered separately.

Episcleritis

This is a relatively common localized inflammation of the episclera. It is unilateral in about two-thirds of cases, and the sex incidence is equal. It may recur at the same or adjacent sites in the palpebral fissure.

The cause is not known, but hypersensitivity reactions may play a role. Certain systemic diseases such as rheumatoid arthritis, Sjögren's syndrome, coccidioidomycosis, syphilis, herpes zoster, and tuberculosis have been associated with episcleritis.

Symptoms of episcleritis include redness, pain, photophobia, tenderness, and lacrimation. Ocular examination reveals localized hyperemia that gives the eyeball a pink or purple color. There is also infiltration, congestion, and edema of the episclera, the overlying conjunctiva, and the underlying Tenon capsule. Two types of episcleritis are recognized: simple and nodular (Fig 10–2). The sclera itself is not involved. About 15% of patients with episcleritis develop mild iritis.

Conjunctivitis is ruled out by the localized nature of episcleritis and the lack of palpebral conjunctival involvement.

The condition is benign, and the course is generally self-limited in 1–2 weeks. However, recurrences may torment the patient for years. Topical therapy with corticosteroids (dexamethasone, 0.1%) resolves the inflammatory changes in 3 or 4 days. Corticosteroids are more effective in simple episcleritis than in nodular episcleritis.

Scleritis

Inflammation of the sclera is less common than episcleritis (Fig 10–3). Scleritis is a relatively rare chronic inflammation of the sclera that is frequently associated with systemic diseases. The causes of scleritis are listed in Table 10–1. The disease may be unilateral or bilateral, and women are more commonly affected than men.

Scleritis is classified according to its clinical and pathologic features. Two types are recognized: anterior and posterior. Anterior scleritis may be subdivided into diffuse, nodular, or necrotizing scleritis with or without adjacent inflammation.

Figure 10–3. Nodular scleritis, left eye, associated with rheumatoid arthritis. (Courtesy of GR O'Connor.)

The symptoms of scleritis include pain, redness, photophobia, tenderness, and lacrimation. Pain is usually more severe than in episcleritis.

Examination reveals an intense violaceous, purple-bluish discoloration that may be diffuse. Episcleral and conjunctival tissues are also involved, and the vessels are characteristically dilated. A practical aid in diagnosis is the topical application of 1 drop of epinephrine, 1:1000, which constricts the superficial vessels but not the deeper scleral vessels. Areas of avascularity may suggest occlusive vasculitis and imply a grave prognosis. Elevated nodules are noted in nodular scleritis. These are often encountered in rheumatoid arthritis as well.

A. Necrotizing Scleritis: The most severe form of scleritis is necrotizing scleritis with adjacent inflammation, otherwise known as **brawny scleritis.** This disorder is characterized by an acute, painful, tender area of localized congestion and necrosis that leads

Table 10–1. Causes of scleritis.

Collagen diseases:
   Ankylosing spondylitis
   Rheumatoid arthritis
   Polyarteritis nodosa
   Relapsing polychondritis
   Wegener's granulomatosis
   Systemic lupus erythematosus
Granulomatous diseases:
   Tuberculosis
   Syphilis
   Sarcoidosis
   Leprosy
Metabolic disorders: Gout, thyrotoxicosis, active rheumatic
   heart disease, psoriatic arthritis
Infections: Onchocerciasis, herpes zoster, herpes simplex
Others:
   Physical (irradiation, thermal burns)
   Chemical (alkali and acid burns)
   Mechanical (penetrating injuries)
Unknown

to thinning and destruction of the scleral collagen fibers. There may be an avascular area in the overlying episcleral tissue. The disease may remain localized or may progress to involve the entire anterior sclera, allowing visualization of the underlying uvea. Elevation of the intraocular pressure may exacerbate scleral ectasia. Corticosteroids may exacerbate both scleral thinning and destruction of collagen fibers.

B. Necrotizing Scleromalacia (Scleromalacia Perforans): This is a rare scleral disease characterized by thinning and melting of the scleral tissue, leading to areas of dehiscence without any history or clinical evidence of inflammation of the sclera. This form of ''scleral melting'' is usually associated with severe forms of rheumatoid arthritis. As is true also of necrotizing scleritis, uveal pigment may be visualized through the areas of scleral thinning. Such thinning may lead to bulging. Rupture of the globe secondary to minor trauma may occur, but this is rare. The prognosis depends on the area of the globe affected but is in general poor. Corticosteroids are contraindicated. In cases of perforation or impending perforation, treatment may consist of repair of the dehiscence with a segment of homologous preserved sclera.

C. Posterior Scleritis: This is an uncommon disorder and is difficult to diagnose because of the absence of signs in the anterior segment. CT scan with contrast medium is valuable in making the diagnosis. The disease should be suspected in patients with pain, proptosis, papilledema, and exudative retinal detachment. The disease is unilateral and is associated with severe pain, a decrease in visual acuity, diplopia, and limitation of ocular movements. Posterior scleritis is usually associated with severe rheumatoid arthritis. Recurrences may lead to extreme thinning of the sclera, giving rise to posterior staphyloma or perforation, especially when intraocular pressure is elevated. Ocular complications other than perforation include keratitis, uveitis, cataract, and glaucoma.

Scleritis is generally resistant to treatment. Topical corticosteroids should be used only with extreme caution because of their potential thinning effects on the scleral tissue and because of the possibility of increasing the intraocular pressure in certain patients. Systemic nonsteroidal anti-inflammatory agents such as salicylates, indomethacin, or ibuprofen appear to be effective in some patients. Systemic immunosuppressive agents are rarely indicated for the treatment of severe resistant forms of scleritis.

INJURIES OF THE SCLERA

The most frequently encountered injuries of the sclera are trauma (penetrating and blunt), physical damage (irradiation, thermal burns), and chemical injuries (alkali and acid burns).

Scleral wounds (lacerations) may result either from blunt trauma or from penetrating trauma caused by sharp instruments or flying objects. Scleral lacerations may be associated with intraocular hemorrhage and injury to other ocular structures. The management of scleral lacerations includes microbiologic control (surface antisepsis and the preparation of a sterile field), suturing of the wound, and excision of any prolapsed uveal tissue. Lacerations of the conjunctiva and Tenon's capsule must be approximated over the scleral wound.

HYALINE DEGENERATION

Hyaline degeneration is a fairly frequent finding in the scleras of persons over age 60. It is manifested by small, round, translucent gray areas that are usually about 2–3 mm in diameter and are located anterior to the insertion of the rectus muscles. They cause no symptoms or complications.

REFERENCES

Cobo M: Inflammation of the sclera. *Int Ophthalmol Clin* 1983;**23**:159.

Foster CS, Forstot SL, Wilson LA: Mortality rate in rheumatoid arthritis patients developing necrotizing scleritis or peripheral ulcerative keratitis: Effects of systemic immunosuppression. *Ophthalmology* 1984;**91**:1253.

Koenig SB, Kaufman HE: The treatment of necrotizing scleritis with an autogenous periosteal graft. *Ophthalmic Surg* 1983;**14**:1029.

Watson PG, Bovey E: Anterior segment fluorescein angiography in the diagnosis of scleral inflammation. *Ophthalmology* 1985;**92**:1.

Young RD, Watson PG: Microscopical studies of necrotising scleritis. 1. Cellular aspects. 2. Collagen degradation in the scleral stroma. *Br J Ophthalmol* 1984;**68**:770, 781.

11

Uveal Tract

The uveal tract is composed of 3 parts: the iris, the ciliary body, and the choroid. It is the middle, vascular layer of the eye, protected externally by the cornea and sclera. It contributes to the blood supply of the retina.

Anatomy of the Iris

The iris is the anterior extension of the ciliary body. It presents a relatively flat surface with a round aperture in the middle called the pupil, which varies in size and has the same form and function as the aperture of a camera. The sphincter and dilator muscles, which serve to constrict and dilate the pupil, are in the iris stroma. The iris lies in contact with the lens and divides the anterior chamber from the posterior chamber, each of which contains aqueous humor.

Because of the presence of a thick collagenous adventitia, normal iris vessels have the histologic appearance of being quite sclerotic. The iris capillaries have an unfenestrated endothelium and hence do not normally leak intravenously injected fluorescein. The 2 layers of epithelium on the posterior surface are heavily pigmented and represent the anterior extension of the pigmented epithelium of the retina as well as the retina proper. The blood supply is from the major circle of the iris (Fig 1–9). The nerve supply is described in Chapter 18.

When the iris is cut, as in doing a small peripheral iridectomy for acute angle-closure glaucoma, it seldom bleeds, and the wound remains permanently with no tendency to heal. Pain fibers are present, as is shown by the pain caused by traction on the iris during surgery.

Anatomy of the Ciliary Body

The ciliary body, roughly triangular in cross section, extends forward from the anterior termination of the choroid to the root of the iris, a distance of about 6 mm. Grossly it consists of 2 zones: the corona ciliaris, the corrugated anterior 2 mm; and the pars plana, the smoother and flatter posterior 4 mm. The surface of the corona ciliaris consists of many elevations and depressions.

There are 2 layers of ciliary epithelium, the external pigmented and the internal nonpigmented, both of which continue as pigmented layers over the posterior surface of the iris. The pigment epithelium represents the forward extension of the pigment epithelium of the retina.

The ciliary muscle consists of longitudinal, radial, and circular portions. Its function is to contract and relax the zonular fibers. This results in altered tension on the capsule of the lens, which gives the lens variable focus for both near and more distant objects in the field of vision. The ciliary processes themselves are composed mainly of capillaries and veins that drain through vortex veins. The capillaries are large and fenestrated and hence leak intravenously injected fluorescein.

The pars plana consists of a thin layer of ciliary muscle and vessels covered by ciliary epithelium. The zonular fibers, which hold the lens in place, originate in the valleys between the ciliary processes (Fig 11–1). The blood vessels to the ciliary body come from the major circle of the iris (Fig 1–9). The sensory nerve supply is through the ciliary nerves.

Anatomy of the Choroid (Fig 11–2)

The choroid (the posterior portion of the uveal tract and the middle coat of the eye) lies between the retina and the sclera. It is largely composed of blood

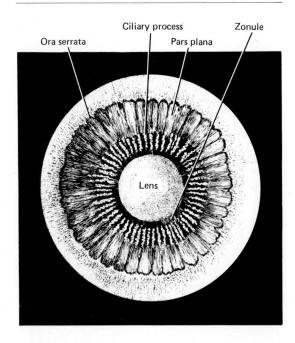

Figure 11–1. Posterior view of ciliary body, zonule, lens, and ora serrata. (Redrawn and reproduced, with permission, from Wolff E: *Anatomy of the Eye and Orbit,* 4th ed. Blakiston-McGraw, 1954.)

vessels. The choroidal vessels are bounded by Bruch's membrane internally and the suprachoroid externally. The avascular suprachoroid is composed of lamellas of collagenous and elastic tissue. Bruch's membrane can be divided into 3 portions: an outer elastic sheath, a middle collagenous sheath, and an inner cuticular sheath. (The latter is actually the basement membrane of the retinal pigment epithelium.)

The lumens of the blood vessels increase the deeper they are located in the choroid. There are 3 layers of blood vessels: large, medium, and small. The innermost layer of small blood vessels is known as the choriocapillaris and consists of large capillaries that nourish the outer portion of the retina. The endothelium of these capillaries is fenestrated and hence leaks intravenously injected fluorescein. Most of the large vessels consist of veins. These coalesce and leave the eye as the 4 vortex veins, one in each of the 4 posterior quadrants. The vessel layers of the choroid also contain some elastic fibers and chromatophores.

The choroid is firmly attached to the margin of the optic nerve posteriorly and extends to the ora serrata anteriorly, where it joins the ciliary body.

Functions of Uveal Structures

The function of the iris is to control the amount of light that enters the eye. This occurs by reflex constriction of the pupil under the stimulus of light and dilatation of the pupil in darkness. The ciliary body forms the root of the iris and serves, through the zonular fibers, to govern the size of the lens in accommodation. Aqueous humor is secreted by the ciliary processes into the posterior chamber. The choroid consists of abundant blood vessels; its function is to nourish the outer portion of the underlying retina.

Physiology of Symptoms

Symptoms of uveal tract disorders depend upon the site of the disease process. For example, since there are pain fibers in the iris, the patient with iritis will complain of moderate pain and photophobia. Inflammation of the iris itself does not cause blurring of vision unless the process is severe or advanced enough to cause clouding of the aqueous humor, cornea, or lens. Choroidal disease itself does not cause pain or blurred vision. Because of the close contact of the choroid with the retina, choroidal disease almost always affects the retina (eg, chorioretinitis). If the macular area of the retina is involved, central vision will be impaired.

The vitreous may also become cloudy as a result of posterior uveitis. The impairment of vision is in proportion to the density of vitreous opacity and is reversible as the inflammation subsides and the vitreous haze clears.

The physician examines for disease of the anterior uveal tract with the flashlight and loupe or slit lamp, and disease of the posterior uveal tract with the ophthalmoscope.

UVEITIS*

Inflammation of the uveal tract has many causes and may involve one or all 3 portions simultaneously. The most frequent form of uveitis is acute anterior uveitis (iritis), usually unilateral and characterized by a history of pain, photophobia, and blurring of vision; a red eye (circumcorneal flush) without purulent dis-

*"Uveitis" is a general term for inflammatory disorders of the uveal tract. "Anterior uveitis" is the preferred general term for iritis and iridocyclitis. "Posterior uveitis" is the preferred term for choroiditis and chorioretinitis. The term "iritis," used above, means acute anterior nongranulomatous uveitis.

Figure 11–2. Cross section of choroid. (Redrawn and reproduced, with permission, from Wolff E: *Anatomy of the Eye and Orbit,* 4th ed. Blakiston-McGraw, 1954.)

Labels in figure: Bruch's membrane; Suprachoroid; Pigment epithelium; Smaller choroidal vessels (choriocapillaris); Larger choroidal vessels; Sclera

Table 11–1. Differentiation of granulomatous and nongranulomatous uveitis.

	Nongranulomatous	Granulomatous
Onset	Acute	Insidious
Pain	Marked	None or minimal
Photophobia	Marked	Slight
Blurred vision	Moderate	Marked
Circumcorneal flush	Marked	Slight
Keratic precipitates	Fine white	Large gray ("mutton fat")
Pupil	Small and irregular	Small and irregular (variable)
Posterior synechiae	Sometimes	Sometimes
Anterior chamber	Flare predominates	Cells predominate
Iris nodules	Sometimes	Sometimes
Vitreous haze	Absent	Sometimes
Site	Anterior tract	Posterior tract (variable)
Course	Acute	Chronic
Prognosis	Good	Fair to poor
Recurrence	Common	Sometimes

charge; and a small pupil. It is important to make the diagnosis early and to dilate the pupil to prevent the formation of permanent posterior synechiae.

Inflammatory disorders of the uveal tract, usually unilateral, are common principally in the young and middle age groups. In most cases the cause is not known. In posterior uveitis the retina is almost always secondarily affected. This is known as chorioretinitis.

Two major types of uveitis may be distinguished upon clinical as well as pathologic grounds: nongranulomatous (more common) and granulomatous (Table 11–1).* Because pathogenic organisms have not been found in the nongranulomatous type and because it responds to corticosteroid therapy, it is thought to be a hypersensitivity phenomenon. Granulomatous uveitis usually follows active microbial invasion of the tissues by the causative organism (eg, *Mycobacterium tuberculosis* or *Toxoplasma gondii*). However, these pathogens are rarely recovered, and a definite etiologic diagnosis is seldom possible. The possibilities can often be narrowed down by clinical and laboratory examination.

Nongranulomatous uveitis occurs mainly in the anterior portion of the tract, ie, the iris and ciliary body. There is an inflammatory reaction, as evidenced by the cellular infiltration of lymphocytes and plasma cells in significant numbers and an occasional mononuclear cell. In severe cases, a large fibrin clot or a hypopyon may form in the anterior chamber.

Granulomatous uveitis may involve any portion of the uveal tract but has a predilection for the posterior uvea. Nodular collections of epithelioid cells and giant cells surrounded by lymphocytes are present in the

*The clinical differentiation of the 2 types is not always clear. In some clinics, this classification has been discarded in favor of an anatomic differentiation into 3 types: anterior, posterior, and diffuse.

affected areas. Inflammatory deposits on the posterior surface of the cornea are composed mainly of macrophages and epithelioid cells. It is possible to make a specific etiologic diagnosis histologically in an enucleated eye by identifying the cysts of *Toxoplasma*, the acid-fast bacillus of tuberculosis, the spirochete of syphilis, the distinctive granulomatous appearance of sarcoidosis and sympathetic ophthalmia, and a few other rare specific causes.

Clinical Findings

A. Symptoms and Signs: In the nongranulomatous form, the onset is characteristically acute, with pain, injection, photophobia, and blurred vision. There is a circumcorneal flush caused by dilated limbal blood vessels. Fine white deposits (keratic precipitates, "KPs") on the posterior surface of the cornea can be seen with the slit lamp or with a loupe. The pupil is small, and there may be a collection of fibrin with cells in the anterior chamber. If posterior synechiae are present, the pupil will be irregular in shape (Figs 11–3 to 11–6). Posterior uveitis is generally classified as granulomatous.

The patient should be asked about previous episodes of arthritis and possible exposure to toxoplasmosis, histoplasmosis, tuberculosis, and syphilis. The remote possibility of a focus of infection elsewhere in the body should also be investigated.

In granulomatous uveitis (which may cause anterior uveitis, posterior uveitis, or both), the onset is usually insidious. Vision gradually becomes blurred, and the affected eye becomes diffusely red with circumcorneal flush. Pain is minimal, and photophobia is less marked than in the nongranulomatous form. The pupil is often constricted and becomes irregular as posterior synechiae form. Large "mutton fat" KPs on the posterior surface of the cornea may be seen

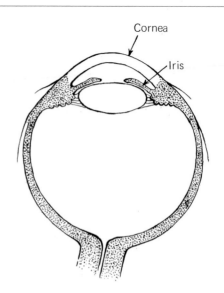

Figure 11–3. Normal anterior chamber.

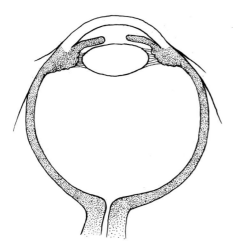

Figure 11–4. Anterior synechiae (adhesions). The peripheral iris adheres to the cornea.

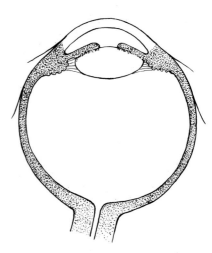

Figure 10–5. Posterior synechiae. The iris adheres to the lens.

with the slit lamp. Flare and cells are seen in the anterior chamber, and nodules consisting of clusters of white cells are seen on the pupillary margin of the iris (Koeppe nodules). These nodules are the equivalent of the mutton fat KPs.

Fresh active lesions of the choroid and retina appear as yellowish-white patches seen hazily with the ophthalmoscope through the cloudy vitreous body. Such posterior cases are generally classified as granulomatous disease. Because of the intimate relationship of the choroid and retina, the retina is nearly always involved (chorioretinitis). As healing progresses, the vitreous haze lessens, and pigmentation occurs gradually at the edges of the yellowish-white spots. In the healed stage, there is usually considerable pigment deposition. If the macula has not been involved, recovery of central vision is complete. The patient is usually not aware of the scotoma in the peripheral field corresponding to the scarred area.

B. Laboratory Findings: Extensive laboratory investigation is usually not indicated in anterior uveitis, particularly if it is nongranulomatous or is readily responsive to nonspecific treatment. In persistent nonresponsive anterior or posterior uveitis, an attempt should be made to arrive at an etiologic diagnosis. Skin tests for tuberculosis and histoplasmosis may be helpful, as well as complement fixation tests and methylene blue dye tests (toxoplasmosis). On the basis of these tests and the clinical appearance, it is often possible to make an etiologic diagnosis.

Differential Diagnosis

In conjunctivitis, vision is not blurred, pupillary responses are normal, a discharge is present, and there is usually no pain, photophobia, or ciliary injection.

In keratitis or keratoconjunctivitis, vision may be blurred and pain and photophobia may be present. Some causes of keratitis such as herpes simplex and

herpes zoster may be associated with a true anterior uveitis.

In acute glaucoma the pupil is dilated, there are no posterior synechiae, and the cornea is steamy.

After repeated attacks, nongranulomatous uveitis may acquire the characteristics of granulomatous uveitis. In recent years there has been less emphasis on this differentiation, and some authorities are disregarding it completely. Nevertheless, the differentiation is still of value as a guide to treatment and prognosis.

Complications & Sequelae

Anterior uveitis may produce peripheral anterior synechiae (Fig 11–4), which impede aqueous outflow at the anterior chamber angle and cause glaucoma. Posterior synechiae can cause glaucoma by impeding the flow of aqueous from the posterior to the anterior chamber. Early and constant pupillary dilatation less-

Figure 11–6. Posterior synechiae (anterior view). The iris is adherent to the lens in several places as a result of previous inflammation, causing an irregular fixed pupil.

ens the likelihood of posterior synechiae. Interference with lens metabolism may cause cataract. Retinal detachment occasionally occurs as a result of traction on the retina by vitreous strands. Cystoid macular edema and degeneration can result from long-standing anterior uveitis.

Treatment

A. Nongranulomatous Uveitis: Symptomatic measures include warm compresses for 10 minutes 3–4 times a day, systemic analgesics as necessary for pain, and dark glasses for photophobia. The pupil must be kept dilated. Atropine is unrivaled in its ability to relieve ciliary spasm. Once relief has been achieved, short-acting dilators such as cyclopentolate (Cyclogyl 1%) should be used to prevent spasm and posterior synechia formation. Local steroid drops are usually quite effective for their anti-inflammatory action. In severe and unresponsive cases, systemic steroids are given also.

B. Granulomatous Uveitis: If the process includes the anterior segment, pupillary dilatation with atropine, 2%, is indicated. Since it is often possible to make a tentative or likely diagnosis of the cause, an attempt at specific therapy is indicated as outlined in Table 11–2.

C. Treatment of Complications: Glaucoma is a common complication. Treatment of the uveitis is of primary importance, particularly dilating the pupil with atropine (not constricting the pupil, as with all forms of primary glaucoma). Carbonic anhydrase inhibitors often effectively reduce intraocular tension by depressing aqueous production. Epinephrine also lowers intraocular pressure by reducing ciliary body secretion of aqueous.

Cataract frequently develops in chronic uveitis. The eye tolerates removal of such cataracts very poorly; but if vision is poor enough, cataract surgery may be essential. Retinal detachment is also very difficult to treat successfully surgically when it occurs in association with uveitis.

Course & Prognosis

With treatment, an attack of nongranulomatous uveitis usually lasts a few days to weeks. Recurrences are common.

Granulomatous uveitis lasts months to years, sometimes with remissions and exacerbations, and may cause permanent damage with marked visual loss despite the best treatment. The prognosis for a focal peripheral chorioretinal lesion is considerably better, often healing well with no significant visual loss.

SPECIFIC TYPES OF UVEITIS
(Uveitis Syndromes)

UVEITIS ASSOCIATED WITH JOINT DISEASE

About 20% of children with the pauciarticular form of **juvenile rheumatoid arthritis** develop a chronic

Table 11–2. Treatment of granulomatous uveitis.

	Anti-infective Chemotherapy	Use of Corticosteroids
Toxoplasmosis	If central vision is threatened, give pyrimethamine (Daraprim), 75 mg orally as a loading dose for 2 days followed by 25 mg once daily for 4 weeks, in combination with trisulfapyrimidines (sulfadiazine, sulfamerazine, and sulfamethazine, 0.167 g of each per tablet), 4 g orally as loading dose followed by 1 g 4 times daily for 4 weeks. If a fall in the white or platelet count occurs during therapy, give folinic acid (leucovorin), 1 mL IM twice weekly or 3 mg orally 3 times a week.	If the response is not favorable after 2 weeks, continue anti-infective therapy and give systemic corticosteroids, eg, prednisolone, 20–25 mg 4 times a day for 1 week, followed by 60–120 mg every other day thereafter,* to protect the macula. Corticosteroids may activate the organisms of toxoplasmosis and tuberculosis but are given as a calculated risk to control the inflammatory response when it threatens vision.
Tuberculosis	Isoniazid, 100 mg 3 times daily, and aminosalicylic acid (PAS), 4 g 3 times daily after meals. If PAS is not tolerated, give streptomycin, 1 g IM twice weekly. Continue treatment for 4–6 months.	If a favorable response does not occur in 6 weeks, continue antimycobacterial therapy and give systemic corticosteroids, eg, prednisolone, 40–80 mg every other day for 2 months.*
Sarcoidosis	Treatment with local corticosteroids and mydriatics and, during active stages, with systemic corticosteroids such as prednisolone, 40–80 mg every other day.* Give supplemental potassium chloride, 2 g 3 times daily. The usual contraindications to systemic corticosteroid therapy apply.	
Sympathetic ophthalmia	Treat with local corticosteroids and mydriatics and systemic corticosteroids in high doses, eg, prednisolone, 40–120 mg every other day.* The usual contraindications to systemic corticosteroid therapy apply, and the drugs may be needed in higher doses and for a longer time. Therefore, management of the side effects is often more difficult. Azathioprine may be helpful in reducing the required dose of corticosteroids. In severe cases that fail to respond to corticosteroids, treatment with cytotoxic agents such as chlorambucil and cyclophosphamide or other immunosuppressants such as cyclosporine has met with some success. *Caution:* White blood counts and platelets must be monitored very carefully in these patients, and these drugs should not be used without careful consideration.	

*Administration every other day has been advocated to minimize the effects of stress and make drug withdrawal easier and safer.

bilateral nongranulomatous iridocyclitis. Females are far more commonly affected than males (4:1). The average age at which the uveitis is detected is 5½ years. In most cases the onset is insidious, the disease being discovered only when the child is noted to have a difference in the color of the 2 eyes, a difference in the size or shape of the pupil, or the onset of strabismus. There is no correlation between the onset of the arthritis and that of the uveitis. The uveitis may precede the arthritis by 3– 10 years. The knee is the most common joint involved. The cardinal signs of the disease are calcific band keratopathy, cells and flare in the anterior chamber, small to medium-sized white KPs with or without flecks of fibrin on the endothelium, posterior synechiae, often progressing to seclusion of the pupil, complicated cataract, variable secondary glaucoma, and macular edema.

Corticosteroids and mydriatics are of value, especially in acute exacerbations, but their long-term effect seems merely to delay the inevitable, ie, severe visual impairment or phthisis bulbi. The prognosis is very poor because of the relentless and progressive character of the disease, which leads to serious complications. These patients tend to do poorly after surgery.

Iridocyclitis occurring in association with adult peripheral rheumatoid arthritis is strictly coincidental. The adult group is more likely to develop scleritis and sclero-uveitis. It is unfortunate that the associated cells and flare in the aqueous humor that accompany the scleritis have been misinterpreted as "iridocyclitis."

About 10– 60% of patients with **Marie-Strümpell ankylosing spondylitis** develop an anterior uveitis. There is a marked preponderance in males. The uveitis presents as a mild to fairly severe nongranulomatous type of iridocyclitis with moderate to severe ciliary injection, pain, blurred vision, and photophobia. It is usually recurrent and eventually may lead to permanent damage if not adequately treated. Histocompatibility antigen HLA-B27 is present in approximately 90% of patients with ankylosing spondylitis.

Ocular examination shows ciliary injection, moderate cells and flare in the anterior chamber, and fine white keratic precipitates located mostly on the inferior cornea. Posterior synechiae, peripheral anterior synechiae, cataracts, and glaucoma are common complications after hyperacute attacks of inflammation. Macular edema occurs in 1% of cases with severe anterior iridocyclitis, which, if persistent, leads to cystoid degeneration and loss of central vision.

Confirmation of the diagnosis is by x-rays of the lumbosacral spine. In about 50% of patients, clinical signs and symptoms may all be absent so that the diagnosis may be made only by the radiologist.

The erythrocyte sedimentation rate, although nonspecific and sometimes normal in mild cases, is elevated in most patients, indicating active disease. The rheumatoid factor test, however, is negative in all but 5% of patients with this disease.

HETEROCHROMIC UVEITIS
(Fuchs's Heterochromic Iridocyclitis)

This disease of unknown cause accounts for about 3% of all cases of uveitis. It is essentially a quiet cyclitis associated with depigmentation of the iris in the affected eye. Pathologically, the iris and ciliary body show moderate atrophy, patchy depigmentation of the pigment layer, and diffuse infiltration of lymphocytes and plasma cells. Involvement is typically unilateral but may be bilateral, and the eyes are of different colors. Early in the course of the disease, the difference in color may not be readily apparent and is best noted in daylight.

The onset is insidious in the third or fourth decade, with no redness, pain, or photophobia; the patient is often unaware of the disorder until cataract formation results in blurred vision.

With the slit lamp (or loupe) one sees fine white deposits on the posterior corneal surface, flare and cells in the anterior chamber, and a slightly atrophic iris. Anterior vitreous floaters may be evident with the ophthalmoscope or slit lamp.

Cataract develops within a few years in about 15% of cases. Glaucoma occurs in 10– 15% of cases. It is usually not necessary to dilate the pupil, as this is one type of uveitis in which posterior synechiae rarely form. The disease does not subside spontaneously, but the visual prognosis is good since the cataract can usually be removed safely despite the low-grade active uveitis.

INTERMEDIATE UVEITIS
(Pars Planitis, Chronic Cyclitis)

The usual patient with pars planitis is a young adult presenting with "floating spots" in the field of vision as the chief complaint. In the majority of cases, both eyes are affected. The sex distribution is equal. Pain, redness, and photophobia do not occur. The patient may be unaware of any ocular problem, but the physician detects vitreous opacities with the ophthalmoscope.

There are few, if any, signs of anterior uveitis. A few cells may occasionally be seen in the anterior chamber; rarely, anterior or posterior synechiae occur. Inflammatory cells are more likely to be seen in the retrolental space or in the anterior vitreous on slit lamp examination. Posterior subcapsular cataract occurs frequently.

Indirect ophthalmoscopy often reveals soft, round, white opacities over the peripheral retina. These cellular exudates may be confluent, often overlying the pars plana. Some of these patients may also have vasculitis, as shown by perivascular sheathing of retinal vessels.

In most patients, the disease remains stationary or gradually improves over a 5- to 10-year period. Some patients develop cystoid macular edema and permanent macular scarring as well as posterior subcapsular cataracts. In severe cases, cyclitic membranes and retinal detachments may occur. Secondary glaucoma is a rare complication.

The cause is unknown. Corticosteroids constitute the only helpful treatment and should only be used in more severe cases, especially when there is decreased vision secondary to macular edema. Topical corticosteroids are used first; if they fail, sub-Tenon or retrobulbar injections of corticosteroids may be effective. Such treatment increases the risk of cataract development. Fortunately, these patients do well following cataract surgery.

LENS-INDUCED UVEITIS

There are no data at present to substantiate the implication that lens material per se is toxic, so that the term phacotoxic uveitis should no longer be used to describe lens-induced uveitis. The terms phacogenic or lens-induced uveitis are more appropriate when referring to an autoimmune disease secondary to lens antigen. The classic case of lens-induced uveitis occurs when the lens develops a hypermature cataract. The lens capsule leaks and lens material passes into the anterior chamber, causing an inflammatory reaction characterized by the accumulation of plasma cells, mononuclear phagocytes, and a few polymorphonuclear cells. The eye becomes red and moderately painful; the pupil is small; and vision is markedly reduced (at times to light perception only). Lens-induced uveitis may also occur following traumatic cataracts.

Endophthalmitis phaco-anaphylactica, the term used for the more severe form of lens-induced uveitis, occurs following an extracapsular lens extraction when the same operation has already been performed on the fellow eye and the patient has been sensitized to his or her own lens material. Many polymorphonuclear leukocytes and mononuclear phagocytes appear in the anterior chamber. The eye becomes red and painful, and vision is blurred. Since most of the lens material has already been removed, treatment is conservative, consisting of corticosteroids locally and systemically plus atropine drops to keep the pupil dilated. If this is ineffective, the cataract incision must be opened and the anterior chamber irrigated.

Glaucoma (phacolytic glaucoma) is a common complication of lens-induced uveitis. Treatment consists of lens extraction after intraocular pressure has been brought under control. If this is done, both the uveitis and the glaucoma are cured, and the visual prognosis is good if the process has not been present for more than 1–2 weeks.

SYMPATHETIC OPHTHALMIA
(Sympathetic Uveitis)

Sympathetic ophthalmia is a rare but devastating granulomatous bilateral uveitis that comes on 10 days

Figure 11–7. Microscopic section of giant cells and lymphocytes in sympathetic ophthalmia involving the choroid. (Courtesy of R Carriker.)

to many years following a perforating eye injury in the region of the ciliary body, or following retained foreign body. The cause is not known, but the disease is probably related to hypersensitivity to some element of the pigment-bearing cells in the uvea. It very rarely occurs following uncomplicated intraocular surgery for cataract or glaucoma.

The injured (exciting) eye becomes inflamed first and the fellow (sympathizing) eye second. Pathologically, there is a diffuse granulomatous uveitis. The epithelioid cells, together with giant cells and lymphocytes (Fig 11–7), form noncaseating tubercles. From the uveal tract the inflammatory process spreads to the optic nerve and to the pia and arachnoid surrounding the optic nerve.

The patient complains of photophobia, redness, and blurring of vision. If a history of trauma is obtained, look for a scar representing the wound of entry in the exciting eye. With the slit lamp or loupe one sees KPs and a flare in the anterior chamber of both eyes. Iris nodules may be present.

Sympathetic ophthalmia may be differentiated from other granulomatous uveitides by the history of trauma or ocular surgery and by the fact that it is bilateral, diffuse, and (usually) acute rather than unilateral, localized, and chronic.

The recommended treatment of a severely injured sightless eye (eg, a penetrating injury through the sclera, ciliary body, and lens, with loss of vitreous) is immediate enucleation to prevent sympathetic ophthalmia, and every effort must be made to secure the patient's informed consent to the operation. If enucleation can be performed within 10 days after injury, there is almost no chance that sympathetic ophthalmia will develop. However, when the inflammation in the sympathizing eye is advanced, it is wise not to enucleate the injured eye, since it may eventually prove to be the better of 2 very bad eyes.

If inflammation appears in the sympathizing eye, treat at once with local corticosteroids and atropine. Systemic corticosteroids or cytotoxic drugs may be required. Cyclosporine has also proved useful in intractable cases. (See Table 11–2.)

Without treatment, the disease progresses slowly but relentlessly over a period of months or years to complete bilateral blindness.

TUBERCULOUS UVEITIS

Tuberculosis causes a granulomatous type of uveitis. Tuberculous uveitis is diagnosed clinically far more often than the disease can be proved by positive identification of tubercle bacilli in the tissues. Although the infection is said to be transmitted from a primary focus elsewhere in the body, uveal tuberculosis is rare in patients with active pulmonary tuberculosis.

Tuberculous uveitis may be diffuse but is characteristically localized in the form of a severe caseating granulomatous chorioretinitis. The tubercle itself consists of giant cells and epithelioid cells. Caseation necrosis commonly occurs.

The patient complains of blurred vision, and the eye is moderately injected. If the anterior segment is involved, iris nodules and "mutton fat" KPs are visible on slit lamp examination. If the choroid and retina are primarily affected, one can see a localized yellowish mass partially obscured by a hazy vitreous.

The nodules and the localized nature of tuberculous uveitis help to make a clinical differentiation from sympathetic ophthalmia, and the caseation necrosis differentiates it pathologically from sympathetic ophthalmia and Boeck's sarcoid.

The pupil should be kept dilated with atropine, 1%, 1 drop 2–3 times daily. Antituberculosis drugs should be prescribed systemically if a reasonably certain clinical diagnosis can be made. (See Table 11–2.)

After a prolonged course of several months, the disease usually resolves, leaving permanently damaged tissue and blurred vision because of scarring of the retina.

SARCOIDOSIS
(Boeck's Sarcoid)

Sarcoidosis is a chronic granulomatous disease of unknown cause characterized by multiple cutaneous and subcutaneous nodules, with similar invasions in the viscera and bones, and periodic exacerbations and remissions. The onset is usually in the third decade. The tissue reaction is much less severe than in tuberculous uveitis, and caseation does not occur. The tuberculin skin test is usually negative or only faintly positive. When the parotid glands are involved, the disease is called uveoparotid fever (Heerfordt's disease); when the lacrimal glands are involved, it is called Mikulicz's syndrome.

Thirty percent of cases are complicated by chronic bilateral anterior uveitis, whereas posterior uveitis is far less common. Anterior uveitis is nodular, and in prolonged cases it may lead to severe visual impairment due to cataract and secondary glaucoma. Posterior uveitis is characterized by multiple whitish-yellow retinal exudates and perivasculitis.

Diagnosis is best aided by positive biopsy of the cutaneous nodules. In a small number of cases, typical nodules were also found on the tarsal or bulbar conjunctiva.

Corticosteroid therapy (Table 11–2) given early in the disease may be effective, but recurrences are common and the long-term visual prognosis is poor.

TOXOPLASMIC UVEITIS

Toxoplasmosis is primarily an inflammation of the central nervous system caused by *T gondii*, a protozoan parasite. In congenital toxoplasmosis, chorioretinitis is almost invariably present. Toxoplasmosis acquired in later life does not usually involve the eye in the acute stage, but chorioretinitis may occur in the chronic form.

The disease is more common in tropical countries.* Pathologically, there is a granulomatous retinochoroiditis. The retina is characteristically necrotic, and *Toxoplasma* organisms are found in the retinal tissues. The clinical picture is variable, but typically there is a chorioretinal lesion or lesions, usually in the macular area, which in the early stages appear as elevated white masses partially obscured by a hazy vitreous. In the later stages, a punched-out pigmented chorioretinal lesion develops through which the sclera may be clearly visible. The methylene blue dye test on the patient's serum is positive, ie, antibodies in the serum prevent the dye from staining *Toxoplasma* organisms.

Although the pathology of the retinochoroiditis is essentially the same, there are 2 distinct clinical types of ocular toxoplasmosis: congenital and acquired. The congenital type is due to intrauterine infection. As in the acquired (adult) type, the chorioretinitis is usually confined to the macular area. The inflammatory process is more severe in congenital than in acquired toxoplasmosis and is frequently bilateral. Cerebral involvement, with radiopaque calcification and mental deficiency, is present in 10% of cases of the congenital type.

Acquired ocular toxoplasmosis is usually milder than congenital toxoplasmosis. It may appear at any

---

*The cat is the definitive host of *T gondii*. The parasite is a coccidian undergoing typical schizogonic cycles and gametogony in the intestinal epithelial cells of the cat. Intermediate hosts such as rodents, birds, or humans become infected by ingestion of the oocysts passed in cat feces. Additional means of transmission among intermediate hosts include carnivorousness with ingestion of cysts present mainly in brain and muscle tissue. The ingestion of raw meat is an established source of the disease.

Figure 11–8. *Toxoplasma* cysts in the retina. (Courtesy of K Tabbara.)

age, is often unilateral, and frequently occurs in the absence of central nervous system involvement. The patient complains of blurred vision if the macula is involved.

For treatment, see Table 11–2.

Clindamycin, a chlorinated lincomycin derivative, appears to hold great promise for the treatment of ocular toxoplasmosis. A combination of subconjunctival and intramuscular injections of clindamycin phosphate has brought about rapid healing of the ocular lesions in rabbits and has made it impossible to recover *Toxoplasma* organisms from the minced tissues of experimentally infected eyes. It appears also that clindamycin may be able to penetrate *Toxoplasma* cysts (Fig 11–8). In clinical studies, clindamycin has been used successfully both alone and in combination with sulfonamides and pyrimethamine. Its major drawback is the risk of pseudomembranous colitis; if this occurs, clindamycin must be discontinued and vancomycin must be given orally.

Although the search for new, more efficacious drugs for the treatment of ocular toxoplasmosis will continue, many investigators believe that the ultimate cure of the disease must come from destruction of the organism by macrophages. Research on ways to promote or augment the effects of activated macrophages on *Toxoplasma* continues.

The chorioretinitis progresses to a healed stage, leaving a scarred retina and choroid. If the macula has been involved, loss of central vision is permanent.

HISTOPLASMOSIS

In some areas of the USA where histoplasmosis is endemic (eg, Cincinnati, Baltimore), the diagnosis of choroiditis presumably due to histoplasmosis is being made with increasing frequency. The patient usually has a positive skin test to histoplasmin and demonstrates "punched-out" spots in the peripheral fundus. These spots are small, irregularly round or oval, depigmented areas, sometimes with a fine pigmented border. They are smaller and have less pigment than the usual healed chorioretinal lesion. Peripapillary atrophy and hyperpigmentation are usually present. Macular lesions that begin as small edematous areas and may progress to hemorrhagic detachments are the most visually threatening feature of the disease. Vitreous haze does not occur.

It has been postulated that in areas where histoplasmosis is endemic, many persons develop a benign form of asymptomatic peripheral chorioretinitis. These lesions soon heal, leaving "histo" spots. This exposure sensitizes the choroid. A later antigenic insult to the choroid results in the observed macular changes. However, this hypothesis has not been verified.

Many types of treatment have been advocated, including systemic corticosteroids, amphotericin B (Fungizone), antihistamines, intradermal desensitization with histoplasmin, and photocoagulation of areas of perimacular leakage. The results have been questionable in all cases, and treatment with amphotericin B is now contraindicated.

Xenon and laser photocoagulation can be effective treatment for those paramacular lesions that cause leaks demonstrable by fluorescein angiography. This form of treatment has limited application since most lesions involve the macula directly and are thus not suitable for coagulation.

TOXOCARIASIS

Toxocara canis and *Toxocara cati* are common dog and cat ascarids that can cause uveitis, usually in children, and nearly always unilaterally. The ova are excreted in the feces of affected animals and contaminate dirt. They are then ingested, usually by children who have handled the contaminated soil. The ova hatch in the intestine and burrow into the intestinal wall to reach the bloodstream, which can carry the organism to any part of the body, including the eye.

The ocular involvement most often takes the form of a localized choroidal granuloma, but a chronic endophthalmitis can occur. Such extensive involvement can closely resemble retinoblastoma, Coats's disease, bacterial or fungal endophthalmitis, or exudative retinitis, thus making differential diagnosis most important.

There is no effective treatment.

REFERENCES

Abrams J, Schlaegel TF Jr: The role of the isoniazid therapeutic test in tuberculous uveitis. *Am J Ophthalmol* 1982;**94**:511.

Akstein RB, Wilson LA, Teutsch SM: Acquired toxoplasmosis. *Ophthalmology* 1982;**89**:2133.

Gass JD: Observation of suspected choroidal and ciliary body melanomas for evidence of growth prior to enucleation. *Ophthalmology* 1980;**87**:523.

Gass JDM: Sympathetic ophthalmia following vitrectomy. *Am J Ophthalmol* 1982;**65**:53.

Kaplan HJ, Waldrep JC: Immunologic insights into uveitis and retinitis: The immunoregulatory circuit. *Ophthalmology* 1984;**91**:655.

Karcioglu ZA, Brear R: Conjunctival biopsy in sarcoidosis. *Am J Ophthalmol* 1985;**99**:68.

Lakhanpal V, Schocket SS, Nirankari VS: Clindamycin in the treatment of toxoplasmic retinochoroiditis. *Am J Ophthalmol* 1983;**95**:605.

Macular Photocoagulation Study Group: Argon laser photocoagulation for ocular histoplasmosis: Results of a randomised clinical trial. *Arch Ophthalmol* 1983;**101**:1347.

Newman PE et al: The role of hypersensitivity to *Toxoplasma* antigens in experimental ocular toxoplasmosis in non-human primates. *Am J Ophthalmol* 1982;**94**:159.

Noble KG, Carr RE: *Toxoplasma* retinochoroiditis. *Ophthalmology* 1982;**89**:1289.

Nussenblatt RB et al: S-antigen uveitis in primates: A new model for human disease. *Arch Ophthalmol* 1981;**99**:1090.

O'Connor GR: Current concepts in ophthalmology: Uveitis and the immunologically compromised host. *N Engl J Med* 1978;**299**:130.

O'Connor GR: Factors related to the initiation and recurrence of uveitis. *Am J Ophthalmol* 1983;**96**:577.

Ohno S et al: Vogt-Koyanagi-Harada syndrome. *Am J Ophthalmol* 1977;**83**:735.

Olk RJ, Burgess DB, McCormick PA: Subfoveal and juxtafoveal subretinal neovascularization in the presumed ocular histoplasmosis syndrome: Visual prognosis. *Ophthalmology* 1984;**91**:1592.

Rollins DF et al: Minocycline in experimental ocular toxoplasmosis in the rabbit. *Am J Ophthalmol* 1982;**93**:361.

Scharf Y, Zonis S: Histocompatibility antigens (HLA) and uveitis. *Surv Ophthalmol* 1980;**24**:220.

Shields JA et al: The differential diagnosis of posterior uveal melanoma. *Ophthalmology* 1980;**87**:518.

Smith RE, Godfrey WA, Kimura SJ: Chronic cyclitis. 1. Course and visual prognosis. *Trans Am Acad Ophthalmol Otolaryngol* 1973;**77**:OP760.

Smith RE, O'Connor GR: Cataract extraction in Fuchs syndrome. *Arch Ophthalmol* 1974;**91**:39.

Stephens RF, Shields JA: Diagnosis and management of cancer metastatic to the uvea: A study of 70 cases. *Ophthalmology* 1979;**86**:1336.

Tabbara KF, O'Connor GR: Treatment of ocular toxoplasmosis with clindamycin and sulfadiazine. *Ophthalmology* 1980;**87**:129.

Weinreb RN, Kimura SJ: Uveitis associated with sarcoidosis and angiotensin converting enzyme. *Am J Ophthalmol* 1980;**89**:180.

12

Lens

John P. Shock, MD

ANATOMY & FUNCTION

The lens is a biconvex, avascular, colorless and almost completely transparent structure, about 4 mm thick and 9 mm in diameter. It is suspended behind the iris by the zonule, which connects it with the ciliary body. Anterior to the lens is the aqueous; posterior to it, the vitreous. The lens capsule (see below) is a semipermeable membrane (slightly more permeable than a capillary wall) that will admit water and electrolytes.

A subcapsular epithelium is present anteriorly (Fig 12–1). The lens nucleus is harder than the cortex. With age, subepithelial lamellar fibers are continuously produced, so that the lens gradually becomes larger and less elastic throughout life. The nucleus and cortex are made up of long concentric lamellas. The suture lines formed by the end-to-end joining of

these lamellar fibers are Y-shaped when viewed with the slit lamp (Fig 12–2). The Y is erect anteriorly and inverted posteriorly.

Each lamellar fiber contains a flattened nucleus. These nuclei are evident microscopically in the peripheral portion of the lens near the equator and are continuous with the subcapsular epithelium.

The lens is held in place by a suspensory ligament known as the zonule (zonule of Zinn). This is composed of numerous fibrils that arise from the surface of the ciliary body and insert into the lens equator.

The primary function of the lens is to focus light rays upon the retina. In order to focus light from a distant object, the ciliary muscle relaxes, tautening the zonular fibers and reducing the anteroposterior diameter of the lens to its minimal dimension; in this position the refractive power of the lens is minimized, and parallel rays are thus focused upon the retina. In

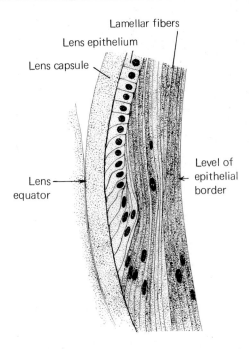

Figure 12–1. Magnified view of lens showing termination of subcapsular epithelium (vertical section).

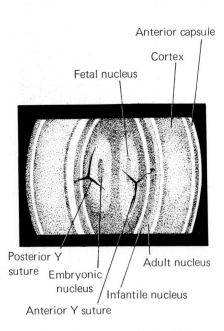

Figure 12–2. Zones of lens showing Y sutures.

[Figs 12–1 and 12–2 are redrawn from Duke-Elder WS: *Textbook of Ophthalmology.* Vol 1. Mosby, 1942. Drawings first appeared in Salzmann M: *Anatomy and Histology of the Human Eyeball in the Normal State.* Univ of Chicago Press, 1912.]

order to focus light from a near object, the ciliary muscle contracts, pulling the choroid forward and releasing the tension on the zonules. The elastic lens capsule then molds the lens into a more spherical body with correspondingly greater refractive power. The physiologic interplay of the ciliary body, zonule, and lens that results in focusing near objects upon the retina is known as **accommodation.** As the lens ages, its accommodative power is gradually reduced.

Composition

The lens consists of about 65% water, about 35% protein (the highest protein content of any tissue of the body), and a trace of minerals common to other body tissues. Potassium is more concentrated in the lens than in most tissues. Ascorbic acid and glutathione are present in both the oxidized and reduced forms.

There are no pain fibers, blood vessels, or nerves in the lens.

Physiology of Symptoms

Disorders of the lens include opacification, distortion, dislocation, and geometric anomalies. Patients with these conditions have blurred vision without pain. Examination for diseases of the lens is by visual acuity testing and by viewing the lens with a slit lamp, ophthalmoscope, hand flashlight, or loupe, preferably through a dilated pupil.

CATARACT

A cataract is a lens opacity. Cataracts vary markedly in degree of density and may be due to a variety of causes but are usually associated with aging. Some degree of cataract formation is to be expected in persons over age 70. Most are bilateral, although the rate of progression in each eye is seldom equal. Traumatic cataract, congenital cataract, and other types are less common.

Cataractous lenses are characterized by lens edema, protein alteration, necrosis, and disruption of the normal continuity of the lens fibers. In general, lens edema varies directly with the stage of cataract development. The immature (incipient) cataract is only slightly opaque. A completely opaque mature (moderately advanced) cataractous lens is somewhat edematous. If the water content is maximal and the lens capsule is stretched, the cataract is called intumescent (swollen). In the hypermature (far-advanced) cataract, water has escaped from the lens, leaving a relatively dehydrated, very opaque lens and a wrinkled capsule.

Most cataracts are not visible to the casual observer until they become dense enough (mature or hypermature) to cause blindness. However, a cataract in its earliest stages of development can be observed through a well-dilated pupil with an ophthalmoscope, loupe, or slit lamp.

The ocular fundus becomes increasingly more difficult to visualize as the lens opacity becomes denser, until the fundus reflection is completely absent. At this stage the cataract is usually mature and the pupil may be white.

The clinical degree of cataract formation, assuming that no other eye disease is present, is judged primarily by the visual acuity. Generally speaking, the decrease in visual acuity is directly proportionate to the density of the cataract. However, some individuals who have clinically significant cataracts when examined with the ophthalmoscope or slit lamp see well enough to carry on with their normal activities. Others have a decrease in visual acuity out of proportion to the degree of lens opacification. This is due to distortion of the image by the partially opaque lens.

Cataract formation is characterized chemically by a reduction in oxygen uptake and an initial increase in water content followed by dehydration. Sodium and calcium content is increased; potassium, ascorbic acid, and protein content is decreased. Glutathione is not present in cataractous lenses. Attempts to accelerate or retard these chemical changes by medical treatment have not been successful, and their causes and implications are not known.

During the past few years, there has been increasing evidence implicating ultraviolet radiation as a significant factor in the occurrence of senile cataracts. Epidemiologic investigations have shown that for persons age 65 years or older there is an increased incidence of cataracts in geographic areas where there are long periods of strong sunlight. Further investigation of the effects of ultraviolet light on the lens is warranted.

AGE-RELATED CATARACT (Senile Cataract)

Age-related cataract (Figs 12–3 to 12–5) is by far the most common type of cataract. Increasingly blurred vision and visual distortion are the only symptoms. Paradoxically, although distant vision is blurred in the incipient stage of cataract formation, near vision may improve slightly, so the patient will read better without glasses ("second sight"). This artificial myopia is due to the greater convexity of the lens in the incipient stage.

There is no medical treatment for cataract. Lens extraction (see Cataract Surgery, below) is indicated when visual impairment interferes with the patient's normal activities. If glaucoma secondary to lens swelling (intumescent lens) occurs, surgical extraction of the lens is indicated.

Glaucoma and lens-induced uveitis are uncommon complications. Lens-induced uveitis requires surgical extraction of the lens to remove the source of the offending lens products.

Senile cataract is usually slowly progressive over

Figure 12–3. Cataract types. *Above, left:* Senile cataract, "coronary" type: club-shaped peripheral opacities with clear central lens; slowly progressive. *Above, right:* Senile cataract, "cuneiform" type: peripheral spicules and central clear lens; slowly progressive. *Left:* Senile cataract, "morgagnian" type (hypermature lens); the entire lens is opaque, and the lens nucleus has fallen inferiorly. (Reproduced, with permission, from Cordes FC: *Cataract Types,* 3rd ed. American Academy of Ophthalmology and Otolaryngology, 1954.)

Figure 12–4 (at right). Mature senile cataract viewed through a dilated pupil. (Courtesy of A Rosenberg.)

Figure 12–5. Senile cataract. In the photo at right the scene shown at left is reproduced as if seen by a person with a moderately advanced senile cataract (opacity denser centrally). (Courtesy of E Goodner.)

years, and death may occur before surgery becomes necessary. If surgery is indicated, lens extraction definitely improves visual acuity in well over 90% of cases. The remainder of patients either have preexisting retinal damage or develop serious postsurgical complications such as glaucoma, retinal detachment, vitreous hemorrhage, infection, or epithelial downgrowth into the anterior chamber, which prevent significant visual improvement.

Intraocular lenses and corneal contact lenses have made adjustment following cataract operation much easier than was the rule when only thick cataract glasses were available.

CONGENITAL CATARACT
(Figs 12–6, 12–7)

Congenital cataracts are common but usually do not cause significant visual loss. Most are bilateral and are probably genetically determined. They occasionally occur as a consequence of maternal rubella during the first trimester of pregnancy. Only those congenital cataracts that cause a marked loss of vision are discussed here.

The parent notices that the child does not see well during the first few months or years of life. The pupil may be white. The opacities vary greatly in density.

If the cataracts are bilateral and dense enough so that the retinas are not clearly visible, lens extraction through a small limbal incision (2–6 mm) by aspiration, irrigation, or ultrasonic fragmentation or with a motor-driven lens and vitreous cutter should be done in one eye by the age of 2 months to permit normal development of vision and prevent nystagmus. Many surgeons also perform anterior vitrectomy at the time of cataract removal. If surgery on the first eye has been successful, surgery on the second eye can be performed soon after. Otherwise, surgery on the second eye should be delayed 1–2 years until the eye is larger and there is less risk of operative complications.

Months or years following surgery, vitreous strands may develop and contract to produce retinal detachment. Retinal detachment may be successfully treated by surgery in the majority of such cases. Recent improved techniques of aspiration and irrigation have materially reduced the incidence of vitreous loss and therefore the late complication of retinal detachment.

Most congenital cataracts are not dense enough to blur the vision significantly and are not progressive.

Figure 12–6 (at left). Congenital cataract.

Figure 12–7. Congenital cataract, zonular type. One zone of lens involved. The cortex is relatively clear. (From Cordes FC: See next page.)

sion. The eye becomes red, the lens opaque, and there may be an intraocular hemorrhage. If aqueous or vitreous escapes from the eye, the eye becomes extremely soft. Complications include infection, uveitis, retinal detachment, and glaucoma.

A magnetic intraocular foreign body should be removed without delay.

Antibiotics and corticosteroids should be given systemically and locally over a period of several days to minimize the chance of infection and uveitis. Atropine sulfate, 1%, 1 drop 3 times daily, is recommended to keep the pupil dilated and to prevent the formation of posterior synechiae.

The cataract can be removed at the same time the foreign body is removed or after the inflammation subsides. If glaucoma occurs during the waiting period, cataract surgery should not be delayed even though inflammation is still present. Some time after cataract surgery, a thin opaque membrane may occur, in which case discission (needling) may be necessary to improve vision. The same techniques utilized for removal of congenital cataracts are generally used for the removal of traumatic cataracts, especially in patients under 30 years of age.

Others progress slowly and may not require surgery until the child is 10–15 years of age.

The visual prognosis for congenital cataract patients requiring surgery is not as good as that for patients with senile cataract. The complications of the operation, associated amblyopia, and occasional associated anomalies of the optic nerve or retina lower the degree of useful vision obtainable in this group of patients. The prognosis for improvement of visual acuity is worst following surgery for unilateral congenital cataracts and best for incomplete bilateral congenital cataracts that are slowly progressive.

TRAUMATIC CATARACT

Traumatic cataract (Figs 12–8 to 12–10) is most commonly due to a foreign body injury to the lens or blunt trauma to the eyeball. BB shot is a frequent cause; less frequent causes include arrows, rocks, contusions, overexposure to heat ("glassblower's cataract"), x-rays, and radioactive materials. Most traumatic cataracts are preventable. In industry, the best safety measure is a good pair of safety goggles.

The lens becomes white soon after the entry of the foreign body since the interruption of the lens capsule allows aqueous and sometimes vitreous to penetrate into the lens structure. The patient is often an industrial worker who gives a history of striking steel upon steel. A minute fragment of a steel hammer, for example, may pass through the cornea and lens at a tremendous rate of speed and lodge in the vitreous, where it can usually be seen with the ophthalmoscope.

The patient complains immediately of blurred vi-

CATARACT SECONDARY TO INTRAOCULAR DISEASE ("Complicated Cataract")

Cataract may develop as a direct effect of intraocular disease upon the physiology of the lens (eg, severe recurrent uveitis). The cataract usually begins in the posterior subcapsular area and eventually involves the entire lens structure. Intraocular diseases commonly associated with the development of cataracts are chronic or recurrent uveitis, glaucoma, retinitis pigmentosa, and retinal detachment.

These cataracts are usually unilateral. The visual prognosis is not as good as in ordinary senile cataract.

CATARACT ASSOCIATED WITH SYSTEMIC DISEASE

Bilateral cataracts may occur in association with the following systemic disorders: diabetes mellitus (Fig 12–11), hypoparathyroidism, myotonic dystrophy, atopic dermatitis, galactosemia, and Lowe's, Werner's, and Down's syndromes.

TOXIC CATARACT

Toxic cataract is uncommon. Many cases appeared in the 1930s as a result of ingestion of dinitrophenol, a drug taken to suppress appetite. Other offenders are triparanol (MER/29) and corticosteroids administered over a long period of time. It has been suggested that echothiophate iodide, a strong miotic used in the treatment of glaucoma, may cause cataracts.

Figure 12–8. Traumatic "star-shaped" cataract in the posterior lens. This is usually due to ocular contusion and is only detectable through a well-dilated pupil.

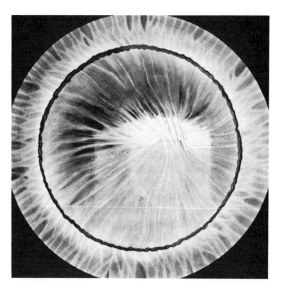

Figure 12–9. Traumatic cataract with wrinkled anterior capsule.

Figure 12–10. "Vossius' ring." Traumatic cataract caused by the imprint of the iris pigment on the anterior surface of the lens. The remainder of the lens is clear, and vision is not impaired.

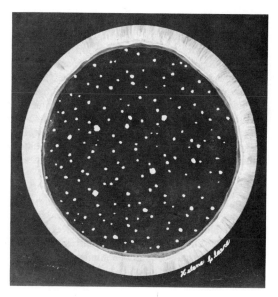

Figure 12–11. Punctate dot cataract. This type of cataract is sometimes seen as an ocular complication of diabetes mellitus. It may also be congenital.

[Figs 12–7 to 12–12 are reproduced, with permission, from Cordes FC: *Cataract Types,* 3rd ed. American Academy of Ophthalmology and Otolaryngology, 1954.]

AFTER-CATARACT
(Secondary Membrane)

After-cataract (Fig 12–12) denotes opacification of the posterior capsule due to partially absorbed traumatic cataract or following extracapsular cataract extraction.

Persistent subcapsular lens epithelium may attempt regeneration of lens fibers, giving the posterior capsule a "fish egg" appearance (Elschnig's pearls). The proliferating epithelium may produce multiple layers, leading to frank opacification. These cells may also undergo myofibroblastic differentiation. Their contraction produces numerous tiny wrinkles in the posterior capsule, resulting in visual distortion. All of these factors may lead to reduced visual acuity following extracapsular cataract extraction.

After-cataract has become a significant problem in that almost all pediatric patients and approximately half of adult patients develop an opaque secondary membrane after extracapsular cataract extraction. Before the neodymium-YAG laser came into use, this condition was treated by performing a small capsulotomy with a needle knife or barbed 27-gauge needle, either at the time of the original operation or as a secondary procedure.

In recent years, the neodymium-YAG laser has gained popularity as a noninvasive method for discission of the posterior capsule. Pulses of laser energy cause small "explosions" in target tissue, creating a small hole in the posterior capsule in the pupillary axis. Complications of this technique include a transient rise in intraocular pressure, damage to the intraocular lens, and rupture of the anterior hyaloid face with forward displacement of vitreous into the anterior chamber. The rise in intraocular pressure is usually detectable within 3 hours posttreatment and resolves within 1 week with treatment. Rarely, the pressure

Figure 12–12. After-cataract.

may not return to normal for several weeks. One group has found that the rise in intraocular pressure is significantly greater in aphakic eyes than in pseudophakic eyes. Small pits or cracks may occur on the intraocular lens, but they usually have no effect on visual acuity. In the aphakic eye, rupture of the vitreous face with anterior displacement of vitreous may predispose to development of rhegmatogenous retinal detachment or cystoid macular edema. Current studies indicate that no significant damage is done to corneal endothelium with the neodymium-YAG laser.

CATARACT SURGERY

Cataract surgery has been changing over the past 10–15 years, principally as a result of introduction of the operating microscope, better instrumentation, improved suture material, and refinement of the intraocular lens. In cataract surgery, the lens is removed from the eye (lens extraction) by either an intracapsular or extracapsular procedure. **Intracapsular extraction** consists of removing the lens in toto, ie, within its capsule, through a 140- to 160-degree superior limbal incision. In **extracapsular extraction,** a superior limbal incision is also made; the anterior portion of the capsule is ruptured and removed; the nucleus is extracted; and the lens cortex is either irrigated or aspirated from the eye, leaving the posterior capsule behind. Some patients develop a secondary opacity of the posterior capsule that requires discission (see After-Cataract, above). **Phacofragmentation** and **phacoemulsification** with irrigation and aspiration are extracapsular techniques that utilize ultrasonic vibrations to remove the nucleus and cortex through a small limbal incision (3–5 mm), thus facilitating postoperative wound healing. These techniques are most useful in congenital, traumatic, and some senile cataracts. They are less effective with dense senile cataracts, and the advantage of a small limbal incision is somewhat negated if an intraocular lens is to be inserted, although flexible intraocular lenses that can be inserted through such small incisions are currently being developed.

Over the past 5 years, extracapsular operations have replaced intracapsular procedures by a large percentage as the most common type of cataract surgery. The principal reason is that an intact posterior capsule allows the surgeon to insert a posterior chamber intraocular lens. The incidence of postoperative complications, such as retinal detachment and cystoid macular edema, also seems to be less when the posterior capsule is intact.

Intraocular Lens

Over 75% of all cataract operations in the USA— or over 0.5 million per year—involve intraocular lens implantation. Refinements in surgical technique and improved lens implants have played major roles in this advance. However, the major stimulus has been the inherent disadvantages of aphakic spectacles, including image magnification, spherical aberrations, limited visual field, and no chance of binocular vision if the other eye is phakic.

About two-thirds of implants are in the posterior chamber and one-third in the anterior chamber. Other less commonly used techniques are iris fixation and iridocapsular lens implantation. There are many styles of lenses, but all consist of 2 basic parts: a spherical optic, usually made of polymethylmethacrylate; and footplates or haptics to maintain the optic in position.

Posterior chamber lenses are generally used in extracapsular procedures. This combination is preferred over anterior chamber or iris fixation lenses because of a lower incidence of sight-threatening complications such as hyphema, secondary glaucoma, macular edema, and pupillary block. There is also a lower incidence of corneal endothelial damage and subsequent pseudophakic bullous keratopathy in patients with posterior chamber lenses. Anterior chamber lenses are used for patients undergoing intracapsular surgery or when the posterior capsule has been inadvertently ruptured in extracapsular surgery.

Contraindications to intraocular lens implantation include recurrent uveitis, proliferative and preproliferative diabetic retinopathy, rubeosis iridis, and neovascular glaucoma. Patients with open-angle glaucoma and ocular hypertension may receive an intraocular lens, but posterior chamber lenses are preferred. Age is considered by many to be a relative contraindication, but younger and younger patients are receiving intraocular lenses each year.

An effective alternative to the intraocular lens is the contact lens—in particular, the continuous-wear soft contact lens, which can be worn day and night for weeks to months at a time. Such a lens offers the same advantages as the intraocular lens when compared to aphakic glasses, but many elderly patients are unable to tolerate them or insert them easily.

Postoperative Care (Senile Cataract)

If a small-incision technique is used, the postoperative recovery period is usually shortened. The patient may be ambulatory on the day of surgery but is advised to move cautiously and avoid straining or heavy lifting for about a month. The eye can be bandaged for a few days, but if the eye is comfortable, the bandage can be removed and the eye protected by spectacles or by a shield during the day. Protection at night by a metal shield is required for several weeks. Temporary glasses can be used a few days after surgery, but usually the patient sees well enough through the intraocular lens to wait for permanent glasses (usually provided 6–8 weeks after surgery).

DISLOCATED LENS
(Ectopia Lentis)

Partial or complete lens dislocation (Fig 12–13) may be hereditary or may result from trauma.

Hereditary Lens Dislocation

Hereditary lens dislocation is usually bilateral and may be associated with coloboma of the lens, homocystinuria, Marfan's syndrome, and Marchesani's syndrome. The vision is blurred, particularly if the lens is dislocated out of the line of vision. If dislocation is partial, the edge of the lens and the zonular fibers holding it in place can be seen in the pupil. If the lens is completely dislocated into the vitreous, it can be seen with the ophthalmoscope.

A partially dislocated lens is often complicated by cataract formation. If so, the cataract may have to be removed, but this should be delayed as long as possible because vitreous loss, predisposing to subsequent retinal detachment, is prone to occur during surgery. If the lens is free in the vitreous, it may lead in later life to the development of glaucoma of a type that responds poorly to treatment.

If dislocation is partial and the lens is clear, the visual prognosis is good.

Traumatic Lens Dislocation

Partial or complete traumatic lens dislocation may occur following a contusion injury such as a blow to the eye with a fist. If the dislocation is partial, there may be no symptoms; but if the lens is floating in the vitreous, the patient has blurred vision and usually a red eye. **Iridodonesis,** a quivering of the iris when the patient moves the eye, is a common sign of lens dislocation and is due to the lack of lens support. This is present both in partially and completely dislocated lenses but is more marked in the latter.

Iritis and glaucoma are common complications of dislocated lens, particularly if dislocation is complete.

If there are no complications, dislocated lenses are best left untreated. If uncontrollable glaucoma occurs, lens extraction must be done despite the poor results of this operation. The technique of choice is pars plana lensectomy using a motor-driven lens and vitreous cutter.

Figure 12–13. Dislocated lens.

REFERENCES

Apple DJ et al: Complications of intraocular lenses: A historical and histopathological review. *Surv Ophthalmol* 1984;**29**:1.

Frayer WC: What's new in surgery? Ophthalmic surgery. *Bull Am Coll Surg* 1982;**67**:32.

Heller R, Giacometti L, Yuen K: Sunlight and cataract: An epidemiologic investigation. *Am J Epidemiol* 1977;**105**:450.

Irvine AR: Extracapsular cataract extraction and pseudophakos implantation in primates: A clinico-pathologic study. *Ophthalmic Surg* 1981;**12**:27.

Jaffe NS, Clayman HM, Jaffe MS: Cystoid macular edema after intracapsular and extracapsular cataract extraction with and without an intraocular lens. *Ophthalmology* 1982;**89**:25.

Jaffe NS, Clayman HM, Jaffe MS: Retinal detachment in myopic eyes after intracapsular and extracapsular cataract extraction. *Am J Ophthalmol* 1984;**97**:48.

Kraff MC, Sanders DR, Lieberman HL: Intraocular pressure and the corneal endothelium after neodymium-YAG laser posterior capsulotomy. *Arch Ophthalmol* 1985;**103**:511.

Lerman S: Ultraviolet radiation photodamage to the ocular lens: Diagnosis and treatment. *Ann Ophthalmol* 1982;**14**:411.

McDonnell PJ, Zarbin MA, Green WR: Posterior capsule opacification in pseudophakic eyes. *Ophthalmology* 1983;**90**:1548.

Percival SPB, Anand V, Das SK: Prevalence of aphakic retinal detachment. *Br J Ophthalmol* 1983;**67**:43.

Radius RL et al: Pseudophakia and intraocular pressure. *Am J Ophthalmol* 1984;**97**:738.

Rice NSC: Congenital cataract: A cause of preventable blindness in children. *Br Med J* 1982;**285**:581.

Shock JP: Phacofragmentation and irrigation. *Ann Ophthalmol* 1976;**8**:591.

Stark WJ et al: Cystoid macular edema in pseudophakia. *Surv Ophthalmol* 1984;**28(Suppl)**:442.

Stark WJ et al: The FDA report on intraocular lenses. *Ophthalmology* 1983;**90**:311.

Stark WJ et al: Trends in cataract surgery and intraocular lenses in the United States. *Am J Ophthalmol* 1983;**96**:304.

Straatsma BR et al: Diabetes mellitus and intraocular lens implantation. *Ophthalmology* 1983;**90**:336.

Taylor DM, Sachs SW, Stern AL: Aphakic cystoid macular edema: Longterm clinical observations. *Surv Ophthalmol* 1984;**28(Suppl)**:437.

Taylor DM et al: Pseudophakic bullous keratopathy. *Ophthalmology* 1983;**90**:19.

Terry AC et al: Neodymium-YAG laser for posterior capsulotomy. *Am J Ophthalmol* 1983;**96**:716.

Vitreous

13

Conor O'Malley, MD

COMPOSITION & ANATOMY

The vitreous is about 99% water. The remaining 1% includes 2 components, collagen and hyaluronic acid, which give it its specific physical character.

The vitreous owes its gel-like form and consistency to a loose syncytium of long-chain collagen molecules capable of binding about 200 times their own weight in water.

The hyaluronic acid molecules are very large, loose skeins capable of binding about 60 times their weight in water. Combined with the collagen element, they account for the physical characteristics of normal vitreous.

The vitreous is a clear, avascular, gelatinous body that comprises two-thirds of the volume and weight of the eye. It fills the space bounded by the lens, retina, and optic disk (Fig 13–1). Since it is quite inelastic and impervious to cells and debris, it plays an important role in maintaining the transparency and form of the eye. If the vitreous were removed, the eye would collapse. When the vitreous is replaced by saline, as in certain forms of vitreous surgery, cellular matter and particulate debris are free to migrate into the optical pathway.

The outer surface of the vitreous—the hyaloid membrane—is normally in contact with the following structures: the posterior lens capsule, the zonular fibers, the pars plana epithelium, the retina, and the optic nerve head. The base of the vitreous maintains a firm attachment throughout life to the pars plana epithelium and the retina immediately behind the ora serrata. The attachment to the lens capsule and the optic nerve head is firm in early life but soon disappears. This is the principal reason that intracapsular

cataract extraction without vitreous prolapse or "loss" is possible in adults and not in children. In addition, the vitreous is prone to vitreoretinal adhesions at the site of lattice degeneration of the retina, congenital retinal rosettes, meridional retinal folds, vitreoretinal scars, and new retinal blood vessels, as in diabetes and central retinal vein occlusion.

The hyaloid canal (Cloquet's canal), which in the fetus contains the hyaloid artery, passes anteroposteriorly from the lens to the optic nerve head. The hyaloid artery usually disappears soon after birth, but the hyaloid canal remains throughout life. It is not visible ophthalmoscopically. A rudimentary portion of the hyaloid artery occasionally remains and can be seen floating in the vitreous with its anterior portion attached to the posterior surface of the lens. This point of attachment can be seen as a black dot (Mittendorf's dot) with the ophthalmoscope.

EXAMINATION OF THE VITREOUS

Slit Lamp Examination

Normal vitreous is not visible by either direct or indirect ophthalmoscopy. The numerous ophthalmoscopically visible features are anomalies attributable either to structural changes, such as the floaters of syneresis and the ringlike form associated with posterior vitreous detachment (Fig 13–2), or to invasive elements, such as blood, white blood cell masses, or fibrovascular proliferations from adjacent tissues. Normal vitreous in situ and many important anomalies (eg, the retraction, condensation, and shrinkage of vitreous characteristic of diabetes or injury) can be viewed only with a slit lamp. **Slit lamps** are microscopes with specialized illuminating systems that make transparent and near-transparent ocular fluids and tissues visible. Although slit lamp examination of the vitreous is quite easy to learn and plays an important role in the management of vitreous disease, too few ophthalmologists make optimal use of this instrument.

Contact Lenses as Aid in Vitreous Examination

The anterior central vitreous is the only part of the inner eye (behind the lens) that can be seen with the slit lamp alone. In order to view other areas, special contact lenses must be placed in the patient's eye (1) to modify the light-focusing power of the aqueous lens and the lens lens (see p 353) and (2) to expand the limited range through which the illumination beam

Figure 13–1. Normal: vitreous gel fills inner eye.

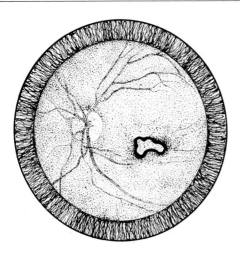

Figure 13–2. Vitreous detachment as seen with the +8 lens of the ophthalmoscope.

of the slit lamp can be angulated with respect to the visual axis of the eyeball.

A relatively thin contact lens with a flat front surface will neutralize the light-bending property of the eye, so that tissues *on and near the visual axis of the eye*—the optic disk, the posterior retina and choroid, and the axial vitreous—can be illuminated in 3-dimensional detail. Much thicker contact lenses with built-in mirrors and a flat front surface can be used to displace the illumination and viewing pathways of the slit lamp with respect to the visual axis of the eyeball, so that much of the nonaxial retina and vitreous can be seen.

These special contact lenses are also used in therapeutic procedures. Fundus contact lenses with built-in mirrors are widely used in laser surgery for panretinal photocoagulation of the peripheral retina. This prevents vitreous hemorrhage that may result from the retinal neovascularizations of diabetic retinopathy (see p 167), retinal vein occlusions (see p 165), and (rarer) sickle cell anemia (p 272). The thinner contact lenses are sometimes used in ablation of macular lesions associated with age-related macular degeneration and histoplasmosis (see p 178).

Use of special contact lenses, whether for diagnostic or therapeutic procedures, requires maximum dilation of the pupil with a combination of mydriatic and cycloplegic solutions (see p 18); use of a topical anesthetic to make the patient more comfortable; and use of a clear viscous solution of methylcellulose to prevent air from entering the lens-cornea interface.

B-Scan Ultrasonography

B-scan ultrasonography is an important diagnostic and prognostic tool used in many posterior segment problems associated with gross vitreous opacification (Fig 13–3). Where light-dependent ophthalmoscopes and slit lamps are of limited value, skillful use of B-scan ultrasonography can provide much information about the vitreous and adjacent structures. For example, it is possible to identify and locate vitreous membranes (Fig 13–4), vitreoretinal relationships and retinal detachments greater than 1 mm in depth (Figs 13–4 to 13–6), scleral ruptures, and intraocular foreign bodies (even nonlucent plastic and glass).

Figure 13–3. Vitreous hemorrhage limited to posterior vitreous region in aphakic eye. (Reproduced, with permission, from Coleman DJ: Ultrasound in vitreous surgery. *Trans Am Acad Ophthalmol Otolaryngol* 1972;**76**:469.)

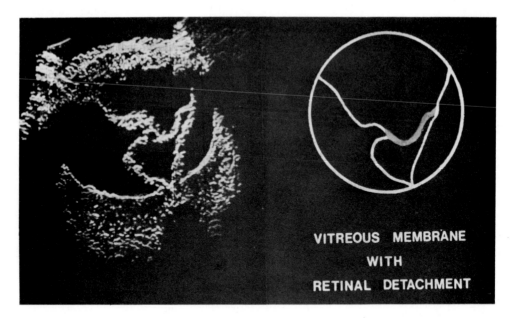

Figure 13–4. Total retinal detachment viewed horizontally below iris plane. A vitreous membrane connecting 2 leaves of retina is clearly demonstrated. (Reproduced, with permission, from Coleman DJ: Ultrasound in vitreous surgery. *Trans Am Acad Ophthalmol Otolaryngol* 1972;**76**:474.)

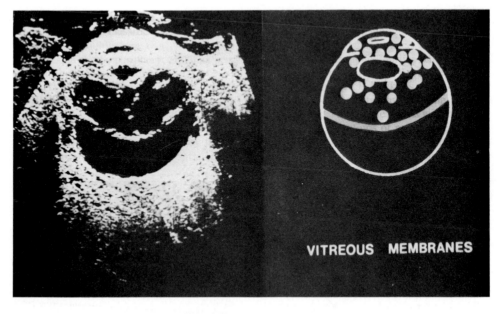

Figure 13–5. Vitreous membrane extending along posterior limiting membrane of vitreous from ora to ora. Retina is in place. (Reproduced, with permission, from Coleman DJ: Ultrasound in vitreous surgery. *Trans Am Acad Ophthalmol Otolaryngol* 1972;**76**:473.)

Figure 13–6. Vitreous membrane connecting 2 leaves of detached retina. Lens is normal. (Reproduced, with permission, from Coleman DJ: Ultrasound in vitreous surgery. *Trans Am Acad Ophthalmol Otolaryngol* 1972;**76**:474.)

DISORDERS OF THE VITREOUS

"FLASHING LIGHTS"

"Flashing lights" are a common symptom of an abnormal relationship between the retina and the vitreous. The patient is aware of a localized "light," "glow," "streak of light," or "flashing" (as of a neon tube) in the field of vision in the absence of a corresponding light source in the environment. The patient can usually point to the area of the disturbance and often describes an arc-shaped flicker in the periphery of one or 2 quadrants. The light seldom persists for more than a fraction of a second. It frequently recurs at short intervals for a few minutes and then disappears for hours, days, or even weeks. It is most readily identified on moving the eye and when illumination is dim or absent. Bilateral episodes may occur simultaneously but more commonly are separated by an interval of days to many years.

The light represents a cerebral awareness of the initial physical traction on and excitation of the sensory retina by abnormal vitreous. It is most commonly associated with recent collapse and detachment of the vitreous due to synersis with focal vitreous traction on vitreoretinal lesions such as lattice degeneration, meridional folds, congenital rosettes, and other visually subclinical vitreoretinal adhesions. A careful history will readily distinguish the light from the scin-

tillating scotoma of migraine, which is characterized by a symmetric quivering scotoma usually in both eyes, of predictable configuration and progression, accompanied by variable nausea or headache.

The vitreoretinal traction may require no treatment. However, as it can induce retinal tears, retinal detachment (Fig 13–7), or vitreous hemorrhage, every new case requires a survey of the vitreoretinal relationship, especially in the periphery.

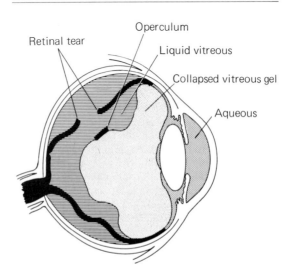

Figure 13–7. Schematic representation of vitreous collapse causing the retina to tear and detach.

VITREOUS FLOATERS

Vitreous floaters are by far the most common symptom of abnormal vitreous. A given floater represents the patient's awareness of the shadow of a mobile vitreous opacity cast upon the retina. The mind projects the corresponding dark form onto the appropriate area of the visual field.

The term vitreous floaters denotes a common, potentially serious symptom that was formerly called *muscae volitantes*—Latin for flies that flit, flutter, or fly to and fro.

The onset may be either insidious or acute and unilateral or bilateral. The patient is aware of one or more (or even many) fine, dark forms in the field of vision. Their configuration is usually so pronounced that the patient spontaneously classifies them as "spots," "soot," "particles," "spiders," "cobwebs," "threads," "worms," "dark streaks," "a ring," etc. Combinations are often reported. The objects continue to migrate after the eye comes to rest—hence the name floaters.

Central, relatively immobile floaters are visually annoying and may even be disabling. Peripheral ones are readily overlooked, as they are intermittent and require large eye motion or special positions merely to be seen. Unlike "flashing lights," they are most readily seen against bright lights or a uniform light background. They are extremely common in myopes and people with syneresis.

Floaters are commonly caused by small hemorrhages into the vitreous due to retinal tears or hemorrhagic diseases such as diabetic retinopathy, hypertension, leukemia, old retinal branch vein occlusion, Eales' disease, Coats' disease, and subacute bacterial endocarditis. Individual red cells are seen as small round black spots. Recent hemorrhages are often seen as black streaks or cobwebs that later break up into small round spots.

White cell invasion of the vitreous gel associated with pars planitis may also cause "spots before the eyes."

Vitreous floaters due to pigment are usually a consequence of long-standing tear-induced detachment of the retina that has not yet reached the macula.

Vitreous floaters should never be dismissed as harmless or imaginary. A careful survey of the vitreous and retina is always indicated in order to identify the nature and origin of floaters and to decide on management. Failure to make such an examination not infrequently leads to missed diagnosis. In the absence of a serious causative pathologic process, the patient may be reassured that the condition is harmless.

ASTEROID HYALOSIS

Asteroid hyalosis is an uncommon condition that occurs in otherwise healthy eyes in elderly people. Unilateral cases are 3 times as common as bilateral cases. Hundreds of small yellow spheres consisting of calcium soaps are seen in the vitreous. These move when the eyes move but always return to their original positions because they are attached to interlacing fibers. There are no related ocular or systemic diseases. The opacities have little or no effect upon vision but reflect the examiner's light very strongly. If there are enough asteroid bodies, the fundus is not viewable by ophthalmoscopy.

ACUTE VITREOUS COLLAPSE

The vitreous cavity is bounded by the retina, optic disk, pars plana, zonule, and crystalline lens. Normal vitreous fills this cavity (Fig 13–1) and remains firmly attached to the retina and pars plana near the ora serrata.

All types of gels, whether vitreous or gelatin, become increasingly prone with the passage of time to a degenerative process known as **syneresis**, involving drawing together of particles of the dispersed medium, separation of the medium, and shrinkage of the gel. Syneresis affects at least 65% of persons over 60 years of age. Myopes are especially susceptible, even in childhood.

With age, the center of the vitreous may undergo syneresis and become filled with liquid breakdown

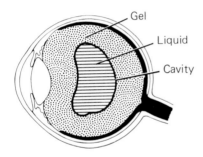

Figure 13–8. Large intravitreal cavity filled with liquid breakdown products of syneresis.

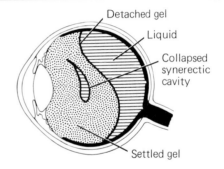

Figure 13–9. Posterior vitreous detachment.

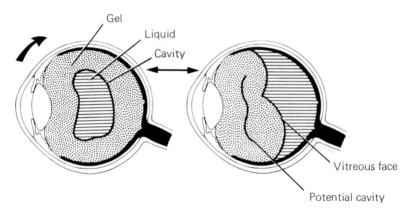

Figure 13-10. Liquid vitreous tends to be drawn into intravitreal cavity on abrupt eye motion *(left)* and expelled at rest *(right)*.

products of the degenerated gel (Fig 13–8). The liquid contents of the cavity can migrate into the preretinal space. The more solid, heavier vitreous gel collapses downward and forward to create a posterior vitreous detachment (Fig 13–9). The dynamic forces that accompany this collapse can rupture the last vestiges of the adhesions that once connected the vitreous to the disk, blood vessels, and sensory retina in childhood.

The patient and examiner can often see portions of the adhesions that remain attached to the collapsed vitreous as opacities. If they arise from the disk margin, the patient and examiner may note a ring-shaped opacity on the back of the vitreous.

Since the front of the vitreous is attached to the globe and the back of the vitreous is collapsed in on itself, abrupt motions of the eye transmit a whiplike force to the back of the vitreous. The vitreous tends to fill out toward its normal configuration; liquid vitreous is drawn into the synerectic cavity, and the posterior separation tends to disappear (Fig 13–10).

The whiplike motions of the vitreous can give rise to **photopsia** (an appearance of sparks or flashes) by causing stimulation of the vitreoretinal juncture and may cause a characteristic floating motion of posterior vitreous opacities, or floaters. The floaters move with the eye and float to a resting position after the eye comes to rest.

Since acute vitreous collapse can also cause asymptomatic retinal tears or detachment, *it should be assumed that patients with new floaters or photopsia have retinal tears or detachment until proved otherwise by thorough examination of the peripheral retina with an indirect ophthalmoscope.*

RETINAL TEARS
(See also Chapter 14.)

While retinal tears can be caused by trauma, vitreous shrinkage, or proliferative vitreoretinopathy,

most are caused by acute vitreous collapse. Tears following acute vitreous collapse are the result of a dynamic interaction between a focal vitreoretinal adhesion, collapsed mobile vitreous, and normal eye movement (Fig 13–11).

Since the gel and liquid components of the collapsed vitreous are structurally relatively independent of the retina, they do not move synchronously with the retina. When the eye (and hence the retina) moves, the gel and liquid tend to lag behind the retina, and when the eye stops moving, the gel and liquid tend to continue in motion. The vitreous gel and liquid are said to exhibit inertial lag with respect to the retina. Inertial lag of the gel can cause the vitreous to tear the friable sensory retina at the point where they adhere to each other (Fig 13–12). With the ophthalmoscope, the torn retina is seen to be pulled inward as a flap or a detached operculum (Fig 13–13). If retinal vessels are broken, they bleed briefly. A variable amount of blood accumulates in the vitreous cavity.

Some patients are not aware of the onset of retinal tears but often complain of photopsia and floaters. Some present with gross vitreous hemorrhage. Many

Figure 13-11. Local vitreoretinal adhesion.

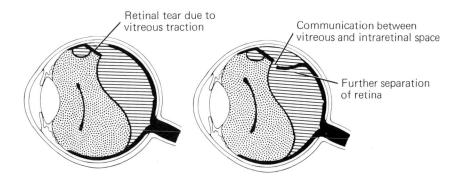

Figure 13–12. *Left:* Retinal tear. *Right:* Retinal detachment.

Figure 13–13. *Left:* Ophthalmoscopic view of retinal tear. *Right:* Ophthalmoscopic view of retinal detachment.

retinal tears never lead to retinal detachment, but recent symptomatic tears, especially those with symptomatic vitreous hemorrhage, have a strong tendency to cause retinal detachment days to years later. Patients with symptoms of acute vitreous collapse or vitreous hemorrhage should therefore undergo careful examination of the retina from the optic disk to the ora serrata to rule out one or more tears. Management of tears by prophylactic laser therapy or cryopexy is relatively simple and very effective compared to the performance of silicone buckling once retinal detachment has occurred.

Retinal tears are usually located anterior to the equator and are more often in the upper quadrants (Fig 13–13 left).

VITREOUS HEMORRHAGE

Vitreous hemorrhage can occur whenever the sensory retina is torn. Retinitis proliferans, central vein occlusion, branch vein occlusion, and hypertension are also frequent causes of vitreous hemorrhage. Acute collapse of the vitreous with posterior vitreous detachment will sometimes cause bleeding without tear formation. The patient often complains of floaters that suggest red blood cells, a sudden shower of small

black dots, or even tiny ringlike forms with clear centers. Visual loss ranges from imperceptible to gross.

The appearance of the retina and its visibility vary with the cause and amount of bleeding in the vitreous cavity (see Chapter 14). Fresh blood is red and tends to be located behind the vitreous gel or within a synerectic cavity (Fig 13–14). Within weeks to months, the blood tends to break down, becomes a pale color, and migrates into the gel (Fig 13–15).

Vitrectomy may be indicated to facilitate surgical reattachment of the retina. For example, vitreous hemorrhage following recent retinal detachment (diagnosed possibly by ultrasonography) may be extensive enough to hamper retinal surgery, which may need to be performed promptly to prevent irreversible macular atrophy.

Vitrectomy is not indicated for 3–6 months if treatment of the underlying cause can wait, as the vitreous may clear adequately without surgery.

RETINAL DETACHMENT
(See also Chapter 14.)

In the normal eye, the intact sensory retina is kept opposed to the pigment epithelium by the suction the latter exerts on the watertight space between them. If

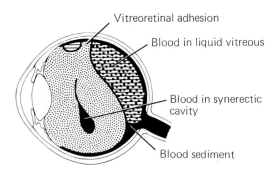

Figure 13-14. Acute vitreous hemorrhage: a retinal vessel ruptures due to vitreous traction.

Figure 13-15. Chronic vitreous hemorrhage.

a retinal tear is present, rapid eye motions and sudden rotation of the globe can readily generate enough inertial force to initiate retinal detachment (Fig 13–16). The space between the 2 layers of the retina fills with liquid vitreous, and eddy currents develop in this space, further accelerating the detachment process (Fig 13–17). Almost invariably, detachment continues until it is total.

Surgery with cryopexy and silicone buckling is required (1) to close the hole in the retina, reestablishing a watertight intraretinal space; (2) to restrict the inertial lag of the liquid and gel with respect to the retina; and (3) to approximate and seal together the 2 layers of the retina around the tear to counter the effects of eddy currents in the vitreous cavity. (See also Chapter 14.)

TRACTION RETINAL DETACHMENT

Traction retinal detachment is detachment of the sensory retina without retinal tears. The most common cause is long-standing diabetes. The detachment is typically found posterior to the equator and is due to vitreous traction on an area of retinitis proliferans (Fig 13–18).

Reattachment by vitrectomy is indicated only if there is clear-cut recent extension of the detachment into the macula.

PROLIFERATIVE VITREORETINOPATHY

A considerable number of abnormal conditions of the vitreous and retina are characterized by contractile membranes arising metaplastically from abnormally located retinal pigment epithelial cells and retinal glial cells. The membranes can occur on either the inner or outer surface of the sensory retina or on several vitreous surfaces. The membranes may be weak and subtle or strong, easily seen, and capable of causing great distortion of the host tissues.

The causal retinal pigment epithelial cells and retinal glial cells are pluripotential cells, with great meta-

plastic potential. They may proliferate at remote sites and take on the characteristics of myofibroblasts. These myofibroblastlike cells readily form contractile membranes that may deform the inner and outer surfaces of the retina and the posterior vitreous surfaces (Fig 13–19).

The basic process, or its outcome, is known as massive vitreous retraction, preretinal traction, preretinal vitreous membrane (see Chapter 14), subretinal fibrosis, macular pucker, or surface wrinkling retinopathy.

Proliferative vitreoretinopathy requires no treatment unless it causes surface wrinkling retinopathy of the macula (also known as macular pucker) or unduly complicates therapy for retinal detachment. While research holds some promise for an antiproliferative pharmaceutical agent, current treatment involves a special surgical procedure that employs distention, severing, or removal of vitreous tissue (see below).

INJURY TO THE VITREOUS

Contusion

Because the vitreous is inelastic compared with the adjacent tissues, contusions that abruptly though briefly alter the shape of the eye are apt to cause injuries where the vitreous is adherent.

Disinsertion of the vitreous base is not uncommon. It is frequently associated with tearing of the pars plana or retina, vitreous hemorrhage, or detachment of the retina—as long as 20 years later.

Less commonly, "flashing lights," vitreous floaters, and even vitreous hemorrhage or detachment of the retina may result from stress behind the vitreous base. The affected sites may be previously subclinical anomalous vitreoretinal adhesions (eg, lattice degeneration) or areas of frank vitreoretinal disease such as diabetic retinopathy.

Rupture of the Globe

Rupture of the globe is always a serious injury that may result in early or late blindness or even loss

Figure 13–16. Abrupt rotation of globe generates eddy currents in liquid vitreous, a result of inertial lag *(left),* that tends to lift the retinal flap and surrounding sensory retina *(right).*

Figure 13–17. Enlargement of retinal detachment due to inertial lag of liquid vitreous within the retina.

Figure 13–18. Traction detachment of retina.

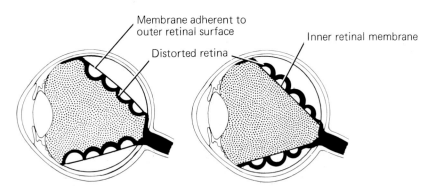

Figure 13–19. Proliferative vitreoretinopathy. *Left:* Contracture of membrane adherent to outer retinal surface. *Right:* Contracture of inner retinal membrane.

of the eyeball. Prolapse of the vitreous through the wound is a severe complication often associated with acute secondary tearing or detachment of the retina. A seemingly uncomplicated prolapse may be followed by late retinal detachment with or without tears due to fibrous ingrowth from the orbit and subsequent contraction. The latter may be visible as membranes or bands in the vitreous. Various forms of vitreous surgery are used to prevent or treat such complications.

Penetration of the Globe

An almost endless variety of material may accidentally penetrate the globe. Common examples are needles, BB shot, and small particles of metal, stone, or plastic that fly into the eye at high velocity.

Prolapse of the vitreous may occur at the site of entry or exit or both. The part traversed by the foreign body is permanently damaged and is often marked by visible condensation, shrinkage, or fibrous elements. Vitreous surgery is increasingly used to prevent or treat complications such as retinal detachment with or without tears.

Vitreous Loss

Vitreous loss is an iatrogenic complication. The vitreous gel prolapses through a surgical wound, usually at (but not limited to) the corneal limbus during the course of operating on the lens, iris, or cornea.

Fibrous tissue invasion and contraction are fre-quent sequels that are prone to cause traction complications involving the retina. Corneal edema and iris displacement (eg, "updrawn pupil") may also occur. An acute prolapse can be effectively excised. An old prolapse may require surgery for release of vitreous traction.

VITREOUS INFLAMMATION

Vitreous inflammation includes a wide spectrum of disorders ranging from a few scattered white cells to abscess formation. Most commonly, one or more focal inflammatory lesions in the choroid or retina—as in chorioretinitis or retinitis—are responsible for a secondary cellular invasion of the liquid vitreous or relatively resistant gel. There may be a mild localized blurring of the fundus landmarks and lesions that provoke little or no visual complaint except for a possible vitreous floater effect. With greater infiltration, vision is decreased and the fundus is invisible or almost so. The condition may be so marked that the red reflection is lost and the vitreous appears opaque and white. Since these conditions spare the anterior segment, there is no pain and the external eye appears normal. The prognosis and treatment depend upon the underlying condition. The vitreous usually clears when the primary defect is quiescent. Vitreous surgery is used to remove gross residual opacities that show no sign of clearing spontaneously.

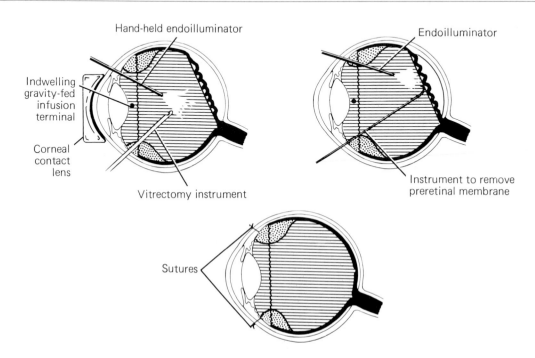

Figure 13–20. Vitreous surgery. *Top left:* Position of corneal contact lens and intraocular devices. *Top right:* Removal of preretinal membrane. *Bottom:* Placement of sutures at completion of procedure.

Vitreous abscess (or **endophthalmitis***) is a rare, painful condition associated with photophobia as well as redness and edema of the conjunctiva and lids. It is a unilateral infection usually caused by *Bacillus subtilis*, a common barnyard contaminant. In most

*If all 3 coats of the eye as well as the vitreous are involved by an inflammatory process, the condition is known as panophthalmitis. The line of demarcation between endophthalmitis and panophthalmitis is usually obscure.

reported cases, the organism has been introduced by a penetrating injury. The vitreous is an excellent culture medium for this organism, and the abscess characteristically progresses rapidly to destroy the eye despite injections of antibiotics into the vitreous. In rare instances, vitreous abscess is the result of blood-borne infection.

The treatment of hospital-acquired endophthalmitis following surgery for cataract or glaucoma is summarized on p 377.

Figure 13–21. Scope of vitreous surgery. *Top:* Removal of vitreous hemorrhage. Residual hemorrhage will clear in time from vitreous remnants. *Middle:* Reattachment of traction retinal detachment following vitrectomy. *Bottom:* Vitreous contracture complicating retinal detachment. Removal of vitreous and repair of retinal detachment.

VITREOUS SURGERY

Vitreous surgery is useful for a broad spectrum of intraocular disorders. Airtight and watertight incisions measuring 1–4 mm are made in the pars plana and sclera (Fig 13–20). One incision is used for an indwelling gravity-fed infusion terminal, which maintains the desired tension and configuration of the globe. Surgical gases and medications are also instilled through this terminal. Another incision is used for a hand-held endoilluminator, which illuminates the contents and all of the walls of the vitreous cavity. The illuminated structures are viewed microscopically through the pupil with the aid of a corneal contact lens that neutralizes the light-focusing power of the eye. The remaining incision is used to allow for instrumentation (severing or removal of tissue), diathermy, and laser photocoagulation (Fig 13–20).

Vitreous surgery provides access to virtually all of the intraocular tissues between the endothelium of the cornea and the retinal pigment epithelium. Surgery is most commonly done (1) to remove vitreous opacified by blood (Fig 13–21 top), (2) to remove shrunken vitreous causing traction retinal detachment (Fig 13–21 middle), (3) to treat vitreous contracture complicating retinal detachment (Fig 13–21 bottom) (see preretinal membranes), (4) to remove metaplastic membranes that deform or detach the sensory retina (Figs 13–19 and 13–20), (5) to create an optical opening in recalcitrant pupillary membranes, and (6) to remove infected vitreous in endophthalmitis (so as to dilute the organismal toxins and reduce the population of causal organisms and to instill therapeutic solutions). Vitreous surgery is frequently combined with scleral buckling for retinal detachment.

REFERENCES

Charles S: *Vitreous Microsurgery.* Williams & Wilkins, 1981.

Constable IJ et al: Clinicopathological correlation of vitreous membranes. Page 245 in: *Retina Congress (Proceedings): Boston, 1972.* Pruett RC, Regan CDJ (editors). Appleton-Century-Crofts, 1974.

Lincoff H, Kreissig I: The conservative management of vitreous hemorrhage. *Trans Am Acad Ophthalmol Otolaryngol* 1973; **79:**858.

Machemer R: Massive periretinal proliferation: A logical approach to therapy. *Trans Am Ophthalmol Soc* 1977;**75:**556.

Machemer R, Aaberg TM: *Vitrectomy,* 2nd ed. Grune & Stratton, 1979.

O'Malley C et al: Closed eye intraocular microsurgery. Pages 39–216 in: *Highlights of Ophthalmology.* Vol 1. Boyd B (editor). Highlights of Ophthalmology Press, 1981.

Peyman GA, Sanders DR: *Advances in Uveal Surgery, Vitreous Surgery, and Treatment of Endophthalmitis.* Appleton-Century-Crofts, 1975.

Ryan SJ: The pathophysiology of proliferative vitreoretinopathy in its management. *Am J Ophthalmol* 1985;**100:**188.

Retina

14

The retina covers the inner aspect of the posterior two-thirds of the wall of the globe. A fundus photo of the posterior pole of a normal retina is shown in Fig 14–1. The principal landmarks of the retina are illustrated and labeled in Fig 3–2.

The retina is a multilayered sheet of neural tissue closely applied to a single layer of pigmented epithelial cells, which in turn is attached to Bruch's membrane (Fig 14–2). The anterior extremity of the retina is firmly bound to the pigment epithelium. Posteriorly, the optic nerve fixes the retina to the wall of the globe. Elsewhere, the retina and the pigment epithelium are easily separated. In adults, the ora serrata—the partly serrated anterior end of the retina—is about 6.5 mm behind Schwalbe's line on the temporal side of the eye and 5.7 mm behind it nasally.

The retina is 0.1 mm thick at the ora serrata and 0.23 mm thick at the posterior pole. It is thinnest at the fovea centralis, the center of the macula. The retina is normally transparent, and some of the incident light is reflected at the vitreoretinal interface. The resulting sheen is especially noticeable when young, heavily pigmented patients are examined with an indirect ophthalmoscope. On examination with the direct ophthalmoscope, the concave foveal surface produces a clearly visible inverted image of the lamp. Absence of this foveal reflection may indicate disease, but the reflection may be absent in blond or elderly patients even though the retina is normal.

The fovea centralis, which lies about 3.5 mm lateral to the optic disk, is specialized for fine visual discrimination. In the fovea, the receptors are all cones; the outer nuclear layer is thinned; the other parenchymal layers are displaced centrifugally; and the internal limiting membrane is thin. Throughout most of the retina, the axons of the receptor cells pass directly to the inner side of the outer plexiform layer, where they connect with dendrites of horizontal and bipolar cells, which extend outward from the inner nuclear layer. In the macula, however, the receptor cell axons follow an oblique course and are called the Henle fiber layer. The normally empty extracellular space of the retina is potentially greatest at the macula, and diseases that lead to accumulation of extracellular material cause considerable thickening of this area.

The axons of the bipolar cells are connected with amacrine and ganglion cells in the densely woven inner plexiform layer. The long axons of the ganglion cells pass in the nerve fiber layer to the optic nerve.

The retina receives its blood supply from 2 sources.

The choriocapillaris is a single layer of closely spaced capillaries intimately attached to the outer surface of Bruch's membrane. The choriocapillaris supplies the outer third of the retina, including the outer plexiform and outer nuclear layers, the photoreceptors, and the pigment epithelium. The inner two-thirds of the retina receive branches of the central retinal artery. As the choriocapillaris is the only blood supply to the fovea centralis, this, the most important part of the retina, is susceptible to irreparable damage when the retina is detached.

PHYSIOLOGY

The optical system of the eye focuses a miniature image of the world upon the outer segments of the rods and cones, where the light starts a complex chain of chemical reactions beginning with a light-sensitive pigment composed of a small molecule, retinal (vitamin A aldehyde), bound to a large protein, opsin. The retinal is the same in both rods and cones, but the opsin differs. Light isomerizes the retinal from the 11-cis to an all-trans shape, so that it no longer remains adherent to the opsin. The liberated all-trans retinal may be metabolized to the 11-cis form and reattached to opsin, or it may be stored as vitamin A to be used later as the need arises.

The chemical sequence following the isomerization of retinal produces a transient excitation of the receptor that is propagated along its axon. A complex system of interconnections between the receptor axon and the cell processes of the horizontal and bipolar cells begins the process of analyzing the raw data from the receptors. The bipolar cells transmit this refined information to the inner plexiform layer, where it is once more modified through connections between amacrine, bipolar, and ganglion cells. The ganglion cells pass this reanalyzed information to the brain.

The cones are used for detailed vision (eg, reading) and color perception (Fig 14–3). They predominate at the macula, the center of visual attention; and they alone are present at the fovea, the site of best visual acuity. The rods, which predominate elsewhere, function best in reduced illumination. The principal roles of the extramacular retina are night vision and visual orientation. Examples of the latter are the ability to walk without tripping over objects or to fix one's gaze on a moving object.

Figure 14–1. Ophthalmoscopic view of a normal retina. Note deep physiologic cup. (Courtesy of S Mettier, Jr.)

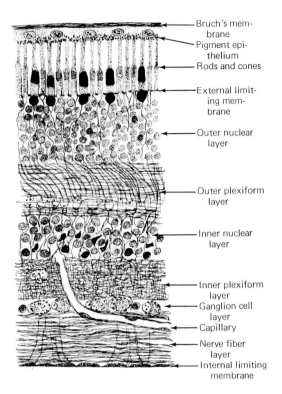

Figure 14–2. Layers of the retina. (Redrawn and reproduced, with permission, from Wolff E: *Anatomy of the Eye and Orbit,* 4th ed. Blakiston-McGraw, 1954.)

Physiology of Symptoms

The function of the retina is to receive visual images, to partly analyze them, and to dispatch this modified information to the brain. In the absence of refractive errors or opacities of the media, the images are seen in sharp focus. If the macular area of the retina is diseased, the patient's central visual acuity is affected, causing difficulty in reading and in discerning small objects in the distance (eg, street signs). If the peripheral portion of the retina is diseased, side vision is impaired but the patient continues to read well. With extreme contraction of peripheral visual field, the patient can read the finest print but bumps into large objects such as chairs and desks.

The retina has no pain nerve fibers, so that diseases of the retina are painless. In addition, they do not cause the eye to become red. The clinical evaluation of patients with retinal disease includes history, visual acuity, refraction, biomicroscopy, ophthalmoscopy, visual fields, color vision tests, and fluorescein angioscopy. Other helpful diagnostic tests in the study of retinal disorders include fluorescein angiography, electroretinography (ERG), electro-oculography (EOG), dark adaptation, and ultrasonography. (See Chapter 3.)

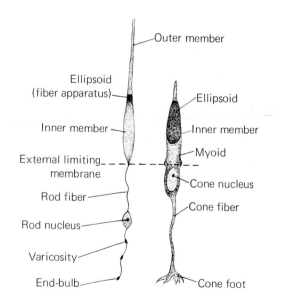

Figure 14–3. Rod *(left)* and cone *(right).* (Redrawn and reproduced, with permission, from Wolff E: *Anatomy of the Eye and Orbit,* 4th ed. Blakiston-McGraw, 1954.)

DISEASES OF THE RETINA

RETINAL ARTERY OCCLUSION

Blockage of the central retinal artery or one of its branches is an uncommon unilateral disorder of older patients. The obstruction may be due to an embolus or may be caused by intimal atherosclerosis. When the central retinal artery is affected, the result is sudden complete or almost complete loss of vision. Ophthalmoscopic examination within 2 hours of the occlusion shows segmentation of the blood column. Later, the vessel may appear normal, but emboli are often visible at its bifurcations. The posterior retina is pale and opaque because of changes in the axons of the nerve fiber layer (Fig 14–4). Lacking the inner retinal layers, the fovea remains transparent with the choroid showing through as a cherry-red spot. The direct pupillary response is absent. The consensual light reaction is normal.

One should attempt to restore the blood flow if the patient is seen within 2 hours of the onset of symptoms. The suggested treatment is massaging the globe and anterior chamber paracentesis. The globe is massaged by pressing firmly through the closed lids for several seconds and then abruptly releasing the pressure. This maneuver is repeated several times.

Anterior chamber paracentesis is performed after anesthesia is achieved by instillation of drops and by local infiltration of the conjunctiva. The conjunctiva is held with a forceps, and a short 30-gauge needle, which is not attached to a syringe, is passed obliquely through the limbus at 4:30 or 7:30 o'clock. The needle is aimed at the 6 o'clock chamber angle so as to avoid the lens. One or 2 drops of aqueous are expressed through the needle by pressing on the globe, and the needle is removed. The rationale of the procedure is that the sudden lowering of the intraocular pressure might allow the blood in the central retinal artery to dislodge the embolus to a more peripheral branch of the vessel.

There is experimental evidence that 100% oxygen at atmospheric pressure may prolong retinal survival. However, if complete loss of vision persists for more than 2 hours, the value of therapy is questionable.

RETINAL VEIN OCCLUSION

1. CENTRAL RETINAL VEIN OCCLUSION (Fig 14–5)

Central retinal vein occlusion is an uncommon, usually monocular condition in which the retina and disk are swollen, the retinal veins are dilated and tortuous, and there are many retinal hemorrhages with a variable number of cotton wool patches. These findings, which are due to blockage of the central retinal vein at the level of the lamina cribrosa or behind it, are most prominent in the posterior pole and are less intense in the peripheral retina. The choriocapillaris protects the retina from ischemic death.

The patient generally presents with a slow, painless loss of vision. Predisposing systemic diseases are hypertension, diabetes, and conditions that slow venous blood flow. Many patients have elevated intraocular tension in both eyes.

One may divide the patients into 2 fairly distinct subgroups. In the less severely affected group, the retinal bleeding is mild and there are few, if any, cotton wool patches. The visual acuity is generally no worse than 6/24 (20/80) and the peripheral visual field is relatively normal. A few of the patients in this group may get worse, so that they will be included

Figure 14–4. Twenty-four hours after left central retinal artery occlusion. Ischemic changes have made the nerve fiber layer pale and opaque. Because the fovea lacks this layer, the choroid can be seen as a cherry-red spot.

Figure 14–5. Central retinal vein occlusion. (Courtesy of University of California, San Francisco.)

in the more severely affected group, but most dry out spontaneously when, in the course of weeks or months, the shunt vessels enlarge. Many regain normal vision, although some, in whom the fovea is permanently damaged by the edema, have a persistent central scotoma.

The usually older patients in the more severely affected subgroup are felt to have a deficient retinal arterial supply compounding the venous obstruction. In these patients, whose condition is sometimes labeled hemorrhagic retinopathy—as opposed to the name, venous stasis retinopathy, applied to the less severely affected group—the congestion and bleeding of the disk and retina are more pronounced and there may be many cotton wool exudates. These hemorrhagic retinopathy patients have a reduced peripheral visual field. Their visual acuity is 6/60 (20/200) or worse. Fluorescein demonstrates absence of blood flow through the greater part of the retinal capillary bed, and histologically there is no viable retinal vascular endothelium. The protracted course of hemorrhagic retinopathy leads to the following states: cystoid degeneration and irreversible loss of foveal function; alterations of all parts of the retinal parenchyma; degeneration of the pigment epithelium; and liquefaction of the vitreous. When the vitreous is severely liquefied and thus no longer serves as a diffusion barrier to angiogenesis stimuli coming from the retina, new vessels often develop on the surface of the iris and the anterior chamber angle, causing peripheral anterior synechiae and intractable glaucoma.

Treatment

Many of the patients with venous stasis retinopathy recover spontaneously and require no treatment. Failing this, steroids may be considered.

Some practitioners advocate photocoagulation for those with hemorrhagic retinopathy. Anticoagulants, if they do anything, make matters worse.

In the hope of preventing neovascular glaucoma, the iris surface should be periodically checked for new vessels. Fluorescein angiography helps visualize these vessels, which first appear at the pupillary margin. If they occur, panretinal photocoagulation—a polka-dot distribution of coagulations covering areas of the retina other than the macula—usually arrests the process. If the media are too opaque for photocoagulation, the equivalent—transcleral cryotherapy—may help.

The possibilities of systemic vascular occlusive disease or blood sludging problems should be considered.

2. RETINAL BRANCH VEIN OCCLUSION (Fig 14–6)

Retinal branch vein occlusion is more common than central retinal vein occlusion. The obstruction occurs at the site of an arteriovenous crossing. Distal to the obstruction, the vein is engorged and tortuous, the retina is edematous, and there are hemorrhages, microaneurysms, and sometimes cotton wool exu-

Figure 14–6. Inferotemporal branch vein occlusion in right eye. Hemorrhages and cotton wool spots are located distal to the point of obstruction at an arteriovenous crossing (arrow). (Courtesy of E Ai.)

dates. Fluorescein angioscopy emphasizes the venous dilation and demonstrates segmental dilation and leakiness of the retinal capillary bed.

The superior temporal vein is most often affected. When the macular area is involved, the vision is reduced. If one-quarter or less of the macula is edematous, the prognosis for spontaneous recovery is good. If more, the prognosis is poor.

A significant number of patients with occlusion of a branch of the retinal vein will subsequently develop new vessels. These proliferate from the surrounding, relatively normal retinal or disk vessels. If the vitreous still is against the retina, they fan out on its back surface and may bleed both behind the vitreous and into its substance, when eventually the vitreous detaches. Rarely, traction by the vitreous may tear the retina at the site of origin of the neovascular frond.

In the presence of preexisting vitreous detachment, the new vessels present as minute protrusions at the inner retinal surface. Such vessels also may bleed, apparently because the mobile vitreous brushes against them.

Three-fourths of patients with branch vein occlusion have high blood pressure. Diabetes, sickle cell disease, polycythemia vera, lymphoma, leukemia, macroglobulinemia, and multiple myeloma are less common causes.

Treatment

Patients with retinal branch vein occlusion should be evaluated by an internist. If visually significant macular edema does not clear spontaneously, the area of capillary leakage identified by angiography can be treated with argon laser photocoagulation in a grid pattern that spares the fovea. If neovascularization is present, photocoagulation of the involved ischemic retinal sector may cause regression of the new vessels. Vitrectomy may become necessary if vitreous hemorrhage does not clear and obscures the retina.

DIABETIC RETINOPATHY

Diabetic retinopathy continues to be one of the leading causes of blindness in the Western world. Its frequency increases with the duration of the underlying disease. Several studies have suggested a strong correlation between poor antecedent blood glucose control and increased incidence and severity of retinopathy. However, it is unknown if there is a causal relationship or if these are separate manifestations of a more severe form of disease.

In terms of both prognosis and treatment, it is useful to divide diabetic retinopathy into nonproliferative and proliferative forms. The former can be further classified as background diabetic retinopathy or preproliferative retinopathy.

1. NONPROLIFERATIVE DIABETIC RETINOPATHY

Diabetic retinopathy is a progressive microangiopathy characterized by small vessel damage and occlusion. The earliest pathologic changes are thickening of the capillary endothelial basement membrane and reduction in the number of pericytes. **Background diabetic retinopathy** (Fig 14– 7A) is a clinical reflection of the hyperpermeability and incompetence of these vascular walls. The capillaries develop tiny dotlike outpouchings called microaneurysms, while the retinal veins become dilated and tortuous.

Multiple hemorrhages may appear throughout different levels of the retina. Flame hemorrhages are so shaped because of their location within the horizontally oriented nerve fiber layer, while dot and blot hemorrhages are in the deeper retina, where cells and axons are vertically oriented.

Leaking capillaries produce retinal edema with a predilection for the macula, giving the retina a thickened, cloudy appearance. In areas where serous fluid is resorbed, a yellowish lipid precipitate may remain in the form of "hard" exudate (Fig 14– 7B). Central vision is variably impaired if the fovea becomes edematous or ischemic or contains deposits of hard exudate. Many diabetics will not progress beyond this stage.

With progressive microvascular occlusion, signs of increasing ischemia may be superimposed on the above background picture, producing so-called **preproliferative diabetic retinopathy.** The most typical change would be the appearance of multiple cotton wool spots (incorrectly termed "soft exudates"), which are microinfarcts of the nerve fiber layer (Fig 14– 7C).

Other signs include gross venous abnormalities, such as loops, boxcarlike segmentation, and intraretinal microvascular abnormalities, which consist of irregularly dilated capillary beds and intraretinal shunts. Fluorescein angiography, which best demonstrates the extent of ischemia, shows "capillary nonperfusion," or large filling defects of capillary dropout usually most pronounced in the midperipheral retina.

Treatment

In background diabetic retinopathy, attention is focused on optimizing control of blood glucose and any associated hypertension. Macular edema may spontaneously improve, but if there is a significant loss of vision, laser photocoagulation may be considered if a focal source of leakage can be targeted by the angiogram. Randomly scattered laser therapy for diffuse macular leakage is controversial.

Preproliferative retinopathy is associated with increased risk for development of neovascularization, and these patients require close monitoring, even if they are asymptomatic. The effect of early laser panretinal photocoagulation during this stage and the benefit of laser treatment for macular edema are being evaluated in a national trial.

2. PROLIFERATIVE DIABETIC RETINOPATHY

The most severe complications of diabetic retinopathy are associated with the proliferative phase. Progressive retinal ischemia eventually stimulates the formation of delicate new vessels that leak serum and proteins (and fluorescein) profusely. Neovascularization is frequently located on the surface of the disk and at the posterior edge of peripheral zones of "nonperfusion" (Figs 14– 7D and 14– 8). Iris neovascularization, or rubeosis, can also result.

The fragile new vessels proliferate onto the posterior face of the vitreous and become elevated once the vitreous starts to contract away from the retina. If the vessels bleed, massive vitreous hemorrhage may cause sudden visual loss. As these elevated neovascular fronds undergo fibrous change, they form taut fibrovascular bands that tug on the retina with continued vitreous contraction (Fig 14– 7E). This can cause either a progressive traction retinal detachment (without a hole) or a rhegmatogenous detachment if a tear is produced. A detachment may be concealed by vitreous hemorrhage.

Treatment

Argon laser panretinal photocoagulation is usually indicated in proliferative diabetic retinopathy. Patients at greatest risk are those with preretinal or vitreous hemorrhage or neovascularization of the disk. Panretinal photocoagulation can significantly reduce the chance of massive vitreous hemorrhage and retinal detachment in these patients by causing the regression, and in some cases, the disappearance of new vessels.

The technique involves scattering up to several thousand regularly spaced laser burns throughout the retina, sparing the central region bordered by the disk and the major temporal vascular arcades (Fig 14– 7F). Although the mechanism is not precisely understood, panretinal photocoagulation presumably works by reducing the angiogenic stimulus from ischemic retina.

If a significant vision-impairing vitreous hemorrhage has not spontaneously cleared by 6 months, vitrectomy may be performed. Operation should be performed immediately if progressive retinal detach-

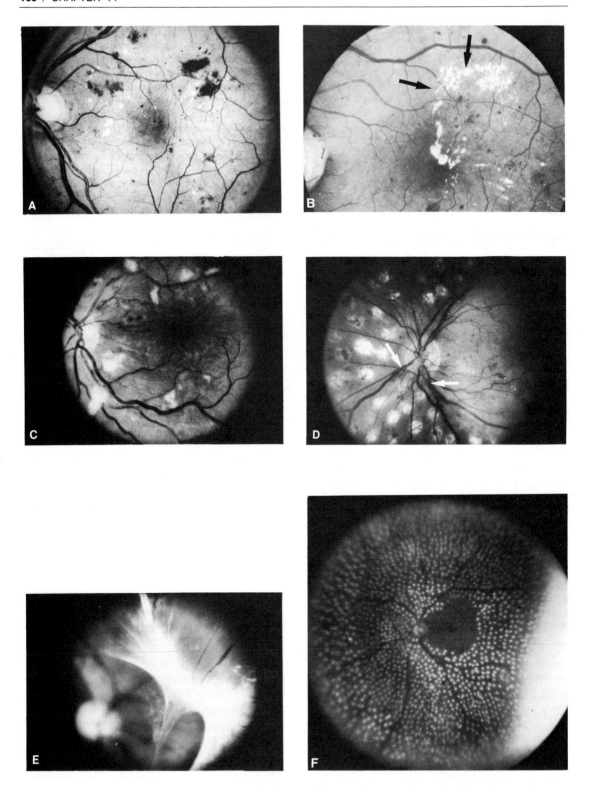

Figure 14–7. *A:* Background diabetic retinopathy. *B:* Background diabetic retinopathy with hard exudate (arrows). (Courtesy of P O'Malley.) *C:* Preproliferative retinopathy with multiple cotton wool spots (incorrectly named "soft exudates"). (Courtesy of E Ai.) *D:* Proliferative diabetic retinopathy with neovascularization of left disk (arrow) and panretinal photocoagulation scars sparing the macula. (Courtesy of E Ai.) *E:* Diabetic traction retinal detachment. (Courtesy of E Ai.) *F:* Wide-angle view of panretinal photocoagulation in left eye. (Reproduced, with permission, from Duane TD [editor]: Diabetic retinopathy. Chap 30, p 17, in: *Clinical Ophthalmology.* Vol 3. Lippincott. Series of 6 vols, 1978–1983.)

Figure 14–8. Proliferative diabetic retinopathy. *A:* Fundus photograph of left eye, showing neovascularization of the disk and along the inferotemporal arcade (arrows). The latter area has bled, producing a preretinal hemorrhage (open arrow). *B:* Fluorescein angiogram (early phase) of the same eye, showing dye filling the area of neovascularization on the disk (arrows). *C:* Mid-phase angiogram, showing dye leakage from the 2 areas of neovascularization. In addition to the irregular venous caliber, extensive ischemic areas of capillary dropout can be seen (arrow). *D:* Late-phase angiogram, showing profuse leakage of fluorescein from the same areas. The retinal vessels are obscured by the preretinal hemorrhage (arrows). (Courtesy of University of California, San Francisco.)

ment is suspected clinically or on ultrasound examination. Traction retinal detachments that involve or threaten the macula are treated by vitrectomy to release the traction and by scleral buckling to help reattach the retina.

The presence of retinal neovascularization alone will not affect vision. In the absence of macular pathology, such patients may be asymptomatic. Because many resulting severe complications can be presented by prompt laser treatment, the importance of early detection and regular monitoring cannot be overemphasized.

EDEMA OF THE RETINA

Between the retinal cells there is a potential space that fills with fluid when the retinal capillaries leak. The accumulation is greatest in the outer part of the outer plexiform layer, less in the outer and inner nuclear layers, and negligible in the remaining tightly woven layers. Because of the oblique course of the receptor cell axons in the Henle fiber layer, the macula swells more than the rest of the retina and the fluid is often visibly loculated in varicose tunnels radiating from the fovea, which itself becomes a single cystlike cavity.

Chronic edema is often accompanied by minute yellow deposits, mainly in the outer plexiform layer or beneath the retina. In the Henle fiber layer, the aggregates have a striking stellate distribution. Elsewhere, a nidus of edema is surrounded by a circular belt of these deposits. If the circinate figure is close to the macula, it spreads along the spaces of the Henle fiber layer, forming one arm of a star figure. Beneath the retina, the fatty material is irregularly clumped like the aggregates sometimes seen when new vessels grow through Bruch's membrane.

The causes of retinal edema include diabetes, retinal vein obstruction, hypertension, retinal angiomas or telangiectases, traction by the vitreous or preretinal membranes, macroaneurysms, and inflammations involving the vitreous or retina. A special case of retinal edema is the **Irvine-Gass syndrome,** which consists of rapid, usually temporary loss of visual acuity in aphakic patients. It occurs more commonly after intracapsular extraction, which allows the vitreous to adhere to the iris. It is probably due to chemicals in the anterior segment having free access to the retina through the liquefied vitreous core.

Clinical Findings

Blurred vision occurs only when the macula is edematous. Visual acuity may be only slightly affected or may be as low as finger counting. The elevation and ground glass appearance of the macular area can be quite striking, and one may discern a cystoid accumulation of fluid. When retinal edema is widespread, with relative sparing of the macula—as can be the case in diabetic patients—the ophthalmoscopic diagnosis is difficult. The only clues are retinal pallor and difficulty in distinguishing details of the pigment epithelium and choroid.

Intravenous fluorescein confirms the diagnosis of retinal edema, because the dye leaks from the normally impermeable vessels and stains the extracellular fluid and because cystoid collections at the macula (which cannot be discerned with the ophthalmoscope) will become easily visible. Later, if there is frank cystoid degeneration, the cavity contents no longer stain. Fluorescein does not stain the waxy yellow deposits observed in chronic edema.

Treatment

If macular edema is due to inflammation, corticosteroids may help when given systemically or by parabulbar injection.

Most patients with the Irvine-Gass syndrome need only explanation and encouragement, since they will improve without treatment. Prophylactic therapy with indomethacin reduces the incidence of this complication. If the vitreous is detached from the retina and is extensively adherent to the iris and the cataract incision, the macular edema often persists until the fovea is irreversibly damaged. Patients with these developments are sometimes helped by vitrectomy.

Focal edema due to vasculopathies—including diabetic retinopathy—may respond to photocoagulation.

Prognosis

Persistent macular edema may eventually become transformed into cystoid generation, with irreversible loss of central vision. In some cases, this is compounded by development of an atrophic hole at the fovea.

RETINAL MACROANEURYSMS

Sometimes, patients with hypertension or other systemic vascular diseases develop focal aneurysmal dilation of a retinal arteriole.

The aneurysm may bleed, but this usually clears spontaneously.

Surrounding the aneurysm is a ring of retinal edema. If this is away from the macula, nothing need be done, for it will clear on its own. If the exudate encroaches on the macula, however, it reduces the visual acuity and usually causes irreversible cystoid degeneration before resorbing. Photocoagulation helps if done before the macula is irreparably damaged.

RETINOPATHY OF PREMATURITY

Retinopathy of prematurity (formerly known as retrolental fibroplasia) is a bilateral retinal disease of premature infants. It was first reported in 1942 and caused total blindness in a large number of patients until 1954, when the usual cause was found to be excessive oxygen given during the first few weeks of life.

A high oxygen concentration causes spasm of the retinal blood vessels. The spasm is followed by edema of the immature peripheral retina with later vascular dilation and fibrovascular proliferation into the vitreous. Total retinal detachment often follows.

Retinopathy of prematurity usually has its onset in the first few days of life and may progress rapidly to blindness over a period of weeks. Once blindness occurs, there is no hope for restoration of sight. In many early cases, there is partial or complete regression in both eyes. Less commonly, the disease process regresses in one eye, allowing it to develop normal vision. Myopia and strabismus are common among those who retain useful vision, and in later life there is a tendency to rhegmatogenous retinal detachment (see p 175).

In advanced cases, one sees in both eyes a white retrolental membrane containing blood vessels. The anterior chamber is shallow, and the pupillary light reflex is absent. The lens is clear, and transillumination is normal. The contracting retrolental tissue draws the ciliary processes inward so that they can be seen at the periphery of the dilated pupil.

Differentiation from persistent hyperplastic vitreous usually is not difficult, since the latter condition is unilateral. Retinoblastoma has a later onset, may not transilluminate, and has an anterior chamber of normal depth. If bilateral, the tumor is usually more advanced in one eye.

Glaucoma, uveitis, cataract, or phthisis bulbi frequently occurs months or years after the onset of retinopathy of prematurity.

Infants of low birth weight and infants who require supplemental oxygen should have their pupils widely dilated for examination by indirect ophthalmoscopy and scleral depression in order to detect the earlier stages of retinopathy of prematurity. At first there is avascularity of the (usually temporal) peripheral retina. Later, a discrete intraretinal band appears at the junction of the vascular and avascular retina, with dilated retinal vessels and arteriovenous shunts behind this junction. Subsequently, new vessels grow into the vitreous at this site. It is the contraction of this fibrovascular tissue that causes the serious complications to the vitreous and retina. If the condition is aborted in the earlier stages, spontaneous regression may be quite complete. Regression is signaled by vessels growing into the previously avascular peripheral retina.

RETINITIS PIGMENTOSA

Retinitis pigmentosa is a group of hereditary dystrophies of the retinal receptors transmitted as autosomal recessive, autosomal dominant, or X-linked traits. The rods slowly degenerate, with secondary atrophy of the remainder of the retina and the pigment epithelium. Cells filled with epithelial pigment aggregate along the retinal vessels to give the typical bone corpuscular appearance (Fig 14–9). These changes begin in the mid periphery, sparing the macular and peripheral regions until later. The retinal problems are often associated with deafness, mental retardation, and other systemic findings, making several distinct syndromes. The most common of these is Laurence-Moon-Biedl syndrome, which combines retinitis pigmentosa, obesity, mental retardation, polydactyly, and hypogenitalism.

Night blindness—the first symptom of retinitis pigmentosa—usually occurs in early youth. Thereafter, the visual fields gradually constrict ("gun barrel vision") to become disabling in the fifth or sixth decade, at which time macular vision may also be lost. The fundi may appear normal at first. Later, most patients have the typical scattered black pigmentary disturbance. The retinal arterioles become attenuated, and the disk becomes pale and waxy. In rare instances, the disease may affect only one eye or just one sector of an eye.

The electroretinogram is reduced or absent, and the electro-oculogram gives a flat curve. Commonly associated eye findings are myopia, posterior polar cataract, and glaucoma.

In rare instances where retinitis pigmentosa is due to abetalipoproteinemia (Bassen-Kornzweig syndrome: steatorrhea, ataxia, and retinitis pigmentosa), its progress may be arrested in the early stages by massive doses of vitamin A. There is no specific therapy for the other causes of retinitis pigmentosa. Genetic counseling should be offered in an attempt to prevent propagation of the disease.

PERIPHERAL CYSTOID DEGENERATION

Cystoid degeneration of the retina consists of the permanent accumulation between the neural elements of a clear material that compresses the glial tissue into columns separating cystlike spaces. Some degree of cystoid degeneration is present in the peripheral retina of many infants and of everybody over age 8. It invariably begins at the ora serrata and progresses backward as a maze of contiguous varicose tunnels. It can extend behind the equator in later life, but not to the point where it causes symptoms or encroaches significantly on the peripheral field of vision.

 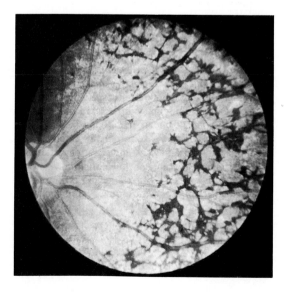

Figure 14 –9. Retinitis pigmentosa. *Left:* Typical "bone spicule" arrangement of pigmentary changes. *Right:* Clumped, scattered pigment, attenuated arteries, and choroidal sclerosis. (Photos by L Arlinghaus.)

Close to the ora serrata, the cystoid cavities are large and often cause the retina to have a moth-eaten appearance. Otherwise, the low magnification of the indirect ophthalmoscope does not normally allow the examiner to see this essentially innocuous condition.

SENILE RETINOSCHISIS

Peripheral cystoid degeneration may lead to splitting of the retina into 2 layers. Such "senile" retinoschisis occurs in about 3% of the population, increasing in frequency from the second decade onward.

The bulging internal wall of the cavity is thin and immobile and often has a "beaten metal" appearance. The thick external wall is hard to see in its usual position against the pigment epithelium, but there are often defects in it—in contrast to the inner layer, which usually is intact. Further diagnostic features include a band of prominent cystoid degeneration separating the cavity from the ora serrata and the presence of other areas of retinoschisis in the temporal half of the same eye or of the fellow eye.

If the contents of the cavity leak through a hole in the outer wall, a self-limited, usually harmless retinal detachment results. Rhegmatogenous detachment may develop when there is a hole in both walls. This rare complication is the only serious consequence of senile retinoschisis.

The bulging internal wall must not be mistaken for a retinal detachment and treated as such. Only when rhegmatogenous detachment has occurred or is imminent is it warranted to intervene with light coagulation, cryothermy, diathermy, or scleral buckling. In extremely rare instances, the retinal splitting threatens the macula and should be treated.

PAVING STONE DEGENERATION OF THE RETINA

Paving stone degeneration is a striking but harmless condition of the peripheral retina in which the pigment epithelium and outer retinal layers are damaged or absent. The intact inner retina is adherent to the exposed Bruch's membrane and also to the pigment epithelium at the edge of the lesion. The vitreous and the outer choroidal structures are normal.

The sharply outlined, rounded lesions are pale yellow, often with a partial rim of increased pigmentation. They range in size up to 1 disk diameter and may occur singly or in clusters. Several lesions may coalesce to form a circumferential band with a scalloped margin.

The process occurs mainly in the lower quadrants, though it is found in any part of the peripheral fundus. It is fairly common in young adults, and its incidence and the frequency of bilateral occurrence increase with age. It is quite innocuous, and the patient is unaware of its presence.

LATTICE DEGENERATION

Lattice degeneration (Fig 14–10) of the retina is characterized by elongated, excavated troughs in the peripheral retina. The lesions are surrounded by a distinct narrow rim, which projects above the level of the normal adjacent retina. The vitreous is firmly adherent to the rim and forms a canopy, which envelops a pocket of fluid lying in the trough. Close to their insertion, the vitreous fibrils are condensed and may be visible as a white frill.

Glistening white spots are common on the retinal surface, giving a snail-track appearance to some lattice areas. Although the pigment epithelium beneath the lesions may appear normal, it is often disturbed and may vary from subtle disarray to gross disorganization. The walls of the retinal vessels are thickened where they cross the abnormal retina in over 10% of lesions. These sclerosed vessels form a white latticework that inspired the name.

The above features are often not visible on routine inspection, and areas of lattice might be missed were it not for the edge-on view afforded by scleral depression. With this aid to examination, the sharp rim and roughened, depressed surface of the trough are readily seen.

The individual lesions are about one-third disk diameter in width and one-half disk diameter to 1 quadrant long. They generally lie parallel to the ora serrata, are confined to the equatorial and oral zones, and are concentrated toward the vertical meridian. There may be as many as 20 lesions in one eye forming 2 or more parallel rows. Both eyes are affected in about a third of cases.

About 8% of the population have lattice degeneration, and the incidence is constant in each age group

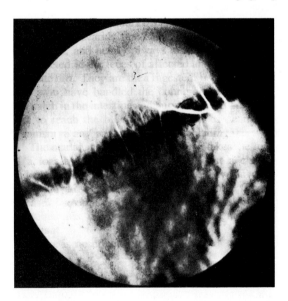

Figure 14–10. Lattice degeneration. (Reproduced, with permission, from O'Malley C, O'Malley P: *The Peripheral Fundus of the Eye.* Medcom, 1973.)

after 10. Surprisingly, teenagers may have heavily pigmented lesions with extreme thinning of the retina, whereas septuagenarians will often have rather superficial nonpigmented lesions. Atrophic round holes are common in all age groups.

Lattice degeneration is an etiologic factor in about one-third of all cases of rhegmatogenous retinal detachment. One of 2 distinct mechanisms is responsible for the detachment. In one group of patients, the leakage is through an atrophic hole. This may result in tiny localized areas of detachment that rarely spread and require no treatment other than periodic observation. In younger patients, such a detachment sometimes spreads slowly, with multiple demarcation lines, and surgery is required.

The more common mechanism by which lattice degeneration leads to retinal detachment derives from the fact that owing to their posterior location, about two-thirds of the lesions have established a firm vitreoretinal adhesion behind the vitreous base. If the vitreous detaches posteriorly, the stress at the ends and the posterior border of the lattice may be enough to produce a tear. The break is in the relatively normal retina beneath the rim and not through the thinned retina. Small lesions far back may be completely avulsed. Much more often, the tear is J-shaped and located at one end of the lattice. As the vitreous continues to tug on the retina, these tears usually cause extensive retinal detachment.

The threat of retinal detachment has given lattice degeneration notoriety in excess of what it deserves. Most people with this condition enjoy a normal asymptomatic existence. They should, however, be checked periodically, and they must be seen immediately if they report symptoms suggestive of vitreous detachment. If it is obvious that retinal detachment is likely—because of retinal detachment in the fellow eye, a family history of retinal detachment, or local findings—then one should perform prophylactic cryothermy or photocoagulation.

RETINAL HOLES

Retinal holes are either tears, which have an operculum (lid) of retinal tissue, or atrophic holes, which do not. The fovea and the peripheral retina are the sites of predilection for retinal holes. In both places, the internal limiting membrane and retinal parenchyma are thin. Extramacular tears and holes are described here. (For macular holes, see p 180.)

1. RETINAL TEARS
(Fig 14–11)

The retina is torn by mechanical force, usually vitreous traction (see also Chapter 13). The distinctive feature of a retinal tear is an operculum of avulsed tissue. The size of the tear may vary tremendously.

When the retina is torn, metaplastic pigment epithelial cells may enter the vitreous. If these tobacco-

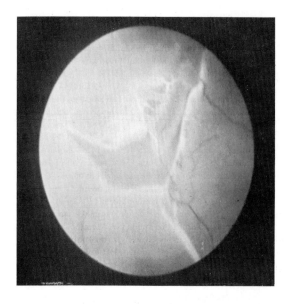

Figure 14–11. Retinal tear at an area of lattice degeneration. Operculum still attached to retina. (Reproduced, with permission, from O'Malley C, O'Malley P: *The Peripheral Fundus of the Eye.* Medcom, 1973.)

dustlike cells are found, a retinal tear is almost certainly present and must be sought.

Retinal tears may be due to constant or intermittent vitreous traction.

Tears due to constant vitreous traction. Proliferative diabetic retinopathy, penetrating injuries, and a variety of other disorders cause scarring of the vitreous. Contraction of the scarred vitreous may tear the retina at its point of attachment. Only a small percentage of retinal tears occurs by this mechanism, but it is important to recognize and treat them promptly for they may lead to extensive retinal detachment.

Tears due to intermittent vitreous traction. When the vitreous is partly liquefied and detached from the retina, acceleration or deceleration of the globe—either as a result of normal eye movements or trauma—will cause whiplike motions of the gel that may exert sufficient stress to tear the retina at normal and abnormal points of vitreoretinal attachments. The latter may be due to a number of anatomic anomalies and pathologic processes that may not be recognizable before the tear appears.

The greater the space inside the eye, the greater the force that can be exerted to tear the retina. This may explain why aphakia, the large globe commonly associated with myopia, forward displacement of the lens by miotics, and localized scleral ectasia predispose to retinal tears.

The operculum of most tears retains a partial attachment at the anterior margin of the break, so that the vitreous continues to tug on the retina. Even so, such retinal tears should be watched and not treated unless (1) the vitreous cavity is unduly large; (2) the holes are multiple, large, or far behind the ora serrata; (3) there is a history of retinal detachment in the fellow eye or a family history of retinal detachment; or (4) there are recent symptoms of vitreous detachment. In these situations, the danger of retinal detachment outweighs the small risk of complications from prophylactic therapy.

Retinal tissue may be torn completely free if the area of vitreoretinal adhesion is small. Such tears are generally round or oval and rarely exceed the diameter of the disk. They are much less likely to lead to retinal detachment than if the operculum is still adherent to the retina.

Relationship of Blood Vessels to Retinal Tears

At the time the retina is torn, capillaries are often ruptured and the patient reports a shower of black spots that represent shadows on the macula caused by red blood cells in the retrovitreal space. If a larger vessel is broken, the subvitreal bleeding may be so severe that the retina is obscured. A few hours of bed rest with bilateral eye patches and elevation of the head will generally allow the blood to settle enough to permit visualization of the retina.

As a rule, the larger vessels do not break, so that the retina either continues to tear beyond the vessel and a segment of the vessel is elevated off the retina or the vessel arrests the shearing force.

In younger patients, the acquired posterior extension of the vitreous base is narrow, so that tears may occur close to the ora serrata. Since the mechanical reinforcement of the retinal vessels is lacking here, the rip can extend a considerable distance around the circumference of the globe.

Causes of Retinal Tears

Vitreous traction, either intermittent or constant, accounts for the vast majority of retinal tears. This usually happens spontaneously, but indirect trauma occasionally precipitates a retinal tear in a predisposed individual.

Direct trauma deforms the globe transiently and can cause conventional tears, giant tears at the posterior margin of the vitreous base, or tears in the nonpigmented epithelium of the pars plana at the anterior margin of the vitreous base (see p 181).

Anomalous zonular attachments to the retina are also believed to cause tears. The detaching retina (for whatever reason) may also tear at the site of chorioretinal adhesions resulting from previous therapy, paving stone degeneration, or chorioretinitis, but this is rare. In these latter cases, the torn fragment remains adherent to the external structure—not in its usual location at or central to the detached retina.

2. ATROPHIC RETINAL HOLES

In addition to the atrophic holes associated with lattice degeneration and retinoschisis, about 1% of people have small, round, nonoperculated holes of unknown cause in the peripheral retina. These are usually close to the ora serrata and rarely cause significant retinal detachment, though a tiny self-limiting detachment is often present.

Most atrophic retinal holes are asymptomatic. Some are accompanied by symptoms of vitreous detachment (see Chapter 13).

Treatment

The greatest problem in treating retinal holes is deciding whether or not treatment is necessary. Unfortunately, the decision must be made with an inadequate knowledge of the natural history of most types of holes and almost total ignorance of the qualitative and quantitative parameters of vitreous traction. However, careful observation does give some clues, for with the passage of time the lips of a retinal hole become white and rounded because of gliosis; opercula slowly shrink; the subjacent pigment epithelium is often altered; and a ring of pigment epithelial reaction may appear at the edge of the narrow halo of retinal detachment, which often accompanies even innocuous holes. In the absence of frank retinal detachment, these findings tell the examiner that the potentially dangerous lesion has been present for some time without causing trouble; thus, a conservative attitude toward prophylactic therapy is required.

The objective of prophylactic treatment is to establish a firm chorioretinal bond around the retinal break. The scar should be broader on the side nearest the ora serrata, since this is usually the site of greatest vitreous pull. Indeed, it is often safest to treat forward to the vitreous base to forestall future vitreous traction.

There are 3 ways to seal a retinal hole: freezing, burning by light, or burning by electricity. The mechanism in each case is to cause an inflammatory response of the retina and choroid that subsequently binds them together.

A. Cryothermy: A supercooled metal probe is placed on the conjunctiva in an area corresponding to the borders of the retinal hole. The instrument must have an adequate heat sink to propagate a dome of ice through the wall of the eye. The surgeon ophthalmoscopically controls the freezing, which selectively destroys cells but leaves the fibrous structures intact.

B. Photocoagulation: A bright light focused on the pigment epithelium will coagulate it and the overlying retina. One may use a xenon arc or argon laser as the light source. This form of therapy is excellent for posterior lesions but is awkward to administer anterior to the equator.

C. Diathermy: The energy of a high-frequency current, when applied to the sclera, is transformed to heat, which coagulates choroid and retina.

RETINAL DETACHMENT

Because the retina is only loosely adherent to the pigment epithelium, the 2 may separate, allowing fluid to accumulate between them. The fluid usually comes from the vitreous, having passed through a hole in the retina. Less often, it leaks from blood vessels, as happens with central serous retinopathy, choroidal tumors, some inflammatory conditions, malignant hypertension, or when vitreous traction creates a subretinal space without perforating the retina. (See also Chapter 13.)

Mechanism of Rhegmatogenous Retinal Detachment

Rhegmatogenous (tear-induced) retinal detachment is dependent upon 3 factors: (1) a retinal hole, (2) liquid in the vitreous compartment with free access to the hole, and (3) a force sufficient to break the bond between the retina and the pigment epithelium and transfer fluid from in front of to behind the retina. The vitreous supplies this force in essentially the same way as it causes retinal tears (see p 174).

Until one or more of these factors is nullified, the detachment will continue to spread. Most of the retina may become detached in a few hours, or it may take years for this to happen.

Clinical Findings

The common sequence is for the symptoms of vitreous detachment (see Chapter 13) to be followed minutes to years later by a "shadow" or "curtain" spreading across the field of vision. When the detachment spreads very slowly, the patient may be unaware of any problem until the macula is affected.

On ophthalmoscopic examination, the detached retina bulges inward and is gently rippled or thrown into folds (Figs 14–12 to 14–16). It is translucent, obscuring the details of the pigment epithelium and choroid, and trembles with each movement of the eye. A careful search will almost always reveal one or more holes. If the detachment is of long standing, the retina will usually be more transparent and a characteristic demarcation line of pigment epithelial disturbance separates detached from normal retina.

The other eye must be examined, since it often has retinal holes or vitreoretinal adhesions that might lead to tears. These should be mapped carefully and treated prophylactically.

Differential Diagnosis

One must consider senile retinoschisis, choroidal detachment, and malignant melanoma of the choroid. The retinoschisis cavity has a thin, immobile inner wall. The honeycomb appearance and large breaks of the outer wall are pathognomonic but are not always present. There may be other areas of retinoschisis on the temporal side of the same or fellow eye.

A detached choroid is not limited by the ora serrata but is prevented from spreading where the vortex vessels enter the sclera. The pigment epithelium is still visible, but the choroidal structures are not.

In malignant melanoma of the choroid, the subretinal fluid shifts on changing the patient's position. The tumor usually does not transilluminate, and its position disregards both ora serrata and vortex vessels.

Treatment

Surgical repair is mandatory in the treatment of rhegmatogenous retinal detachment, since spontaneous reattachment is extremely rare. The first step is ophthalmoscopic examination of the entire retina and construction of a detailed map showing each hole and each area of vitreoretinal traction. The goal is to seal the holes and prevent further holes from developing. By reducing the volume of the vitreous compartment and distorting it in various ways, vitreous traction is relieved. The retina is thus placed in contact with choroid, and the tissues are stimulated by diathermy, cryothermy, or photocoagulation to establish a permanent chorioretinal bond around the hole.

Course & Prognosis

With care, 90% of retinal detachments can be repaired by one operation. Subsequent procedures salvage another 6%. If the retina is still in place after 6 months, it is unlikely to become detached again.

The fovea may suffer irreparable damage in a brief period of separation from its only blood supply, the choriocapillaris. By contrast, on reattaching the retina, extrafoveal function may recover to a remarkable degree even after several months of detachment.

PRERETINAL MEMBRANES

These thin sheets of contractile tissue on the inner retinal surface are produced by glia or by pigment epithelium that has undergone metaplasia. They arise in association with a variety of conditions, including spontaneous vitreous detachment, retinal tears with or without retinal detachment, diabetic retinopathy, occlusion of retinal veins, and penetrating injuries. The associated condition apparently provides a vitreous-free retinal surface in combination with a break in the inner limiting lamina, or a full-thickness retinal hole through which the offending cells migrate.

In the beginning, the membrane, which covers part or all of the retina behind the vitreous base, is composed of elongated cells and delicate supportive tissue; later it contracts, exerting traction through scattered focal retinal attachments. This causes retinal folds if the retina is detached and mobile or if it causes the lips of a retinal tear to roll inward. If a large area of detached retina is involved, the condition is called **massive preretinal retraction.** In contrast, there is very little puckering when the retina is attached— whence the name **surface wrinkling retinopathy.** (See also Chapter 13.)

Clinical Findings

Vision is rapidly lost when a contracting preretinal membrane in the presence of a retinal hole causes retinal detachment. At the opposite end of the spectrum, if the retina is attached and a membrane is some distance from the macula, the patient is asymptomatic. If the macula is wrinkled, however, visual acuity may be reduced to less than 6/60 (20/200).

Figs 14–12 to14–16 are reproduced, with permission, from Arruga H: *Detachment of the Retina.* Salvat, 1936.

Figure 14–12. Tear in retina causing retinal detachment (microscopic section). Also shows cystoid degeneration of retina.

Figure 14–13. Retinal detachment 3 days after onset with crescent-shaped retinal tear.

Figure 14–15. Appearance of retinal detachment 40 days after onset.

Figure 14–14. Retinal detachment and retinal tear 6 days after onset.

Figure 14–16. Operative cure of retinal detachment. Appearance of retina 2 months after surgical repair.

It is usually impossible to detect an early preretinal membrane with the ophthalmoscope, since it is virtually transparent. When the membrane contracts, it may become visible, especially with the aid of red-free light. The membrane is slightly opaque, with an irregular, ill-defined outline. It bridges the apexes of the retinal folds when the retina is detached and is at the focus of the retinal wrinkles and has a shiny surface when the retina is attached.

Treatment

Treatment is usually not necessary for surface wrinkling retinopathy. However, if severe visual loss occurs, one may attempt the hazardous task of surgically cutting the membrane on the surface of the retina. If retinal detachment is present, scleral buckling and sometimes vitrectomy are indicated.

THE MACULA

CENTRAL SEROUS CHORIORETINOPATHY (Fig 14–17)

This disorder occurs at any age past the early teens and affects males more often than females. Although it is usually monocular, both eyes may be affected either concurrently or sequentially. One or more small defects appear in the pigment epithelial layer of an otherwise normal-appearing fundus, and fluid leaks from the choriocapillaris to the subretinal space. This transudate is either clear or partly opaque. The resulting smooth retinal detachment may extend up to 6 disk diameters in circumference.

The main symptom is blurred vision, and—as with most macular problems—exposure to bright light makes this worse. Visual acuity is reduced to a variable degree, and there is a slight shift toward hyperopia. Ophthalmoscopic and slit lamp examinations reveal a shallow retinal detachment with loss of the foveal reflection. Intravenous fluorescein demonstrates the site of leakage. Because the fresh fluorescein-stained fluid is warm, it rises by convection in the cooler preexisting fluid. The new fluid eventually becomes mixed with the old, and detectable fluorescence persists for about 30 minutes.

In most cases the leak closes spontaneously, and the subretinal fluid is resorbed within 3 months of the onset of the disease. Most of these patients recover good vision. Sometimes the detachment persists longer, increasing the likelihood of secondary cystoid degeneration of the macula. Permanent damage to the retina is also more likely if there are repeated episodes of central serous detachment.

If the pigment epithelial leakage persists longer than 3 months and if it is not directly beneath the fovea, photocoagulation is indicated. This seals the leakage site and the subretinal fluid is resorbed, with improvement in vision.

Although central serous chorioretinopathy appears to be a distinct entity, it must be stressed that any condition damaging Bruch's membrane and the pigment epithelium may cause leakage of serous fluid beneath the central retina. The differential diagnosis thus includes age-related macular degeneration, angioid streaks, tumors such as choroidal angioma, ne-

Figure 14–17. Central serous chorioretinopathy. *Left:* Fundus photo of a 34-year-old man with serous detachment of the macula (arrows). *Right:* Fluorescein angiogram showing leakage of fluid into the subretinal space. (Reproduced, with permission, from Gass J: *Stereoscopic Atlas of Macular Diseases.* Mosby, 1970.)

vus, and malignant melanoma, familial drusen, high myopia, and trauma.

Very rarely, a pit of the optic nerve may be associated with detachment in the posterior polar retina. In these cases, there is no demonstrable leak in the pigment epithelium, and it is thought that the fluid may originate from the vitreous.

AGE-RELATED MACULAR DEGENERATION (Involutional or Senile Macular Degeneration)

Age-related macular degeneration is the leading cause of permanent blindness in the elderly. The exact cause is unknown, but the incidence increases with each decade over the age of 50. Other associations besides age include race (usually Caucasian), sex (slight female predominance), family history, and a history of cigarette smoking. Age-related macular degeneration includes a broad spectrum of clinical and pathologic findings, which can be classified into 2 groups: nonexudative ("dry") and exudative ("wet"). Although both types are progressive and usually bilateral, they differ in terms of their manifestations, prognosis, and management. The more severe exudative form accounts for approximately 90% of all cases of legal blindness due to age-related macular degeneration.

1. NONEXUDATIVE AGE-RELATED MACULAR DEGENERATION

Nonexudative age-related macular degeneration is characterized by variable degrees of atrophy and degeneration of the outer retina, retinal pigment epithelium, Bruch's membrane, and choriocapillaris (Fig 14–2). Of the ophthalmoscopically visible changes in the retinal pigment epithelium and Bruch's membrane, **drusen** are the most typical. These appear as variably sized, yellowish round spots that are located deep to the retina and scattered throughout the macula and posterior pole. With time, they may enlarge, coalesce, calcify, and increase in number (Fig 14–18).

Microscopically, drusen are small mounds of amorphous material deposited within Bruch's membrane by retinal pigment epithelial cells. Other types of drusen can occur in younger patients and in dominantly inherited patterns, but these differ ultrastructurally from the age-related type. In addition to drusen, clumps of pigment irregularly interspersed with depigmented areas of atrophy may progressively appear throughout the macula. The level of associated visual impairment is variable and may be minimal. Fluorescein angiography demonstrates the irregular patterns of retinal pigment epithelial hyperplasia and thinning. Drusen hyperfluoresce owing to overlying retinal pigment epithelial attenuation.

Treatment

There is no known means of treatment or preven-

Figure 14–18. *A:* Nonexudative age-related degeneration, showing multiple drusen in the macula. (Reproduced, with permission, from Wilmer L: *Atlas Fundus Oculi.* Macmillan, 1934.) *B:* Fluorescein angiogram, showing dye filling a subretinal neovascular membrane beneath the macula (arrows). (Courtesy of E Ai.) *C:* Cicatricial stage, showing subretinal hemorrhage and a disciform macular scar (arrows). (Courtesy of E Ai.)

tion for this stage of the disease. Fortunately, progression of the atrophic changes is slow and may stabilize. However, the exudative stage may suddenly develop at any time, and in addition to regular ophthalmic examinations, patients are given an Amsler grid (see Chapter 3) to help monitor themselves for any symptomatic changes.

2. EXUDATIVE AGE-RELATED MACULAR DEGENERATION

The impairment of Bruch's membrane as a barrier between the retinal pigment epithelium and the choriocapillaris gives rise to the complications of "wet" age-related macular degeneration. Serous fluid or blood from the choroid can leak through small defects in the collagenous membrane, causing a focal dome-shaped elevation of the pigment epithelium, or so-called retinal pigment epithelial detachment (Fig 14–19). Additional fluid may lead to further separation of the overlying sensory retina, and vision usually decreases if the fovea becomes detached. Retinal pigment epithelial detachments may spontaneously flatten, with variable visual results, and may leave a geographic area of depigmentation at the involved site.

The prognosis is much worse if a subretinal neovascular membrane is present. Degenerative breaks in Bruch's membrane provide a pathway through which choroidal neovascularization can proliferate beneath the retinal pigment epithelium. The stimulus for the growth of the vessels is unknown. They may behave in a variety of patterns, remaining unnoticed in a dormant "subclinical" state or actively leaking or bleeding while exhibiting amazingly rapid growth. Although fluorescein angiography may fail to detect occult neovascularization, this technique usually identifies these membranes, which are typically lacy, delicate vascular networks that leak dye profusely (Figs 14–18 and 14–19).

A leaking macular subretinal neovascular membrane may produce **metamorphopsia** (wavy distortion of vision), a blurred scotoma, or decreased central acuity. Any of these symptoms may develop suddenly. Funduscopic signs of subretinal neovascularization include subretinal hemorrhage, sub- and intraretinal hard exudate, overlying detachments of the retinal pigment epithelium and sensory retina, and the appearance of a "dirty gray" subretinal membrane, occasionally surrounded by a pigmentary ring.

Although some neovascular membranes may occasionally regress, the natural course of age-related macular degeneration associated with subretinal neovascularization is usually one of progressive, severe worsening. The time span is variable, but a rapid decline can occur within days. The sensory retina may be damaged by long-standing edema, detachment, or subretinal hemorrhage. Furthermore, a hemorrhagic detachment of the retina may undergo fibrous metaplasia and organization, resulting in an elevated subretinal mass called a **disciform scar.** This fixed, but variably sized, fibrovascular mound represents the cicatricial stage of exudative age-related macular degeneration. If centrally located, it results in permanent loss of central vision (Fig 14–18).

Treatment

In the absence of subretinal neovascularization, laser treatment of serous retinal pigment epithelial detachments is of no proved benefit. However, if a subretinal neovascular membrane is present and has not yet involved the fovea, laser photocoagulation offers hope for stabilization or improvement.

An angiogram is used to define the precise location and borders of the neovascular membrane, which is then completely ablated by heavy confluent laser burns. Photocoagulation destroys the overlying retina as well but is worthwhile if the subretinal membrane can be halted short of the fovea. The opportunity for treat-

Figure 14–19. Early-phase *(left)* and late-phase *(right)* angiograms of the same eye, show a serous retinal pigment epithelial detachment on the right, adjacent to a subretinal neovascular membrane on the left (arrows). Note the irregular pattern of fluorescence of the neovascular membrane in contrast to the homogeneous pattern of the serous detachment. A subretinal hemorrhage is seen at the inferior edge of the membrane. (Courtesy of E Ai.)

ment is lost once the fovea is involved; this under-scores the importance of prompt detection and evaluation.

The argon blue-green laser was the first to be proved successful in the treatment of subretinal neovascular membranes located at least 200 μm away from the center of the fovea. Because of the particular absorption characteristics of this technique, it is not as safe for treatment closer to the fovea. For the photocoagulation of juxtafoveal membranes, 3 other laser wavelengths—red and yellow krypton and argon green—appear safer and are being clinically evaluated. Treatment is not indicated for subfoveal neovascularization.

Even when successfully treated, subretinal neovascular membranes can recur, either adjacent to the initial area or at new sites within the same or fellow eye. The incidence of membranes occurring in the fellow eye may be as high as 12–15% per year. Thus, careful monitoring with Amsler grids, ophthalmoscopy, and angiography is essential. Once both foveas have been damaged, the only helpful measures are low-vision aids and magnifiers.

ANGIOID STREAKS
(Fig 14–20)

Linear breaks in the fibroelastic layer of Bruch's membrane may ophthalmoscopically resemble blood vessels, for which reason they are called angioid streaks. They are brown, irregular bands radiating from the disk. Associated findings are pseudoxanthoma elasticum (Groenblad-Strandberg syndrome), sickle cell disease, and Paget's disease (osteitis deformans). From a practical point of view, the lacquer

breaks of high myopia and traumatic ruptures of Bruch's membrane can be grouped with angioid streaks. The pigment epithelium overlying all of these lesions slowly degenerates, and new vessels sometimes grow through the defect in Bruch's membrane to cause a disciform lesion in a manner similar to that which occurs in age-related macular degeneration.

In the absence of neovascularization, angioid streaks are usually asymptomatic. If new vessels are present, photocoagulation occasionally helps.

PRESUMED HISTOPLASMOSIS SYNDROME

A considerable number of patients from the eastern half of the USA have combinations of the following findings: positive skin test for histoplasmosis, miliary opacities of the lungs, tiny choroidal scars, peripapillary disruption of the choroid, and exudation or bleeding from subretinal neovascular lesions at or near the macula. Except for the macular complications, the condition is asymptomatic and benign. Once disciform changes commence, the prognosis is very poor. Photocoagulation usually arrests the course of active lesions that are eccentric to the fovea.

MACULAR HOLE

As in the retinal periphery, the parenchyma and internal limiting membrane at the avascular fovea are thin and prone to hole formation (Fig 14–21). These atrophic macular holes are fairly common and can be caused by prolonged macular edema or traction by a preretinal membrane. In older patients, they may develop spontaneously.

The loss of vision is proportionate to the size of the hole and the associated findings. If the retina is flat, it is often difficult to tell if the macula is really perforated. However, one can be reasonably confident of the diagnosis if the view of the underlying pigment

Figure 14–20. Retinal photograph showing angioid streaks in retina. (Courtesy of M Hogan and S Aiken.)

Figure 14–21. Macular hole. (Courtesy of E Ai.)

epithelium is sharp, the hole margin is rounded and more opaque than the contiguous retina, and the background choroidal fluorescence shows through clearly.

There is no effective treatment for macular atrophic holes. They very rarely lead to retinal detachment and should merely be watched.

HEREDITARY DISEASES OF THE MACULA

The hereditary diseases of the macula—all of which are untreatable—can be loosely divided into those that involve primarily the choriocapillaris and those that initially affect the pigment epithelium.

Central areolar choroidal sclerosis is an example of the former group. This autosomal dominant or recessive disease leads to slow loss of central vision in middle life. Abnormalities of the choriocapillaris and pigment epithelium are apparent early. By the time symptoms occur, there may be complete atrophy of the central pigment epithelium.

Stargardt-Behr disease and Best's disease are examples of macular diseases primarily affecting the pigment epithelium. Stargardt-Behr disease is usually transmitted in an autosomal recessive manner. Commencing at different ages, the macular pigment epithelium slowly degenerates. The intensity of the pigment epithelial changes and the degree of visual loss vary from family to family.

In Best's vitelliform macular degeneration, there is a diffuse abnormality of the pigment epithelium, but the visible changes are confined to the macula. Initially in this autosomal dominant disease—though the vision is good—there are deposits in the pigment epithelium, giving the appearance of a poached egg "sunny side up." Later, when the yolk of the egg appears scrambled, macular vision is seriously reduced.

TRAUMA

Though the eye as a whole must be considered when dealing with an injury (see Chapter 24), some details particular to the retina are described here.

BLUNT TRAUMA

A nonpenetrating injury to the globe may tear the retina or produce commotio retinae, or it may indirectly damage the retina as a result of fracturing Bruch's membrane.

Traumatic Retinal Tears

The severe, almost instantaneous distortion of the globe caused by blunt trauma can tear the retina, primarily because of the different rates at which the vitreous and the eye wall change shape. The non-uniform structure of the vitreous and the attachments of the vitreous to the retina dictate where the tears will occur. Thus, the vitreous base, the ribbon of very firm vitreoretinal adhesion extending 1–2 mm in front of and behind the ora, may be disinserted, or the tears may be confined to the retina at the posterior margin of the vitreous base or the nonpigmented epithelium of the pars plana at its anterior margin. Such tears can lead to retinal detachment and usually require treatment.

Trauma may prematurely cause a posterior vitreous detachment, such as normally happens as an aging phenomenon to most people. On detaching, the vitreous may tear the retina at focal vitreoretinal adhesions situated behind the vitreous base. These tears and the associated bleeding into the vitreous are handled the same way as those that occur spontaneously.

Commotio Retinae (Berlin's "Edema")

A blow to the front of the eye can sometimes avulse the outer segments of the retinal receptor cells in a discrete area at the back of the eye. In the following weeks, this debris is phagocytosed by the pigment epithelium. At first, the white subretinal material is easily visible. Eventually, little ophthalmoscopic evidence of it remains other than a localized mild disturbance of the underlying pigment epithelium. There is a permanent scotoma in the affected area. When it includes the macula, the symptoms are distressing. Otherwise, the loss of visual field may go unnoticed.

With involvement of the peripheral retina or the fovea, where the retina and its internal limiting membrane are thinnest, an atrophic retinal hole may later develop at the site of the contrecoup injury (Fig 24–3). Such holes rarely cause a significant retinal detachment.

Fracture of Bruch's Membrane

Blunt trauma will sometimes cause one or more easily visible linear fractures of Bruch's membrane, which are usually accompanied by subretinal bleeding. The break may occur anywhere. Those in the posterior pole are curved and are concentric with the optic nerve head. In the course of time, the subretinal blood resorbs, but the pigment epithelium bordering the fracture atrophies over the areas of choriocapillaris supplied by the affected ciliary arterioles. Later still, new vessels may grow into the subretinal space through the breaks in Bruch's membrane (see Exudative Age-Related Macular Degeneration, above).

If they are some distance from the macula, fractures of Bruch's membrane and possible complications are of little consequence to the patient. However, a fracture beneath the fovea usually causes permanent loss of function, though vision sometimes improves when the subretinal blood is resorbed. Late involvement of the macula by a disciform lesion usually causes permanent loss of macular vision. These disciform cases are occasionally helped by photocoagulation. (See Fig 24–4.)

PENETRATING INJURY

At the time of a penetrating injury, the retina may be directly damaged by the penetrating object or indirectly damaged through traction on the vitreous. The findings are protean and are handled surgically according to the anatomic situation.

Quite often, an injury involving the vitreous will cause late traction on the retina owing either to contraction of fibrous tissue, which grows along the penetration tract, or to the delayed detachment of the vitreous, which was initiated by the injury. In either case, the retina may be distorted or detached and may require surgical intervention.

INJURY DUE TO EXPOSURE TO ELECTROMAGNETIC ENERGY
Orson W. White, MD

Damage to retinal elements caused by exposure to excessive electromagnetic energy, including light, has occurred with increasing frequency in recent years. Causes include increased retinal exposure during operations with the operating microscope, prolonged and repeated retinal examinations, repeated retinal photographs, and therapeutic and accidental exposure to lasers.

The energy from light and other forms of radiomagnetic energy can be calculated with the following equation:

Energy = Planck's constant $\times$ Number of photon $\times$ Frequency

A deer struck by an automobile and one struck by a bullet from a high-powered rifle delivering the same amount of energy on impact would suffer different injuries. In similar fashion, the effect on the molecule or atom varies with the frequency (wavelength) of the energy absorbed. With a transition from the relatively longer wavelengths of radio waves, microwaves, and infrared rays, through the visible spectrum and ultraviolet light, to the shorter wavelength x-rays and gamma rays, there are qualitative differences in the damage caused.

It is important to be aware that excessive electromagnetic energy, including light energy, can result in permanent visual damage.

COLOR VISION & COLOR BLINDNESS

Light may be defined as that portion of the electromagnetic spectrum (400– 700 nm) that readily stimulates human retinal receptors. To other species, ''light'' may encompass a different set of wavelengths.

The cones mediate color vision. In order to be stimulated, they require a greater intensity of light than the rods. Thus, one cannot detect color in moonlight. Each cone has one of 3 distinct spectral sensitivity patterns. These curves are overlapping, with maxima at red, green, or blue. A given light elicits different degrees of response in each type of cone. This generates data which the neural computer interprets as a specific color.

Color is dependent upon hue, saturation, and brightness. Objects appear to have a particular **hue** primarily because they reflect, irradiate, or transmit light of certain wavelengths. The addition of black to a given hue produces the various **shades.**

Saturation is an index of purity of a hue. For example, scarlet is more saturated than pink because pink is made up of red and white mixed together.

Brightness is that aspect of perception most closely related to light intensity.

Color blindness is a misleading term, since most color-blind people have normal visual acuity. According to Marriott, 8% of men and 0.4% of women interpret colors differently than the rest of humanity. They are classified as follows:

(1) Cone monochromats: These individuals have only one type of cone. The incidence is about 1:1,000,000.

(2) Dichromats: Persons having 2 rather than 3 types of cones. They are divided into 3 groups: Protanopes, or red-blind subjects, are insensitive to deep red light. Deuteranopes confuse shades of red, green, and yellow. Tritanopes are blue-blind subjects who confuse blue and green shades and, generally, orange and pink shades.

(3) Anomalous trichromats: This is by far the largest group. Protans have similar but milder defects than occur in protanopia; deutans have similar but milder defects than occur in deuteranopia; and tritans have similar but milder defects than occur in tritanopia.

(4) Rod monochromats: Rod monochromatism is a very rare disorder in which there is complete lack of cone function. It is always associated with photophobia, nystagmus, and poor visual acuity.

The common types of color blindness are inherited as X-linked characteristics. Acquired causes of color blindness include retinal disease and poisoning. In the acquired cases, the patient may be color-blind in only one area of the visual field.

The detection of color blindness is described in Chapter 3. Because of the relationship to choice of occupation, color vision testing should be done early in life (eg, age 8– 12). However, the physician must be wary of attributing too much importance to a hereditary anomaly that in its more common milder forms is little more than an occasional social inconvenience.

Treatment is of no value.

REFERENCES

The Branch Vein Occlusion Study Group: Argon laser photocoagulation for macular edema in branch vein occlusion. *Am J Ophthalmol* 1984;**98**:271.

Bresnick GH: Diabetic maculopathy: A critical review highlighting diffuse macular edema. *Ophthalmology* 1983;**90**:1301.

Brown GC, Magargal LE: Central retinal artery obstruction and visual acuity. *J Am Acad Ophthalmol* 1982;**89**:14.

Byer NE: The natural history of asymptomatic retinal breaks. *Ophthalmology* 1982;**89**:1033.

Byer NE: The natural history of senile retinoschisis. *Trans Am Acad Ophthalmol Otolaryngol* 1976;**81**:459.

Clarkson JG, Altman RD: Angioid streaks. *Surv Ophthalmol* 1982;**26**:235.

Cunha-Vas JG et al: A follow-up study by vitreous fluorophotometry of early retinal involvement in diabetics. *Am J Ophthalmol* 1978;**86**:467.

The Diabetic Retinopathy Study Research Group: Photocoagulation treatment of proliferative diabetic retinopathy: Clinical application of diabetic retinopathy study (DRS) findings, DRS report number 8. *Ophthalmology* 1981;**88**:583.

Doft BH et al: The association between long-term diabetic control and early retinopathy. *Ophthalmology* 1984;**91**:763.

Foos RY: Vitreoretinal junction: Topographical variations. *Invest Ophthalmol* 1972;**11**:801.

François J: Metabolic tapetoretinal degenerations. *Surv Ophthalmol* 1982;**26**:293.

Galainena MC: Solar retinopathy. *Ann Ophthalmol* 1976;**8**:304.

Gass JDM: *Stereoscopic Atlas of Macular Diseases,* 2nd ed. Mosby, 1977.

Gass JDM: Treatment of retinal vascular abnormalities. *Trans Am Acad Ophthalmol Otolaryngol* 1977;**83**:432.

Hayreh SS: Classification of central retinal vein occlusion. *Ophthalmology* 1983;**90**:458.

Heller MD, Straatsma BR, Foos RY: Detachment of the posterior vitreous in phakic and aphakic eyes. *Mod Probl Ophthalmol* 1972;**10**:23.

Hilton GF, McLean EB, Norton EWD: *Retinal Detachment,* 4th ed. American Academy of Ophthalmology, 1981.

Irvine AR: Diabetic retinopathy pathogenesis as a guide to therapy. *Ann Ophthalmol* 1980;**12**:13.

Jaffe NS, Clayman HM, Jaffe MS: Cystoid macular edema after intracapsular and extracapsular cataract extraction with and without an intraocular lens. *J Am Acad Ophthalmol* 1982;**89**:25.

Kalina RE, Karr DJ: Retrolental fibroplasia: Experience over two decades in one institution. *J Am Acad Ophthalmol* 1982;**89**:91.

Kearns TP: Differential diagnosis of central retinal vein obstruction. *Ophthalmology* 1983;**90**:475.

Kohner EM: Symposium on retinal vascular disease. 1. Morphological, circulatory and histopathologic response to retinal vein occlusion: Pathophysiology of retinal vein occlusion. *Trans Ophthalmol Soc UK* 1976;**96**:189.

Kreissig I, Lincoff H: Mechanism of retinal attachment after cryosurgery. *Trans Ophthalmol Soc UK* 1975;**95**:148.

Lincoff J, Gieser R: Finding the retinal hole. *Arch Ophthalmol* 1971;**85**:565.

Machemer R: The importance of fluid absorption, traction, intraocular currents, and chorioretinal scars in the therapy of rhegmatogenous retinal detachments: The 41st Edward Jackson Memorial Lecture. *Am J Ophthalmol* 1984;**98**:681.

Macular Photocoagulation Study Group: Argon laser photocoagulation for senile macular degeneration. *Arch Ophthalmol* 1982;**100**:912.

Maumenee AE, Emery JM: An anatomic classification of diseases of the macula. *Am J Ophthalmol* 1972;**74**:594.

Merin S, Auerbach E: Review: Retinitis pigmentosa. *Surv Ophthalmol* 1976;**20**:303.

Michels RG: *Vitreous Surgery.* American Academy of Ophthalmology, 1982.

Michels RG, Rice TA, Rice EF: Vitrectomy of diabetic traction detachment involving the macula. *Am J Ophthalmol* 1983;**95**:22.

Michels RG, Rice TA, Rice EF: Vitrectomy for diabetic vitreous hemorrhage. *Am J Ophthalmol* 1983; **95**:12.

O'Malley P et al: Paving-stone degeneration of the retina. *Arch Ophthalmol* 1965;**73**:169.

Palestine AG, Robertson DM, Goldstein BG: Macroaneurysms of the retinal arteries. *Am J Ophthalmol* 1982;**93**:164.

Patz A: Clinical and experimental studies on retinal neovascularization: The 29th Edward Jackson Memorial Lecture. *Am J Ophthalmol* 1982;**94**:715.

Patz A: Observations on the retinopathy of prematurity. *Am J Ophthalmol* 1985;**100**:164.

Patz A et al: Diseases of the macula: Diagnosis and management of choroidal neovascularization. *Trans Am Acad Ophthalmol Otolaryngol* 1977;**83**:468.

Ryan SJ: The pathophysiology of proliferative vitreoretinopathy in its management. *Am J Ophthalmol* 1985;**100**:188.

Schatz H et al: *Interaction of Fundus Fluorescein Angiography.* Mosby, 1977.

Schlagel TF Jr: The presumed ocular histoplasmosis syndrome. Pages 720–731 in: *Controversy in Ophthalmology.* Brockhurst RJ et al (editors). Saunders, 1977.

Sipperly JO, Quigley HA, Gass JD: Explanation of commotio retinae: Traumatic retinopathy in primates. *Arch Ophthalmol* 1978;**96**:2267.

Spencer WH (editor): *Ophthalmic Pathology: An Atlas and Textbook.* Vol 2. *Vitreous and Retina.* Saunders, 1985.

Straatsma BR et al: Lattice degeneration of retina: The 30th Edward Jackson Memorial Lecture. *Trans Am Acad Ophthalmol Otolaryngol* 1974;**78**:87.

Trempe CL et al: Macular photocoagulation: Optimal wavelength selection. *Ophthalmology* 1982;**89**:721.

Virdi PS, Hayreh SS: Ocular neovascularization with retinal vascular occlusion. *Arch Ophthalmol* 1982;**100**:331.

Walsh JB: Hypertensive retinopathy: Description, classification, and prognosis. *Ophthalmology* 1982;**89**:1127.

Yannuzzi LA, Gitter KA, Schatz H: *The Macula: A Comprehensive Text and Atlas.* Williams & Wilkins, 1978.

Glaucoma

15

Glaucoma includes a complex of disease entities that have in common an increase in intraocular pressure sufficient to cause degeneration of the optic disk and defects in the visual field. An estimated 50,000 persons in the USA are blind as a result of glaucoma. The incidence of glaucoma in unselected persons over age 40 is about 1.5%. The disease is particularly common in black individuals. In black persons age 45–65, the prevalence is 15 times that of whites in the same age group.

The chief threat of chronic (open-angle) glaucoma is insidious visual impairment. The degree of interference with vision varies from slight blurring to complete blindness. The disease is bilateral and is genetically determined, probably by multifactorial or polygenic inheritance. Infantile glaucoma usually has an autosomal recessive mode of inheritance, whereas some specific glaucoma syndromes are transmitted as autosomal dominant diseases. Acute glaucoma (angle-closure glaucoma) comprises less than 5% of primary glaucoma cases.

In most cases, blindness can be prevented if treatment is instituted early. The objective of therapy is to facilitate the outflow of aqueous through existing drainage channels by the use of miotics and in some cases to inhibit the secretion of aqueous by the ciliary processes, using systemically and topically administered drugs. The most commonly used miotic is pilocarpine. The most commonly used secretory suppressants are epinephrine and timolol maleate, which are applied topically, and acetazolamide, which is given orally. Increase in outflow can also be accomplished by laser trabeculoplasty. Operative treatment is sometimes indicated in the later stages of glaucoma when medical management is no longer sufficient to control the intraocular pressure.

The management of glaucoma is best left to the ophthalmologist, but all physicians should participate in the diagnosis by making ophthalmoscopy and tonometry a part of the routine physical examination of all patients old enough to cooperate. This is especially important in patients with a family history of glaucoma. The physician should learn to recognize optic nerve changes associated with glaucoma as seen with the ophthalmoscope. Doubtful cases should be referred to an ophthalmologist for confirmation and management.

AC = anterior chamber	I = iris	S = sclera	TM = trabecular meshwork
C = cornea	I-C = iris-corneal angle	SC = Schlemm's canal	TPB = trabecular pigment band
CB = ciliary body	IP = iris processes	SL = Schwalbe's line	
CP = ciliary process	P = pupil	SP = scleral spur	

Figure 15–1. Composite illustration showing anatomic *(left)* and gonioscopic *(right)* view of normal anterior chamber angle. (Courtesy of R Shaffer.)

Classification

A generally accepted classification of glaucoma is as follows:

A. Primary Glaucoma:

1. Open-angle glaucoma—Also called simple glaucoma, chronic simple glaucoma. The most common form.
2. Angle-closure glaucoma—Also called narrow-angle glaucoma, closed-angle glaucoma.
   a. Acute.
   b. Subacute or chronic.
   c. Plateau iris.

B. Congenital Glaucoma:

1. Primary congenital glaucoma, infantile glaucoma, trabeculodysgenesis.
2. Glaucoma associated with congenital anomalies—
   a. Pigmentary glaucoma.
   b. Aniridia.
   c. Axenfeld's syndrome.
   d. Sturge-Weber syndrome.
   e. Infantile glaucoma developing late.
   f. Marfan's syndrome.
   g. Neurofibromatosis.
   h. Lowe's syndrome.
   i. Microcornea and megalocornea.

C. Secondary Glaucoma:

1. Due to changes of the lens—
   a. Dislocation.
   b. Intumescence.
   c. Phacolytic.
   d. Exfoliative syndrome (pseudoexfoliation of lens capsule, glaucoma capsulare).
2. Due to changes of the uveal tract—
   a. Peripheral anterior synechiae (PAS) (angle closure without pupillary block).
   b. Iridocyclitis.
   c. Tumor.
   d. Essential iris atrophy (iridocorneoendothelial [ICE] syndrome).
3. Due to trauma—
   a. Massive hemorrhage into the anterior chamber.
   b. Massive hemorrhage into the posterior chamber.
   c. Corneal or limbal laceration with iris prolapse into the wound.
   d. Retrodisplacement of iris root following contusion (angle recession).
4. Following surgical procedures—
   a. Epithelial ingrowth into the anterior chamber.
   b. Failure of prompt restoration of the anterior chamber following cataract extraction.
5. Associated with rubeosis (diabetes mellitus and central retinal vessel occlusion).
6. Associated with pulsating exophthalmos.
7. Associated with topical corticosteroids.
8. Other rare causes of secondary glaucoma.

D. Absolute Glaucoma: The end result of any uncontrolled glaucoma is a hard, sightless, and often painful eye.

PHYSIOLOGY

Aqueous Humor

The intraocular pressure is determined by the rate of aqueous production by the ciliary body epithelium and the resistance to outflow of aqueous from the eye. Some knowledge of the physiology of aqueous is necessary to an understanding of glaucoma.

A. Composition of Aqueous: The aqueous is a clear liquid that fills the anterior and posterior chambers of the eye. Its volume is about 125 μL. The osmotic pressure of aqueous is slightly higher than that of plasma. The total protein content is 0.02%. The albumin-globulin ratio is the same as that of blood serum (2:1). In general, the same electrolytes and other components are found in the aqueous as in plasma, although the concentrations differ.

Intraocular inflammation and surgical or traumatic emptying of the anterior chamber cause the formation of plasmoid aqueous, which closely resembles blood serum and has a much higher protein concentration than normal aqueous.

B. Formation and Flow of Aqueous: A great deal is known about the dynamics of aqueous humor, but the exact mechanism of production and elimination of aqueous is not completely understood. Water, electrolytes, and nonelectrolytes enter and leave the eye at varying rates. Water enters both by diffusion from the ciliary body and by secretion from the epithelium of the ciliary processes. From the posterior chamber the fluid passes through the pupil into the anterior chamber (Fig 15–1). The flow in the anterior chamber is peripheral, toward the filtering trabecular meshwork and into Schlemm's canal. Efferent channels from Schlemm's canal (about 30 collector channels and about 12 aqueous veins) conduct the fluid into the venous system. There is also a constant exchange of nonelectrolytes as well as a major exchange of water in and out of the iris stroma. A small amount of aqueous leaves the eye through the uveal vessels and the sclera (uveoscleral flow) (Fig 15–2).

Pressure Dynamics*

Intraocular pressure is such an important feature of glaucoma that a review of pressure dynamics is desirable.

A. Pressure-Tension-Strain Relationships: The terms pressure, tension, and strain are frequently used interchangeably and are listed as synonyms in some dictionaries. However, the precise distinctions and interactions between these related but different terms

*This section on pressure dynamics by Orson W. White, MD, presents important new information that should be carefully studied by all persons interested in the pathophysiology of glaucoma.

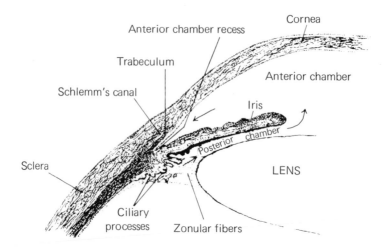

Figure 15–2. Anterior segment structures. Arrows indicate direction of flow of aqueous.

must be appreciated before pressure dynamics in glaucoma can be understood.

1. Pressure–Hydrostatic pressure is the force per unit area exerted by a fluid (gas or liquid). With the eye, as with other pressure vessels, the pressure force is exerted normal to the structural wall (in the eye, this is the corneoscleral wall). Hydrostatic pressure per se causes no damage to the delicate neurons paralleling the scleral wall, even at high levels. A neuron in the eye may be compared to a diver resting on the ocean bottom; at a depth of 43 meters (1693 ft), the diver will experience no discomfort, even though at this depth, the total force being exerted on the body is about 9000 kg (10 tons). The concept that intraocular pressure damages neurons by pushing them against the sclera is false.

The unit of pressure in the International System of Units (SI) is the pascal (Pa), which is 1 newton per square meter (N/m²). To convert millimeters of mercury to kilopascals (kPa), divide millimeters of mercury by 7.5. However, for calculation of pressure within the eye, it is helpful to convert millimeters of mercury to grams per square centimeter. Multiply millimeters of mercury by 1.36 to obtain grams per square centimeter, which is also the pressure in centimeters of water. One may thus determine the pressure effect in millimeters of mercury of an infusion bottle infusing the eye by measuring the height in centimeters from the eye to the top of the fluid in the bottle and dividing by 1.36. A satisfactory approximation is to double the height in inches; thus, a 12-inch-high infusion bottle creates an intraocular pressure of about 24 mm Hg.

2. Tension (tensile stress)–A jack supporting a car is subjected to compressive stress. A towline pulling a car is subjected to tensile stress, or tension. Stresses are assigned a magnitude of force per unit area. Tensile stress, or the tension force vector, acts parallel to the scleral wall (attempting to pull the sclera apart). In the same way, the pressure of the abdomen at right angles to a belt is almost analogous to intraocular pressure, while the tension along the belt acting to pull the belt apart is analogous to scleral tension.

Trampolines and drumheads are examples of pure tension without pressure. The pressure is the same on either side of the tensed membrane. Tension levels in the sclera, cornea, and lamina cribrosa are not equal. The tension equation for thin-walled spheres can be used to obtain a close approximation of tensions in various parts of the corneoscleral wall of the eye. Tension in the sclera is directly proportional to the intraocular pressure multiplied by the radius of curvature of the sclera and inversely proportional to twice the thickness of the sclera:

$$\text{Tension} = \frac{\text{Pressure} \times \text{Radius}}{2 \times \text{Thickness}}$$

An inflated surgical glove or balloon (Fig 15–3) illustrates this relationship. The palm of the glove has relatively high tension and the thumb has relatively low tension, though the pressure within the glove is equal at all locations. The thumb has low tension because the radius of curvature is small and the thickness large relative to the same factors at the palm. In the eye, tension is lower in the cornea or optic cup than in the sclera.

An eye under slowly increasing pressure usually ruptures beneath the lateral rectus, as the tension equation would suggest. The 43 meters' sea depth used in the example of harmless pressure was chosen because this same pressure within the eye residing at atmospheric pressure results, via tension and strain, in rupture of the eye. A precipitous pressure rise due to trauma (eg, a blow from a club) frequently ruptures the eye at the limbus owing to the anvil effect of the more viscous vitreous.

3. Strain–Strain is stretch or displacement per unit length. A strain gauge measures displacement. Strain can result in damage, and in the body can cause both

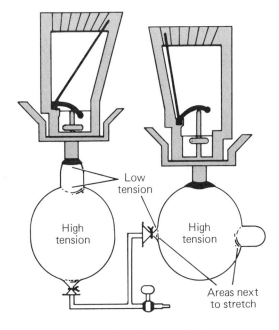

Figure 15–3. Equal-pressure balloons.

pain and damage. Using the belt analogy, strain is the stretch per unit length of the belt resulting from the tension in the belt caused by the pressure of the abdomen.

To calculate the strain or stretch of a substance at a given pressure or tension, one of 3 moduli of elasticity is used. Each modulus is appropriate for a different type of structure. Thomas Young (1773–1829), an English physician, clarified these complex relationships as follows:

a. Young's modulus E–Young's modulus E is used for determining the elastic properties of structures such as cables, pressure vessels, submarines, *and eyes*. E is defined as the tension required to stretch a material of unit cross section to double its original length. This is represented by the following equation:

$$E = \frac{\text{Change in tension in sclera}}{\text{Change in length of sclera per unit length}}$$

Thus, the stretch of the sclera per unit length (strain) is given by dividing the change in tension of the sclera by Young's modulus of the sclera E.

b. Shear modulus G–The shear modulus G is used for determining the elastic properties of structures such as drive shafts and bolts. G should not concern us in the discussion of elasticity of the eye. It is sometimes called the modulus of rigidity, and the unfortunate term "scleral rigidity" may have originated from inappropriate use of the shear modulus in ocular calculations.

c. Bulk modulus K–The bulk modulus K also should not concern us in our discussion of elasticity of the eye. The bulk modulus is the hydrostatic pressure (compressive stress) required to compress (strain) a solid material to half its original volume.

The empirical "scleral rigidity" equation found in some glaucoma literature resembles the bulk modulus equation. However, using the bulk modulus for the eye would be valid only if the eye were solid sclera and subjected to external hydrostatic pressure. However, the eye is a nearly spherical shell of elastic sclera filled with fluid under pressure and is therefore appropriately described only by Young's modulus, as are other thin-walled pressure vessels.

The belt analogy may now be used to illustrate the way in which neurons are damaged in glaucoma. Envision a very obese person wearing a large belt (sclera) with a delicate cloth liner (neurons). After fasting for several days, the obese subject feasts heavily, with the result that there is some ripping of the delicate cloth liner. The progression of the damage process is as follows: (1) The expanding abdomen (intraocular pressure) exerts gentle pressure at right angles to the belt, producing a summation tension parallel to the belt (sclera) tending to pull the belt apart. (2) The tension leads to stretching (strain) of the belt, following the rules of Young's modulus. (3) The stretching (strain) results in damage to the delicate cloth liner (neurons).

B. Devices for Measuring Ocular Tension and Pressure: The Goldmann applanation device is designed to measure intraocular pressure, with results recorded in millimeters of mercury. The Schiotz device is a true tonometer, primarily measuring tension. Recordings should be in tension units or scale units, as originally proposed by Schiotz, but they are commonly converted to millimeters of mercury (a pressure unit, not a tension unit).

C. Local Exceptions to the Mathematical Theory of Elasticity: The tension and strain exerted on areas of discontinuity, such as the optic disk and the limbal area, are not easy to calculate. These relationships can be studied by various methods of photoelasticity on models or actual eyes. Note in the balloon model (Fig 15–3) that the area next to stretch occurring when the pressure in the balloon is increased is analogous to the disk and limbal areas of the eye.

D. Biologic Exceptions to the Mathematical Theory of Elasticity: Living tissue reacts in the same way as nonliving material to brief changes in tension and strain. However, long-term tensions and strains have a unique effect on living tissue, causing changes in growth, shape, and strength. This is the basis of the "orthodontic shift" of teeth and the way in which deformities of the head, face, and foot have been created in some cultures over the course of history. The cupping of the disk may be a response to long-term tension and strain. *Nerve damage in glaucoma is not due directly to intraocular pressure on the neurons but may be due to deformation and stretching, caused by long-term tension-strain effects.*

SPECIAL DIAGNOSTIC TECHNIQUES (See also Chapter 3.)

A number of special diagnostic tests have been developed to help detect, classify, and follow the course of glaucoma.

Tonometry

This is an important test in establishing the diagnosis of glaucoma. A single normal reading either with the Schiotz or applanation tonometer does not rule out glaucoma, however, as the intraocular pressures may vary within wide limits. A single "high normal" reading (24– 32 mm Hg) is suggestive of glaucoma but always requires repeated testing before a definite diagnosis can be made.

Gonioscopy

Visualization of the anterior chamber angle differentiates angle-closure from open-angle glaucoma, demonstrates the extent of peripheral anterior synechiae, and offers the only means of detecting an impending angle closure before there is any rise in intraocular pressure. It is an essential part of any glaucoma evaluation.

Ophthalmoscopy

Direct visualization of the optic disk is the single most important test in diagnosing glaucoma and evaluating the response to treatment. A patient with elevated intraocular pressure (eg, 32 mm Hg) and normal-appearing optic disks may not require active treatment but only periodic examinations.

Provocative Tests

A. Open-Angle Glaucoma: Provocative tests are not helpful in predicting what pressure level will damage the individual patient's optic nerve, which is the important consideration. Therefore, provocative tests are of little help in open-angle glaucoma.

B. Narrow-Angle Glaucoma:

1. Dark room test of Seidel–The patient sits in a dark room for 1 hour without going to sleep. A rise in intraocular pressure of more than 8 mm suggests that iris blockage is impeding outflow when the pupil is relatively dilated. Positive results must be confirmed by gonioscopic evidence of angle closure. A negative result does not rule out a future attack of angle-closure glaucoma.

2. Prone position test–If a patient lies in a prone position and the intraocular pressure rises 8– 10 mm Hg, this may indicate angle-closure glaucoma. As with test 1 (above), gonioscopy is necessary to confirm the angle closure if the pressure rises. This may be used in conjunction with the dark room test.

Visual Fields in Glaucoma

The visual field test is most important in detecting open-angle glaucoma and in following the course of visual deterioration caused by the disease. The tangent screen, the Goldmann perimeter, and various automated perimeters give important information. Small extensions of the blind spot or early nerve fiber bundle defects not necessarily connected to the blind spot are noted early in the disease. Ideally, the diagnosis is made before visual field loss occurs. Under these circumstances, medical control can usually prevent significant visual loss.

The nerve fibers are arranged in the retina as indicated in Fig 15– 4. Increased intraocular pressure will gradually destroy the function of a bundle of these fibers, and the resulting visual field defect is spoken of as a "nerve fiber bundle defect." As the nerve fiber bundle defect enlarges, it takes an arcuate shape from the blind spot encircling the fixation area. It arches into either the superior or inferior field and ends at the horizontal meridian (Bjerrum scotoma). A double arcuate scotoma (one in the superior and one in the inferior field) forms a full-ring scotoma around the central fixation area.

Loss of peripheral field occurs later in the course of the disease. The nasal and superior fields are usually lost first. The last remnant of the visual field is usually a temporal island.

The field of vision may slowly contract in some cases down to 5 degrees from fixation, leaving the patient with good central vision but no peripheral vision. Central visual acuity, therefore, is not a reliable index of the progress of the disease. There is no substitute for careful periodic study of the visual field, applanation tonometry, and, most importantly, ophthalmoscopic visualization of the optic disks.

OPEN-ANGLE GLAUCOMA

At least 90% of cases of primary glaucoma are of the open-angle type. Open-angle glaucoma is bilateral, insidious in onset, and slowly progressive. There are no symptoms until visual impairment occurs, often too late to salvage useful vision. It is therefore the physician's responsibility to diagnose glaucoma before irreversible optic nerve damage has occurred. Early treatment prevents or delays visual deterioration.

Significant advances in the understanding of the course of open-angle glaucoma have been made in recent years, but unsolved problems remain and there are still differences of opinion among authorities on some issues. It now seems certain that increased intraocular pressure is caused by interference with aqueous outflow due to degenerative changes in the trabeculum, Schlemm's canal, and adjacent channels (see below). Increased pressure, whether caused by obstructed outflow or increased production of aqueous, affects primarily the retina and optic nerve, the functional elements of the eye.

Some authorities feel that in open-angle glaucoma, there is also a primary degenerative disorder of the optic nerve due to mechanical distortion of the lamina cribrosa, vascular insufficiency, or both. This view is supported by the observation that loss of function

Baring of the blind spot. The earliest nerve fiber bundle defect.

Incipient double nerve fiber bundle defect (Bjerrum scotoma).

Bjerrum scotoma isolated from blind spot.

End stages in glaucoma field loss. Remnant of central field still shows nasal step.

Fully developed nerve fiber bundle defect with nasal step (arcuate scotoma).

Peripheral depression with double nerve fiber bundle defect. Isolation of central field.

The basic visual field loss in glaucoma is the nerve fiber bundle defect with nasal step and peripheral nasal depression. It is here shown superimposed upon the nerve fiber layer of the retina and the retinal vascular tree. All perimetric changes in glaucoma are variations of these fundamental defects.

Double arcuate scotoma with peripheral breakthrough and nasal step.

Nasal depression connected with arcuate scotoma. Nasal step of Rönne.

Peripheral breakthrough of large nerve fiber bundle defect with well developed nasal step.

Seidel scotoma. Islands of greater visual loss within a nerve fiber bundle defect.

Figure 15–4. Visual field changes in glaucoma. (Reproduced, with permission, from Harrington DO: *The Visual Fields: A Textbook and Atlas of Clinical Perimetry,* 5th ed. Mosby, 1981.)

Figure 15–5. Cross section of an eye with open-angle glaucoma. Note open anterior chamber angle (peripheral iris is not in contact with the posterior corneal surface). Deep glaucomatous cupping ("bean-pot" appearance) shows the process to be well advanced. (Courtesy of R Carriker.)

early open-angle glaucoma reveal primary degeneration in the trabecular meshwork, degeneration of the collagen and elastic fibers of the trabeculum, and endothelial proliferation and edema. The trabecular spaces tend to be obliterated. The collector channels also undergo degenerative changes.

If the pressure remains elevated, gross damage to the eye occurs. The optic nerve undergoes degeneration, often assuming a typical bean-pot cupping appearance (Figs 15– 5 and 15– 6). There is degeneration of ganglion cells and nerve fibers in the retina. The iris and ciliary body become atrophic, and the ciliary processes show hyaline degeneration.

Genetic aspects. Open-angle glaucoma is a familial, genetically determined disorder, probably multifactorial or polygenic in origin. In any case, family history and routine systematic testing of relatives are most important in glaucoma detection.

Clinical Findings

Open-angle glaucoma causes no early symptoms. Subjective visual loss is nearly always a late finding. Although the disease is nearly always bilateral, one eye is frequently involved earlier and more severely than the other.

Optic disk changes are the most important early findings. The temporal disk margin thins (Fig 15– 7), and the cup gradually becomes wider and deeper. The large vessels become nasally displaced, and the affected area of the disk becomes atrophic (light gray or white rather than pink). The lamina cribrosa becomes more exposed.

The intraocular pressure is increased. The anterior chamber angle may be normal on gonioscopy. The loss of visual function from glaucoma can best be determined by repeated studies of the visual fields.

sometimes continues to progress even after the intraocular pressure has been normalized by miotic therapy or surgery. Also, patients with systemic disease (eg, diabetes, arteriosclerosis) are more likely than others to suffer optic nerve damage as a result of ocular hypertension.

There are few detectable histologic changes in the early stages. Nonspecific changes common to all forms of primary glaucoma occur in later stages. Studies of

Figure 15–6. Glaucomatous ("bean-pot") cupping of the optic disk.

Figure 15–7. Typical glaucomatous cupping. Note the nasal displacement of the vessels and hollowed-out appearance of the optic disk except for a thin border. (Courtesy of S Mettier Jr.)

Treatment

A. Medical Treatment: Miotics facilitate aqueous outflow by increasing the efficiency of the outflow channels. The exact mechanism of their effect is not understood. The drug of choice is pilocarpine, 1–4%, instilled in each eye up to 5 times daily. Carbachol, 0.75–3%, may be effective when pilocarpine fails or in patients who are allergic to pilocarpine. These are cholinergic drugs.

Anticholinesterase drugs are the longest-acting miotics available. These include demecarium bromide (Humorsol), 0.06–0.25%, and echothiophate (Phospholine) iodide, 0.03–0.25%. These drugs are primarily useful in aphakic glaucoma. *Caution:* These drugs should not be used in the presence of a narrow anterior chamber angle or in chronic angle-closure glaucomas since the extreme miosis increases relative pupillary block and can lead to angle closure. They also have cataractogenic properties and therefore should be avoided, if possible, in the phakic eye. They may cause iritis, bleeding, and excessive conjunctival scarring if used before surgery. Also, systemic effects have been noted in children who receive succinylcholine during anesthesia. Because of their high complication rate, their use is generally reserved for patients with open-angle glaucoma who are not good surgical candidates or who are aphakic.

Miotics frequently cause dimness of vision for 1–2 hours after instillation due to pupillary constriction, and younger glaucoma patients often have accommodative spasm with induced myopia. Side effects can be reduced by the use of a membrane-controlled delivery system (Ocusert) that permits continuous diffusion of active drug for approximately 1 week. A pilocarpine gel, Piloplex, is now available that can be used once or twice a day to provide the same control as 4% pilocarpine used every 6 hours.

Timolol maleate (Timoptic), a beta-adrenergic blocking agent, lowers intraocular pressure by decreasing aqueous production. It is available in 2 strengths, 0.25% and 0.5%, for use as eye drops instilled twice daily. Timolol can be used alone or in combination with other drugs. This drug has been used worldwide for over 5 years and continues to gain acceptance. Although side effects of timolol are rare, they can be serious; the action of the beta blockade slows the heart rate and lowers the blood pressure. The drug is contraindicated in chronic obstructive lung diseases, particularly asthma. Depression, confusion, and fatigue may occur. Patients should be taught to occlude the tear ducts after instillation to reduce systemic absorption.

Betaxolol (Betoptic) is a promising new alternative to timolol in the treatment of glaucoma. It is also a beta-adrenergic blocking agent with comparable effects on intraocular pressure, but it has the added advantage of β_1-receptor selectivity. Thus, systemic side effects are less likely to include bronchoconstriction, particularly the exacerbation of reactive airway disease, as demonstrated in a number of clinical trials. Cardiac or metabolic side effects may still occur. At present, clinical experience with betaxolol is limited.

Epinephrine, 0.5–2% instilled 1–2 times daily, decreases aqueous production and increases aqueous outflow. No miosis or myopia is induced, and it has a longer action than the miotics. For these reasons, epinephrine is often used as the primary drug in open-angle glaucoma (do not use in narrow angle eyes), with miotics and carbonic anhydrase inhibitors added later as necessary to lower the intraocular pressure.

Epinephrine instilled once or twice daily dramatically reduces the intraocular pressure in selected cases of aphakic glaucoma. Watch for macular edema as a complication.

Dipivefrin (Propine) is a prodrug of epinephrine that is metabolized intraocularly to its active state. This decreases the side effects of the epinephrine.

Carbonic anhydrase inhibitors such as acetazolamide (Diamox), 125–250 mg 4 times daily, or Diamox Sequels, 500 mg twice daily, are used in open-angle glaucoma if strong antiglaucoma solutions do not adequately control intraocular pressure. Dichlorphenamide (Daranide), methazolamide (Neptazane), and ethoxzolamide are similarly effective carbonic anhydrase inhibitors and, like acetazolamide, usually suppress aqueous production from 40 to 60%. Complications of long-term therapy with carbonic anhydrase inhibitors include renal calculi (see also p 375). Nevertheless, these drugs are indicated to avoid glaucoma surgery.

B. Laser Trabeculoplasty: Treatment of the trabecular meshwork by laser energy will reduce intraocular pressure by almost 25% in 80% of patients. It can be used as an adjunct to medical therapy before resorting to surgery. The initial gratifying decrease in pressure is often lost after a few months or years.

C. Surgical Treatment: (See p 198.) Surgery for open-angle glaucoma may be performed if the intraocular pressure is not maintained within normal limits by medical therapy and there is progressive visual field loss associated with optic nerve damage. There is no operation that can be called uniformly successful in the treatment of open-angle glaucoma. Standard filtration procedures such as trephine, sclerectomy, and thermal sclerostomy all have their advocates. Trabeculectomy and other forms of filtering procedures beneath a scleral flap have recently become popular. This is not because they are more effective but because they have a lower complication rate, since the anterior chamber remains formed following the procedure. The success rate without medication averages about 75%. Cataract formation does not occur as rapidly or as frequently following these latter procedures as it did with standard filtering operations.

If a cataract is present that should be extracted, this alone will help control the glaucoma in some cases. If the glaucoma is difficult to control or is uncontrolled prior to extraction, the cataract operation and trabeculectomy may be done simultaneously. The success rate of glaucoma surgery in the aphakic patient is approximately 60%. If medical therapy fails, however, subscleral filtration procedures may be used. Some authorities still use cyclodialysis.

In patients under 40 years of age, filtration surgery of any type has a low success rate. Standard filtering techniques are somewhat mutilating to the eye. The external trabeculotomy is somewhat more successful in these patients and is less mutilating. In general, surgery is recommended in open-angle glaucoma only when maximum medical therapy has failed to halt the progression of visual field and optic nerve deterioration.

Course & Prognosis

Without treatment, open-angle glaucoma may be insidiously progressive to complete blindness. If antiglaucoma drops control the intraocular pressure in an eye that has not suffered extensive glaucomatous damage, the prognosis is good (although visual field loss sometimes continues to progress in spite of normalized intraocular pressure). When the process is detected early, most glaucoma patients can be successfully managed medically.

LOW PRESSURE GLAUCOMA

This term denotes a number of conditions in which there is evidence of intraocular glaucomatous damage (cupping of the optic disk, visual field defects, etc) with normal or low intraocular pressure. Most such cases can be classified in the following groups:

(1) Cases in which some type of glaucoma, usually secondary, has caused permanent changes and then regressed spontaneously. Tonography may reveal a diminished facility of outflow.

(2) Diurnal variation: The pressure is usually normal when taken but is elevated at other times. This may be due to diurnal variation, so that if the pressure is measured at the same time of day it seems normal. Diurnal pressure curves disclose the real diagnosis.

(3) A variety of miscellaneous cases of damage to the optic nerve and retina, including vascular, congenital, degenerative, and other diseases, or tumors involving the optic chiasm. Some of these are apparently due to reduced blood pressure and blood flow to the optic nerve or perhaps to an easily distorted lamina cribrosa.

ANGLE-CLOSURE GLAUCOMA (Acute Glaucoma)

Angle-closure glaucoma occurs when there is a sudden increase in the intraocular pressure due to a block of the anterior chamber angle by the root of the iris, which cuts off all aqueous outflow, causing severe pain and sudden visual loss.

An acute attack of angle-closure glaucoma can develop only in an eye in which the anterior chamber angle is anatomically narrow. This situation can be easily assessed clinically by estimation of the depth of the anterior chamber, using oblique illumination from a penlight (Fig 15– 8). The following factors may cause further encroachment upon the anterior chamber angle, setting the stage for angle-closure glaucoma.

(1) Physiologic pupillary block: When the anterior chamber angle is narrow; the iris has a relatively large arc of contact with the anterior surface of the lens. This may obstruct the free passage of aqueous from the posterior to the anterior chamber. As pressure builds up in the posterior chamber, the peripheral iris is pushed forward (iris bombé). If the iris is pushed forward far enough so that it lies against the trabeculum, aqueous humor drainage is impeded, resulting in acute angle-closure glaucoma.

(2) Increased size of the lens: Normally, the lens continues to enlarge slightly with age. During the act of accommodation there may be a further increase in the forward displacement of the lens, increasing the relative pupillary block.

Precipitating Factors

The more miotic the pupil, the more tightly the iris is held against the lens, thus increasing pupillary block. If a patient with a narrow angle is given pilocarpine, an acute attack of angle-closure glaucoma may be precipitated. Usually, however, the pull of the sphincter on the peripheral iris will tend to open the angle.

Dilating the pupil has the opposite effect, making it easier for the aqueous humor trapped behind the iris by the relative pupillary block to lift the peripheral iris against the trabecular meshwork. The most dangerous pupillary position in such an eye is mid-dilation. With further dilation, the arc of contact of iris to lens is reduced, lessening pupillary block. It is wise to perform gonioscopy of a shallow-chambered eye

Figure 15–8. Estimation of depth of anterior chamber by oblique illumination (diagram). (Courtesy of R Shaffer.)

whenever the pupil is dilated or contracted, to avoid causing iatrogenic angle-closure glaucoma.

Plateau iris is a rare condition in which the central anterior chamber depth is normal but the angle is very narrow. Such an eye has little pupillary block, but dilation will cause "bunching up" of the peripheral iris, occluding the angle even if peripheral iridectomy has been performed. Miotics or iridoplasty can help open the angle.

A secondary cause of shallow anterior chamber and angle-closure glaucoma is a sudden increase in the volume of the posterior chamber. This can result from subchoroidal hemorrhage, a swollen lens, iris bombé, wound leakage, or ciliary block (malignant) glaucoma or from therapeutic procedures such as panretinal photocoagulation or scleral buckling.

Pathology

The pathologic changes in acute glaucoma include peripheral anterior synechiae and edema and congestion of the ciliary processes and iris. These are secondary to the vascular strangulation that results from the high pressure. Late changes are the result of interference with circulation and the continued high pressure. The iris and ciliary body become atrophic, and the ciliary processes show hyaline degeneration. Chronic edema of the cornea results in loosening of the corneal epithelium and the formation of epithelial bullae (bullous keratopathy). The most important pathologic change is damage to the nerve elements: degeneration of nerve fibers and a loss of substance of the optic cup associated with a backward bowing of the cribriform plate. The ganglion cell layer and the nerve fiber layer of the retina undergo degeneration. Eventually the lens may show cataractous change.

Clinical Findings

Angle-closure (acute) glaucoma is characterized by a sudden onset of blurred vision followed by excruciating pain, and a rainbow-colored halo is seen around lights. Nausea and vomiting are often present. The pain is usually localized in and around the eye. Other findings include markedly increased intraocular pressure, a shallow anterior chamber, an edematous cornea, decreased visual acuity (at times limited to light perception only), a fixed, moderately dilated pupil, and ciliary injection.

Differential Diagnosis

Acute iritis and conjunctivitis must be considered with acute angle-closure glaucoma in the differential diagnosis of any acutely inflamed eye, although they seldom have shallow anterior chambers or increased tension. (1) Acute iritis causes more photophobia and less pain than acute glaucoma. Intraocular pressure may be normal, the pupil is constricted, and the cornea is not edematous. Marked flare and cells are present in the anterior chamber, and there is deep ciliary injection. (2) In acute conjunctivitis there is little or no pain and no visual loss. There is discharge from the eye and an intensely inflamed conjunctiva, but no ciliary injection. The pupillary responses are normal, the cornea is clear, and intraocular pressure is normal. (3) Iridocyclitis with secondary glaucoma occasionally presents a difficult problem of differentiation. Gonioscopy to define the type of angle is most helpful. If corneal or anterior chamber haze prevents good visibility, gonioscopy of the other eye will usually confirm the diagnosis.

Complications & Sequelae

A. Formation of Peripheral Anterior Synechiae:

The peripheral iris adheres to the trabecular meshwork and blocks the outflow of aqueous.

B. Cataract Formation: The lens sometimes swells, and a cataract may develop. The enlarged lens pushes the iris even farther anteriorly; this increases the pupillary block, which in turn increases the degree of angle block.

C. Atrophy of the Retina and Optic Nerve: The nerve elements of the eye withstand the effects of increased intraocular pressure poorly. Glaucomatous cupping of the optic disk and retinal atrophy, particularly of the ganglion cell layer, occur.

D. Absolute Glaucoma: The end result of uncontrolled angle-closure glaucoma is absolute glaucoma. The eye is stony hard, sightless, and often quite painful, in which case enucleation or retrobulbar alcohol injection is necessary.

Prevention

Although miotics can usually widen a narrow angle and break an attack of angle-closure glaucoma, prevention is best accomplished by iridectomy that bypasses the pupillary block permanently. This is best effected by laser.

Treatment

Angle-closure glaucoma is an ophthalmic surgical emergency.

A. Medical Treatment: Before surgery, every effort must be made to reduce the intraocular pressure by medical means. Osmotic agents, miotics, and acetazolamide are usually required. The immediate administration of oral glycerin (glycerol), 1 mL/kg of body weight in a cold 50% solution mixed with chilled lemon juice, nearly always interrupts the acute attack by making the blood hypertonic and drawing fluid from the eye. Pilocarpine 2%, 2 drops every 15 minutes for several hours, will usually constrict the pupil and pull the iris away from the trabeculum, allowing aqueous outflow to be reestablished (unless permanent adhesions have formed).

If treatment with glycerin is not successful or if the patient is nauseated, intravenous hypertonic mannitol (20%) may be effective in total doses of 1.5–3 g/kg. Acetazolamide, 500 mg given intramuscularly if the patient is nauseated, will further reduce intraocular pressure by decreasing aqueous production.

Meperidine, 100 mg intramuscularly, or other systemic analgesic should be given as necessary to relieve pain.

B. Surgical Treatment: (See p 198.) Although surgical intervention can be delayed for several hours to permit clearing of the cornea, surgery is indicated whether or not pressure has been reduced. The safest method of breaking the pupillary block is laser iridectomy.

SUBACUTE OR CHRONIC ANGLE-CLOSURE GLAUCOMA

Chronic angle-closure glaucoma is caused by the same etiologic factors as acute angle-closure glaucoma. The difference is that there is no sudden complete block to aqueous outflow by the iris being pushed against the trabeculum. The iris extends its arc of contact with the trabeculum gradually until an adequate area of angle is no longer available for aqueous outflow. The pressure rises and glaucoma results that may be clinically similar to open-angle glaucoma.

Clinical Findings

Symptoms are minimal or absent. Occasional mild attacks of increased intraocular pressure cause transient blurring of vision, halos around lights, and possibly slight pain in or about the eyes. On examination, one finds a shallow anterior chamber, high intraocular pressure (25–50 mm Hg), and a partially closed chamber angle as seen on gonioscopic examination. The iris is in apposition to the trabeculum except in an area covering one-fifth or less of the chamber angle.

Treatment

Treatment is the same as for acute angle-closure glaucoma. After breaking of the pupillary block by iridectomy, residual glaucoma should be treated in the same way as open-angle glaucoma.

CILIARY BLOCK GLAUCOMA (Malignant Glaucoma)

Surgery upon an eye with markedly increased intraocular pressure and a closed angle can lead to ciliary block glaucoma. Immediately after surgery, the intraocular pressure increases markedly and the lens-iris diaphragm is pushed forward as a result of the collection of aqueous in and behind the vitreous body.

Treatment

Treatment consists of cycloplegics, mydriatics, and hyperosmotic agents. Atropine, 2–4%, should be used topically every 2 hours for the first day and may need to be continued indefinitely on a daily basis thereafter. Phenylephrine, 10%, is used 4 times a day. Hyperosmotic agents are used to shrink the vitreous body and let the lens-iris diaphragm fall posteriorly.

Posterior sclerotomy, vitrectomy, and even lens extraction may be needed.

PRIMARY CONGENITAL OR INFANTILE GLAUCOMA (Trabeculodysgenesis)

Infantile glaucoma is a form of developmental glaucoma with onset in the first year of life. One-fourth of cases are present at birth. A few are diagnosed after the second year of life. The pathologic

Figure 15-9. Infantile glaucoma (buphthalmos).

picture is produced by an arrest in development of the angle structures at about the seventh month of fetal life. The iris is hypoplastic and inserts onto the trabecular surface in front of a poorly developed scleral spur (Fig 15-9).

Clinical Findings

The earliest and most constant symptom is epiphora. Photophobia may be present. Increased intraocular pressure is the cardinal sign. Glaucomatous cupping of the optic disk is a relatively early and most important change. Later findings include increased corneal diameter (above 11.5 mm is considered significant), epithelial edema, tears of Descemet's membrane, and increased depth of the anterior chamber (associated with general enlargement of the anterior segment of the eye), as well as edema and opacity of the corneal stroma. The iris inserts anteriorly onto the trabeculum instead of into the ciliary body.

Differential Diagnosis

Megalocornea, secondary glaucoma, and traumatic corneal haze should be ruled out. Measurement of intraocular pressure, gonioscopy, and evaluation of the optic disk are important in making the differential diagnosis.

Treatment

Unlike open-angle glaucoma, in which the best treatment is often nonsurgical, infantile glaucoma must be treated surgically to obtain lasting results. Medical treatment with miotics is at best a preoperative adjunctive measure.

Goniotomy is the treatment of choice. If repeated goniotomies fail or are not possible due to corneal haze, external trabeculotomy is often effective. Subscleral filtration (trabeculectomy) may be tried if these measures fail. The long-term visual prognosis is then much less favorable.

Course & Prognosis

In untreated cases, blindness occurs early. The eye undergoes marked stretching and may even rupture with minor trauma. Typical glaucomatous cupping occurs relatively soon, emphasizing the necessity of early effective treatment.

The earlier the disease becomes manifest, the less favorable the prognosis, since the early appearance of symptoms implies a more severe defect of aqueous drainage. Over 80% of cases are evident by age 3 months. Goniotomy controls the pressure permanently in 70-80% of cases. The long-term visual prognosis in such cases is good.

DEVELOPMENTAL GLAUCOMA ASSOCIATED WITH OTHER CONGENITAL ANOMALIES*

A number of syndromes characterized by increased intraocular pressure in persons under 40 have been grouped under this broad heading, which includes late-developing infantile glaucoma.

Pigmentary Glaucoma

This syndrome seems to be primarily a degeneration of the pigmented epithelium of the iris and ciliary body. The pigment granules flake off the iris as a result of friction against the underlying packets of zonular fibers, resulting in iris transillumination. The pigment is deposited on the posterior corneal surface (Krukenberg's spindle) and becomes lodged in the trabecular meshwork, impeding the normal outflow of aqueous. The syndrome occurs most often in myopic males between the ages of 25 and 40 who have a deep anterior chamber with a wide anterior chamber angle.

A number of pedigrees of autosomal dominant inheritance of pigmentary glaucoma have been reported. The pigmentary changes may be present without glaucoma, but such persons must be considered "glaucoma suspects."

This type of glaucoma responds to timolol and to epinephrine. Miotics can seldom be used in these young patients because of induced myopia. The prognosis is not favorable if the process is severe enough to require a filtering operation. Laser trabeculoplasty may improve the prognosis.

Aniridia

The distinguishing feature of aniridia, as the name implies, is the vestigial iris. Often, little more than the root of the iris or a thin iris margin is present. Other deformities of the eye may be present, such as congenital cataracts, corneal dystrophy, and foveal hypoplasia. Vision is usually poor. Glaucoma frequently develops before adolescence and is usually refractory to medical or surgical management.

This rare syndrome is genetically determined. Nu-

*Formerly classified as juvenile glaucoma.

merous examples of both autosomal dominant and recessive inheritance have appeared in the literature.

If medical therapy is ineffective, goniotomy or trabeculotomy may occasionally normalize the intraocular pressure. Often, filtering operations are necessary, but the long-term visual prognosis is poor.

Iridocorneal Trabeculodysgenesis (Axenfeld's Syndrome, Peters' Anomaly, Rieger's Syndrome)

These rare diseases represent a spectrum of improper development of the mesodermal structures of the anterior segment. The result is an abnormally developed angle, iris, and cornea. Occasionally, lens changes are present. Usually there is some hypoplasia of the anterior stroma of the iris, with bridging filaments connecting the iris stroma to the cornea. If these bridging filaments occur peripherally and connect to a prominent, axially displaced Schwalbe's line (posterior embryotoxon), the disease is known as **Axenfeld's syndrome.** If adhesions are between the central iris and central posterior surface of the cornea, the disease is known as **Peters' anomaly.** If there are broader iridocorneal adhesions associated with the disruption of the iris with polycoria and, in addition, skeletal and dental anomalies, the disorder is called **Rieger's syndrome.**

These diseases are usually dominantly inherited, although sporadic cases have been reported. Glaucoma occurs in approximately 50% of such eyes. Since no highly effective surgical procedure is available for these syndromes, they are treated as open-angle glaucomas. Filtering surgery or trabeculotomy may be used if medical therapy fails. The prognosis is guarded for long-term retention of good visual function.

SECONDARY GLAUCOMA

Increased intraocular pressure occurring as one manifestation of some other intraocular disease is called secondary glaucoma. These diseases are difficult to classify satisfactorily.

In addition to treatment of the underlying disease, several drugs are of value in control of secondary glaucoma. With moderate elevation of intraocular pressure, reduction of aqueous production with epinephrine or timolol with or without acetazolamide is adequate management. With extreme elevations, osmotic agents are indicated. These ocular antihypertensive drugs may prevent permanent damage due to increased intraocular pressure until the underlying cause of secondary glaucoma can be controlled.

GLAUCOMA SECONDARY TO CHANGES IN THE LENS

Lens Dislocation (Traumatic)

The lens may dislocate anteriorly, pressing the iris against the posterior cornea and blocking aqueous outflow, or it may dislocate posteriorly. Secondary glaucoma is a frequent complication of posterior dislocation of the lens and is not easy to explain. Often it may be due to angle recession or trabecular damage that occurred at the time of the trauma. In other cases pupillary block occurs when a wedge of vitreous curls around the dislocated lens and plugs the pupillary opening. Surgery may be necessary if the intraocular pressure cannot be controlled medically.

Intumescence of the Lens

The lens may take up considerable fluid during cataractous change, increasing its size markedly. It may then encroach upon the anterior chamber and produce a pupillary block, resulting in angle-closure glaucoma. Treatment consists of lens extraction.

Phacolytic Glaucoma

As cataract formation proceeds, the lens cortex elements may undergo liquefaction and seep out through the lens capsule. Lens protein products may cause an inflammatory reaction within the eye. In this case, uveitis occurs, and the protein and cellular debris lodge in the outflow system to obstruct the free passage of aqueous. Edema of the trabeculum itself is probably associated, further decreasing the facility of aqueous outflow. Lens extraction is indicated.

Exfoliative Syndrome (Pseudoexfoliation of the Lens Capsule, Glaucoma Capsulare)

In exfoliative syndrome, deposits of unknown origin and composition are seen on the lens surface, ciliary processes, zonule, posterior iris surface, loose in the anterior chamber, and in the trabecular meshwork. The disease is usually found in patients over the age of 65. Glaucoma and sometimes cataract may eventually develop. Lens extraction has no effect on the glaucoma. Miotics, timolol, and epinephrine are moderately effective, but laser trabeculoplasty or a filtering operation may be necessary.

GLAUCOMA SECONDARY TO CHANGES IN THE UVEAL TRACT

Uveitis

Often the intraocular pressure is below normal early in uveitis. This is because the inflamed ciliary body is functioning poorly and does not secrete the elements that produce the difference in osmotic pressure between aqueous and plasma. There is edema of the trabeculum as well as the ciliary body and iris, and this may result in a decreased facility of aqueous outflow. As long as there is no osmotic difference between blood and aqueous there will be no rise in pressure, but when the ciliary body begins secreting there will be an abrupt rise of pressure unless there has been a simultaneous improvement in the patency of the outflow channels. Long-standing or repeated attacks of iridocyclitis cause permanent anterior synechiae. In these cases, after the inflammatory reaction has subsided, miotics or even filtering procedures may be needed to control the intraocular pressure.

Tumor

Rapidly growing melanomas originating in the uveal tract can cause increased intraocular pressure by volume replacement, by encroachment on the filtration angle, or by blocking of a vortex vein. Enucleation is indicated.

Iridocorneoendothelial (ICE) Syndrome (Essential Iris Atrophy, Iris Nevus Syndrome, Chandler's Syndrome, Cogan-Reese Syndrome)

Slowly progressive atrophy of iris tissue is a rare disorder of unknown cause that is almost always associated with glaucoma. Anterior synechiae form and the degenerated iris elements block the trabecular meshwork, creating a glaucoma that is very difficult to control either medically or surgically. Endothelial degeneration occurs with edema of the cornea at relatively low intraocular pressures. The condition is nearly always unilateral.

GLAUCOMA SECONDARY TO TRAUMA

Massive Hemorrhage Into the Anterior Chamber

Contusion or penetrating injuries of the globe can cause tears in the iris or ciliary body and thus massive hemorrhage into the anterior chamber. The intraocular pressure may be elevated, and blood breakdown products or organized clots lodge in the outflow mechanism. One serious complication is blood staining of the cornea. Once well established, the staining may require several years to absorb. If the intraocular pressure cannot be controlled with systemic hypotensive drugs, the anterior chamber should be lavaged through a limbal incision. Patients with sickle cell trait or disease are at greater risk of developing glaucoma following anterior chamber hemorrhage.

Corneal or Limbal Laceration With Prolapse of Iris Into the Wound

Lacerations of the anterior eye or contusions causing anterior rupture of the eye precipitate a loss of the anterior chamber and the rapid closure of the chamber angle by the adherence of the iris to the cornea. Occasionally, a prolapse of uveal tissue into the wound will seal the defect and maintain the anterior chamber. The primary objective of the treatment is the re-formation of the anterior chamber to prevent permanent anterior peripheral synechiae. Excision of prolapsed uvea, tight closure of the wound, and injection of saline into the anterior chamber are of paramount importance.

Contusion Causing Retrodisplacement of the Iris Root & Deepening of the Anterior Chamber Angle (Angle Recession Glaucoma)

A number of clinicians have called attention to this type of trauma-induced unilateral secondary glaucoma. Following a contusion injury, the anterior chamber may be significantly deeper than in the uninjured eye. Gonioscopically, one sees a recession of the angle and a torn ciliary body. Glaucoma occurs if there is sufficient associated damage to the trabecular meshwork to interfere with aqueous outflow. The condition often responds to standard open-angle glaucoma therapy, although occasionally a filtering operation is necessary.

GLAUCOMA FOLLOWING SURGERY

Epithelial Ingrowth Into the Anterior Chamber

Following cataract surgery with resultant poor healing of the wound edges, epithelium may grow into the anterior chamber and eventually line the anterior chamber angle structures, preventing normal outflow of aqueous. This is a difficult complication to treat once it is well established. An effort can be made to scrape the newly deposited epithelium off the angle structures. Corneal transplant may be beneficial. The problem is primarily one of prevention.

Flat Anterior Chamber Following Cataract Surgery

Following cataract surgery, aqueous may escape through an imperfectly closed wound resulting in a flat (absent) anterior chamber. If the chamber fails to re-form within 1–3 days, repair of the wound is required to avoid anterior synechiae and endothelial damage.

GLAUCOMA SECONDARY TO RUBEOSIS IRIDIS

Rubeosis often follows central vessel occlusion and occurs frequently in advanced diabetes mellitus. Small vessels grow on the anterior surface of the iris and into the anterior chamber angle, interfering with normal aqueous outflow. Miotics are of little value. Cyclocryosurgery is the best therapeutic technique available, but results are poor. Early panretinal photocoagulation can arrest the blood vessel proliferation. Filtering surgery can then be successful in some cases.

GLAUCOMA SECONDARY TO ARTERIOVENOUS FISTULAS

Pulsating exophthalmos from arteriovenous fistula is usually accompanied by a slightly elevated intraocular pressure due to increased venous pressure. Treatment is directed at the underlying condition.

GLAUCOMA SECONDARY TO THE USE OF TOPICAL CORTICOSTEROIDS

Much interest has been aroused by the observation that topically administered corticosteroids may produce a type of glaucoma that simulates open-angle glaucoma. Most persons do not develop significant intraocular pressure elevations while on such treatment. In those who do, withdrawal of the medication eliminates the glaucoma; but permanent damage can occur if the condition goes unrecognized too long. If topical steroid therapy is absolutely necessary, miotics or other open-angle glaucoma therapy usually will control the glaucoma. It is imperative that patients receiving long-term topical steroid therapy have periodic tonometry and ophthalmoscopy. It is equally important to beware of topical administration of corticosteroids in the eyes of patients known to have glaucoma or a family history of glaucoma. Less commonly, glaucoma can occur in patients being given long-term systemic corticosteroids over prolonged periods. Injections of corticosteroids under the conjunctiva and under Tenon's capsule may cause elevated intraocular pressure for several months. Surgical excision of the residual steroid deposit may allow the pressure to return to normal.

OCULAR HYPERTENSION

Ocular hypertension is the term coined to denote an elevated intraocular pressure (above the statistically normal level of 10–25 mm Hg) without evidence of anatomic or functional damage to the eye. The diagnosis changes to glaucoma if there is asymmetry of the disk cups (cup in one eye larger than the cup in the other) or increase of the size of the disk cup over a period of time. Obviously, functional loss represents visual field defects specific for glaucoma.

The patient with ocular hypertension should be considered a glaucoma suspect. Although no evidence of damage from the elevated intraocular pressure may be apparent, there is as yet no sure means of predicting which patient will subsequently develop damage. Frequent observation (1–3 times yearly) of the optic disk, tonometry, and visual field testing are indicated in order to make certain that proper treatment is initiated immediately if the optic nerve appears threatened.

SURGICAL PROCEDURES USED IN THE TREATMENT OF THE GLAUCOMAS

PERIPHERAL IRIDECTOMY

In acute or chronic angle-closure glaucoma when extensive peripheral anterior synechiae have not formed, peripheral iridectomy is the operation of choice. It offers the one hope of a permanent cure by reestablishing ready communication between the posterior and anterior chambers. This relieves pupillary block and allows the iris root to drop away from the filtration angle, thus reestablishing the outflow of aqueous by normal channels.

In recent years, the laser has been used for most peripheral iridectomies. The risk of intraocular surgery and the expense of hospitalization are avoided.

LASER TRABECULOPLASTY

When maximal medical therapy fails to control the pressure of open-angle glaucoma, laser trabeculoplasty is usually indicated before filtration surgery is considered. Laser energy is focused through a goniolens onto the trabecular meshwork. Intraocular pressure is reduced by improved aqueous outflow in about 80% of cases. Medications must usually be continued. The effect of the laser decreases with time. The procedure may be repeated but with much less effectiveness.

FILTRATION SURGERY

When pressures cannot be maintained at a safe level in open-angle glaucoma despite the use of medications and laser therapy, filtration surgery is indicated. The variety of procedures available indicates that none is perfect. In "full-thickness" operations (trephine, thermal sclerostomy, posterior lip sclerectomy), a channel is created from the anterior chamber into the subconjunctival space. There, the aqueous is absorbed by the lymphatics and blood vessels and via transudation through the conjunctiva. In about 25% of cases, postoperative scarring closes the opening, and reoperation becomes necessary.

In recent years, a protected filtration operation, trabeculectomy, has achieved universal popularity. A half-thickness scleral flap is sutured over the limbal opening in addition to closure of the conjunctival flap. Complications are reduced, but pressure reduction is somewhat less than with the unprotected methods.

CYCLOCRYOTHERMY

Cyclocryothermy has generally replaced cyclo-diathermy in the treatment of aphakic glaucoma. It has the advantage of destroying the ciliary body without causing damage to either the conjunctiva or the sclera. No cutting is required. The highly vascular reaction in the ciliary body leads to fibrosis, decreased ciliary body function, and consequent decreased aqueous production.

Laser trabeculoplasty (see above) can also be tried in aphakic glaucoma, with an approximate success rate of 40%.

GONIOTOMY

Infantile glaucoma is best treated by goniotomy. This procedure was introduced for treatment of in-fantile glaucoma by Otto Barkan in 1938 and changed the prognosis of the disease from very bad to good (70–80% cure). The operation aims to establish normal aqueous outflow through physiologic channels.

THERAPEUTIC ULTRASOUND

This promising new noninvasive treatment of all types of glaucoma was introduced by Dr. Jackson Coleman of the Cornell Medical Center. To date, it has been used only in advanced cases, with a success rate of more than 50%. High-frequency sound waves are focused on the ciliary body and targeted through the sclera near the limbus. The damaged ciliary body produces less aqueous, and the weakened sclera allows seepage of aqueous.

REFERENCES

Abraham RK, Miller GL: Argon laser iridectomy for angle-closure glaucoma. (Letter.) *Ann Ophthalmol* 1973;**5**:613.

Abraham RK, Miller GL: Argon laser iridectomy for angle-closure glaucoma. Presented at the American Society for Contemporary Ophthalmology, Miami Beach, March 2, 1973.

Anderson DR: Pathology of the glaucomas. In: Cambridge Ophthalmological Symposium—Perrers Taylor Memorial (Sept 1971). *Br J Ophthalmol* 1972;**56**:146.

Armaly MF: Glaucoma: Annual review. *Arch Ophthalmol* 1975;**93**:146.

Becker B, Kolker AE: Glaucoma: A classic treatise. (7 parts.) *Eye Ear Nose Throat Mon* 1975;**54**:350, 379, 431, 460 and 1976;**55**:15, 58, 89.

Carpel EF et al: Normal cup-disk ratio. *Am J Ophthalmol* 1981;**91**:588.

Chandler PA et al: *Glaucoma*, 2nd ed. Lea & Febiger, 1980.

Coleman DJ et al: Therapeutic ultrasound in the treatment of glaucoma. 1. Experimental model. 2. Clinical applications. *Ophthalmology* 1985;**92**:339, 347.

David R et al: Genetic markers in glaucoma. *Br J Ophthalmol* 1980;**64**:227.

Drance SM et al: Multivariate analysis in glaucoma. *Arch Ophthalmol* 1981;**99**:1019.

Edwards RS: Behaviour of the fellow eye in acute angle-closure glaucoma. *Br J Ophthalmol* 1982;**66**:576.

Glaucoma: 1984 Annual Meeting of the American Academy of Ophthalmology, Atlanta, November 11–15. *Ophthalmology* 1984;**91**:307, 1005. [Entire issues.]

Glaucoma: 1985 Annual Meeting of the American Academy of Ophthalmology, San Francisco, September 29–October 3. *Ophthalmology* 1985;**92**:853. [Entire issue.]

Harrington DO: *The Visual Fields: A Textbook and Atlas of Clinical Perimetry*, 5th ed. Mosby, 1981.

Hayreh SS: Pathogenesis of cupping of the optic disc. *Br J Ophthalmol* 1974;**58**:863.

Hetherington J: Treatment of juvenile glaucoma: Commentary. In: Cambridge Opthalmological Symposium—Perrers Taylor Memorial (Sept 1971). *Br J Ophthalmol* 1972;**56**:262.

Hoskins HD Jr, Gelber EC: Optic disk topography and visual field defects in patients with increased intraocular pressure. *Am J Ophthalmol* 1975;**80**:284.

Hoyt WF: Ophthalmoscopy of the retinal nerve fibre layer in neuro-ophthalmologic diagnosis. *Aust J Ophthalmol* 1976; **4**:14.

Jocson VL, Sears ML: Channels of aqueous outflow and related blood vessels. 1. *Macaca mulatta* (rhesus). 2. *Cercopithecus ethiops. Arch Ophthalmol* 1968;**80**:104 and 1969;**81**:244.

Kitazawa Y, Horie T: Diurnal variation of intraocular pressure in primary open-angle glaucoma. *Am J Ophthalmol* 1975; **79**:557.

Kolker AE, Hetherington J: *Becker-Shaffer's Diagnosis and Therapy of the Glaucomas*, 5th ed. Mosby, 1983.

LeBlanc RP et al: Timolol. *Ophthalmology* 1981;**88**:244.

Miller SJH: Glaucoma simplex and the management of first-degree relatives. In: Cambridge Ophthalmological Symposium—Perrers Taylor Memorial (Sept 1971). *Br J Ophthalmol* 1972;**56**:284.

Quigley HA: Early detection of glaucomatous damage. 2. Changes in the appearance of the optic disk. *Surv Ophthalmol* 1985;**30**:111.

Quigley HA et al: Optic nerve damage in human glaucoma. *Arch Ophthalmol* 1982;**100**:135.

Shaffer RN et al: The use of diagrams to record changes in glaucomatous discs. *Am J Ophthalmol* 1975;**80**:460.

Spencer WH: Microsurgery of the outflow channels: Histologic evaluation of microsurgical glaucoma techniques. (Symposium.) *Trans Am Acad Ophthalmol Otolaryngol* 1972;**76**:389.

Van Buskirk EM, Fraunfelder FT: Ocular beta-blockers and systemic effects. (Editorial.) *Am J Ophthalmol* 1984;**98**:623.

Watson PG: Surgery of the glaucomas. In: Cambridge Ophthalmological Symposium—Perrers Taylor Memorial (Sept 1971). *Br J Ophthalmol* 1972;**56**:299.

Watson PG et al: The place of trabeculectomy in the treatment of glaucoma. *Ophthalmology* 1981;**88**:197.

Werner EB, Drance SM: Early visual field disturbances in glaucoma. *Arch Ophthalmol* 1977;**95**:1173.

Williams MT: Community screening for glaucoma and diabetes. *Sight Sav Rev* 1974;**44**:79.

Wise J: Long-term control of adult open-angle glaucoma by argon laser treatment. *Ophthalmology* 1981;**88**:197.

Zimmerman TJ: Medication versus surgery: Are we doing it wrong? (Editorial.) *Ann Ophthalmol* 1981;**13**:783.

Strabismus

Howard M. Eggers, MD

Under normal binocular viewing conditions, the image of the object of regard falls simultaneously on the fovea of each eye (bifoveal fixation), and the vertical retinal meridians are both upright. Either eye can be misaligned, so that only one eye at a time views the object of regard. Deviation from perfect alignment (strabismus) may be in any direction—inward, outward, up, down, or in a rotary direction about the line of sight. The amount of deviation is the angle by which the deviating eye is misaligned. Strabismus present under binocular viewing conditions is called manifest strabismus, heterotropia, or tropia. Deviation present only after binocular vision has been interrupted (ie, deviation controlled by binocular vision) is called latent strabismus, heterophoria, or phoria.

Strabismus is present in about 2% of children. Treatment should begin as soon as the diagnosis is made in order to ensure the best possible visual acuity and binocular visual function. It is extremely rare for true strabismus to be outgrown.

ANATOMY

Muscles

Six extraocular muscles control the movement of each eye: 4 rectus and 2 oblique muscles.

A. Rectus Muscles: The 4 rectus muscles originate at a common ring tendon (annulus of Zinn) surrounding the optic nerve at the posterior apex of the orbit. They are named according to their insertion into the sclera on the medial, lateral, inferior, and superior surfaces of the eye. The muscles are about 40 mm long, becoming tendinous 4–6 mm from insertion, and are about 10 mm wide at the point of insertion. The approximate distances of insertion from the corneal limbus are as follows: medial rectus, 5 mm; inferior rectus, 6 mm; lateral rectus, 7 mm; and superior rectus, 8 mm (Fig 16–1). With the eye in primary position, the vertical rectus muscle makes an angle of 23 degrees with the optic axis.

B. Oblique Muscles: The 2 oblique muscles control primarily torsional movement and, to a lesser

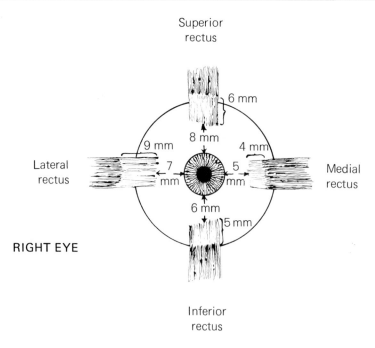

Figure 16–1. Approximate distances of the rectus muscles from the limbus, and the approximate lengths of tendons.

extent, upward and downward movement. The inferior oblique muscle arises from the nasal orbital wall several millimeters behind the orbital rim; it passes under the inferior rectus and curves around the eyeball, making a large arc of scleral contact, and inserts in the posterior lateral quadrant of the eye just lateral to the fovea. The main muscle body of the superior oblique muscle originates from the annulus of Zinn just above the origin of the superior rectus muscle and passes to the cartilaginous pulley (trochlea) attached to the nasal side of the superior orbital rim. At the pulley it is reflected downward, outward, and posteriorly, passing under the tendon of the superior rectus muscle to insert into the sclera. In the primary position, the muscle plane of the superior and inferior oblique muscles forms an angle of 51–54 degrees with the optic axis.

Innervation

The abducens nerve innervates the lateral rectus muscle; the trochlear nerve innervates the superior oblique muscle; and the oculomotor nerve innervates the other 3 rectus muscles and the inferior oblique muscle.

Fascia

The rectus and oblique muscles are ensheathed by fascia. Near the points of insertion of these muscles the fascia is continuous with Tenon's capsule, which is between the sclera and conjunctiva. Fascial condensations to adjacent orbital bony structures serve as check ligaments for the extraocular muscles and limit ocular rotation (Figs 16–2 and 16–3).

DEFINITIONS

Angle kappa: The angle between the visual axis and the central pupillary line. When the eye is fixing a light, if the corneal reflection is centered on the pupil, the visual axis and the central pupillary line coincide and the angle kappa is zero. Ordinarily, the light reflex is 2–4 degrees nasal to the pupillary center, giving the appearance of slight exotropia (positive angle kappa). A negative angle kappa gives the false impression of esotropia.

Conjugate: Movement of the eyes in the same direction at the same time.

Ductions: (Fig 16–4.) Monocular rotations with no consideration of the position of the other eye.

Adduction: Inward rotation.

Abduction: Outward rotation.

Sursumduction (elevation): Upward rotation.

Infraduction (depression): Downward rotation.

Fusion: Formation of one image from the 2 images seen simultaneously by the 2 eyes. Fusion has 2 aspects:

Motor fusion: Adjustments made by the brain in innervation of extraocular muscles in order to bring both eyes into bifoveal and torsional alignment.

Sensory fusion: Integration in the visual sensory areas of the brain of images seen with the 2 eyes into one sensory percept.

Heterophoria (phoria): Latent deviation of the eyes held in check by binocular vision.

Esophoria: Tendency for one eye to turn inward.

Exophoria: Tendency for one eye to turn outward.

Hyperphoria: Tendency for one eye to deviate upward.

Hypophoria: Tendency for one eye to deviate downward.

Heterotropia (tropia):

Strabismus: Manifest deviation of the eyes uncontrolled by binocular vision.

Esotropia: Convergent manifest deviation ("crossed eyes").

Exotropia: Divergent manifest deviation ("wall-eyes").

Hypertropia: Manifest deviation of one eye upward.

Hypotropia: Manifest deviation of one eye downward. By convention, in the absence of specific pathologic disease to explain the low visual direction of one eye, vertical deviations are named according to the high eye.

Incyclotropia: Rotation of one eye about the line of sight to produce a convergence of the 12 o'clock meridians of the 2 eyes.

Excyclotropia: Rotation of one eye about the line of sight to produce a convergence of the 6 o'clock meridians of the 2 eyes.

Orthophoria: The absence of any tendency of either eye to deviate when fusion is suspended. This state is rarely seen clinically. A small degree of phoria is normal.

Primary deviation: The deviation measured with the normal eye fixing and the eye with the paretic muscle deviating.

Prism diopter (Δ): A unit of angular measurement used to characterize ocular deviations. One centimeter subtends 1 prism diopter at 1 meter. This is along a tangent scale, so that with larger angles, each incremental prism diopter is progressively smaller. A 1-diopter prism deflects a ray of light toward the base of the prism by 1 centimeter at 1 meter. One degree of arc equals approximately 1.7 Δ. (For technique of measurement, see p 206.)

Secondary deviation: (Fig 16–5.) The deviation measured with the paretic eye fixing and the normal eye deviating.

Torsion: Rotation of the eye about its anteroposterior axis.

Intorsion (incycloduction): Rotation of the 12 o'clock meridian of the eye toward the midline of the head.

Extorsion (excycloduction): Rotation of the 12 o'clock meridian of the eye away from the midline of the head.

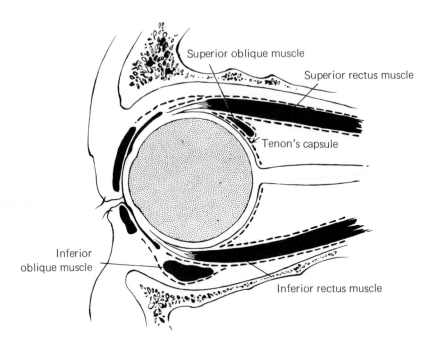

Figure 16–2. Fascia about muscles and eyeball (Tenon's capsule).

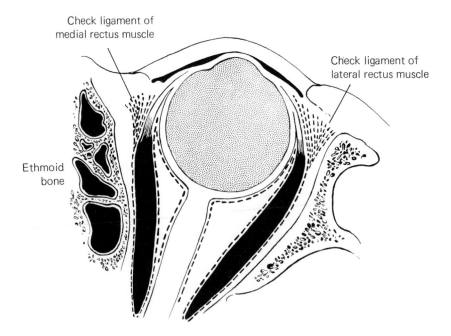

Figure 16–3. Check ligaments of medial and lateral rectus muscles, right eye (diagrammatic).

Figure 16–4. Ductions (monocular rotations), right eye.

Primary deviation
(left eye fixing)

Secondary deviation (right eye fixing;
"inshoot" of sound left eye)

Figure 16–5. Paresis of horizontal muscle (right lateral rectus). Secondary deviation is greater than primary deviation because of Hering's law. With the left eye fixing, the right eye is deviated inward because of the paretic right lateral rectus. For the right eye to fix, the paretic right lateral rectus muscle must receive excessive stimulation. The yoke muscle, the left medial rectus, also receives the same excessive stimulation (Hering's law), which causes "inshoot" shown above.

Vergences (disjunctive movements): Movement of the 2 eyes in opposite directions.

Convergence: The eyes turn inward.

Divergence: The eyes turn outward.

Versions: Binocular rotations of the eyes in qualitatively the same direction.

Dextroversion (levoversion): Movement of the eyes to the right (or left).

Supraversion (infraversion): Movement of the eyes up (or down).

Dextrocycloversion: Torsional movement of both eyes to the right (clockwise).

Levocycloversion: Torsional movement of both eyes to the left (counterclockwise).

PHYSIOLOGY

1. MOTOR ASPECTS

Individual Muscle Functions (Table 16–1)

Each of the 6 extraocular muscles plays a role in positioning the eye about 3 possible axes of rotation. The primary action of a muscle is the principal effect it has on eye rotation. Lesser effects are called secondary or tertiary actions. The exact action of any muscle depends on the direction of the eye in space.

The medial and lateral rectus muscles adduct and abduct the eye, respectively, with little effect on elevation or torsion. The vertical rectus and oblique muscles have vertical rotation and torsion as their chief functions. In general terms, the vertical recti are the main elevators and depressors of the eye, and the obliques are mostly involved with torsional positioning. The vertical effect of the superior and inferior recti is greater in abduction than in adduction. The vertical effect of the obliques is greater in adduction than in abduction.

Field of Action

The position of the eye is determined by the equilibrium position achieved by the pull of all 6 extraocular muscles. In any direction of gaze, the agonist muscles contract to pull the eye into that direction and the antagonist muscles relax. When the eye is at rest in any direction of fixation, the pull exerted by the agonist muscles is exactly equal to that of the antagonist muscles plus the load of deflecting the eye from

primary position. The field of action of a muscle is the direction of gaze in which that muscle has its greatest contraction as agonist, eg, the lateral rectus undergoes the greatest contraction in abducting the eye. The fields of action of the vertical rectus and oblique muscles overlap to some extent.

Donder's Law

The orientation of the eye about the fixation axis is determined by the direction of gaze (Donder's law). The eye has 3 degrees of rotational freedom in space; one degree is constrained by the innervation pattern of the 6 extraocular muscles, and 2 degrees are independent rotational coordinates.

Synergistic & Antagonistic Muscles (Sherrington's Law)

Synergistic muscles are those having the same field of action. Thus for vertical gaze, the superior rectus and inferior oblique muscles are synergists. Muscles synergistic for one function may be antagonistic for another. The superior rectus and inferior oblique muscles are antagonists for torsion, the superior rectus causing intorsion and the inferior oblique extorsion. The extraocular muscles, like skeletal muscles, show reciprocal innervation of antagonistic muscles (Sherrington's law). Thus, in dextroversion (right gaze), the right medial and left lateral rectus muscles are inhibited in proportion to the gaze effort.

Yoke Muscles (Hering's Law)

For movements of both eyes in the same direction, the corresponding agonist muscles receive approximately similar innervation (Hering's law). The pair of agonist muscles with the same primary action is called a yoke pair. The right lateral rectus and the left medial rectus muscles are a yoke pair for right gaze. The right inferior rectus and the left superior oblique muscles are a yoke pair for gaze down to the right. Table 16–2 lists the yoke muscle combinations.

Development of Binocular Movement

Eye movements in the infant are strongly dependent on the amount of illumination. In bright light, the eyes are fully or partially closed much of the time and there is more nystagmus on lateral gaze. In dim illumination, the eyes are opened and the infant scans the environment. The eyes linger over areas rich in

Table 16–1. Functions of the ocular muscles.

Muscle	Primary Action	Secondary Action
Lateral rectus	Abduction	None
Medial rectus	Adduction	None
Superior rectus	Elevation	Adduction, intorsion
Inferior rectus	Depression	Adduction, extorsion
Superior oblique	Depression	Intorsion, abduction
Inferior oblique	Elevation	Extorsion, abduction

Table 16–2. Yoke muscle combinations.

Cardinal Direction of Gaze	Yoke Muscles
Eyes up, right	Right superior rectus and left inferior oblique
Eyes right	Right lateral rectus and left medial rectus
Eyes down, right	Right inferior rectus and left superior oblique
Eyes down, left	Right superior oblique and left inferior rectus
Eyes left	Right medial rectus and left lateral rectus
Eyes up, left	Right inferior oblique and left superior rectus

visual contours, such as a face. Eye control is better in dim illumination. The eye movements of the infant are generally conjugate, although the control of convergence is inexact until 3–4 months of age. Transient exodeviations may be seen and are of no great import, since they tend to disappear with maturation. Esodeviations are more significant and tend to be permanent. An infant can be productively examined at any age and should be brought to an ophthalmologist as soon as any abnormality is suspected.

2. SENSORY ASPECTS

Binocular Vision

In each eye, whatever is imaged on the fovea is seen subjectively as being straight ahead. Thus, if 2 dissimilar objects were imaged on the 2 foveas, the 2 objects would be seen superimposed, but the dissimilarities would prevent fusion into a single impression. Because of the different vantage point in space of each eye, the image in each eye is actually slightly different from that in the other. Sensory fusion and stereopsis are the 2 different physiologic processes that are responsible for binocular vision.

A. Sensory Fusion: Sensory fusion is the process whereby dissimilarities between the 2 images are not appreciated. On the peripheral retina of each eye, there are **corresponding points** that in the absence of fusion localize stimuli in the same direction in space. In the process of fusion, the direction values of these points can be modified. Thus, each point of the retina in each eye is capable of fusing stimuli that strike sufficiently close to the corresponding point in the other eye. This region of fusible points is called **Panum's area.**

B. Stereopsis: While fusion is possible because subtle differences between the 2 images are ignored, stereopsis, or binocular depth perception, is possible because of recognition of these very same differences. When disparate retinal points are stimulated at the same time, fusion of the different images results in perception of an object in 3 dimensions.

Sensory Changes in Strabismus

Up to age 7 or 8 the brain may develop several responses to abnormal binocular vision that cannot occur later in life.

A. Diplopia: If strabismus is present, each fovea receives a different image. The objects imaged on the 2 foveas are seen in the same direction in space. This process of localization of spatially separate objects to the same location is called **visual confusion.** The object viewed by one of the foveas is imaged on a peripheral retinal area in the other eye. The foveal image is localized straight ahead, while the peripheral image of the same object in the other eye is localized in some other direction. Thus, the same object is seen in 2 places (diplopia).

B. Suppression: Under binocular viewing conditions, the images seen by one eye become predominant and those seen by the other eye are not perceived (suppression). Suppression takes the form of a **scotoma** (an area of depressed vision within the visual field, surrounded by an area of less depressed or normal vision) in the deviating eye only under binocular viewing conditions. Suppression scotomas in esotropia are usually approximately elliptical in shape, extending on the retina from just temporal to the fovea to the point in the peripheral retina where the object of regard for the other eye is imaged. In exotropia, the suppression area tends to be larger and extends from the fovea to usually the entire temporal half of the retina. When fixation shifts to the other eye, the suppression scotoma also switches to the newly deviating eye. In the absence of strabismus, a blurred image in one eye may also lead to suppression. The lack of simultaneous perception in the central retina prevents fine stereopsis, although crude stereopsis from the peripheral retina may still be present.

C. Amblyopia: Prolonged abnormal visual experience may also lead to amblyopia (reduction in visual acuity in the absence of detectable organic disease). The 2 clinical contexts in which amblyopia occurs are strabismus and disorders producing degradation of retinal image quality in one eye, such as **anisometropia.** In strabismus, the eye used habitually for fixation retains normal acuity and the nonpreferred eye becomes amblyopic. If spontaneous alternation of fixation is present, there is usually no amblyopia. Suppression and amblyopia are different processes. While amblyopia usually occurs in the presence of suppression, suppression may occur without amblyopia (eg, in strabismic patients with alternating fixation).

Anomalous Retinal Correspondence

In strabismus under binocular viewing conditions, the peripheral retinal areas outside the suppression scotoma may take on new direction values shifted in space by the amount of deviation. There is thus an anomalous correspondence of direction values between the retinal points in the 2 eyes. The direction values in the deviating eye are remapped just enough to avoid diplopia. Stereopsis is not possible under these conditions, and the new direction values may be labile, readjusting themselves from moment to moment as the exact deviation changes with direction of gaze. Should fixation shift to the opposite eye, the anomalous direction values also shift eyes. On monocular testing, the direction values are normal.

Eccentric Fixation

In eyes with sufficiently severe amblyopia, an extrafoveal retinal area may be used for fixation under monocular viewing conditions. It is only a sign of severe amblyopia and does not depend on anomalous retinal correspondence. The area used instead of the fovea may be the area of best remaining visual acuity. The eccentric fixation point is usually but not necessarily displaced in a direction appropriate to the direction of strabismus (eg, the nasal retina in esotropia). Gross eccentric fixation can be readily identified clinically by occluding the dominant eye and directing the patient's attention to a light source held directly in front. An eye with gross eccentric fixation will not point toward the light source but will appear to be looking in a different direction. More subtle degrees of eccentric fixation may be detected by an ophthalmoscope that projects a small fixation target onto the retina. The area of the retina used for fixation may then be directly observed.

EXAMINATION

History

A careful history is of great aid in the diagnosis, prognosis, and treatment of strabismus.

A. Family History: Strabismus is frequently present; autosomal dominant inheritance is common.

B. Age at Onset: This is the single most important factor in prognosis. The earlier the onset, the worse the prognosis for fusion.

C. Type of Onset: The onset may be gradual, sudden, intermittent, or associated with systemic disease.

D. Type of Deviation: Under what conditions does the patient notice strabismus? When viewing near objects? When tired? Is the amount of deviation constant? Does the patient shut one eye in the sunlight? It is most important to know if the eyes are straight at any time.

E. Fixation: Is it always the same eye that deviates? Is there alternating strabismus?

Visual Acuity

Visual acuity must be evaluated, even if only a rough approximation or comparison of the 2 eyes is possible. Each eye must be evaluated by itself, as binocular testing will not reveal poor vision in one eye. For the very youngest children, sometimes all that can be established is that the eye can fixate or follow a target. The target should be made as small as is compatible with the child's age, interest, and level of alertness. If occlusion of one eye produces resistance but occlusion of the other eye does not, poor vision may be present in the eye that can be occluded without provoking a response. A dot test, in which the child puts its finger on a dot of calibrated size, is the earliest quantitative test done routinely (starting at 2– 2½ years). At 2½– 3 years, it is possible to perform recognition testing of small pictures (Allen card). At age 3, many children will play the "E" game: a conventional Snellen chart with "E's" pointing in various directions is used, and the child points a hand in the direction of the "E."

Visual acuity and other visual capabilities of infants can be determined by preferential looking methods, which rely on the infant's habit of looking at a patterned field in preference to a uniform field. (See also Chapters 3 and 21.)

Determination of Refractive Error

It is very important to determine the cycloplegic refractive error by retinoscopy (see p 359). The standard of comparison for producing complete cycloplegia is atropine. This may be given as a drop or ointment, 0.5 or 1%, several times a day for several days to produce complete cycloplegia. It is much less desirable to use atropine in older children, since the prolonged cycloplegia, lasting up to 2 weeks, can interfere with schoolwork. At all ages, homatropine, 5%, or cyclopentolate, 1 or 2%, may also be used successfully.

Inspection

Inspection alone may show whether the strabismus is constant or intermittent, alternating or nonalternating, and variable or constant. Associated ptosis and abnormal position of the head may also be noted. The quality of fixation of each eye separately and both eyes together is important. Nystagmoid movements indicate poor fixation and reduced visual acuity.

Prominent epicanthal folds commonly confuse laymen as well as some physicians. The folds obscure a portion of the nasal sclera and may give the child the appearance of esotropia ("pseudoesotropia"). This pitfall can be avoided if the positions of the corneal reflections are noted. When the child is observing a light source, the corneal reflection of this light should be centered in the 2 pupillary areas. Prominent epicanthal folds usually disappear by 4 or 5 years of age.

Determination of Angle of Strabismus (Angle of Deviation)

A. Prism and Cover Tests: (Fig 16– 6.) Cover tests consist of 3 parts: (1) the cover test, (2) the uncover test, and (3) the alternate cover test. In all 3 tests the patient looks intently at a target, which may be in any direction of gaze, distance or near.

1. Cover test–As the examiner observes one eye, a cover is placed in front of the other eye so as to block its view of the target. If the observed eye moves to take up fixation, it clearly is not also fixating the target, and manifest deviation (strabismus) is present. The direction of movement reveals the direction of deviation (eg, the eye moves laterally if there is esotropia).

2. Uncover test–As the cover is removed from the eye following the cover test, the eye emerging from under cover is observed. If the position of the eye changes, interruption of binocular vision has allowed it to deviate, and heterophoria is present. The direction of corrective movement shows the type of heterophoria.

3. Alternate cover test–The cover is alternately placed in front of one eye and then the other. This tends to break up the control of heterophoria that may last through a single cover-uncover cycle. This test shows the total deviation of heterotropia plus heterophoria.

4. Prism plus cover testing–To quantitatively measure the deviation, prisms are placed in front of

Eyes straight (maintained in position by fusion).

Position of eye under cover in orthophoria (fusion-free position). The right eye under cover has not moved.

Position of eye under cover in esophoria (fusion-free position). Under cover, the right eye has deviated inward. Upon removal of cover, the right eye will immediately resume its straight-ahead position.

Position of eye under cover in exophoria (fusion-free position). Under cover, the right eye has deviated outward. Upon removal of the cover, the right eye will immediately resume its straight-ahead position.

Figure 16–6. Cover testing. The patient is directed to look at a target at eye level 6 m (20 ft) away. *Note:* In the presence of heterotropia, the deviation will remain when the cover is removed.

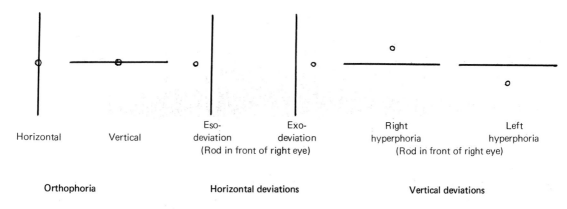

Horizontal	Vertical	Eso-deviation	Exo-deviation	Right hyperphoria	Left hyperphoria

(Rod in front of right eye)   (Rod in front of right eye)

Orthophoria   Horizontal deviations   Vertical deviations

Figure 16–7. Maddox rod test. Normal and abnormal responses. (Subjective view of the patient.)

one or both eyes so as to slightly reverse the direction of the refixation movements produced by the cover. For example, to measure the full esodeviation, the cover is alternated, and prisms of increasing base-out strength are placed in front of one or both eyes until the lateralward refixation movement of the deviated eye is reversed to a just observable movement in a medial direction. The threshold for naked eye observation of eye movements is generally considered to be about 2 prism diopters, so 2 prism diopters are then subtracted from the prism strength to obtain the final deviation. Prism measurements are done either as simultaneous prism and cover measurements, using the cover test, to determine the manifest deviation; or as prism and alternate cover measurements, to record the total deviation in the fusion-free position.

B. Maddox Rod Test: (Fig 16–7.) This test is an accurate method of measuring a deviation if normal retinal correspondence is present. It is particularly useful for measurement of heterophoria but can also be used in heterotropia. A Maddox rod consists of a series of thin red glass cylinders placed side by side, usually mounted in a circular holder that can be held before the eye. When a target light is seen through the Maddox rod, its image is a red focal line perpendicular to the axes of the cylinders. Thus, one eye sees the light directly while the other views its image through the Maddox rod. In orthophoria the red line appears to run through the light. When the Maddox rod is held so that the cylinders are horizontal, a vertical red line is seen that in cases of horizontal deviation is displaced laterally. A prism can be held in front of one eye so that the red line appears to "run through the light." The strength of such a prism measures the angle of deviation. By rotating the Maddox rod 90 degrees, a horizontal line is produced (cylinders of the rod are vertical). Its displacement can also be measured by prisms as described for horizontal deviations.

C. Objective Tests: Prism and cover measurements are objective in the sense that no report of sensory observations is required from the patient. However, cooperation and some degree of vision are required. The Maddox rod test is more subjective because the end point of the measurement is based on a report of sensory observations by the patient. Confused, obtunded, or immature patients may be unable or unwilling to cooperate sufficiently. Clinical determinations of eye position that require no sensory observation by the patient (objective tests) are considerably less accurate, although still useful at times. Two methods commonly used depend on observing the position of the corneal reflection of a light. Results by both methods or any objective method must be modified by allowing for the angle kappa.

1. Hirschberg method–The patient fixes a light at a distance of about 33 cm (13 inches). The decentering of the light reflection is noted in the deviating eye. By allowing 15 diopters for each millimeter of decentration, an estimate of the angle of deviation can be made.

2. Prism reflex method (modified Krimsky test)–The patient fixes a light at any distance. A prism is placed before the fixing eye, and the strength of the prism required to center the corneal reflection of the deviating eye measures the angle of deviation.

Ductions (Monocular Rotations)

With one eye covered, the other eye follows a moving light in all directions of gaze, so that any weakness of rotation can be noted. Such a weakness can be due to muscle paralysis or to a mechanical anatomic anomaly.

Versions (Conjugate Ocular Movements)

According to Hering's law, yoke muscles receive equal stimulation during any conjugate ocular movement. The versions are tested by having the eyes follow a light at 33 cm in the 9 diagnostic positions: primary—straight ahead; secondary—right, left, up, and down; and tertiary—up and right, down and right, up and left, and down and left. Apparent rotation of one eye relative to the other is noted as overaction or underaction. By convention, in the tertiary positions, the oblique muscles are said to be overacting or underacting with respect to the yoke rectus muscle. Fixation in the field of action of a paretic muscle results in overaction of the yoke muscle, since greater innervation is required for contraction (Figs 16–8 and 16–9). Conversely, fixation by the normal eye will lead to underaction of the paretic muscle.

Disjunctive Movements

A. Convergence: (Fig 16–10.) As the eyes follow an approaching object, they must turn inward in order to maintain alignment of the visual axes with the object of regard. The medial rectus muscles are contracting and the lateral rectus muscles are relaxing under the influence of neural stimulation and inhibition. (Neural pathways of supranuclear control are discussed in Chapter 18.)

Convergence is an active process with a strong voluntary as well as involuntary component. An important consideration in evaluating the extraocular muscles in strabismus is convergence.

To test convergence, a small object or light source is slowly brought toward the bridge of the nose. The patient's attention is directed to the object by saying, "Keep the light from going double as long as possible." Convergence can normally be maintained until the object is nearly to the bridge of the nose. An actual numerical value is placed on convergence by measuring the distance from the bridge of the nose (in millimeters) at which the eyes "break" (ie, when the nondominant eye swings laterally so that convergence is no longer maintained). This point is termed the **near point of convergence,** and a value of up to 50 mm (2 inches) is considered within normal limits.

B. Divergence: Electromyography has established that divergence is an active process, not merely a relaxation of convergence as previously believed by some authorities. Clinically, this function is seldom

Eyes Up Right
   Right superior rectus
   Left inferior oblique

Eyes Up Left
   Right inferior oblique
   Left superior rectus

Eyes Right
   Right lateral rectus
   Left medial rectus

Primary Position

Eyes Left
   Right medial rectus
   Left lateral rectus

Eyes Down Right
   Right inferior rectus
   Left superior oblique

Eyes Down Left
   Right superior oblique
   Left inferior rectus

Figure 16–8. Normal version movement (binocular rotations). Pairs of yoke muscles concerned with ocular movement in various directions are shown.

Eyes Up Right (Right Eye Fixing). Shows upshoot of left eye, indicating overaction of left inferior oblique. The fixating eye determines the innervation level to the yoke pair of right superior rectus and left inferior oblique. The left eye overacts because the paretic superior oblique does not load or resist the inferior oblique, which then rotates the left eye further than it ordinarily would.

Eyes Up Right (Left Eye Fixing). Shows relative underaction of right superior rectus. The fixating left eye determines the innervation level. Since the superior oblique is paretic, the inferior oblique rotates further at any innervation level than it otherwise would. Since the innervation level is less than normally required, the right superior rectus rotates less than normally. On duction testing, it will rotate fully.

Figure 16–9. Testing versions. Example of paretic left superior oblique.

Figure 16–10. Convergence. The normal position of the eyes at the near point of convergence (NPC) is shown above. The break point is within 50 mm of the bridge of the nose.

tested except in considering the amplitude of fusion (see below).

Sensory Examination

Many tests of the status of binocular vision have been devised, only a few of which can be mentioned here. The chief tests are for stereopsis, suppression, and anomalous retinal correspondence. They all require the simultaneous presentation of 2 targets separately to the 2 eyes.

A. Stereopsis Testing: Most stereopsis testing is done with polaroid glasses and targets to separate the stimuli. The monocularly observed targets have nearly imperceptible clues to depth. **Random dot stereograms** have no monocular depth clues. A field of random dots is seen by each eye, but the dot-to-corresponding-dot correlation between the 2 targets is such that if stereopsis is present, a form is seen standing out from the background.

B. Suppression Testing: The presence of suppression is readily demonstrated with the **Worth 4-dot test.** Glasses containing a red lens over one eye and a green lens over the other are placed on the patient. A flashlight containing red, green, and white spots is viewed. The color spots are markers for perception through each eye, and the white dot, potentially visible to each eye, can indicate the presence of diplopia. The separation of the spots and the distance at which the light is held determine the size of the retinal area tested. Foveal and peripheral areas may be tested at distance and near.

C. Anomalous Retinal Correspondence Testing: Anomalous retinal correspondence may be demonstrated in 2 ways: (1) by showing that one of the foveas does not have straight-ahead localization or (2) by showing that a peripheral retinal point in one eye shares a common visual direction with the fovea of the other eye.

1. After-image test–The first method is used in the after-image test and various projection methods. A bright line with a centered fixation gap is used to produce a vertical after-image in one eye and a horizontal after-image in the other eye. The gaps superimpose in the after-images if the 2 foveas have the same visual direction.

2. Bagolini striated glass test–The Bagolini striated glass test uses the second testing method. Clear glasses containing fine striations in a different direction for each eye are placed in front of the eyes. The test conditions are as close as possible to natural vision. A point source of light is viewed, and streaks of light perpendicular to the direction of striation are seen with each eye. If peripheral retinal elements in the deviated eye localize the streak through the light, anomalous retinal correspondence is present.

OBJECTIVES & PRINCIPLES OF THERAPY OF STRABISMUS

The main objectives of strabismus treatment in children are (1) reversal of the deleterious sensory effects of strabismus (amblyopia, suppression, and loss of stereopsis) and (2) maintenance of improvement through medical or surgical straightening of the eyes. In adults with acquired strabismus, the aims are to alleviate diplopia and restore a range of binocular single vision.

Timing of Treatment in Children

A child can be productively examined at any age, and treatment for amblyopia or strabismus should be instituted as soon as the diagnosis is made. Neurophysiologic studies in animals have shown that the infant brain is very responsive to sensory experience, and the quality of function possible later in life is determined by the quality of early life experiences. It is generally believed that a better long-term result is obtained if the eyes are made as straight as possible by age 2 years. This is not a magic cutoff age by any means, and good results can be obtained later; however, improvements in brain function and modifications in synaptic connections become more difficult as time passes. By age 8 in most children, no permanent changes can be established. Treatment of amblyopia must be started as soon as possible; after age 8, efforts are usually futile.

Goals of Treatment

The 2 goals of eliminating suppression and restoring stereopsis are achieved by restoring alignment of the 2 eyes. Prisms can be useful in diagnosis or treatment (usually as a temporary measure) of deviation. Treatment of anomalous retinal correspondence by itself is not necessary. It disappears with improvement in eye position, and in cases with unimproved position, it is protective against diplopia.

Medical Treatment

Nonsurgical treatment of strabismus is achieved through treatment of amblyopia and the use of optical devices (prisms and glasses), pharmacologic agents, and various eye exercises.

A. Treatment of Amblyopia: The elimination of amblyopia is crucial in the treatment of strabismus and is always one of the first goals. Occasionally, strabismus will disappear entirely once amblyopia is cured. The deviation to be operated on can change considerably following treatment of amblyopia, and surgical results tend to be better.

1. Occlusion therapy–The mainstay of amblyopia treatment and the standard of comparison for all other treatments is occlusion therapy. In its simplest form, the sound eye is covered with a patch, and all seeing must be done with the amblyopic eye. Partial occlusions may also be created with plastic membranes, tape, blurring lenses, or alternate patching in various patterns. Sometimes an eye is blurred only for distance or only for near. All amblyopia treatment assumes that any refractive error has been determined with cycloplegic refraction and correction has been made, usually with spectacles if the refractive error is sufficient. Of particular importance is refractive asymmetry between the eyes. A very small refractive difference can produce amblyopia.

Two stages in amblyopia treatment can be distinguished: initial improvement and maintenance treatment.

a. Initial stage–Full-time occlusion is the standard initial treatment. Sometimes only partial occlusion is used at the beginning if the amblyopia does not seem to be too severe. As a rule of thumb, full-time occlusion may be done for as many weeks as the child's age in years without damaging the vision in the sound eye. If vision in the sound eye drops more than a line or 2, a brief vacation from patching may be given or a less vigorous patching regimen selected. Occlusion treatment is continued in some form as long as vision continues to improve (sometimes for 2 or more years). Six months of full-time occlusion with no improvement at all is a treatment failure, and in such cases, it is usual to look again for any detectable organic lesion to explain the lack of response. Amblyopia is functional by definition (ie, there is no identifiable lesion). In most cases, if treatment is begun soon enough, substantial improvement or complete normalization of visual acuity can be achieved. Occasionally, there is no improvement and no reason can be found. Poor compliance with treatment (peeking around or through a patch by the child or inadequate enforcement of patching by the parents) must always be ruled out in these cases.

b. Maintenance stage–Maintenance treatment consists of intermittent patching continued after the improvement phase, with the goal of preserving improvement to beyond an age when amblyopia can be reacquired (about age 8 years). Whenever treatment is discontinued, there may be some loss of acuity. Later in life, acuity can be recovered to the best level achieved with occlusive treatment.

2. Other therapies–Other forms of amblyopia therapy mostly require periods of attentive vision, with variable patching regimens. With brief periods of intense visual effort, acuity can sometimes be improved with only minimal occlusion. Devices that have been employed are video games, rotating gratings (Cam stimulator), red filters, and games with small drawings. No method has been shown to be more effective than patching, and most are frequently less effective.

B. Optical Devices:

1. Spectacles–The most important optical device in the treatment of strabismus is accurate spectacles. The clarification of the retinal image produced by glasses allows the natural fusion mechanisms to operate to the fullest. Small refractive errors need not be corrected. If there is significant hyperopia and esotropia, the esotropia probably is at least partially due to the hyperopia (accommodative esotropia). The prescription should take into account the full cycloplegic findings. If a bifocal lens permits sufficient relaxation of the near synkinesis to allow fusion at near, it may also be prescribed.

2. Prisms–Prisms produce an optical redirection of the line of sight. Corresponding retinal elements are brought into line, and binocular diplopia is alleviated if the prism strength is correct. Correct sensory alignment of the eyes is also a form of antisuppression treatment. Used preoperatively, prisms can simulate the sensory effect of surgery and predict whether symptoms will be improved. In patients with horizontal deviation, prisms will show the patient's ability to fuse a simultaneous small vertical deviation, thereby indicating whether surgery also needs to be done for the vertical deviation. In children with esotropia, prisms can be used preoperatively to predict a postoperative shift in position that might nullify the surgical result, and the planned surgery can be modified accordingly (prism adaptation test).

Prisms can be implemented in several ways. A particularly convenient form is the plastic Fresnel press-on prism. These inexpensive plastic membranes can be placed on the glasses without the help of an optician and are very useful for diagnostic and temporary therapeutic purposes. For permanent wear, prisms are best ground into the spectacle prescription.

C. Pharmacologic Agents: The conventional pharmacologic agents used to treat strabismus are of 2 types: cycloplegic agents and miotics. A recently introduced pharmacologic substitute for surgical muscle-weakening procedures is the injection of botulinum toxin into the extraocular muscle.

1. Cycloplegic agents–Cycloplegic agents paralyze the ciliary muscle through a competitive inhibition of acetylcholine at the neuromuscular junction and thus prevent accommodation. They are most useful in the treatment of amblyopia, to allow clearer vision with the glasses on than is provided by peeking over the lenses. Another use is to provide blurred vision at near in the sound eye, so that all near vision must be performed with the amblyopic eye. The long-acting cycloplegic agent used for these purposes is atropine solution or ointment, usually 0.5 or 1% concentration. Weak short-acting cycloplegic agents have been used to stimulate accommodation in exotropia in an attempt to reduce the deviation.

2. Miotics–Miotics are used to reduce excess convergence at near in esotropia, referred to as a high accommodative convergence to accommodation ratio, or AC/A ratio. The agents usually used are echothiophate iodide (Phospholine Iodide) or isoflurophate (Floropryl), both of which irreversibly inactivate acetylcholinesterase at the neuromuscular junction and thus potentiate the effect of every nerve impulse. Accommodation should therefore be more effective with respect to convergence than before treatment. Since accommodation drives the near synkinesis (the triad of accommodation, convergence, and miosis), less convergence will be invoked with accommodation at near. Treatment with miotics is useful only if esodeviation is substantially reduced. Miotic treatment can be continued for years.

3. Botulinum toxin–The injection of botulinum toxin A into an extraocular muscle produces a dose-dependent depth and duration of paralysis of that muscle. The injection is given under electromyographic position control of the needle, and the toxin is tightly bound to the muscle tissue. The doses used are so small that systemic toxicity does not occur. Paralysis typically lasts for several months. The eye shifts into the field of action of the antagonist muscle and then starts to return to its original position as the injected muscle recovers its strength. During the time the eye is deviated, the tissues about the eye become adapted to the new position and apply a force opposing the returning muscle force. Frequently, multiple sequential injections must be given to obtain a lasting effect. The end result is a small net shift in position.

The method is useful for single-muscle weakening. If a muscle needs to be strengthened, the direction of action of a muscle shifted, adhesions lysed, or the strength of several muscles modified, surgery must be done instead. Botulinum toxin is useful in treating symptomatic heterophorias, shifting blind eyes (because it can be so readily repeated), or fine-tuning the results of surgery and whenever a small correction in position achieved by muscle weakening is needed to correct the deviation. Occasionally, botulinum toxin is used to correct larger deviations, but the results are not consistent. As with surgery, the best results are obtained in patients with good binocular function.

D. Eye Exercises: Various sensory exercises are sometimes used. These are best done by the patient at home. Exercises requiring fine vision can be used in treating amblyopia. Antisuppression exercises may also be done at home. These are most useful in intermittent exotropia to try to eliminate the facile suppression that prevents the patient from being aware that the eye has drifted out and correcting it voluntarily. The amplitudes of fusional vergence may be increased by exercising with prisms. Progressively larger prisms are placed in front of one or both eyes and the separated images re-fused. Poor convergence can also be exercised. This can be combined with antisuppression treatment, ie, a card having large colored spots on each side is placed in the midline sagittal plane in front of the nose. The task is to see the dots singly while being aware of the color rivalry. So-called pencil push-ups, in which an approaching rod is kept single, can also be of some help. It is important

that accommodation be controlled during convergence exercises.

Exercises for intermittent exotropia are rarely curative—only delaying—and patients who have been taught to inappropriately converge their eyes have a much higher incidence of postoperative overcorrection when they finally do come to surgery. Finally, the richness and variety of naturally occurring stimuli provide a rather complete repertoire of tasks for the visual system. The most effective exercises are those that can be performed naturally during daily oculomotor behavior or done at home. Exercise sessions in the physician's office are costly and rarely have any lasting effect.

Surgical Treatment (Figs 16–11 and 16–12)

A. Surgical Procedures: A variety of changes in the rotational effect of an extraocular muscle can be achieved with surgery.

1. Resection and recession–Conceptually, the simplest procedures are strengthening and weakening. A muscle is strengthened by a procedure called resection. The muscle is detached from the eye, stretched out longer by a measured amount, and then resewn to the eye, usually at the original insertion site. The small amount of extra length is trimmed off. Recession is the standard weakening procedure. The muscle is detached from the eye, freed from fascial attachments, and allowed to retract. It is resewn to the eye a measured distance behind its original insertion.

The superior oblique is strengthened by tucking its tendon. This can be done by a graded amount. Superior oblique weakening is limited to the all-or-none procedure of cutting through its tendon (tenotomy). Attempts at measured recessions of the superior oblique tendon have been made. There is no effective strengthening procedure on the inferior oblique. The inferior oblique can be weakened by recession, myectomy, or disinsertion, with generally equivalent results.

2. Shifting of point of muscle attachment–In addition to simple strengthening or weakening, the point of attachment of the muscle can be shifted; this may give the muscle a rotational action it did not have before. For example, a vertical shift of both horizontal rectus muscles affects the vertical position of the eye. Shifts of the horizontal recti in opposite vertical directions affect the horizontal position in upgaze and downgaze. This is done for ''A'' or ''V'' patterns, in which the horizontal deviation is more of an esodeviation in upgaze or downgaze, respectively. The torsional effect of a muscle can also be changed. Tightening of the anterior fibers of the superior oblique tendon gives that muscle enhanced torsional action.

3. Faden procedure–A special procedure for muscle weakening is called the Faden procedure (Fig 16–12) after the German word for ''thread.'' In this operation, a new insertion for the muscle is created far in the back of the eye by suturing the muscle to

Exposure of lateral rectus

Recession

← Muscle stump

← Sclera

Resection

Figure 16–11. Surgical correction of strabismus (right eye).

the sclera, so that it cannot unwrap as the eye rotates into its field of action. This weakens the muscle only in its field of action and not in primary position. When combined with a muscle recession operation, the Faden operation can have a profound weakening effect on a muscle. This procedure is used in dissociated vertical divergence, nystagmus, high AC/A ratio, and miscellaneous other disorders.

B. Choice of Muscles to Be Corrected: Deciding which muscles to correct and how much correction to make is a technical decision based on measurements of the deviation in various directions of gaze. The usual positions measured are distance and near in primary position, secondary gaze directions at distance, and tertiary gaze directions at near, as well as lateral gaze to either side at near. Frequently, the near deviation is also measured with the patient looking down while wearing bifocals. In choosing which muscles to correct, both the primary and secondary actions of the muscles must be taken into account. Lateral or vertical incomitances must be planned for. To avoid a deviation in gaze away from primary position, the gaze effort required by the 2 eyes must be matched.

For this, the strength of the 2 muscles in a yoke pair is balanced. With regard to near or distance positions, the medial recti have more effect at near and the lateral recti more effect at distance. For esotropia greater at near, both medial rectus muscles would be weakened. For exotropia greater at distance, both lateral recti would be weakened. For deviation the same at distance and near, both the medial and lateral recti of one eye may be corrected. Both eyes may be corrected if the deviation is large or if there is lateral incomitance requiring treatment of a pair of yoke muscles.

The same operation performed on 2 different people will give somewhat different results because of the varying mechanical properties of the muscles and surrounding soft tissues. Prior to operation, it is not known exactly how much of a deviation is due to abnormal muscle force and how much to abnormal surrounding tissues, such as adhesions or fibrous bands, or to abnormal points of muscle insertion. Consequently, several operations are frequently required to obtain a satisfactory position.

C. Adjustable Sutures: (Fig 16–13.) The development of adjustable sutures has been a great boon

Figure 16–12. Faden procedure. The rectus muscle is tacked to the sclera far posterior to its insertion. This prevents unwrapping of the muscle as the eye turns into the muscle's field of action. The muscle is progressively weakened in its field of action. If this procedure is combined with recession, the alignment in primary position is also affected.

Figure 16–13. Adjustable suture. The suture is placed on the sclera at any point that will be accessible to the surgeon the next day. The bow is untied and the position of the muscle changed as desired.

in muscle surgery and the greatest advance in the field in the past decade. During operation, the muscles are reattached with a bow knot placed so that it is accessible to the surgeon. The next day, a topical anesthetic drop is placed in the eye, and the sutures can be tightened or loosened to change the eye position as necessary, under the guidance of prism and cover measurements.

The operation can be done effectively a second time, as long as approximately the correct procedure was done the first time. Adjustable sutures can be used on any rectus muscle for either recession or resection and on the superior oblique muscle for correction of torsion. Any patient willing to cooperate is suitable. With care in selection, even 5-year-old children can undergo suture adjustment without any special anesthetic measures, although the method is commonly not used for children age 12 or under.

CLASSIFICATION OF STRABISMUS

Classification of strabismus is based on the forms that are found to occur most commonly in practice.
  A. Esotropia.
  1. Nonparetic.
    a. Nonaccommodative.
    b. Accommodative.
    c. Partially accommodative.
  2. Paretic.
  B. Exotropia.
  1. Intermittent.
  2. Constant.
  C. "A" and "V" Syndromes.
  D. Hypertropia.
  1. Nonparetic.
  2. Paretic.

ESOTROPIA
(Convergent Strabismus, "Crossed Eyes")

Esotropia is the most common type of strabismus. Most cases acquired in adulthood are paretic, caused by lateral rectus weakness following injury to the sixth cranial nerve. Esotropia in childhood is usually, but not always, nonparetic. The most common forms of childhood esotropia are infantile esotropia, accommodative esotropia, and partially accommodative esotropia.

I. NONPARETIC ESOTROPIA

NONACCOMMODATIVE ESOTROPIA

1. INFANTILE ESOTROPIA

The most common form of nonparetic, nonaccommodative esotropia is infantile esotropia. By convention, the onset must be before 6 months of age to qualify under the definition. The cause is not established.

Clinical Findings

The deviation is usually large (≥ 50 degrees) and usually comitant. Abduction may be somewhat limited but can be demonstrated. Vertical deviations are frequently observed (commonly, dissociated vertical divergence; sometimes, overaction of the inferior oblique muscle). Either of these deviations may produce an upshoot in adduction. Nystagmus, manifest or latent, is frequently present. The commonest refractive error is low-to-moderate hyperopia (< 3 diopters). Amblyopia may occur, especially if there is anisometropia.

The eye that appears to be straight is the eye used for fixation. Almost without exception, it is the eye with better vision or lower refractive error, or both. If there is anisometropia, there will probably be some amblyopia as well. If at various times either eye is used for fixation, the patient is said to show spontaneous alternation of fixation; in this case, vision will be nearly equal in both eyes. Sometimes, the eye preference is determined by the direction of gaze. For example, with large-angle esotropia, there is a tendency for the right eye to be used in left gaze and the left eye to be used in right gaze (cross fixation).

Treatment

Congenital esotropia almost invariably requires surgical correction. Nonsurgical treatment is aimed at correcting refractive errors and treating amblyopia. It is essential that amblyopia be fully treated prior to surgery. Hyperopic refractive errors greater than 2 diopters are worth treating. A miotic agent can substitute for a trial of glasses in an uncooperative infant.

Surgery is indicated after medical therapy and treatment of amblyopia have been tried and there remains a significant deviation. Examination must be performed, and reproducible measurements of deviation must be obtained. There is nothing to be gained by waiting beyond this point, and there is evidence that sensory results are better the sooner surgery is undertaken. Many procedures have been recommended, but the 2 most popular procedures are (1) weakening of both medial rectus muscles and (2) recession of the medial rectus and resection of the lateral rectus on the same eye.

2. ACQUIRED NONACCOMMODATIVE ESOTROPIA

Several types of strabismus are included under this heading, with onset after the age of 6 months.

Basic Esotropia

The onset is in childhood, but there is no accommodative factor. The angle of strabismus is originally much smaller than in congenital esotropia but may increase with time. Treatment is correction of any refractive error and treatment of amblyopia, followed by surgical correction.

Esotropia of Myopia

This typically begins in young adults as diplopia at distance gradually extending to near. It must be distinguished from divergence insufficiency or lateral rectus paresis associated with elevated intracranial pressure. A severe form of esotropia may also be associated with high myopia, in which the medial recti become extremely tight. Prisms for distance vision may help the former type of esotropia for a time. Surgery is otherwise indicated in both conditions.

ACCOMMODATIVE ESOTROPIA

Accommodative esotropia occurs when there is a normal physiologic mechanism of accommodation but insufficient relative fusional divergence to hold the eyes straight. There are 2 pathophysiologic mechanisms at work: (1) sufficiently high hyperopia requiring so much accommodation to clarify the image that esotropia results and (2) a high AC/A ratio, which may be accompanied by refractive error. The 2 mechanisms may be present in the same patient.

Accommodative Esotropia Due to Hyperopia

Accommodative esotropia due to hyperopia typically begins at age 2–3 but may occur in infancy or later in life. Deviation is variable prior to treatment. Treatment is full cycloplegic refraction.

Accommodative Esotropia Due to High AC/A Ratio

In accommodative esotropia due to a high AC/A ratio, a deviation is greater at near than at distance. There is an abnormal convergence response during near synkinesis. The refractive error may not be hyperopic, although moderate hyperopia is frequently found. Treatment is full cycloplegic refraction, amblyopia therapy, and bifocals or miotics, or both, to relieve excess deviation at near.

PARTIALLY ACCOMMODATIVE ESOTROPIA

An accommodative element frequently occurs superimposed onto infantile or basic esotropia. Antiaccommodative therapy is of partial benefit. Surgery is reserved for the nonaccommodative component of the deviation that remains after antiaccommodative therapy and treatment for amblyopia.

II. PARETIC (INCOMITANT) ESOTROPIA (Abducens Palsy) (Fig 16–14)

In incomitant strabismus there are always one or more paretic extraocular muscles. In the case of incomitant esotropia, the paresis is always of one of the lateral rectus muscles, usually as a result of palsy of the abducens nerve. These cases are most often seen in adults who have had cerebrovascular accidents or diabetes, but abducens palsy may occasionally be the first sign of a tumor or of inflammatory disease involving the central nervous system. Head trauma is a frequent cause of abducens palsy.

Incomitant esotropia is also seen in infants and children, but much less commonly than comitant esotropia. These cases result from birth injuries affecting the muscle directly, from injury to the nerve, or, less

Primary position: right esotropia

Left gaze: no deviation   Right gaze: left esotropia

Figure 16–14. Incomitant strabismus (paralytic). Paralysis of right lateral rectus muscle, with left eye fixing.

commonly, from a congenital anomaly of the lateral rectus muscle or its fascial attachments.

Clinical Findings

If the lateral rectus muscle is totally paralyzed, the eye will not abduct past the midline. Esotropia is characteristically greater at distance than at near and greater to one side. Paresis of the right lateral rectus causes esotropia that becomes greater to the right and, if paresis is sufficiently mild, no deviation in far left gaze.

Treatment

A prism may be helpful in milder cases. Any spontaneous improvement should be allowed to develop as far as possible. If there is no improvement by 6 months, it is unlikely that any will occur, and surgery is indicated. Botulinum toxin injections may be helpful or curative in mild cases. More severe cases require surgery in proportion to the amount of deviation. Resection of the paretic muscle along with recession of some or all of the remaining horizontal recti (depending on the measurements) is required. For complete paralysis, the insertions of the superior and inferior rectus muscles may be transferred to the lateral rectus and the other horizontal recti may be recessed. Adjustable sutures allow the titration of surgery to each of the muscles, so that frequently, single vision may be obtained in many fields of gaze. Abduction of the paretic muscle will always be limited. Completely successful results are possible only with mild paresis.

EXOTROPIA
(Divergent Strabismus)

Exotropia is less common than esotropia, particularly in infancy and childhood. Its incidence increases gradually with age. Not infrequently, a tendency to divergent strabismus beginning as exophoria progresses to intermittent exotropia and finally to constant exotropia if no treatment is given. Other cases begin as constant or intermittent exotropia and remain stationary. As in esotropia, there may be a hereditary element in some cases. Exophoria and exotropia (considered as a single entity of divergent deviation) are frequently passed on as autosomal dominant traits, so that one or both parents of an exotropic child may demonstrate exotropia or a high degree of exophoria.

Alternative Classification of Exotropia

Constant or intermittent exotropia can also be classified on a descriptive basis, according to whether there is apparent excess of divergence or insufficiency of convergence. These terms should not be understood to imply the cause.

A. Basic Exotropia: Distance and near deviations are approximately equal.

B. Divergence Excess: Distance deviation is significantly larger than near deviation.

Figure 16–15. Child with intermittent exotropia squinting in sunlight.

C. Convergence Insufficiency: Near deviation is significantly larger than distance deviation.

D. Pseudodivergence Excess: Distance deviation is significantly larger than near deviation; however, use of a 3-diopter lens for near measurement will cause the near deviation to become approximately equal to the distance deviation.

INTERMITTENT EXOTROPIA

Clinical Findings
Intermittent exotropia (Fig 16– 15) comprises well over half of cases of exotropia. The onset of the deviation may be in the first year, and practically all have shown up by age 5. The history reveals that the condition has become progressively worse. A characteristic sign is closing one eye in bright sunlight, as this avoids diplopia. There is usually a manifest exotropia for distance. The patient can fuse for near vision, overcoming moderate- to large-angle exophoria. Convergence is frequently excellent. There is no correlation with a specific refractive error.

Since the child fuses at least part of the time, there is usually no gross sensory abnormality. For distance, with one eye deviated, there is suppression but normal retinal correspondence and no amblyopia.

Treatment
A. Medical Treatment: Nonsurgical treatment is largely confined to refractive correction and amblyopia therapy. If the AC/A ratio is high, the use of minus lenses may delay surgery for a while. Occasionally, antisuppression or convergence exercises may be of some, albeit usually temporary, benefit.

B. Surgical Treatment: Surgery should be considered in adult patients with sufficiently severe symptoms or in children with signs of progression of the deviation (eg, increasing frequency of exotropia [implying loss of fusional control], larger deviation, development of convergence insufficiency or lateral incomitance, or development of suppression [lack of diplopia during the manifest phase of deviation]). The goal of surgery is restoration of normal binocular function.

The choice of procedure depends on the measurements of the deviation. The 2 lateral rectus muscles alone may be corrected in cases in which deviation is mostly at distance. If there is much deviation at near, it is best to perform resection of a medial rectus as well as weakening of a lateral rectus. Both eyes may need to be corrected for larger deviations. Because all exodeviations tend to recur, it is best to produce slight overcorrection at the time of surgery. The use of botulinum toxin injections may help to prevent recurrences.

CONSTANT EXOTROPIA
(Fig 16–16)

Constant exotropia is less common than intermittent exotropia. It may be present at birth or may occur when intermittent exotropia progresses to constant exotropia. Some cases have their onset later in life, particularly following loss of vision in one eye. Except for cases due to loss of vision, the fundamental cause is usually not known.

Clinical Findings
Constant exotropia may be of any degree. With chronicity or poor vision in one eye, the deviation can be quite large. Adduction may be limited; hypertropia may occur along with exotropia; and stereopsis is lost. There is usually extensive suppression if the deviation was acquired by age 6– 8; otherwise, diplopia is present. If exotropia is due to very poor vision, there may be no diplopia, although poor vision per se is not protective against diplopia. Anomalous retinal correspondence is unusual in the presence of extensive suppression. Amblyopia is uncommon in the absence of anisometropia, and spontaneous alternation of the fixating eye is frequently observed.

Figure 16–16. Right exotropia.

Treatment

The best treatment is surgery. Overcorrection is attempted because exotropia frequently recurs. The prognosis for maintenance of the improved position is particularly poor if one eye is blind. Botulinum toxin injections can be useful as primary treatment if the deviation is small or as a backup to surgery if exotropia begins to recur.

"A" & "V" SYNDROMES

A horizontal deviation may be vertically incomitant, ie, the deviation is different in upgaze versus primary position versus downgaze ("A" or "V" pattern). An "A" pattern shows more esodeviation or less exodeviation in upgaze compared to downgaze. A "V" pattern shows less esodeviation or more exodeviation in upgaze compared to downgaze. An "A" pattern is diagnostically significant when greater than 10 Δ and a "V" pattern when greater than 15 Δ. Whether the pattern is clinically significant must be determined from the other findings. When the patient comes to surgery, the procedure is frequently modified to allow for "A" or "V" patterns.

HYPERTROPIA
(Fig 16–17)

Vertical deviations are customarily named according to the high eye, regardless of which eye has the better vision and is used for fixation. Hypertropias are less common than horizontal deviations and are usually acquired after childhood.

There are many causes of hypertropia. Congenital anatomic anomalies may result in muscle attachments in abnormal locations. Occasionally, there are anomalous fibrous bands that attach to the eye. Closed head trauma frequently produces paresis of the superior oblique muscle. Orbital tumors, brain stem lesions, and systemic diseases such as myasthenia gravis, mul-

Figure 16–17. Right hypertropia.

tiple sclerosis, and Graves' disease can all produce hypertropias. Many of these specific entities are discussed in Chapter 18, Neuro-ophthalmology.

Clinical Findings

The clinical findings may vary, depending on the cause. The history is particularly important in diagnosis of hypertropias. Prism and cover measurements are the mainstay of clinical evaluation and may be diagnostic. Observation of ocular rotations for limitations can also be of great value.

Prism and cover measurements must be made in primary position at distance and near, at distance in secondary position, at near in tertiary position, and to the right, left, and down in reading position.

Diplopia is almost invariably present if strabismus develops past age 6–8. As in other forms of strabismus, sensory adaptation occurs if the onset is before this age range. Suppression and anomalous retinal correspondence may be present in gaze directions where there is strabismus. In gaze directions without strabismus, there may be no suppression and normal stereopsis.

There may be head tilt, turn, or abnormal posture of the head. The deviation may be of any magnitude and usually changes with the direction of gaze. Most hypertropias are incomitant. The deviation tends to be greatest in the field of action of one of the 4 vertically acting muscles. There may be associated **cyclotropia,** especially with oblique dysfunction. To measure cyclotropia, a Maddox rod in a trial frame may be rotated in front of each eye in turn, until the observed line is parallel to the subjective horizontal with the head erect. The angle of tilt is then read from the angular scale on the trial frame.

The superior oblique is the most commonly paretic vertical muscle. The vertical rectus muscles are commonly involved in trauma, as with entrapment of the inferior rectus in an orbital floor fracture, and in thyroid eye disease, in which the inferior rectus becomes hypertrophied, inelastic, and fibrotic and pulls the eye downward.

Paresis of the superior oblique may present in several patterns. It is not understood why different patients show different patterns. The simplest pattern is maximum deviation in the field of action of the muscle (ie, the lower field of gaze to the contralateral side). Another pattern is maximum deviation in the field of action of the ipsilateral antagonist, the inferior oblique. Deviation is then maximum in the upper field of gaze to the contralateral side. Deviation in the lower field need not be entirely lateralized and may have spread across to the other side as well. Deviation may also be to one side only without being much greater up or down, or it may be up and down the side and across the bottom as well. Most cases show some degree of excyclotorsion.

The Bielschowsky head tilt test (Fig 16–18) is useful to confirm the diagnosis of superior oblique paresis. The test exploits the differing effects of each vertical muscle on torsion and elevation. Thus, with

Figure 16–18. Head tilt test (Bielschowsky test). Paresis of right superior oblique. *Left:* Hypertropia is minimized on tilting the head to the sound side. The right eye may then extort and the intorting superior oblique and superior rectus relax. *Right:* When the head is tilted to the paretic side, the intorting muscles contract together, but their vertical actions do not cancel out as usual, because of superior oblique paresis. Hypertropia is worse with head tilt to the paretic side.

a paretic right superior oblique when the head is tilted to the right, both muscles that attach to the top of the eye contract to intort the eye and maintain the position of the retinal vertical meridian as much as possible. The superior rectus elevates the eye, and the superior oblique depresses the eye. Because of weakness of the superior oblique muscle, the vertical forces do not cancel out as they normally would, and right hypertropia becomes worse. In head tilt to the left, the intorting muscles for the right eye relax and the inferior oblique and inferior rectus both contract to extort the eye. Both the paretic superior oblique and superior rectus relax, and hypertropia is minimized. Hypertropia should be quantified with prism and cover measurements with the head tilted to either side.

Treatment

A. Medical Treatment: For smaller and less incomitant deviations, a prism may be all that is required. As with any form of strabismus, one eye may be occluded if the patient can function adequately without binocular vision. Many patients find occlusion of an eye with good vision to be unpleasant, if not intolerable. If there is systemic disease, it must be fully treated. Botulinum toxin injections may be of help in some cases, if muscle strengthening is not required.

B. Surgical Treatment: Surgery is the remaining possibility for cases that have not improved with the preceding methods (see p 212). The choice of procedure depends on the cause and the quantitative measurements. The use of adjustable sutures (Fig 16– 13)

is nearly indispensable in vertical muscle surgery, because the precision of the required result is greater than in horizontal rectus surgery.

DUANE'S RETRACTION SYNDROME

Duane's retraction syndrome is typically characterized by marked limitation of abduction, mild limitation of adduction, retraction of the globe and narrowing of the palpebral fissure on attempted adduction, and, frequently, upshoot or downshoot of the eye in adduction. Usually, only the left eye is affected. Most cases are sporadic, although some families with dominant inheritance have been described. A variety of other anomalies may be associated, such as dysplasia of the iris stroma, heterochromia, cataract, choroidal coloboma, microphthalmos, Goldenhar's syndrome, Klippel-Feil syndrome, cleft palate, and anomalies of the face, ear, or extremities. The causes of the motility defects are varied, and some anomalies of the muscles have been found. Most cases can be explained by an inappropriate innervation pattern to the lateral rectus and sometimes other muscles as well. Sherrington's law of reciprocal innervation is not obeyed, because nerve fibers to the medial rectus also go to the lateral rectus. Cases with proved absence of the abducens nucleus and nerve have been found.

Treatment

Treatment for the abnormal motility pattern is surgical. Traditionally, for a typical case, only recession of the medial rectus on the affected side has been done if esotropia is present in primary position. Care must be taken to preserve good binocular function if it exists. For more complicated cases, the technique must be adjusted for each individual.

SPECIAL FORMS OF VERTICAL STRABISMUS

1. DISSOCIATED VERTICAL DIVERGENCE

Dissociated vertical divergence is frequently associated with congenital and rarely with otherwise normal muscle balance. The exact cause is not known, although it can be said to be supranuclear.

Clinical Findings

Each eye drifts upward under cover, frequently with extorsion and small exotropic shift, and then returns close to its resting binocular position when the cover is removed. Sometimes the eye rests in a hypotropic position and comes up to assume fixation when the other eye is covered. Most cases are bilateral, although asymmetry of involvement is usual. There are usually no symptoms in children, but later in life there are occasionally strange, indescribable, sometimes annoying sensations produced when one eye is dissociated upward. Rarely, there is diplopia.

Treatment

Treatment is indicated if the problem is symptomatic or disfiguring. Nonsurgical treatment is limited to refractive correction to maximize the potential of motor fusion and therapy for amblyopia. Surgical results have traditionally been variable and somewhat disappointing. Currently, the most popular and successful procedures are very large recession of the superior rectus or recession of the superior rectus combined with the Faden procedure (see p 212).

2. BROWN'S SUPERIOR OBLIQUE TENDON SHEATH SYNDROME

Brown's syndrome is due to fibrous adhesions in the superonasal quadrant of the eye, which mechanically limit elevation of the eye when in an adducted position. Differential diagnosis is concerned mainly with paresis of the inferior oblique muscle. When inferior oblique paresis is present, a forced duction test will show free rotation of the eye into elevation in adduction; this will not be seen with Brown's syndrome. There is hypertropia of the other eye on gaze to the uninvolved side, which increases on upgaze and may extend to primary position. The condition may be idiopathic or may be due to trauma or systemic inflammatory disorders.

After appropriate therapy for any systemic illness, the only remaining treatment is surgery. The general strategy is to free the mechanical adhesion. Restoration of full mobility is seldom achieved.

HETEROPHORIA

Heterophoria is deviation of the eyes that is held in check by binocular vision. Almost all individuals have some degree of heterophoria, and small amounts are considered normal. Larger amounts may or may not cause symptoms, depending on the level of effort required by the individual to control latent muscle imbalance.

Clinical Findings

The symptoms of heterophoria may be clear-cut (intermittent diplopia) or vague ("eyestrain" or asthenopia). Diplopia may come on only with fatigue or with poor lighting conditions, as in night driving. Usage requirements for the eyes and personality type are additional variable factors. Thus, there is no degree of heterophoria that is clearly abnormal, although larger amounts are more likely to be symptomatic. Except for hyperopia, high AC/A ratios, and mild cases of muscle paresis not resulting in frank heterotropia, the fundamental causes of heterophorias are unknown.

Asthenopia is sometimes caused by uncorrected refractive errors as well as by muscle imbalance. One possible mechanism is **aniseikonia,** in which an image seen by one eye is a different size and shape from that seen by the other eye. Because it is difficult to prove that aniseikonia is a cause and because of the variability of patient responses in treating symptomatic disease, the diagnosis of aniseikonia has been made infrequently in recent years. Spectacles with unequal lens power in the 2 eyes can cause asthenopia by creating prismatic displacement of the image in one eye for gaze away from the optic axis that is too large to control (induced prism). Another mechanism that may produce symptoms is a change in space perception due to the curvature of the lenses or astigmatic corrections.

The symptoms encountered in asthenopia take a wide variety of forms. There may be a feeling of heaviness, tiredness, or discomfort of the eyes, varying from a dull ache to deep pain located in or behind the eyes. Headaches of all types occur. Easy fatigability, blurring of vision, and diplopia, especially after prolonged use of the eyes, also occur. Symptoms are more common for near visual work than for distance. Frequently, an aversion to reading develops. Symptoms can be brought on by fatigue or illness or following the ingestion of medications or alcohol.

Diagnosis

The diagnosis of heterophoria is based on prism and cover measurements. Heterophoria or intermittent heterotropia must be present before a diagnosis of asthenopia can be justified. The relative fusional vergence amplitudes should be measured. While the patient views an accommodative target (ie, a target that calls for a performance that tests visual acuity and thus controls the level of accommodation) at distance or reading position, prisms of increasing strength are placed in front of one eye to displace the image. The fusional vergence amplitude is then the amount of prism the patient is able to overcome and still maintain single vision. This measurement is done both at distance and at near with base-out and base-in prisms. The prisms may also be placed vertically to measure positive vertical vergence with the right eye directed upward and negative vergence with the left eye directed upward. Absolute fusional vergence amplitudes measured on a light are more indicative of the maximum effort that can be put forth than what happens under normal physiologic conditions. The important feature is the size of the amplitudes in comparison to the angle of heterophoria. While one cannot give exact norms for normal relative fusional vergences, guidelines for typical normal findings are as follows: at distance, convergence is 14 Δ, divergence is 6 Δ, and vertical is 3 Δ; at near, convergence is 25 Δ, divergence is 15 Δ, and vertical is 3 Δ.

Treatment

Heterophoria requires treatment only if symptomatic. Untreated heterophoria or asthenopia does not cause any permanent damage to the eyes. Treatment methods are all aimed at reducing the effort required to achieve fusion or at changing muscle mechanics so that the muscle imbalance itself is reduced.

A. Medical Treatment:

1. Accurate refractive correction–Occasionally, poor visual acuity is found in the presence of symptomatic heterophoria. Spectacles providing clear vision are sometimes all that is needed to alleviate symptoms. The clearer image allows the patient's fusional capacity to function to its fullest.

2. Manipulation of accommodation–The general principle is that esophorias are treated with antiaccommodative therapy and exophorias by stimulating accommodation. Plus lenses for near work will reduce the accommodative load and the accompanying convergence. A high AC/A ratio may be treated with plus lenses or miotics.

In exophoria, minus lenses may be used to stimulate accommodation. This works only in young children; otherwise, presbyopia may be produced. A weak cycloplegic drop applied in the morning may also stimulate accommodation. This produces other undesirable symptoms in adults but may be helpful in children.

3. Prisms–The use of prisms requires the wearing of glasses; for some patients, this is unacceptable. A trial of plastic Fresnel press-on prisms should be made before expensive ground-in prisms are ordered. For optical reasons, larger amounts of prismatic correction produce distortions of the geometry of space. Furthermore, very thick lenses can result. The usual practice is to prescribe about one-third to one-half of the measured deviation. This should lessen the work load on the visual system while keeping the fusional amplitudes built up, minimizing the tendency for frank diplopia due to reduced fusional amplitudes when the glasses are not being worn. Prisms are useful for esophoria, exophoria, and vertical phorias, as well.

4. Botulinum toxin injection– (See above.) This new treatment is well suited to producing small shifts in ocular alignment. It may be used as a substitute for small-to-moderate amounts of surgical weakening of one muscle. One disadvantage is that results may not be known for many months. In time, this method may prove to be quite useful in treating heterophorias.

B. Surgical Treatment: Surgery should be the last resort after medical methods have been tried. As in strabismus, muscles are chosen for correction according to the measured deviation at distance and near in various directions of gaze. Sometimes, only one muscle needs to be corrected, although a new incomitant deviation may then be created. Adjustable sutures are very helpful (Fig 16–13).

REFERENCES

Cross HE, Pfaffenbach DD: Duane's retraction syndrome and asociated congenital malformations. *Am J Ophthalmol* 1972; **73**:442.

Duke-Elder S, Wybar K: Ocular motility and strabismus. In: *System of Ophthalmology*. Vol 6. Duke-Elder S (editor). Mosby, 1973.

Eggers HM: Functional anatomy of the extraocular muscles. Chapter 31 in: *Biomedical Foundations of Ophthalmology*. Duane T (editor). Harper & Row, 1982.

Foster RS, Paul TO, Jampolsky A: Management of infantile esotropia. *Am J Ophthalmol* 1976;**82**:291.

Helveston EM: *Atlas of Strabismus Surgery*, 2nd ed. Mosby, 1977.

Huber A: Electrophysiology of the retraction syndrome. *Br J Ophthalmol* 1974;**58**:293.

Ing MR: Early surgical alignment for congenital esotropia. *Trans Am Ophthalmol Soc* 1981;**79**:625.

Ingram RM: Refraction as a basis for screening children for squint and amblyopia. *Br J Ophthalmol* 1977;**61**:8.

Knapp P: Diagnosis and surgical treatment of hypertropia. *Am Orthop J* 1971;**21**:29.

Lennarstrand G, Bach-y-Rita P (editors): *Basic Mechanisms of Ocular Motility and Their Clinical Implications*. Pergamon, 1975.

New Orleans Academy of Ophthalmology: *Symposium on Strabismus*. Mosby, 1971, 1978.

Parks MM: The monofixation syndrome. *Trans Am Ophthalmol Soc* 1969;**67**:609.

Robinson DA: A quantitative analysis of extraocular muscle cooperation and squint. *Invest Ophthalmol* 1975;**14**:801.

Romano PE, Robinson JA: General anesthesia morbidity and mortality in eye surgery at a children's hospital. *J Pediatr Ophthalmol Strabismus* 1981;**18**:17.

Scott AB: Botulinum toxin injection of eye muscles to correct strabismus. *Trans Am Ophthalmol Soc* 1981;**79**:734.

Scott AB: Ocular motility. Chapter 21 in: *Physiology of the Human Eye and Visual System*. Records R (editor). Harper & Row, 1979.

Stockbridge L, Moore S: Prisms to determine the importance of a vertical component associated with esotropia. Page 213 in: *Orthoptics: Past, Present, Future*. Moore S, Mein J, Stockbridge L (editors). Stratton, 1976.

von Noorden GK: *Burian–von Noorden's Binocular Vision and Ocular Motility*, 3rd ed. Mosby, 1985.

von Noorden GK: *von Noorden–Maumenee's Atlas of Strabismus*, 3rd ed. Mosby, 1977.

Orbit

17

John H. Sullivan, MD

ANATOMY
(Figs 17–1 to 17–6)

The orbital cavity is schematically represented as a pyramid of 4 walls that converge posteriorly. The medial walls of the right and left orbit are parallel and are separated by the nose. In each orbit the lateral and medial walls form an angle of 45 degrees, which results in a right angle between the 2 lateral walls. The orbit is compared to the shape of a pear, with the optic nerve representing its stem. The anterior circumference is somewhat smaller in diameter than the region just within the rim, which makes a sturdy protective margin.

The orbits are related to the frontal sinus above, the maxillary sinus below, and the ethmoid and sphenoid sinuses medially. The thin orbital floor is easily damaged by direct trauma to the globe, resulting in a "blowout" fracture with herniation of orbital contents into the maxillary antrum. Infection within the sphenoid and ethmoid sinuses can erode the paper-thin medial wall (lamina papyracea) and involve the contents of the orbit. Erosion of the roof (eg, neuro-fibromatosis) may result in visible pulsations of the globe transmitted from the brain.

Orbital Walls

The roof of the orbit is composed principally of the orbital plate of the **frontal bone.** The lacrimal gland is located in the lacrimal fossa in the anterior lateral aspect of the roof. Posteriorly, the lesser wing of the **sphenoid bone** containing the optic canal completes the roof.

The lateral wall is separated from the roof by the superior orbital fissure, which divides the lesser from the greater wing of the **sphenoid bone.** The anterior portion of the lateral wall is formed by the orbital surface of the **zygomatic (malar) bone.** This is the strongest part of the bony orbit. Suspensory ligaments, the lateral palpebral tendon, and check ligaments have their connective tissue attachment to the lateral orbital tubercle.

The orbital floor is separated from the lateral wall by the inferior orbital fissure. The orbital plate of the **maxilla** forms the large central area of the floor and is the region where blowout fractures most frequently

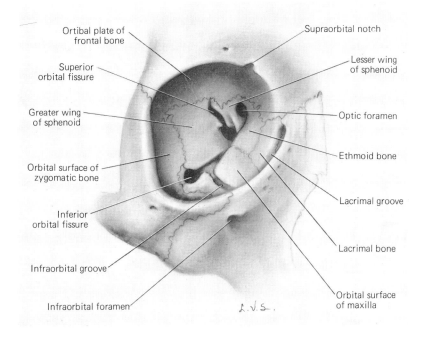

Ortibal plate of frontal bone

Superior orbital fissure

Greater wing of sphenoid

Orbital surface of zygomatic bone

Inferior orbital fissure

Infraorbital groove

Infraorbital foramen

Supraorbital notch

Lesser wing of sphenoid

Optic foramen

Ethmoid bone

Lacrimal groove

Lacrimal bone

Orbital surface of maxilla

Figure 17–1. Anterior view of bones of right orbit.

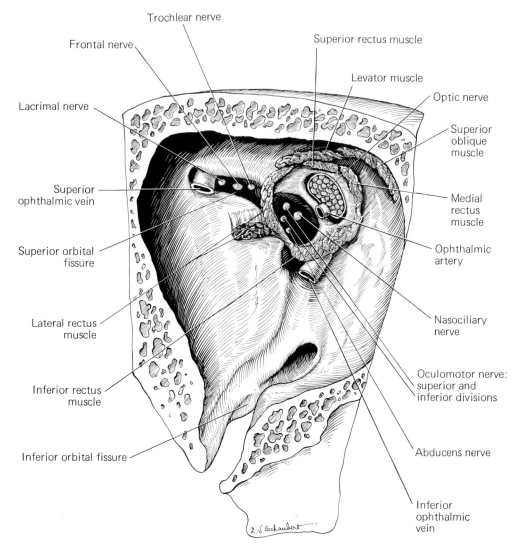

Figure 17–2. Anterior view of apex of right orbit.

occur. The frontal process of the **maxilla** medially and the **zygomatic bone** laterally complete the inferior orbital rim. The orbital process of the **palatine bone** forms a small triangular area in the posterior floor.

The boundaries of the medial wall are less distinct. The **ethmoid** bone is paper-thin but thickens anteriorly as it meets the **lacrimal bone.** The body of the **sphenoid** forms the most posterior aspect of the medial wall, and the angular process of the **frontal bone** forms the upper part of the posterior lacrimal crest. The lower portion of the posterior lacrimal crest is made up of the **lacrimal bone.** The anterior lacrimal crest is easily palpated through the lid and is composed of the frontal process of the **maxilla.** The lacrimal groove lies between the 2 crests and contains the lacrimal sac.

Contents of the Orbit

The volume of the adult orbit is approximately 30 mL, and the eyeball occupies only about one-fifth of the space. Fat and muscle account for the bulk of the remainder.

The anterior limit of the orbital cavity is the **orbital septum.** It is a thin sheet of fascia extending from the orbital rim to the tarsus in the lower lid and to a point slightly above the border of the tarsus in the upper lid. The orbital septum acts as a barrier between the eyelids and the orbit. The extraocular muscles are described and discussed in Chapter 16.

The principal arterial supply of the orbit and its structures derives from the **ophthalmic artery,** the first major branch of the intracranial portion of the internal carotid artery. This branch passes beneath the

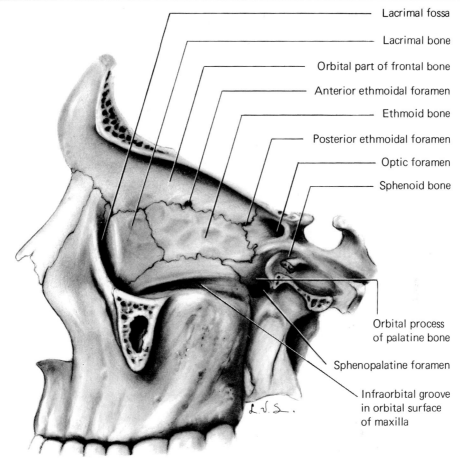

Figure 17–3. Medial view of bony wall of left orbit.

Lacrimal fossa
Lacrimal bone
Orbital part of frontal bone
Anterior ethmoidal foramen
Ethmoid bone
Posterior ethmoidal foramen
Optic foramen
Sphenoid bone
Orbital process of palatine bone
Sphenopalatine foramen
Infraorbital groove in orbital surface of maxilla

optic nerve and accompanies it through the optic canal into the orbit. The first intraorbital branch is the central retinal artery, which enters the optic nerve about 8– 15 mm behind the globe. The ophthalmic artery also sends branches to the lacrimal gland as well as to the intraocular structures via the short, long, and anterior ciliary arteries. The most anterior branches contribute to the formation of the arterial arcades of the eyelids, which make an anastomosis with the external carotid circulation via the facial artery.

The venous drainage of the orbit is primarily through the superior and inferior orbital veins. The superior orbital vein is important because it drains the skin of the periorbital region directly to the cavernous sinus. This forms the basis of the potentially lethal septic cavernous sinus thrombosis resulting from a superficial infection in this region.

The apex of the orbit is the entry portal for all nerves and vessels to the eye and the site of origin of all extraocular muscles except the inferior oblique. Expanding lesions of the apex result in a predictable neurologic deficit known as the orbital apex syndrome. The nerves enter the orbit through the **superior orbital fissure.** In its pathway to the cavernous sinus, the superior ophthalmic vein usually crosses at the highest point of the superior orbital fissure. Beneath the skin of the eyelid, this vein makes an anastomosis with the angular vein. The blood thus may drain posteriorly through the orbit or anteriorly to the facial vein.

The upper lateral aspect of the superior orbital fissure carries the **lacrimal nerve,** a branch of the first (ophthalmic) division of the trigeminal nerve. This small twig remains outside the area of origin of the rectus muscles (annulus of Zinn) and continues its lateral course in the orbit to terminate in the lacrimal gland, providing its sensory innervation. Slightly medial to the lacrimal nerve within the superior orbital fissure is the **frontal nerve,** which is the largest of the first division of branches of the trigeminal nerve. It also crosses over the annulus of Zinn and follows a course over the levator to the medial aspect of the orbit, where it divides into the supraorbital and supratrochlear nerves. These provide sensation to the brow and forehead. The only other nerve to enter the orbit outside the annulus of Zinn is the **trochlear nerve.** Although the thinnest of the cranial nerves, the trochlear nerve has the longest intracranial course, and it is also the only nerve to originate on the dorsal surface of the brain stem. The fibers decussate before

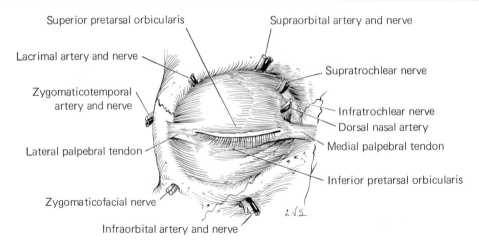

Figure 17–4. Vessels and nerves to extraocular structures.

they emerge from the brain stem just before the inferior colliculi, where they are subject to injury from the tentorium. The nerve pierces the dura behind the sella turcica and travels within the lateral wall of the cavernous sinus to enter the superior orbital fissure medial to the frontal nerve. From this point it travels within the periorbita of the roof over the levator muscle to the upper surface of the superior oblique muscle.

The rectus muscles originate from a fibrous ring (the annulus of Zinn), which surrounds the remainder of the superior orbital fissure as well as the optic canal. The superior division of the **oculomotor nerve** is adjacent to the trochlear nerve but lies within the annulus of Zinn at its highest point. The oculomotor nerve originates from between the cerebral peduncles and passes near the posterior communicating artery of the circle of Willis. Lateral to the pituitary gland, it is closely approximated to the optic tract, and here it pierces the dura to course in the lateral wall of the cavernous sinus. As the nerve leaves the cavernous sinus, it divides into superior and inferior divisions. The superior division enters high within the annulus of Zinn and passes over the optic nerve to innervate the levator and superior rectus muscles. The inferior division enters the annulus of Zinn low and passes below the optic nerve to supply the medial and inferior rectus muscles. A large branch from the inferior division extends forward to supply the inferior oblique. A small twig from the proximal end of the nerve to the inferior oblique carries parasympathetic fibers to the ciliary ganglion.

Between the superior and inferior divisions of the oculomotor nerve within the annulus of Zinn lie the last 2 orbital nerves. On the lateral aspect is the **abducens nerve,** and medially the **nasociliary nerve.** The abducens originates between the pons and medulla and pursues an extended course up the clivus to the posterior clinoid, penetrates the dura, and passes within the cavernous sinus. (All other nerves course through the lateral wall of the cavernous sinus.) After passing through the superior orbital fissure within the annulus of Zinn, the nerve continues laterally to innervate the lateral rectus muscle.

The nasociliary nerve is the third branch of the first (ophthalmic) division of the trigeminal nerve and is the sensory nerve of the eye. The trigeminal nerve originates from the pons, and its sensory roots form the trigeminal ganglion. The first of the 3 divisions passes through the lateral wall of the cavernous sinus and divides into the lacrimal, frontal, and nasociliary nerve. The nasociliary nerve, after entering through the annulus of Zinn, lies between the superior rectus and the optic nerve. It sends a branch to the ciliary ganglion and other branches to supply the cornea (the posterior ciliary nerves), eventually terminating near the tip of the nose. Thus, the skin on the tip of the nose may be affected with vesicular lesions prior to the onset of herpes zoster ophthalmicus.

The second (maxillary) division of the trigeminal nerve passes through the foramen rotundum and enters the orbit through the inferior orbital fissure. It passes through the infraorbital canal and exits via the infraorbital foramen, supplying sensation to the lower lid and adjacent cheek. It is frequently damaged in fractures of the orbital floor.

PHYSIOLOGY OF SYMPTOMS

Owing to the rigid bony structure of the orbit, with only an anterior opening for expansion, any increase in the orbital contents taking place to the side of or behind the eyeball will displace that organ. Pressure behind the eyeball will push it forward (proptosis). Pressure on one side will displace the eyeball to the other side.

With the change in position of the eyeball, especially if it takes place rapidly, there may be enough interference with the movement of the eye to cause dissociation of ocular movements and diplopia (double

Figure 17–5. Normal CT scan showing the anatomy of the orbit. Axial CT sections, thickness 1.5 mm. *A,* lowest section; *H,* highest section. Note clear delineation of individual muscles, optic nerve, and major veins within the orbital fat.

Figure 17–6. Coronal computer reconstructions from axial CT sections. *A,* most anterior section; *H,* most posterior section. Note detailed demonstration of ocular and orbital structures.

vision). Pain is absent unless there is extreme swelling of the tissues or unless the eyelids are unable to protect the cornea adequately and there is irritation from exposure.

EXOPHTHALMOS
(Proptosis)

Etiology & Classification

Exophthalmos may be due to any of the following factors: (1) a space-occupying lesion in the rigid bony orbit, displacing the only movable tissue, the eyeball; (2) swelling of the retrobulbar tissues through edema or hemorrhage, pushing the eyeball forward; (3) relaxation of the retracting effect of the extraocular muscles through paralysis or trauma; and (4) the apparent forward displacement (pseudoexophthalmos) seen with lid retraction (Graves' disease) and large eye (myopia, macrophthalmos).

A. Acute Exophthalmos:
1. Emphysema due to rupture of the medial orbital wall, allowing air from the sinus to enter the orbit.
2. Hemorrhage (traumatic or spontaneous).
3. Orbital cellulitis.

B. Pulsating Exophthalmos:
1. Carotid–cavernous sinus fistula.
2. Vascular tumors or aneurysms.
3. Cerebral pulsations due to a defect in the orbital roof.

C. Unilateral Exophthalmos:
1. Inflammatory—Cellulitis, pseudotumor of orbit, abscess, tenonitis, lacrimal gland inflammation, panophthalmitis, cavernous sinus thrombosis (may become bilateral).
2. Vascular—Hemorrhage, traumatic or spontaneous; varicosities, aneurysms.
3. Traumatic—Fracture, hemorrhage, rupture of the extraocular muscles, emphysema from sinuses, aneurysms.
4. Tumors—Primary, from the eye or orbital contents; spread from surrounding structures, metastatic.
5. Cysts—Congenital dermoid, parasitic, mucocele from surrounding sinuses.
6. Relaxation of retractors of eyeball, as with paralysis of the extraocular muscles.
7. General disease—Leukemia, lymphoma (frequently bilateral).

D. Bilateral Exophthalmos:
1. Endocrine—(Sometimes begins as unilateral exophthalmos.) Orbital Graves' disease.
2. Pseudoexophthalmos—Congenital macrophthalmos, high myopia, lid retraction (Graves' disease).

The most frequent primary orbital tumor in adults is cavernous hemangioma; the prognosis with surgery is good. The most common cause of proptosis—unilateral or bilateral—is orbital Graves' disease. Mild exophthalmos and lid retraction associated with hyperthyroidism are usually completely reversible with appropriate medical therapy. Malignant exophthalmos is a progressive, more severe form. Eye signs may occur years before any detectable physical or biochemical abnormality. Tissue changes consist of lymphocytic infiltration and orbital edema. Massive hypertrophy of the extraocular muscles begins in the inferior oblique and inferior rectus. The resultant limitation of movement often becomes permanent when fibrosis ensues. Restricted upgaze with vertical diplopia is characteristic. In severe cases, there is intractable diplopia, corneal ulceration from inability to close the eyelids, and occasionally optic neuropathy from orbital compression. These changes are generally believed to be due to an immunologic disorder involving both cellular and humoral elements. The diagnosis is made by demonstration of muscular hypertrophy on ultrasonography or CT scan.

Treatment of malignant exophthalmos is difficult. High doses of systemic corticosteroids are sometimes effective. Orbital radiation has also been used with some success in selected cases. Lubrication of the cornea, particularly at night, may prevent serious damage. Optic neuropathy is an indication for surgical decompression of the orbit using the antral, temporal, or transcranial approach. Once the condition has stabilized, lid retraction can be corrected by retractor recession, scleral grafting, and tarsorrhaphy.

Sudden onset of unilateral proptosis in childhood is most frequently from malignant rhabdomyosarcoma. Bilateral proptosis in a child is usually a result of metastatic neuroblastoma. Optic nerve glioma also presents in children and is sometimes associated with café au lait spots.

Lymphomatous orbital tumors and most metastatic tumors occur after middle age and are usually suspected because of systemic involvement. Tumors originating from the lacrimal gland should be excised in toto rather than subjected to biopsy. Fifty percent of these tumors are malignant, and an incisional biopsy is associated with tumor seeding. When there is good evidence of a primary malignant lacrimal gland tumor, it is preferable to take a biopsy specimen through an incision of the eyelid to prevent seeding within the orbit. Exenteration plus x-ray therapy offers the only chance for survival of these highly malignant tumors.

A skilled clinician may suspect the diagnosis in a patient with proptosis but is greatly assisted by CT scan and ultrasonography. Venography is useful in the diagnosis of an orbital varix. Air or positive contrast orbitography is seldom indicated.

ENOPHTHALMOS

Retraction of the eye into the orbit is a normal change in elderly people that is due to senile atrophy of the orbital fat. Enophthalmos before age 25 occurs rarely as part of Horner's syndrome or because of atrophy of the orbital fat in hemifacial atrophy or following surgery.

The most common cause of enophthalmos is trauma. Fracture of the orbital floor results in herniation into the maxillary sinus. After severe contusion, orbital fat may absorb slowly for many months.

INFLAMMATORY ORBITAL DISEASES

ORBITAL CELLULITIS
(Fig 17–7)

Orbital cellulitis is usually caused by *Haemophilus influenzae*, pneumococci, streptococci, or staphylococci, the same organisms that cause acute sinusitis. They enter the orbit by direct extension or through the vascular channels between the orbital contents and infected ethmoid, sphenoid, maxillary, or frontal sinuses.

Swelling and redness of the eyelids, chemosis, exophthalmos of varying degrees, and dull pain are usually present in mild cases. The onset is often sudden. More severe involvement may cause pain on rotation of the eyeball. Occasional intraocular hemorrhage and inflammatory signs are probably due to involvement of the vessels of the retina or choroid. Constitutional symptoms vary, according to the severity of the infection, from mild fever, malaise, and leukocytosis to high fever and marked debility. Infection may spread to the cavernous sinuses or meninges.

Orbital cellulitis must be differentiated from tenonitis, orbital periostitis, and cavernous sinus thrombosis. In children, rhabdomyosarcoma must be ruled out.

Almost all cases respond well to large doses of antibiotics. Hot compresses are useful to localize the inflammatory reaction. Unless the condition is growing steadily worse, surgical drainage should be delayed until absolutely necessary.

If antibiotics fail to bring the condition under control after a vigorous trial of 2–3 days, surgical drainage must be employed. The safest method is to make an incision into the area of greatest fluctuation—avoiding, if possible, the areas of the trochlea of the superior oblique muscle and the lacrimal gland recess.

The response to antibiotics is generally good. If not, the infection may localize anteriorly and rupture or require drainage, or it may extend posteriorly, causing cavernous sinus thrombosis, meningitis, or brain abscess. Optic neuritis with secondary atrophy may follow severe inflammatory reactions. The visual prognosis is excellent in the absence of complications.

CAVERNOUS SINUS THROMBOSIS

Orbital signs and symptoms are usually associated with thrombosis of the cavernous sinus. Exophthalmos with edema of the orbit and eyelids, diminished or absent pupillary reflexes, impaired visual acuity, and papilledema are usually present. Since the third, fourth, and sixth cranial nerves and the ophthalmic division of the fifth cranial nerve traverse the cavernous sinus, involvement of these nerves leads to paresis of the respective muscles and limitations of ocular movement. Fever is of the septic type.

Thrombosis of the cavernous sinus is usually due to infection spreading along the venous channels that drain the orbit, central face, throat, and nasal cavities.

Differentiation from orbital cellulitis is sometimes necessary. Cavernous sinus thrombosis may be bilateral, whereas orbital cellulitis is almost always unilateral. In cellulitis the pupillary reflexes remain normal, there is no papilledema, and pain and tenderness are more severe.

Massive doses of systemic antibiotics are necessary. Prophylactic chemotherapy and avoidance of manipulation of pyogenic infections, which may drain into the cavernous sinus, are of the greatest importance.

Since the pyogenic bacteria are usually responsible, most patients can be saved with good visual recovery. Before the antibiotics became available, all patients died.

PSEUDOTUMOR OF ORBIT

Pseudotumor of the orbit is an uncommon inflammatory reaction, usually unilateral, that clinically resembles a neoplasm. The histopathologic features may vary from vasculitis to a generalized lymphocytic inflammation. Exophthalmos is a prominent clinical finding. Many bacteria, viruses, parasites, and other possible causes have been investigated, but the cause has not been determined.

Figure 17–7. Orbital cellulitis. Abscess draining through upper eyelid.

Inflammatory pseudotumor is characterized by restriction of ocular movement, exophthalmos with occasional lateral displacement, swelling of the lids, and resistance to retrodisplacement of the eye with finger pressure. Pain and diplopia are present in about one-half of cases. The onset is usually gradual, and other signs of inflammation such as are seen with the more acute orbital cellulitis are not present.

The resemblance of pseudotumor to neoplasm may lead to exploratory orbital surgery; biopsy of the tissue reveals only signs of chronic inflammation or granuloma.

Treatment is often difficult. Anti-infective chemotherapeutic and antibiotic drugs and x-ray radiation have been tried without effect. Systemic steroids in high doses have proved to be effective in many cases. Therapy may have to be continued for weeks or months to prevent serious relapse. If the swollen, chronically inflamed tissues impinge upon the optic nerve, there may be permanent damage to the optic nerve. Corticosteroid therapy decreases the chances of optic atrophy.

A significant number of patients with orbital pseudotumor later manifest systemic neoplastic disease.

REFERENCES

Beard C, Quickert MH: *Anatomy of the Orbit.* Aesculapius, 1969.

Converse JM, Smith B: On the treatment of blowout fractures of the orbit. (Editorial.) *Plast Reconstr Surg* 1978;**62**:100.

Fraunfelder FT et al: No-touch technique for intraocular malignant melanomas. *Arch Ophthalmol* 1977;**95**:1616.

Garner A: Pathology of "pseudotumors" of the orbit: A review. *J Clin Pathol* 1973;**26**:639.

Grove AS: Evaluation of exophthalmos. *N Engl J Med* 1975; **292**:1005.

Henderson JW: *Orbital Tumors,* 2nd ed. Saunders, 1980.

Hurbli T et al: Radiation therapy for thyroid eye diseases. *Am J Ophthalmol* 1985;**99**:633.

Jakobiec FA: *Ocular and Adnexal Tumors.* Aesculapius, 1978.

Jones IS, Jakobiec FA: *Diseases of the Orbit.* Harper & Row, 1979.

Kincaid MC, Green WR: Diagnostic methods in orbital diseases. *Ophthalmology* 1984;**9**:719.

Koornneef L: Orbital septa: Anatomy and function. *Ophthalmology* 1979;**86**:876.

Krohel GB, Krauss HR, Winnick J: Orbital abscess: Presentation, diagnosis, therapy, and sequelae. *Ophthalmology* 1982;**89**:492.

Leone CR Jr: The management of ophthalmic Graves' disease. *Ophthalmology* 1984;**91**:770.

Moseley I, Sanders M: *Computerized Tomography in Neuro-ophthalmology.* Saunders, 1982.

Ogura JH, Pratt LL: Transantral decompression for malignant exophthalmos. *Otolaryngol Clin North Am* 1971;**4**:193.

Sassani JW, Osbakken MD: Anatomic features of the eye disclosed with nuclear magnetic resonance imaging. *Arch Ophthalmol* 1984;**102**:541.

Stewart WB, Krohel GB: Evaluation of orbital diseases. Page 302 in: *Ophthalmic Plastic and Reconstructive Surgery.* American Academy of Ophthalmology Manuals Program, 1984.

Trokel SL, Jakobiec FA: Correlation of CT scanning and pathologic features of ophthalmic Graves' disease. *Ophthalmology* 1981;**88**:553.

Unsöld R, Newton TH, De Groot J: CT-evaluation of extraocular muscles: Anatomic-CT-correlations. *Albrecht Von Graefes Arch Klin Exp Ophthalmol* 1980;**214**:155.

Warwick R: *Eugene Wolff's Anatomy of the Eye and Orbit,* 7th ed. Saunders, 1976.

Weiss A et al: Bacterial periorbital and orbital cellulitis in childhood. *Ophthalmology* 1983;**90**:195.

Zimmerman RA et al: Orbital magnetic resonance imaging. *Am J Ophthalmol* 1985;**100**:312.

18

Neuro-ophthalmology

The eyes are intimately related to the brain and frequently give important diagnostic clues to central nervous system disorders. Indeed, the optic nerve is a part of the central nervous system. Intracranial disease frequently causes visual disturbances because of destruction of or pressure upon some portion of the optic pathways. Cranial nerves III, IV, and VI, which control ocular movements, may be involved, and nerves V and VII are also intimately associated with ocular function.

See Fig 18–1 for magnetic resonance imaging (MRI) of the normal brain.

THE SENSORY VISUAL PATHWAY

Topographic Overview
(Fig 18–2)

The second cranial nerve subserves the special sense of vision. Light is detected by the rods and cones of the retina, which may be considered the special sensory end organ for vision. The cell bodies of these receptors extend processes that synapse with the bipolar cell, the second neuron in the visual pathway. The bipolar cells synapse, in turn, with the retinal ganglion cells. Ganglion cell axons comprise the nerve fiber layer of the retina and converge to form the optic nerve. The nerve emerges from the back of the globe and travels posteriorly within the muscle cone to enter the cranial cavity via the optic canal.

Intracranially, the 2 optic nerves join to form the optic chiasm. At the chiasm, more than half of the fibers (those from the nasal half of the retina) decussate and join the uncrossed temporal fibers of the opposite nerve to form the optic tracts. All of the fibers receiving impulses from the right half of the visual field thus make up the left optic tract and project to the left cerebral hemisphere. Similarly, the left half of the visual field projects to the right cerebral hemisphere. Each optic tract sweeps around the cerebral peduncle toward the lateral geniculate nucleus. Twenty percent of the fibers in the tract subserve pupillary function. These fibers leave the tract just anterior to the nucleus and pass via the brachium of the superior colliculus to the midbrain. The remaining fibers synapse in the lateral geniculate nucleus. The cell bodies of this structure give rise to the geniculocalcarine tract. This tract passes through the posterior limb of the internal capsule and then fans into the optic radiations that traverse parts of the temporal and parietal lobes en route to the occipital cortex.

Analysis of Visual Fields in Localizing Lesions in the Visual Pathways

In clinical practice, lesions in the visual pathways are localized by means of central and peripheral visual field examination. The technique (perimetry) is discussed on p 18. Fig 18–3 shows the types of field defects caused by lesions in various locations of the pathway. Lesions anterior to the chiasm (of the retina or optic nerve) cause unilateral field defects; lesions anywhere in the visual pathway posterior to the chiasm cause contralateral homonymous defects. These may be congruent (ie, identical in size, shape, and location) or incongruent. Chiasmal lesions usually cause bitemporal defects.

Multiple isopters (field tests with several objects of different sizes) should be used in order to evaluate the defects thoroughly. A field defect shows evidence of actively spreading disease when there are areas of "relative scotoma" (ie, a larger field defect for a smaller test object). Such visual field defects are said to be "sloping." This is in contrast to vascular lesions with steep borders (ie, the defect is the same size no matter what size test object is used).

Another important generalization is that the more congruous the homonymous field defects (ie, the more similar the 2 fields), the farther posterior the lesion is in the visual pathway. A lesion in the occipital region causes identical defects in each field, whereas optic tract lesions cause incongruous (dissimilar) homonymous field defects. Also, the more posterior the lesion, the more likely macular sparing and, therefore, maintenance of good visual acuity.

THE OPTIC NERVE

Anatomy (Fig 18–4)

The optic nerve is a trunk containing about 1.1 million axons arising from the ganglion cells of the retina. The nerve emerges from the back of the globe through a short, circular opening (0.7 mm long, 1.5 mm in diameter) in the sclera situated 1 mm below and 3 mm nasal to the posterior pole of the eye. The orbital portion is 25–30 mm long and travels posteriorly within the muscle cone. The nerve then passes via the bony optic canal into the cranial cavity. This intracanalicular portion measures 4–9 mm. After a 10-mm intracranial course, the nerve joins the opposite optic nerve to form the optic chiasm.

The nerve fibers become myelinated upon leaving the eye; this increases the diameter from 1.5 mm (within the sclera) to 3 mm (within the orbit). Since the ganglion cells of the retina and their axons that make up the optic nerve are actually extensions of the central nervous system, they have no capacity to regenerate if severed.

Sheaths of the Optic Nerve (Fig 18–4)

The fibrous wrappings that ensheathe the optic nerve are continuous with the meninges. The pia mater is loosely attached about the nerve near the chiasm and only for a short distance within the cranium, but it is closely attached around most of the intracanalicular and all of the intraorbital portions. The pia consists of some fibrous tissue with numerous small blood vessels (Fig 18– 5). It divides the nerve fibers into bundles by sending numerous septa into the nerve substance. The pia continues to the sclera, with a few fibers running into the choroid and lamina cribrosa.

The arachnoid comes in contact with the optic nerve at the intracranial end of the optic canal and accompanies the nerve to the globe, where it ends in the sclera and overlying dura. This sheath is a diaphanous connective tissue membrane with many septate connections with the pia mater, which it closely resembles. It is more intimately associated with pia than with dura.

The dura mater lining the inner surface of the cranial vault comes in contact with the optic nerve as it leaves the optic canal. As the nerve enters the orbit from the optic canal, the dura splits, one layer (the periorbita) lining the orbital cavity and the other forming the outer dural covering of the optic nerve. The dura becomes continuous with the outer two-thirds of the sclera. The dura consists of tough, fibrous, relatively avascular tissue lined by endothelium on the inner surface.

The subdural space is between the dura and arachnoid; the subarachnoid space is between the pia and the arachnoid. Both are more potential than actual spaces under normal conditions but are direct continuations of their corresponding intracranial spaces. Subarachnoid or subdural fluid under sufficient pressure will fill these potential spaces about the optic nerve. The meningeal layers are adherent to each other and to the optic nerve and the surrounding bone within the optic foramen, making the optic nerve resistant to traction from either end.

Figure 18–1. Magnetic resonance imaging (MRI) of normal brain in sagittal section *(upper left),* coronal section *(upper right),* and axial section *(lower left).* The white arrows indicate the chiasm. The future impact of this technique on localization of lesions affecting the intracranial visual and ocular motor pathways will be profound.

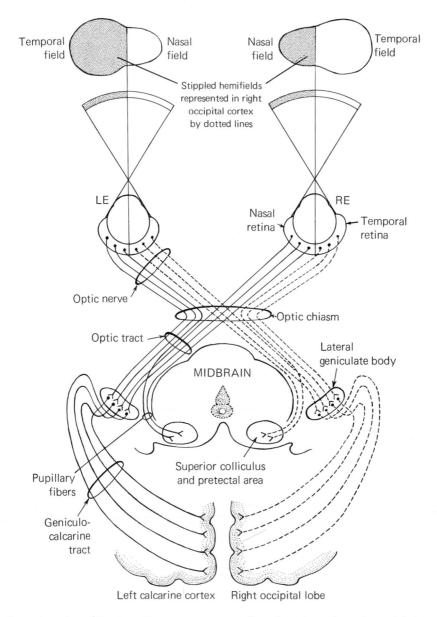

Figure 18–2. The optic pathway. The dotted lines represent nerve fibers from the retina to the occipital cortex that carry visual and pupillary afferent impulses from the left half of the visual field.

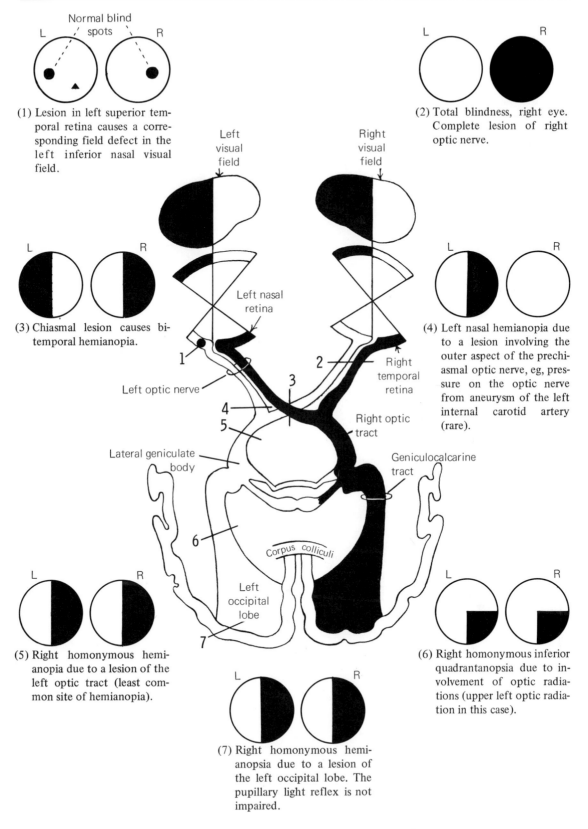

(1) Lesion in left superior temporal retina causes a corresponding field defect in the left inferior nasal visual field.

(2) Total blindness, right eye. Complete lesion of right optic nerve.

(3) Chiasmal lesion causes bitemporal hemianopia.

(4) Left nasal hemianopia due to a lesion involving the outer aspect of the prechiasmal optic nerve, eg, pressure on the optic nerve from aneurysm of the left internal carotid artery (rare).

(5) Right homonymous hemianopia due to a lesion of the left optic tract (least common site of hemianopia).

(6) Right homonymous inferior quadrantanopsia due to involvement of optic radiations (upper left optic radiation in this case).

(7) Right homonymous hemianopsia due to a lesion of the left occipital lobe. The pupillary light reflex is not impaired.

Figure 18–3. The visual system; topographic diagnosis.

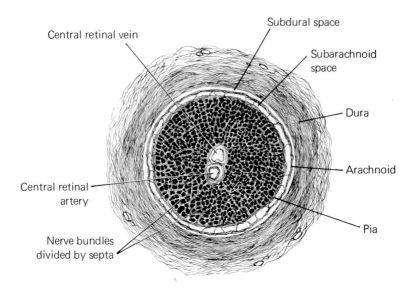

Figure 18–4. Cross section of the optic nerve. (Redrawn and reproduced, with permission, from Wolff E: *Anatomy of the Eye and Orbit,* 6th ed. Blakiston-McGraw, 1968.)

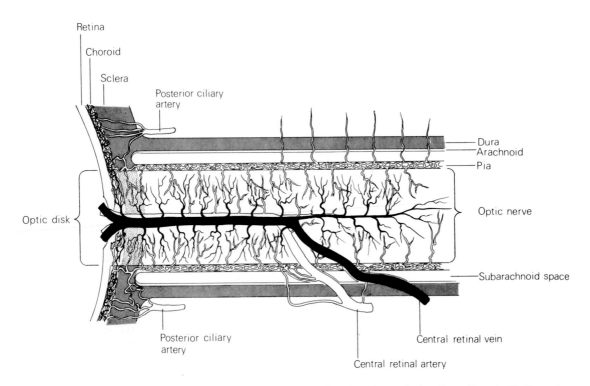

Figure 18–5. Blood supply of the optic nerve. (Redrawn and reproduced, with permission, from: Hayreh SS: *Trans Am Acad Ophthalmol Otolaryngol* 1974;**78**:240.)

DISEASES OF THE OPTIC NERVE

Etiologic Classification

A. Idiopathic optic neuritis.

B. Demyelinating Diseases:
1. Multiple sclerosis.
2. Other rare demyelinating syndromes–Neuromyelitis optica (Devic's disease).

C. Viral Infections:
1. Postviral optic neuritis (measles, mumps, chickenpox, influenza).
2. Postinfectious encephalomyelitis.
3. Polyradiculoneuronitis (Guillain-Barré syndrome).
4. Infectious mononucleosis.
5. Herpes zoster.

D. Local Extension of Inflammatory Disease:
1. Sinusitis.
2. Intracranial–Meningitis, encephalitis.
3. Orbital–Cellulitis, vasculitis.
4. Intraocular–Chorioretinitis, endophthalmitis, iridocyclitis.

E. Systemic Infections and Inflammation:
1. Syphilis.
2. Tuberculosis.
3. Cryptococcosis.
4. Coccidioidomycosis.
5. Infective endocarditis.
6. Sarcoidosis.

F. Nutritional and Metabolic:
1. Diabetes mellitus.
2. Dysthyroidism.
3. Vitamin deficiencies–Beriberi, pellagra.

G. Toxic:
1. Tobacco-alcohol amblyopia.
2. Heavy metal–Arsenic, lead, thallium.
3. Drugs–Ethambutol, isoniazid, streptomycin, disulfiram, digitalis, chloramphenicol, chloroquine, chlorpropamide, halogenated hydroxyquinones (eg, iodochlorhydroxyquin).
4. Methanol.

H. Hereditary Optic Atrophy:
1. Leber's disease.
2. Dominant (juvenile) optic atrophy.
3. Recessive (infantile) optic atrophy.
4. Behr's syndrome.

I. Vascular Disease:
1. Cranial arteritis.
2. Arteriosclerosis (anterior ischemic optic neuropathy).
3. Polyarteritis nodosa.
4. Takayasu's disease.

J. Neoplastic:
1. Direct infiltration of optic nerve, leukemic or malignant.
2. Compressive neuropathy.
3. Paraneoplastic syndrome.

K. Trauma.

L. Radiation neuropathy.

1. OPTIC NEURITIS
(Fig 18–6)

Optic neuritis (papillitis) is a broad term denoting inflammation, degeneration, or demyelinization of the optic nerve. A wide variety of diseases can cause optic neuritis. Loss of vision is the cardinal symptom and serves to differentiate optic neuritis from papilledema, which it may resemble on ophthalmoscopic examination.

Retrobulbar neuritis is optic neuritis that occurs far enough behind the optic disk so that no early changes of the optic disk are visible by means of the ophthalmoscope. Visual acuity is markedly reduced. ("The patient sees nothing and the doctor sees nothing.")

The most frequent cause of retrobulbar neuritis is multiple sclerosis. A diagnosis of multiple sclerosis is eventually made in 25–50% of patients between 20 and 45 years of age who have an attack of retrobulbar neuritis. Other causes are late neurosyphilis, toxic amblyopias, other demyelinating diseases, Leber's optic atrophy, diabetes mellitus, and vitamin deficiency. If the process is sufficiently destructive, retrograde optic atrophy results. The disk loses its normal pink color and becomes pale. In very severe cases a chalky-white disk with sharp outlines in a blind eye results.

Clinical Findings

There is usually a temporary but severe loss of vision. There may be pain in the region of the eye, especially upon movement of the globe. Vision characteristically improves dramatically within 2–3 weeks.

Central scotomas are the most common visual field defect. They are usually circular, varying widely in size and density. Almost any unilateral field change is possible. The pupillary light reflex is sluggish.

Ophthalmoscopically, hyperemia of the optic disk and distention of large veins are early signs. Blurred disk margins and filling of the physiologic cup are common. The process may advance to marked edema of the nerve head, but elevations of more than 3 diopters (1 mm) are unusual. Extensive surrounding retinal

Figure 18–6. Mild disk swelling in optic neuritis.

edema may be present. Flame-shaped hemorrhages may occur in the nerve fiber layer near the optic disk.

Differential Diagnosis

Papilledema is the most common differential diagnostic problem. In papilledema there is often greater elevation of the optic nerve head, nearly normal visual acuity, normal pupillary response to light, associated increased intracranial pressure, and no visual field defect except an enlarged blind spot unless the visual pathway has been interrupted intracranially. Papilledema is usually bilateral, whereas papillitis is usually unilateral. Despite these obvious differences, differential diagnosis continues to be a problem because of the similarity of the ophthalmoscopic findings.

Treatment

Ideally, treatment is directed toward the underlying cause. If the cause cannot be effectively treated or is not known, treatment is often unsatisfactory. Systemic corticosteroids have not been proved to be helpful in persistent optic neuritis due to any cause. Since the tendency is in the direction of improvement, many drugs have been reported to be "successful" in the treatment of this disorder.

Course & Prognosis

Loss of vision occurs within the first few hours after onset and is maximal within several days. Visual acuity usually begins to improve 2–3 weeks after onset and sometimes returns to normal in a few days.

Improvement may continue slowly over a period of several months. The appearance of optic atrophy indicates some permanent destruction of nerve fibers with permanent loss of function. Optic neuritis associated with systemic or local inflammatory disease or of unknown cause does not usually recur. Optic neuritis in demyelinating disease has a favorable prognosis without treatment for an individual attack, but over a period of years significant visual loss is the rule since permanent damage results from recurrent attacks.

2. MULTIPLE SCLEROSIS (Fig 18–7)

Multiple sclerosis is a chronic, relapsing demyelinating disorder of the central nervous system of unknown cause. Onset is usually in young adult life; this disease rarely begins before 15 years or after 55 years of age. There is a tendency to involve the optic nerves and chiasm, brain stem, cerebellar peduncles, and spinal cord, although no part of the central nervous system is invulnerable. The peripheral nervous system is not often involved. Clinically, there are a variety of symptoms and signs that may vary in number and character from time to time. In addition to ocular disturbances, there may be muscle weakness, ataxia, urinary disturbances, paresthesia, dysarthria, intention tremors, sensory disturbances, and pyramidal signs.

Figure 18–7. Retinal nerve fiber layer in demyelinative optic neuropathy of multiple sclerosis. The upper temporal nerve fiber bundles show multiple slitlike areas of thinning (arrows) representing retrograde axonal atrophy from subclinical disease in the optic nerve. Vision in the eye was 6/6 (20/20).

Pathologically, multiple areas of demyelination are present in the white matter. Early, there is degeneration of the myelin sheaths and a relative sparing of the axons. Glial tissue overgrowth and complete nerve fiber destruction with some round cell infiltrations are seen later. The disease has a predilection for the optic nerve and chiasm.

Patients may first complain of blurring of vision, as if a mist or film covers the eye. This is due to optic neuritis (especially retrobulbar neuritis) and is characterized by acute unilateral loss of vision with a tendency toward recovery. Because of the transient nature of the visual defect and the absence of physical findings, the complaint is sometimes discussed as being of hysterical origin. The other eye is involved eventually. With each attack, there may be some residual permanent damage (eg, loss of visual acuity or defective color vision).

Because of the tendency toward selective involvement of the papillomacular bundle within the optic nerve, central scotoma is by far the most common visual field defect during the acute stage.

The pupil reacts sluggishly to light. If the optic neuritis is severe, there may be atrophy of the optic disk that is ophthalmoscopically visible as the so-called temporal pallor.

Diplopia is a frequent early symptom of extraocular muscle involvement, due most frequently to internuclear ophthalmoplegia. This condition, caused by a lesion of the medial longitudinal fasciculus, is characterized by paresis of one or both of the medial rectus muscles on conjugate lateral gaze to the opposite side and symptoms in the opposite (abducting) eye; medial rectus function is normal for convergence. Ptosis may also occur; less commonly, weakness of the lateral rectus or other muscles, singly or together, occurs.

Nystagmus is a common early sign, and—unlike most manifestations of the disease (which tend toward remission)—it is often permanent (70%).

Retinal vessel vasculitis and low-grade uveitis are occasionally associated with multiple sclerosis.

The cerebrospinal fluid gamma globulin concentration is frequently high, but some patients with multiple sclerosis have no spinal fluid abnormalities.

The visual evoked response (VER) may help confirm involvement of the visual pathway. The VER has been reported to be abnormal in 80% of definite, 43% of probable, and 22% of suspected cases of multiple sclerosis. A normal VER in suspected multiple sclerosis makes the diagnosis questionable.

There is no specific therapy for multiple sclerosis. Treatment is symptomatic and supportive. The course of the disease is unpredictable, and remissions and exacerbations may occur. The prognosis for vision in retrobulbar neuritis is fairly good, but with successive attacks there may be an increased permanent defect. Complete blindness may occur when there is severe optic atrophy. Death may occur within a decade, but survival for 25–30 years is not uncommon.

3. NEUROMYELITIS OPTICA (Devic's Disease)

This rare demyelinating disease of the central nervous system (considered by many to be a severe form of multiple sclerosis) is characterized by bilateral optic neuritis and paraplegia. The cause is not known. There is usually a subacute onset of blindness in one eye, followed soon by blindness in the other eye and paraplegia. There is only a moderate tendency to recovery of both elements of the disease. The mortality rate is 50% in some series. There is no treatment.

PAPILLEDEMA (Figs 18–8 to 18–11)

Papilledema (choked disk) is a noninflammatory congestion of the optic disk associated with increased intracranial pressure. Papilledema will occur in any intracranial pressure. Papilledema will occur in any condition causing persistent increased intracranial pressure; the most common causes are cerebral tumors, abscesses, subdural hematoma, hydrocephalus, and malignant hypertension. An important factor in the mechanism of papilledema is obstruction to the venous flow caused by pressure on the central retinal vein where it leaves the optic nerve and passes through the subarachnoid and subdural spaces.

OPTIC NERVE ATROPHY (Figs 18–12 to 18–15)

Etiologic Classification

A. Vascular: Occlusion of the central retinal vein or artery; arteriosclerotic changes within the optic nerve itself, disturbing its normal nutrition; or posthemorrhagic, due to sudden massive blood loss (eg, bleeding peptic ulcer).

B. Degenerative: Consecutive atrophy secondary to retinal disease, with destruction of ganglion cells (eg, retinitis); or as part of a systemic degenerative disease (eg, cerebromacular degeneration).

C. Secondary to Papilledema: See p 239.

D. Secondary to Optic Neuritis (Including Retrobulbar Neuritis): See p 237.

E. Pressure Against the Optic Nerve: Aneurysm of the anterior circle of Willis, bony pressure at the optic foramen (eg, osteitis deformans), intracanalicular or parasellar tumors.

F. Toxic: End result of toxic amblyopia (see pp 256–258).

G. Metabolic: Eg, diabetes, ganglioside disease.

H. Traumatic: Direct injury to a nerve (ie, severing, avulsion, or contusion).

I. Glaucomatous: See Chapter 15.

Clinical Findings

Loss of vision is the only symptom. Pallor of the optic disk and loss of pupillary reaction are usually proportionate to visual loss.

Figure 18–8. Early papilledema. The disk margins are blurred superiorly and inferiorly by the thickened layer of nerve fibers entering the disk.

Figure 18–10. Fully developed papilledema. The disk tissue is swollen, elevated, and congested, and the retinal veins are markedly dilated.

Figure 18–9. Papilledema with opaque (white) patches of swollen nerve fibers and hemorrhages.

Figure 18–11. Chronic atrophic papilledema in a child with a cerebellar medulloblastoma. The disk is pale and slightly elevated and has blurred margins. The white areas surrounding the macula are reflected light from the vitreo-retinal interface. The inferior temporal nerve fiber bundles are partially atrophic (arrows).

Figure 18–12. Optic nerve hypoplasia. The disk border (arrows) is small in circumference. Note the disproportion between the small disk and the normal-sized central retinal vessels.

Figure 18–13. Chronic ischemic optic atrophy with loss of neuroglial tissue and exposure of the lamina cribrosa. The pale disk has a shallow cup without nasal displacement of the central retinal vessels. Multiple dark holes are present in the disk surface. The disk is ringed by a zone of choroidal atrophy. The retinal arterioles are narrowed irregularly.

Figure 18–14. Large path of myelinated nerve fibers originating from superior edge of disk. Another smaller patch is present near inferior nasal border of disk. (Right eye.)

Treatment, Course, & Prognosis

It is rarely possible to treat the underlying cause effectively. Changes in visual function occur very slowly over weeks or months. It is difficult to assess prognosis on the basis of ophthalmoscopic findings alone. Atrophic cupping, attenuation and reduced number of vessels on the disk, and pallor with papilledema are unfavorable prognostic signs. Optic atrophy secondary to vascular, traumatic, degenerative, and some toxic causes usually has a very bad prognosis. Visual loss due to pressure on the optic nerve may be reversed, particularly if the cause is relieved early.

GENETICALLY DETERMINED OPTIC ATROPHY

Leber's Optic Neuropathy

This rare disease, characterized by sequential, rapidly progressive optic neuropathy, occurs in young men age 20– 30 (very rarely in women). It has classically been considered to be due to an X-linked recessive gene, but its real mode of inheritance must still be considered to be in doubt. Vision is not totally lost. There is no known treatment. Other types of central nervous system involvement can be present and may cause confusion with multiple sclerosis.

Figure 18–15. Examples of optic atrophy. *Upper left:* Primary optic atrophy due to nutritional amblyopia. *Upper right:* Secondary optic atrophy with optociliary shunts (arrows) due to optic nerve sheath meningioma. *Lower left:* Optic atrophy with optic disk drusen. *Lower right:* Pallor (atrophy) of right optic disk due to nerve compression by sphenoid meningioma. The left disk is normal.

Congenital or Infantile Hereditary Optic Atrophy

This occurs in a severe autosomal recessive form and a milder autosomal dominant form. The recessive form is present at birth or within 2 years and is accompanied by nystagmus. The more common dominant form has an insidious onset in childhood, with little progression thereafter. There is characteristically a centrocecal scotoma with variable loss of central visual acuity.

Behr's Hereditary Optic Atrophy

This rare autosomal recessive disease is characterized by (1) bilateral optic atrophy, rarely complete; and (2) associated neurologic findings such as mild ataxia, a positive Babinski sign, clubfoot, mental deficiency, nystagmus, and other findings, at times with generalized slow progression to a static condition by late adolescence. There is no known treatment.

THE OPTIC CHIASM

Anatomy (Fig 18–16)

The optic chiasm is variably situated near the top of the diaphragm of the sella turcica (most often posteriorly, projecting over the dorsum sellae) and usually separated from it by several millimeters of subarachnoid space. Above, the lamina terminalis forms the anterior wall of the third ventricle. The internal carotid arteries lie just laterally, adjacent to the cavernous sinuses. The chiasm is made up of the junction of the 2 optic nerves and provides for crossing of the nasal fibers to the opposite optic tract and the passage of temporal fibers to the ipsilateral optic tract. The macular fibers are arranged similarly to the rest of the fibers except that their decussation is farther posteriorly. In general, lesions of the chiasm cause bitemporal hemianopic defects. These defects are typically incomplete and are often asymmetric. The nasal field may also be involved, and central visual acuity may be decreased.

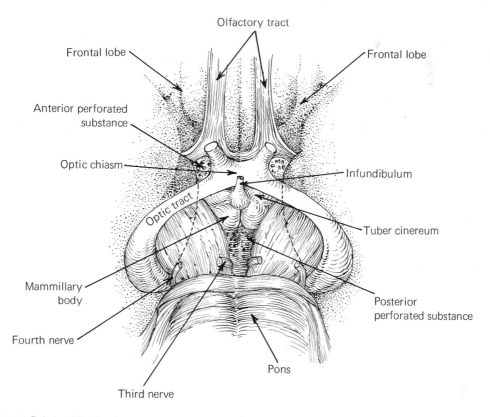

Figure 18–16. Relationship of optic chiasm from inferior aspect. (Redrawn and reproduced, with permission, from Duke-Elder WS: *System of Ophthalmology.* Vol 2. Mosby, 1961.)

Figure 18–17. Pituitary adenoma with suprasellar extension (arrows) causing bitemporal hemianopia. CT scans with contrast enhancement. Sagittal re-formation *(top)*. Coronal re-formation *(bottom)*.

PITUITARY TUMORS

The anterior lobe of the pituitary gland is the site of origin of pituitary tumors (Fig 18–17). Symptoms and signs include loss of vision, field changes, pituitary dysfunction, extraocular nerve palsies, and evidence on CT scan of sellar and suprasellar tumor.

Surgical removal is the usual method of treatment. Visual loss or endocrine dysfunction is an indication for treatment. Visual acuity and visual fields may improve dramatically after pressure has been removed from the chiasm.

CRANIOPHARYNGIOMA

Craniopharyngiomas are a group of tumors arising from epithelial remnants of Rathke's pouch (80% of the population normally have such remnants) and characteristically become symptomatic between the ages of 10 and 25 years. They are usually suprasellar, occasionally intrasellar. The signs and symptoms vary tremendously with the age of the patient and the exact location of the tumor as well as its rate of growth. When a suprasellar tumor occurs, asymmetric chiasmal field defects are prominent. Papilledema is more common than in pituitary tumor. Pituitary deficiency may result, and involvement of the hypothalamus may cause stunted growth. Calcification of parts of the

tumor contributes to a characteristic appearance on CT scan. Treatment consists of surgical removal, if possible, but evacuation of the cystic contents and removal of the cyst wall are often all that can be done.

SUPRASELLAR MENINGIOMAS

Suprasellar meningiomas arise from the meninges covering the tuberculum sella and the planum sphenoidale, with a high proportion of patients being female. The tumor is usually anterior and superior to the chiasm, and visual field changes are frequent. The optic nerves are often involved early (but asymmetrically) in the slowly progressive damage to the visual pathway. CT scans with contrast enhancement easily demonstrate these tumors (see Fig 18–22). Treatment consists of surgical removal.

GLIOMA OF THE OPTIC CHIASM

Optic chiasm glioma is a rare, usually indolent disorder of children that sometimes occurs as part of the clinical picture of neurofibromatosis. Onset may be sudden, with rapid loss of vision. Optic atrophy occurs, and visual field defects reveal a chiasmal syndrome. CT scans may reveal enlarged optic nerves and a mass in the region of the chiasm and hypothalamus. Treatment is by irradiation, since surgical removal usually results in blindness.

THE RETROCHIASMAL VISUAL PATHWAYS

Anatomy

Each optic tract begins at the posterolateral angle of the chiasm and sweeps around the upper part of the cerebral peduncle to end in the lateral geniculate nucleus. Afferent pupillary fibers leave the tract just anterior to the nucleus and pass via the brachium of the superior colliculus to the midbrain. (The pupillary pathway is diagrammed in Fig 18–18.) Afferent visual fibers terminate on cells in the lateral geniculate nucleus that give rise to the geniculocalcarine tract. This tract traverses the posterior limb of the internal capsule and then fans out into a broad bundle called the optic radiation. The fibers in this bundle curve backward around the anterior aspect of the temporal horn of the lateral ventricle and then medially to reach the calcarine cortex of the occipital lobe, where they terminate. The most inferior fibers, which carry the projections from the superior aspect of the contralateral half of the visual field, course anteriorly into the temporal lobe in a configuration known as Meyer's loop. Lesions of the temporal lobe involving these fibers can produce superior quadrantanopic field defects.

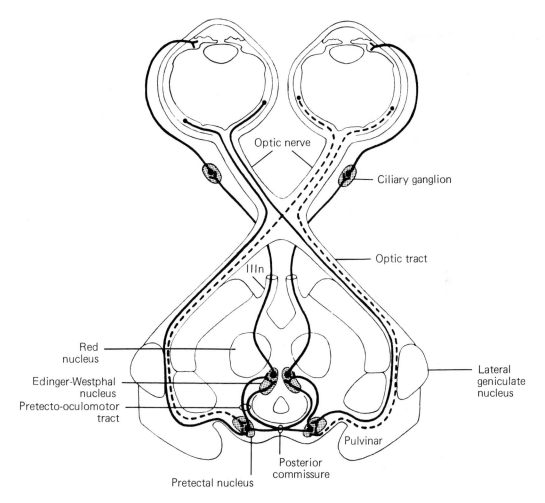

Figure 18–18. Diagram of the path of the pupillary light reflex. (Reproduced, with permission, from Walsh FB, Hoyt WF: *Clinical Neuro-ophthalmology,* 3rd ed. Vol 1. Williams & Wilkins, 1969.)

The primary visual cortex (area 17) occupies the upper and lower lips and the depths of the calcarine fissure on the medial aspect of the occipital lobe. Each lobe receives input from the 2 ipsilateral half-retinas, representing the contralateral half of the binocular visual field. The projection of the visual field onto the visual cortex occurs in a precise and orderly retinotopic pattern. The macula is represented at the posterior pole, and the peripheral parts of the retina project to the most anterior part of the calcarine cortex.

LESIONS OF THE RETROCHIASMAL PATHWAYS

Cerebrovascular disease and tumors are responsible for most lesions of the retrochiasmal visual pathways, although almost any intracranial disease process can involve these structures. The optic tracts and lateral geniculate nucleus are infrequently affected and, when involved, typically produce incongruous homonymous visual field defects. After several weeks, the disks may appear pale, and the retinal nerve fiber layer is deficient.

Lesions involving the geniculocalcarine tract or occipital cortex produce homonymous field defects but do not result in optic atrophy. Generally, the more posterior a lesion is located, the more congruous the homonymous visual field defect. Tumors occur more frequently in temporal and parietal lobes, while occipital lobe lesions are overwhelmingly vascular. Lesions of the temporal and parietal lobes usually result in multiple neurologic deficits, and isolated visual loss is rare. Vascular lesions of the occipital lobe, on the other hand, are common and account for over 80% of isolated homonymous visual field loss in patients over age 50. CT scans demonstrate vascular and neoplastic disease of the occipital lobe with remarkable clarity (Figs 18– 19 and 18– 20).

Figure 18–19. Occipital hematoma (arrow) resulting from a bleeding arteriovenous malformation. This lesion produced homonymous hemianopia and headache.

Figure 18–20. CT scans showing bilateral small infarctions of the visual cortex causing a ringlike scotoma in the middle field of vision. *Top:* Axial section. *Bottom:* Magnified view of the occipital cortex. The infarcted areas appear as zones of low density between the splenium and the occipital pole.

THE PUPIL

The size of the normal pupil varies at different ages and from person to person. The normal pupillary diameter is usually about 3– 4 mm, tending to be larger in childhood and progressively smaller with advancing age. Many normal persons have a slight difference in pupil size (physiologic anisocoria). Occasionally there is a marked difference in pupil size in otherwise normal eyes. Mydriatic and cycloplegic drugs work more effectively on blue eyes than on brown eyes. The function of the pupil is to control the amount of light entering the eye to give best visual function under the various degrees of light intensity normally encountered. The pathways controlling this purely reflex function are described below and are diagrammed in Fig 18– 2.

Neuroanatomy of the Pupillary Pathways

The evaluation of the pupillary reactions is important in localizing lesions involving the optic pathways. A knowledge of the neuroanatomy of the pathway for reaction of the pupil to light and the miosis associated with accommodation is very important.

A. Light Reflex: The pathway for the light reflex is entirely subcortical. The afferent pupillary fibers are included within the optic nerve and pathway until they leave the optic tract just before the visual fibers synapse in the lateral geniculate body. They go to the pretectal area of the midbrain and synapse. Impulses are then relayed by crossed fibers through the posterior commissure to the opposite Edinger-Westphal nucleus. Some fibers also go directly ventral to the ipsilateral Edinger-Westphal nucleus. The efferent pathway is via the third nerve to the ciliary ganglion within the retrobulbar extraocular muscle cone. The postganglionic fiber goes via the short ciliary nerves to innervate the sphincter muscle of the iris.

B. The Near Reflex: When the eyes look at a near object, 3 reactions occur: accommodation, convergence, and constriction of the pupil, bringing a sharp image into focus on corresponding retinal points. There is convincing evidence that the final common pathway is mediated through the oculomotor nerve with a synapse in the ciliary ganglion. The afferent pathway has not been worked out, but there is evidence that it enters the midbrain ventral to the Edinger-Westphal nucleus and sends fibers to both sides of the cortex. Although the 3 components are closely associated, it cannot be considered a pure reflex as each component can be neutralized while leaving the other 2 intact— ie, by prism (neutralizing convergence), by lenses (neutralizing accommodation), and by weak mydriatic drugs (neutralizing miosis).

ARGYLL ROBERTSON PUPIL

A typical Argyll Robertson pupil is very suggestive of central nervous system syphilis associated with tabes dorsalis or general paresis. The pupil is less than 3 mm in diameter (miotic) and does not respond to light stimulation. The pupil does constrict with accommodation. The finding is nearly always bilateral. The pupils are commonly irregular and eccentric and dilate poorly with mydriatics. Less commonly, the sign is incomplete (slow response to light) or unilateral. Some degree of Argyll Robertson pupil is present in over 50% of patients with central nervous system syphilis. A wide variety of other central nervous system diseases infrequently cause incomplete Argyll Robertson pupil. These include diabetes, chronic alcoholism, encephalitis, multiple sclerosis, central nervous system degenerative disease, and tumors of the midbrain. The site or sites of the central nervous system lesion are not definitely known.

TONIC PUPIL

Tonic pupil occurs because of an abnormal pupillary constrictor mechanism, in which the sphincter muscle contracts slowly (tonically) to near stimulation and not at all to direct light stimulation. It may be associated with loss of tendon reflexes (Adie's syndrome). It results from damage to the ciliary ganglion. A weak (0.25%) solution of pilocarpine instilled into the conjunctival sac causes a tonic pupil to constrict; normal pupils are not affected. The tonic pupil dilates slowly in the dark and reacts promptly to mydriatics.

HORNER'S SYNDROME

Horner's syndrome is caused by a lesion of the sympathetic pathway in the brain stem, upper spinal cord, or peripheral sympathetic chain. Unilateral miosis, ptosis, and absence of sweating on the ipsilateral face and neck make up the complete syndrome. Causes of Horner's syndrome include cervical vertebral fractures, tabes dorsalis, syringomyelia, cervical cord tumor, apical bronchogenic carcinoma,

aneurysm of the carotid or subclavian artery, neck injuries, and injuries to the carotid artery high in the neck.

EXTRAOCULAR MOVEMENTS

This section deals with the neural apparatus that controls the movements of the eyes and causes them to move simultaneously in tandem up or down and side to side as well as in convergence or divergence.

THE SUPRANUCLEAR PATHWAYS

The supranuclear neural pathways of the extraocular muscles innervate conjugate lateral and vertical gaze as well as the disjunctive movements of convergence and divergence. They consist of central nervous system connections to the nuclei of cranial nerves III, IV, and VI located in the midbrain. The highest centers for these functions are located in the frontal lobe (voluntary or command movement) and the occipital lobe (involuntary or fixation movement).

Anatomy of Voluntary Conjugate Movements

A. Horizontal: The location of the cortical center that controls horizontal conjugate movements of the eyes is situated in the frontal lobe. The pathway descends through the basal ganglia into the brain stem and crosses to the opposite side of the pons. Impulses enter the paramedian pontine reticular formation. The ipsilateral lateral rectus and the contralateral medial rectus muscles are stimulated to produce conjugate movement via the medial longitudinal fasciculus (Fig 18–21).

B. Vertical: The centers and pathways are probably the same as for horizontal movement, except that the subcortical pathway terminates in the pretectal area. The impulses then go to the medial longitudinal fasciculus and are distributed to the appropriate oculomotor nuclei to effect vertical gaze.

C. Convergence: It is probable that the supranuclear impulses for convergence travel much the same pathway as do those for conjugate horizontal and vertical gaze, arriving at a midbrain synapse near or in the oculomotor nucleus. From this synapse, stimulating impulses go to each medial rectus, and inhibitory impulses go to each lateral rectus via the medial longitudinal fasciculus.

D. Divergence: Electromyography has established divergence as an active process (not a relaxation of convergence, as was once thought). The supranuclear pathway is probably more or less the same as for convergence, arriving at a midbrain center near the sixth nerve nuclei. Stimulating impulses go to each lateral rectus and inhibitory impulses to each medial

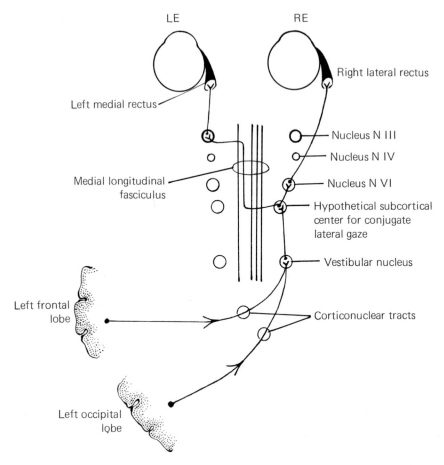

Figure 18–21. Conjugate gaze. The impulses for voluntary conjugate movements in right lateral gaze are initiated in the left frontal lobe. Involuntary conjugate movements in right lateral gaze are initiated in the left occipital lobe or, according to recent reports, the ipsilateral occipital lobe. (After Spiegel and Sommer. Redrawn with modifications and reproduced, with permission, from Moses R: *Adler's Physiology of the Eye,* 5th ed. Mosby, 1970.)

rectus via the medial longitudinal fasciculus as the eyes undergo divergence.

Anatomy of Pursuit Horizontal & Vertical Conjugate Movements

The cortical center is a large ill-defined area of the occipital lobe. The descending pathway is not definitely known, but in general it follows a route similar to the voluntary pathway into the internal capsule, midbrain, and medial longitudinal fasciculus. This pathway carries the impulses of the "following movement" as demonstrated by optokinetic nystagmus. The eyes will "follow" a slowly moving object even when the voluntary pathway is nonfunctioning. When both pathways are intact, the voluntary influence dominates the pursuit influence.

1. LESIONS OF THE SUPRANUCLEAR PATHWAYS

Frontal Lobe

A seizure focus in the frontal lobe may cause involuntary turning of the eyes to the opposite side. Destructive lesions cause transient deviation to the same side, and the eyes cannot be turned voluntarily to the opposite side. This is termed a frontal gaze palsy. Ocular pursuit to the opposite side is retained. There is no diplopia. Exaggerated end point nystagmus can be the first sign of a frontal gaze palsy or may occur as a residuum of a clearing gaze palsy.

Occipital Lobe

Smooth ocular pursuit may be lost with posterior lesions of the hemispheres. The patient is unable to follow a slowly moving object in the direction of the gaze palsy. The command movement is not lost.

2. PARINAUD'S SYNDROME (Pretectal Syndrome)

This syndrome is characterized by loss of voluntary upward gaze and (frequently) loss of the pupillary light response with retention of miosis in response to the near reflex. Nystagmus retractorius, which consists of convergent retraction movements of the globe on attempted upward gaze, is also a feature. There may also be accommodative spasm, a loss of conjugate voluntary downward gaze associated with loss of convergence and accommodation, ptosis or lid retraction, papilledema, or third nerve palsy. Surrounding structures may also be involved depending upon the size and location of the lesion. Conjugate horizontal ocular movements are usually not affected. The syndrome results from tectal or pretectal lesions affecting the periaqueductal area. Pinealomas, infiltrating gliomas, vascular lesions, and trauma may produce this picture.

3. LESIONS OF THE BRAIN STEM

Lesions of the brain stem are the most common causes of gaze palsies. The lesions most often encountered (in order of frequency) are vascular accidents, multiple sclerosis, tumors, and encephalitis.

4. SUPRANUCLEAR SYNDROMES INVOLVING DISJUNCTIVE OCULAR MOVEMENTS

Spasm of the Near Reflex

The near reflex consists of 3 components: convergence, accommodation, and constriction of the pupil. Spasm of the near reflex is usually caused by hysteria, although encephalitis, tabes dorsalis, and meningitis may cause spasm by irritation of the supranuclear pathway. It is characterized by convergent strabismus with diplopia, miotic pupils, and spasm of accommodation.

If hysteria is the cause, atropine, 1%, 2 drops in each eye twice daily, or minus (concave) lenses may give temporary relief. Psychiatric consultation is indicated for treatment of an underlying mental cause.

Convergence Paralysis

Convergence paralysis is characterized by a sudden onset of diplopia for near vision, with absence of any individual extraocular muscle palsy. It is caused by hysteria or destructive lesions of the supranuclear pathway for convergence. Multiple sclerosis, encephalitis, tabes dorsalis, tumors, aneurysms, minor cerebrovascular accidents, and Parkinson's disease are the most common organic causes.

5. SUPRANUCLEAR LESIONS & STRABISMUS

Strabismus is dealt with in Chapter 16, but it should be mentioned here that idiopathic esotropias and exotropias with onset early in life may result from cerebral developmental abnormalities of the supranuclear mechanisms regulating divergence and convergence.

NUCLEAR & INFRANUCLEAR CONNECTIONS

Peripheral & Intermediate Connections of the Nuclei of Cranial Nerves III, IV, & VI

A. Oculomotor (III): The motor fibers arise from a group of nuclei in the central gray matter ventral to the cerebral aqueduct at the level of the superior colliculus. Mainly uncrossed fibers course through the red nucleus and the inner side of the substantia nigra to emerge on the medial side of the cerebral peduncles. The nerve runs alongside the sella turcica, in the outer wall of the cavernous sinus, and through the superior orbital fissure to supply the medial, superior, and inferior rectus muscles and the inferior oblique and levator palpebrae muscles.

The parasympathetics arise from the Edinger-Westphal nucleus just rostrad to the motor nucleus of the third nerve and pass via the inferior division of the third nerve to the ciliary ganglion. From there the short ciliary nerves are distributed to the sphincter muscle of the iris and to the ciliary muscle, which controls the shape of the lens during accommodation.

B. Trochlear (IV): Motor (entirely crossed) fibers arise from the trochlear nucleus just caudal to the third nerve at the level of the inferior colliculus, run posteriorly, decussate in the anterior medullary velum, and wind around the cerebral peduncles. From here the fourth nerve follows the third nerve along the cavernous sinus to the orbit, where it supplies the superior oblique muscle.

C. Abducens (VI): Motor (entirely uncrossed) fibers arise from the nucleus in the floor of the fourth ventricle in the lower portion of the pons near the internal genu of the facial nerve. Piercing the pons, the fibers emerge anteriorly, the nerve running a long course over the tip of the petrous portion of the temporal bone to the outer wall of the cavernous sinus. It enters the orbit with the third and fourth nerves to supply the lateral rectus muscle.

Central Reflex Connections of the Nuclei of Cranial Nerves III, IV, & VI

The central reflex connections of these nuclei originate in 5 areas: (1) From the pretectal region via the posterior commissure to the Edinger-Westphal nuclei for mediation of ipsilateral and consensual light reflexes. Interruption of this pathway may cause an Argyll Robertson pupil. (2) From the superior colliculi via the tectobulbar tract to the nuclei of cranial nerves III, IV, and VI for the mediation of miosis associated with accommodation. (3) From the inferior colliculi via the tectobulbar tract to the eye muscle nuclei for reflexes correlated with hearing. (4) From the vestibular nuclei via the medial longitudinal fasciculus for reflex gaze movement correlated with equilibrium. (5) From the cortex through the corticobulbar tract for mediation of voluntary and involuntary conjugate movements of the eyes.

SUMMARY OF DISORDERS OF CRANIAL NERVES III, IV, & VI

Oculomotor Paralysis (Cranial Nerve III)

A. Complete Oculomotor Paralysis: The lesion involves the third nerve anywhere from the nucleus (midbrain) to the peripheral branches in the orbit. It causes divergent strabismus since the eye is turned out by the intact lateral rectus muscle and slightly depressed by the intact superior oblique muscle. There is a dilated fixed pupil, absent accommodation, and ptosis of the upper lid, often severe enough to cover the pupil. The eye may only be moved laterally. Trauma, carotid aneurysm, and diabetes are the most common causes. In diabetes, the pupillary responses are usually intact; in carotid aneurysm, they almost never are spared.

B. Complete Internal Ophthalmoplegia: This consists of a dilated and fixed pupil and paralysis of accommodation. The lesion is nearly always peripheral in the ciliary ganglion and often results in tonic pupil.

Trochlear Paralysis (Cranial Nerve IV)

Lesions of the fourth nerve are usually traumatic. The nerve is vulnerable to injury at the site of exit from the dorsal aspect of the posterior mid brain stem. Both nerves may be damaged as they decussate in the anterior medullary velum, resulting in bilateral superior oblique palsies. Superior oblique palsy results in upward deviation (hypertropia) of the eye. The hypertropia increases when the patient looks down and with adduction. In addition, there is excyclotropia, and one of the diplopic images will be tilted with respect to the other. Tilting the head toward the involved side increases the deviation. Tilting the head away from the side of the involved eye may relieve the diplopia, and patients frequently present with a head tilt.

Abducens Paralysis (Cranial Nerve VI)

This is the most common single muscle palsy, since one nerve with a long intracranial course supplies one extraocular muscle. Abduction of the eye is absent; esotropia is present in the primary position and increases upon gaze to the affected side. Movement of the eye to the opposite side is normal. Cerebrovascular accidents are a common cause; basilar artery disease, increased intracranial pressure, tumors at the base of the skull, meningitis, diabetes, and trauma are other frequent causes.

Duane's Syndrome

See p 258.

Symptoms & Signs of Extraocular Muscle Palsies

Diplopia occurs when the visual axes are not aligned. This is especially true when the onset of strabismus is after age 6 (suppression and abnormal retinal correspondence do not develop). Dizziness is often associated. Head tilt occurs, especially in paresis of the superior oblique muscle, when the head tilt is to the opposite side to avoid diplopia by moving the eye out of the field of action of the paralyzed muscle.

Ptosis is caused by weakness or paralysis of the levator muscle.

SYNDROMES AFFECTING CRANIAL NERVES III, IV, & VI (Fig 18–22)

Peripheral Involvement of Cranial Nerves III, IV, & VI

A. Gradenigo's Syndrome: This is characterized by pain in the face (from irritation of the trigeminal nerve) and abducens palsy. The syndrome is produced by meningitis at the tip of the petrous bone and most often occurs as a rare complication of otitis media.

B. Cavernous Sinus Syndrome: See p 230.

C. Orbital Fissure Syndrome: All extraocular peripheral nerves pass through the orbital fissure and can be involved by a traumatic bone fracture in this area or by tumor encroaching on the fissure from the orbital or cranial side.

D. Orbital Apex Syndrome: This is similar to the orbital fissure syndrome with the addition of optic nerve signs. It is caused by an orbital tumor or trauma that damages the optic and extraocular nerves.

Chronic Progressive External Ophthalmoplegia*

This rather rare disease involves all 3 extraocular nerves. It is characterized by a slowly progressive inability to move the eyes and very often is associated with severe early ptosis and normal pupillary reactions and accommodation. It may begin at any age and progresses over a period of 5–15 years to complete external ophthalmoplegia. This disease is frequently associated with other abnormalities such as pigmentary degeneration of the retina, deafness, cardiac conduction defects, and peripheral neuropathy. When it is part of a larger constellation of signs and symptoms, it is called **ophthalmoplegia plus,** or Kearns-Sayre syndrome. There is no effective treatment. Cosmetic surgery for strabismus or ptosis is often necessary. Myasthenia gravis is the major differential problem.

---

*"External ophthalmoplegia" is a general term that denotes inability to move the eyes normally as a result of any nuclear or infranuclear involvement of cranial nerves III, IV, or VI; the pupillary reaction and accommodation are normal.

Figure 18–22. CT scans of 4 patients with eye signs of basal cranial tumors. *Upper left:* Optic nerve compression due to thyroid myopathy (black arrows) and meningioma (white arrows). *Upper right:* Sixth nerve palsy due to chordoma of petrous tip (arrow). *Lower left:* Proptosis due to sphenoid ridge meningioma. *Lower right:* Third nerve palsy due to intracavernous aneurysm (black arrow).

NYSTAGMUS

Nystagmus is defined as involuntary, rhythmically repeated oscillations of one or both eyes in any or all fields of gaze. The movements are either pendular, with undulatory movements of equal speed, amplitude, and duration in each direction; or jerky, with slower movements in one direction (slow component) followed by a rapid return to the original position (fast component). The full mechanism is unknown, and the location of the defect cannot usually be specified.

Nystagmus is classified as grade I, present only with the eyes directed toward the fast component; grade II, present also with the eyes in primary position; or grade III, present even with the eyes directed toward the slow component. The movements may be horizontal, vertical, oblique, rotatory, circular, or a combination of these. The direction may change depending upon the direction of gaze. Amplitude refers to the extent of the movement; rate refers to the frequency of oscillation. Generally, the faster the rate, the smaller the amplitude and vice versa.

Known factors relating to ocular movements, malfunction of which can cause nystagmus, are as follows. The labyrinth exerts influence on eye movements by 2 mechanisms: (1) The otolith apparatus influences torsional eye movements in response to head position; (2) the semicircular canals influence eye movements in response to acceleration and deceleration. The gaze mechanism influences the supraconnections of extraocular muscle function (see pp 247–250). These complicated pathways are known in a general but not a complete way. The fixation mechanism also is not completely understood but undoubtedly involves the retina, visual pathways, brain stem, and cerebellum.

Physiology of Symptoms

Reduced visual acuity is caused by inability to maintain steady fixation. False projection is evident in vestibular nystagmus, where past-pointing is present. Head tilting is usually involuntary, to decrease the nystagmus. The head is turned toward the fast components in jerky nystagmus, or set so that the eyes are in a position which minimizes ocular movement in pendular nystagmus. The patient sometimes complains of illusory movements of objects (oscillopsia). This is more apt to be present in nystagmus due to lesions of lower centers, such as the labyrinth, or associated with the sudden onset of nystagmus in an adult. The apparent movement of the environment occurs during the slow component and causes an extremely distressing vertigo, so that the patient is unable to stand. Head nodding is most apt to accompany congenital nystagmus, spasmus nutans, and miner's nystagmus. Nystagmus is noticeable and cosmetically disturbing except when excursions of the eye are very small.

Classification of Nystagmus
A. Physiologic Nystagmus:
  1. End point.
  2. Optokinetic.
  3. Stimulation of semicircular canals.
B. Pathologic Nystagmus:
  1. Congenital–
    a. Sensory defect type.
    b. Motor defect type.
    c. Latent.
  2. Spasmus nutans.
  3. Nystagmus due to neurologic disturbances–
    a. Acquired pendular or jerky nystagmus.
    b. Ocular flutter.
    c. See-saw nystagmus.
    d. Nystagmus retractorius.
  4. Vestibular nystagmus.
  5. Gaze nystagmus.
  6. Voluntary and hysterical nystagmus.

PHYSIOLOGIC NYSTAGMUS

The following 3 types of nystagmus can be elicited in the normal person. Alteration of normal response may be helpful diagnostically.

End Point Nystagmus
A jerky type of nystagmus of small amplitude with the fast component in the direction of gaze commonly occurs in extreme lateral gaze after a latent period of not more than 30 seconds. The nystagmus appears earlier and is of larger amplitude in general fatigue states.

Optokinetic Nystagmus
This is a jerky type of nystagmus which may be elicited in all normal individuals, most easily by means of a rotating drum with alternating black and white lines. The slow component follows the object and the fast component moves rapidly counterwise to fixate each succeeding object. Unilateral or asymmetric hor-

izontal response usually indicates a parietal lobe tumor. Anterior cerebral (ie, frontal lobe) lesions may inhibit this response only temporarily, which suggests the presence of a compensatory mechanism that is much greater than for lesions situated farther posteriorly. Asymmetry of response in the vertical plane suggests a brain stem lesion.

Nystagmus Elicited by Stimulation of Semicircular Canals
A. Bárány Rotating Chair: The horizontal canals are parallel to the floor when the head is tilted 30 degrees forward. Rotation of the subject causes a jerky nystagmus in the direction of the turning. The slow component is in the opposite direction, the same as the flow of endolymph in the semicircular canals.

B. Caloric Stimulation: With the subject supine and the head flexed on the chest, cold water ear irrigation produces nystagmus with the fast component away from the side of irrigation while warm water produces nystagmus with the fast component toward the side of irrigation. (Mnemonic device is COWS: cold—opposite; warm—same.)

PATHOLOGIC NYSTAGMUS

1. CONGENITAL NYSTAGMUS

Sensory Defect Type
Congenital impairment of vision in any part of the eye or optic nerve can result in pendular nystagmus. Causes include corneal opacity, cataract, albinism, posterior polar chorioretinitis, aniridia, and optic atrophy. Oscillations of the head that are synchronous with the nystagmus but in the opposite direction often accompany sensory defect congenital nystagmus.

Motor Defect Nystagmus
This is manifested as a jerky nystagmus on gaze to either side with the fast component in the direction of gaze. The eyes are otherwise normal except when strabismus is associated (20%). There is always a position of relative rest. If this position is with the eyes deviated to one side, the head will be turned toward the opposite side to obtain the best possible vision. This condition shows some spontaneous improvement up to about age 10. The cause is not known, but a lesion of the brain stem is probably responsible. About 20% of cases are inherited as an autosomal recessive trait.

Latent Nystagmus
Latent nystagmus occurs upon occlusion of either eye. The nystagmus is conjugate and jerky, with the fast component toward the side of the covered eye. The condition has no known neurologic significance and is only of consequence when the affected individual loses one eye.

2. SPASMUS NUTANS

This uncommon condition of unknown cause occurs in infants 4– 12 months of age. The nystagmus is of the dissociated vertical or asymmetric horizontal pendular type and is often associated with nonsynchronous head nodding. The prognosis is good; recovery occurs within a few months to 2 years.

3. NYSTAGMUS DUE TO NEUROLOGIC DISTURBANCES

Pendular or Jerky Nystagmus

Acquired pendular or jerky nystagmus is usually horizontal (occasionally vertical) and causes oscillopsia. It is frequently seen in demyelinating disease (occasionally in vascular disease) and is due to a lesion of the brain stem.

Ocular Flutter

Ocular flutter is a sign of cerebellar disease. It consists of a series of rapid to-and-fro horizontal saccadic movements while fixating an object.

See-Saw Nystagmus

This rare type of nystagmus consists of regular reciprocating oscillations in which one eye rises while the other falls. Tumors in the region of the optic chiasm and diencephalon are the most frequent cause.

Nystagmus Retractorius

On attempted upward gaze, convergent nystagmus associated with retraction of the eyes occurs. It is diagnostic of a lesion of the rostral midbrain and is associated with signs of lid retraction, loss of upward gaze (Parinaud's syndrome), and abnormal pupillary reactions.

4. VESTIBULAR NYSTAGMUS

Vestibular nystagmus is always of the jerky type. The slow component is considered to be a response to impulses originating in the semicircular canals; the fast component is a corrective movement. Vestibular nystagmus is not dependent upon visual stimuli, ie, it is present with the lids closed as well as open and can be elicited in blind individuals also. It is inhibited or damped by visual fixation. Rotatory movements are especially characteristic of vestibular nystagmus, but horizontal or vertical vestibular nystagmus also occurs.

Physiologic nystagmus elicited by stimulation of the semicircular canals by means of the Bárány chair or caloric stimulation depends upon normal vestibular function.

The following characteristics of vestibular nystagmus demonstrate its origin in labyrinthine and vestibular nerve disease: (1) Vertigo, tinnitus, and deafness are apt to be associated. (2) Nystagmus is maximal early in the disease and tends to improve or disappear in 2– 3 weeks (unless the vestibular nuclei

are affected directly, in which case nystagmus may be permanent). (3) The lesion is always destructive, and its direction (fast component) is away from the side the lesion is on.

Specific Lesions Causing Vestibular Nystagmus

Vestibular nystagmus may be due to labyrinthitis, Meniere's disease, traumatic (including surgical) destruction of one labyrinth; vascular, inflammatory, or neoplastic lesions of the vestibular nerves; lesions of the vestibular nuclei (encephalitis, multiple sclerosis, syringobulbia, poliomyelitis, thrombosis of the posteroinferior cerebellar artery); or cerebellar tumors and abscesses (probably as a result of pressure on the vestibular pathways). (*Note:* There is some dispute about whether a cerebellar lesion per se can cause nystagmus. Evidence suggests that nystagmus in such cases results from pressure on the vestibular structures. An alternative explanation is that the cerebellar hemispheres exert an inhibitory influence on nystagmus on its own side through the cerebellobulbar tract. Thus a lesion on one side causes nystagmus toward the lesion.)

5. GAZE NYSTAGMUS

Gaze nystagmus is probably the most common nystagmus and often represents the first sign or the residuum of a gaze palsy. These patients have no nystagmus on forward gaze but develop nystagmus in one or more fields of gaze with the fast component in the direction of gaze.

The causes vary and include drug toxicity (especially phenytoin, but barbiturates also) and demyelinating, degenerative, neoplastic, or vascular disease. Gaze nystagmus is of no specific localizing value except that it suggests lesions of the posterior fossa.

6. VOLUNTARY & HYSTERICAL NYSTAGMUS

Voluntary nystagmus is an uncommon "parlor trick." The individual "wills" a rapid horizontal nystagmus of high frequency and low amplitude that can be maintained only a few seconds.

Hysterical nystagmus is similar to voluntary nystagmus. It is particularly common in anxiety neuroses.

CEREBROVASCULAR DISORDERS OF OPHTHALMOLOGIC IMPORTANCE

Vascular Insufficiency & Occlusion of the Internal Carotid Artery

Episodes of amaurosis fugax frequently occur as a result of atherosclerotic lesions of the ipsilateral internal carotid artery. Cerebral and retinal disturbances occur as a result of small emboli breaking loose from the sclerotic plaque and lodging in cerebral or retinal arterioles (occlusion of the central retinal artery or a major branch can occur). These small plaques (Hollenhorst plaques) may be visible with the ophthalmoscope as small glistening yellow spots situated at bifurcations of the retinal arteries. A finding of reduced ophthalmic artery pressure—as determined by ophthalmodynamometry, bruits over the internal carotid artery, and angiography—helps to confirm the diagnosis.

Removal of the plaque by carotid endarterectomy is frequently indicated and may prevent a major stroke or a central retinal artery occlusion.

Occlusion of the Middle Cerebral Artery

This disorder may produce severe contralateral hemiplegia, hemianesthesia, and homonymous hemianopia. The lower quadrants of the visual fields (upper radiations) are most apt to be involved. Aphasia may be present.

Vascular Insufficiency of the Vertebral-Basilar Arterial System

Brief episodes of transient bilateral blurring of vision commonly precede a basilar artery stroke. An attack seldom leaves any residual visual impairment, and the episode may be so minimal that the patient or doctor does not heed the warning. The blurring is described as a graying of vision just as if the house lights were being turned down at a theater. The change seldom lasts more than 5 minutes (often only a few seconds) and may be associated with other transient symptoms of vertebral-basilar insufficiency. Such episodes of visual loss are termed amaurosis fugax.

Occlusion of the Basilar Artery

Complete or extensive thrombosis of the basilar artery nearly always causes death. With partial occlusion or basilar "insufficiency" due to arteriosclerosis, a wide variety of brain stem and cerebellar signs may be present. These include nystagmus, supranuclear oculomotor signs, and involvement of cranial nerves III, IV, VI, and VII.

Prolonged anticoagulant therapy has become the accepted treatment of partial basilar artery occlusion or "insufficiency," but transluminal angioplasty may soon become a common form of therapy.

Occlusion of the Posterior Cerebral Artery

Occlusion of the posterior cerebral artery seldom causes death. Occlusion of the cortical branches (most common) causes homonymous hemianopia, usually superior quadrantic (the artery supplies primarily the visual cortex). Lesions on the left in right-handed persons can cause aphasia and dyslexia. Occlusion of the proximal branches may produce the thalamic syndrome (thalamic pain, hemiparesis, hemianesthesia, choreoathetoid movements) and cerebellar ataxia.

Weber's, Benedikt's, or Parinaud's syndrome may result.

Cavernous Sinus Thrombosis

See p 230.

Subdural Hemorrhage

Subdural hemorrhage results from tearing or shearing of the veins bridging the subdural space from the pia mater to the dural sinus. It leads to an encapsulated accumulation of blood in the subdural space, usually over one cerebral hemisphere. It is nearly always caused by trauma to the head. The trauma may be minimal and may precede the onset of neurologic signs by weeks or even months.

In infants, subdural hemorrhage produces progressive enlargement of the head with bulging fontanelles. The diagnosis is established by the finding of bloody spinal fluid on tapping the subdural space and by enlarged head measurements. Ocular signs include strabismus, pupillary changes, papilledema, and retinal hemorrhages.

In adults, the symptoms of chronic subdural hematoma are severe headache, drowsiness, and mental confusion, usually appearing hours to weeks (or even months) after trauma. Symptomatology is similar to that of cerebral tumors. Papilledema is present in 30–50% of cases. Retinal hemorrhages occur in association with papilledema. Ipsilateral dilatation of the pupil is the most common and most serious pupillary sign and is an urgent indication for immediate surgical evacuation of blood. Unequal, miotic, or mydriatic pupils can occur, or there may be no pupillary signs. Other signs, including vestibular nystagmus and cranial nerve palsies, also occur. Many of these signs result from herniation and compression of the brain stem and therefore often appear late, with stupor and coma.

Skull films may show a shift of a calcified pineal gland. Carotid arteriography frequently confirms the diagnosis.

Treatment of acute subdural hematoma consists of surgical evacuation of the blood. Without treatment, the course is progressively downhill to coma and death. With early and adequate treatment, the prognosis is good except for infants, in whom repeated subdural taps may be only temporarily lifesaving or may result in residual damage (convulsions, low mentality, motor and sensory defects).

Subarachnoid Hemorrhage (Fig 18–23)

Subarachnoid hemorrhage most commonly results from ruptured congenital berry aneurysms of the circle of Willis in the subarachnoid space. It may also result from trauma, birth injuries, intracranial hemorrhage, hemorrhage associated with tumors, arteriovenous malformations, or systemic bleeding disorders.

The most prominent symptom of subarachnoid hemorrhage is sudden, severe headache, usually occipital and often associated with signs of meningeal

Figure 18–23. Subhyaloid hemorrhage around optic disk associated with subarachnoid hemorrhage. (Drawing.)

irritation (eg, stiff neck). Drowsiness, loss of consciousness, coma, and death may occur rapidly. Ocular symptoms are not always present. Extraocular muscle palsies are the most common single ocular sign. An oculomotor palsy with associated numbness and pain in the distribution of the ipsilateral trigeminal nerve is pathognomonic of a supraclinoid, internal carotid, or posterior communicating artery aneurysm. Papilledema usually appears late when it does occur. Various types of retinal hemorrhage occur infrequently (preretinal hemorrhages are the most common). Exophthalmos may occur as a result of extravasation of blood into orbital tissues. Pressure of an aneurysm on the optic nerve may cause blindness in one eye.

Arteriography following injection of radiopaque substances may help to demonstrate and localize the aneurysms. Blood is present in the cerebrospinal fluid.

Ligation of aneurysmal vessels or of parent arterial trunks may be advisable. Supportive treatment, including control of blood pressure, is at times all that can be done.

Migraine

Migraine is a common episodic illness of unknown cause and varied symptomatology characterized by severe unilateral headache, visual disturbances, nausea, and vomiting. It is associated with dilatation and constriction of the external carotid artery and its branches. The neurologic symptoms that usually precede the headache occur in the vasoconstrictor phase; the headache follows in the vasodilative phase. There is usually a family history of a similar disorder. The disease usually becomes manifest between ages 15 and 30. It is more common and more severe in women.

Many factors, particularly emotional ones, may predispose or contribute to attacks. Prodromal symptoms are common and include drowsiness, paresthesias, "scintillating" scotomas, blurred vision, and other symptoms. In some patients, homonymous hemianopia can be accurately recorded on the tangent screen during attacks. There are no other objective findings. Visual symptoms usually last only 15– 30 minutes.

Ergotamine tartrate, when given early in an attack, is often effective. Once the attack is well under way, treatment is of little value. The headaches last from several hours to several days. Bed rest is often helpful if not essential.

MISCELLANEOUS DISEASES OF NEURO-OPHTHALMOLOGIC IMPORTANCE

PHAKOMATOSES

1. NEUROFIBROMATOSIS (Recklinghausen's Disease)

Neurofibromatosis is a generalized hereditary disease characterized by multiple tumors of the skin, central nervous system, peripheral nerves, and nerve sheaths. Other developmental anomalies, particularly of the bones, may be associated. Inheritance is autosomal dominant with incomplete penetrance. Thus, the disease can be quite mild in one generation and appear as a full-blown debilitating disease in the next.

Neurofibromas are made up of randomly oriented or palisaded cells of either fibroplastic or Schwann cell origin. Nerve fibers often course through or over the tumor. The tumors are discrete and benign but may undergo sarcomatous degeneration.

Clinical Findings

Tumors may occur anywhere in the body, including the eye. Café au lait spots (small pigmented areas of skin) tend to enlarge and darken with age. Tumors of the lids are often present. Tumors of the orbital portion of the optic nerve are particularly common, causing papilledema and retrobulbar neuritis early and optic atrophy later in the disease. There may be iris nodules and corneal nerve changes.

Neurofibromatosis of the lid is associated rarely with unilateral infantile glaucoma.

Intracranial gliomas may be associated with neurofibromatosis. Spinal cord neurofibromas frequently occur. The acoustic nerve is the cranial nerve most commonly involved and produces the syndrome of the cerebellopontine angle.

Bone development is affected when the tumor involves periosteum. Pulsating exophthalmos occasionally occurs when an osseous defect of the posterior orbit is present.

Treatment & Prognosis

Orbital or intracranial surgery may be needed to remove tumors for functional or cosmetic reasons.

When lesions are confined to the skin, the prognosis is good. Intracranial and intraspinal lesions are usually multiple and have a bad prognosis. The disease tends to be fairly stationary, with only slow progression over long periods of time.

2. ANGIOMATOSIS RETINAE (Von Hippel-Lindau Disease)

This rare disease occurs most commonly in men in the third decade but can appear at any age up to 60. The earliest signs are dilatation and tortuosity of the retinal vessels, which later develop into an angiomatous formation with hemorrhages and exudates. A stage of massive exudation, retinal detachment, and absolute glaucoma occurs later, and usually destroys the eye within 5–15 years after onset. The disease is unilateral in 65% of cases. In 25% of cases the retinal angiomatosis is associated with a similar generalized process, most often affecting the cerebellum and less commonly the pancreas, kidney, adrenal gland, and other organs. The evidence at present suggests that this is all one genetically determined disease showing autosomal dominant inheritance with variable expression. Several reports of abnormal chromosomal patterns have been reported.

Treatment & Prognosis

Early treatment of retinal lesions with photocoagulation and cryotherapy has been effective in some cases. Cerebral and cerebellar tumors have been successfully removed, but if the central nervous system is involved the prognosis for life is poor. A downhill course and death, usually by middle age, are the rule.

3. STURGE-WEBER SYNDROME

This uncommon disease is recognizable at birth by a characteristic nevus flammeus (port wine stain type of angioma) on one side of the face following the distribution of one or more branches of the fifth cranial nerve. Unilateral infantile glaucoma on the affected side frequently develops if there is extensive involvement of the eye with hemangioma of the choroid. Lid and conjunctival involvement nearly always implies ultimate intraocular involvement and glaucoma. Extensive venous aneurysms in the meningeal sheaths extending into the brain substance account for the high incidence of central nervous system disturbances, of which jacksonian convulsive seizures are the most common. These cranial lesions are on the same side as the skin lesions and usually become manifest within the first decade. Radiographically, calcification in the cerebral cortex is usually present. The disease follows an autosomal dominant hereditary pattern with variable expression. There is at least one study reporting a 22 trisomy on cytogenic study.

Treatment & Prognosis

There is no effective treatment of Sturge-Weber syndrome, although the glaucoma can be controlled in rare cases by cyclodiathermy. Other glaucoma operations have been unsuccessful.

The prognosis for life as well as for sight is poor, with death before age 30 the rule.

4. TUBEROUS SCLEROSIS (Bourneville's Disease)

This is a generalized disease whose manifestations include adenoma sebaceum (85%), central nervous system tumors, retinal tumors (50%), renal tumors (50%), and multiple lung cysts. The signs may be present at birth or may develop within the first few years of life. Onset is with convulsive seizures and mental retardation. The large papular skin lesions have the appearance of overgrown "blackheads" and are often the earliest sign of the disease. The retinal tumors appear as oval or circular white areas in the peripheral fundus and characteristically have a mulberrylike appearance (see Fig 23–12). Histologically, the retinal tumors are composed of hyaline material with areas of calcification.

The disease is inherited as an autosomal dominant with high penetrance. No treatment is available. The prognosis is very poor, with a progressive downhill course and death in adolescence the rule.

AMBLYOPIA DUE TO METHANOL POISONING

Methanol (methyl alcohol, wood alcohol) has long been used as an intoxicating drink, either by mistake or because ethyl alcohol was not available. It may be mixed either accidentally or purposely with ethyl alcohol. Its breakdown product, formaldehyde, can cause severe poisoning marked by gastroenteritis, pulmonary edema, cerebral edema, and extensive retinal damage. There are great individual variations in tolerance; small amounts (30 mL) may cause profound effects in some persons while much larger amounts cause no poisonous effects in others. Significant systemic absorption has been reported from inhaled fumes and, very rarely, through the skin.

There is a marked destruction of the ganglion cells of the retina as well as degeneration of nerve fibers in the optic nerve, occasionally extending well past the optic chiasm in severe cases.

Clinical Findings

A. Symptoms and Signs: Acute symptoms appear within 18 hours of ingestion. Weakness, anorexia, nausea, vomiting, headache, dizziness, Kussmaul respiration, and pain in the back, extremities, and abdomen may occur in succession or almost simultaneously. Extensive exposure will lead to delirium, convulsions, coma, and death.

Visual disturbances range from "spots before the

eyes'' to complete blindness. The field defects are quite extensive and nearly always include the centrocecal area (Fig 18–24).

Hyperemia of the disk is the first ophthalmoscopic finding. Within the first 2 days a whitish, striated edema of the disk margins and nearby retina appears. Papilledema can last up to 2 months and is followed by optic atrophy of mild to severe degree.

Decreased pupillary response to light occurs in proportion to the amount of visual loss. In severe cases the pupils become dilated and fixed. Extraocular muscle palsies and ptosis may also occur.

B. Laboratory Findings: Severe metabolic acidosis results from conversion of methanol→formaldehyde→formic acid. Bicarbonate in extracellular fluid is displaced by the organic acid. Analysis of arterial blood shows a low pH, low bicarbonate, and low P_{CO_2} (from compensatory hyperpnea).

Treatment

If ethanol and methanol are ingested or inhaled simultaneously, the effects of methanol will not become evident until most of the ethanol is excreted. If the patient is seen soon after exposure, gastric lavage should be performed. Acidosis should be controlled with large and repeated doses of bicarbonate. Ethanol inhibits the metabolic oxidation of methanol; therefore, a blood ethanol concentration of 100 mg/dL blood should be maintained until all methanol has been excreted.

Course & Prognosis

Patients with dilated, fixed pupils during the acute attack usually die. If they survive, they have severe visual loss. Patients with retinal edema usually have moderate to marked permanent visual loss. The initial loss of vision shows an early improvement that may be only transitory. Visual improvement occurs only during the first week; if little or no immediate improvement occurs, eventual optic atrophy with very low visual acuity is the rule. Only in mild cases is normal visual function regained.

NUTRITIONAL AMBLYOPIA
(Tobacco-Alcohol Amblyopia)

Nutritional amblyopia is the preferred term for the entity sometimes referred to as tobacco-alcohol amblyopia, tobacco amblyopia, or alcohol amblyopia since they are all the same entity. Persons with poor dietary habits, particularly if the diet is deficient in thiamine, may develop centrocecal scotomas that are usually of constant density. When density of the scotoma varies, the most dense portion usually lies between fixation and the blind spot.

Heavy drinking with or without heavy smoking is most often associated with the poor nutritional state. Occasionally, there is a history of heavy smoking without drinking.

Bilateral loss of central vision is present in over 50% of patients, reducing visual acuity below 6/60 (20/200). Most of the others have severe central loss in one eye with some deficit, often about 6/15 (20/50) visual acuity, in the better eye. Central visual fields reveal scotomas that nearly always include both fixation and the blind spot (centrocecal scotoma) (Fig 18–25). Pallor of the optic disks may be present. Loss of the ganglion cells of the macula and destruction of myelinated fibers of the optic nerve, and sometimes of the chiasm as well, are the main histologic changes.

Chiasmal lesions can cause similar visual field

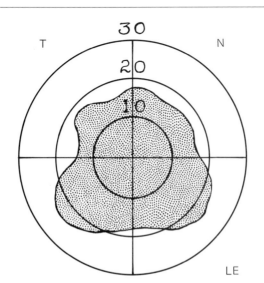

Figure 18–24. Methyl alcohol amblyopia showing very large centrocecal scotoma. VA = hand movements only.

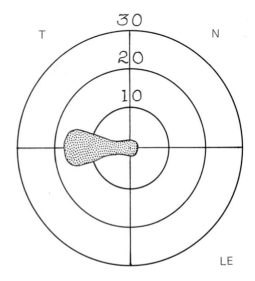

Figure 18–25. Nutritional amblyopia showing centrocecal scotoma. VA = 6/60 (20/200).

changes, but the scotomas generally stop at the midline, allowing differentiation. Rarely, multiple sclerosis, pernicious anemia, methanol poisoning, retrobulbar neuritis, or macular degeneration may cause diagnostic confusion.

Adequate diet plus thiamine, folic acid, and vitamin B_{12} is nearly always effective in completely curing the disease if it is recognized early. Withdrawal of tobacco and alcohol is advisable and may hasten the cure, but innumerable cases are known in which adequate nutrition alone effected the cure despite continued excessive intake of alcohol or tobacco or both. Improvement usually begins within 1–2 months, although occasionally significant improvement may not occur for a year. Visual function may not return to normal; permanent optic atrophy can occur depending upon the stage of disease at the time treatment was started. If there has been neuronal degeneration, permanent dysfunction results.

HERPES ZOSTER
(Shingles)

Infection with herpes zoster virus is characterized by the appearance of vesicles upon the skin in the area of distribution of a nerve. The virus has a predilection for the gasserian ganglion and the first 2 divisions of the fifth cranial nerve. Severe pain over one side of the face may precede by several days the eruption of vesicles on the forehead and eyelids on one side. The vesicles contain clear fluid that rapidly becomes purulent. These rupture, leaving ulcers that usually become secondarily infected and form crusts. Some permanent scarring always results. The eyelids become red and edematous, and there is tearing with scanty discharge. The conjunctiva is red and the cornea shows discrete white subepithelial opacities (involvement of the nasociliary branch of the first division of the fifth cranial nerve). Fine dendritic lesions may occur. Corneal sensitivity is markedly decreased, favoring exposure and secondary infection. The keratopathy lasts several months and may clear with minimal scarring. Complications include secondary glaucoma, iritis, and scleritis. Corneal opacity may persist and markedly reduce vision. Severe, persistent neuralgia may be a late manifestation.

Complete internal and external ophthalmoplegia occurs rarely. Incomplete palsy of the third nerve is the most common type of involvement. Optic neuritis is rare but quite serious, as recovery of function is minimal. Gaze palsies and encephalitis seldom occur.

There is no specific therapy for shingles. Ophthalmologic treatment is directed toward protecting the exposed cornea, combating secondary infection, and lowering the intraocular pressure if there is secondary glaucoma. Antibiotic ointments are used locally. Dilatation of the pupil with homatropine, 2–5%, puts the eye at rest and is particularly useful if iritis is present. Systemic corticosteroids do not help, and there are several reports of death following their administration. Postherpetic neuralgia has been treated with a variety of agents, including the major tranquilizers, with variable reports of success.

The prognosis is good, and recurrences are rare.

NEUROPARALYTIC KERATITIS

Loss of function of the sensory nerve to the cornea (nasociliary branch of the ophthalmic division of the fifth cranial nerve) can lead to trophic changes in the cornea. Punctate epithelial lesions appear first, usually as small vesicles that lead to irritation, photophobia, and ciliary injection. If the process continues, epithelium is lost and a corneal ulcer may develop with secondary infection. Iritis, hypopyon, and, at times, an overwhelming endophthalmitis with loss of the eye can occur.

Neuroparalytic keratitis usually occurs as a complication of section of the sensory fifth nerve root in the treatment of tic douloureux, and it also occurs following herpes zoster keratitis, posterior fossa tumor extirpations, and other rarer conditions.

Protection of the cornea and treatment of secondary infection are the only available measures. Antibiotic ointments should be applied locally, particularly at night. Protective eye shields may be necessary. In well-established cases, suturing the lids together temporarily may be the best way to control keratitis.

MARCUS GUNN PHENOMENON
(Jaw Winking)

This rare congenital condition consists of elevation of a ptotic eyelid upon movement of the jaw. Acquired cases occur after damage to the oculomotor nerve with subsequent abnormal regeneration of nerve fibers. Muscular palsies may be present.

Treatment is surgical. The best results have been obtained by severing the levator muscle completely and then doing a ptosis operation later, utilizing the frontalis muscle.

DUANE'S SYNDROME

This uncommon congenital, stationary, nearly always unilateral condition consists of deficient horizontal ocular motility originally thought to be due to fibrous rectus muscles. Recent evidence based on pathologic studies has determined that Duane's syndrome is a result of congenital absence of the sixth nerve. The lateral rectus is innervated by a branch of the third nerve. Attempted adduction movements result in retraction of the globe and narrowing of the lid fissure. The visual handicap is seldom severe. Visual acuity is normal, and the eye is otherwise normal. Unless the deviation is very large, strabismus surgery is best avoided.

CRANIOSYNOSTOSIS

Under this general heading are grouped a number of rare dysostoses causing distortion of the face and head and having recessive or irregular dominant inheritance. In oxycephaly the sutures of the bones of the face and head close before the brain growth is complete. Continued growth of frontal bone allows for brain expansion, leading to tower skull or other abnormal shapes of the skull. At times the sphenoid bone does not develop properly, leaving an inadequate optic canal and constricting the optic nerve and causing optic atrophy. Increased intracranial pressure may result from the inadequate cranial vault volume. One variant of particular note is gargoylism (Hurler's disease), a form of dwarfism with oxycephaly and hypertelorism (widely spaced eyes). Gargoylism is an autosomal recessive disease due to overproduction of mucopolysaccharides. Acid mucopolysaccharides and glycoproteins are deposited in the cornea, abdominal organs, and central nervous system, causing death before age 20.

WAARDENBURG'S SYNDROME

This rare entity, inherited as an irregular dominant, is distinguished by wide separation of the inner canthi, broad nasal root, heavy eyebrows, heterochromia of the iris, white forelock, and congenital deafness.

MYASTHENIA GRAVIS

This disease, characterized by ease of fatigability of the striated muscles, often is first manifested by weakness of extraocular muscles. Unilateral ptosis is a frequent first sign, with subsequent bilateral involvement of extraocular muscles so that diplopia is often an early symptom. Generalized weakness of the arms and legs, difficulty in swallowing, weakness of jaw muscles, and difficulty in breathing may follow rapidly in untreated cases. There are no sensory changes. The disease is not rare. It usually affects young adults age 20–40, though it may occur at any age.

The onset may follow an upper respiratory infection or an injury and has been noted as a transitory condition in newborn infants of myasthenic mothers. The disease has been associated with hyperthyroidism, collagen disease, and diffuse metastatic carcinoma. Accumulating evidence suggests that an autoimmune mechanism is a significant factor.

The differential diagnosis includes progressive nuclear ophthalmoplegia, brain stem lesions, epidemic encephalitis, bulbar and pseudobulbar palsy, and postdiphtheritic paralysis.

Although substantial neurophysiologic evidence indicates that the site of the disorder is the neuromuscular junction, convincing evidence of morphologic changes has not been presented. It is known that there is insufficient utilization of acetylcholine at the motor end plate. Thymomas have been reported in 25% of myasthenic persons over age 35. About half of patients with thymomas have myasthenia gravis. The 2 diseases must be related, but the mechanism remains obscure.

Cholinesterase destroys acetylcholine at the myoneural junction, and cholinesterase-inhibiting drugs (neostigmine) markedly improve the condition. The edrophonium chloride (Tensilon) test is used in addition to the neostigmine-atropine diagnostic test. Edrophonium, 2 mg (0.2 mL), is given intravenously over 15 seconds. Relief of ptosis constitutes a positive response and confirms the diagnosis of myasthenia gravis. If no response occurs in 30 seconds, an additional 8 mg (0.8 mL) are given. The test is most critical when marked ptosis is present. It is best performed with the patient looking upward, as this most effectively demonstrates improvement in levator action (30–60 seconds after injection).

Neostigmine bromide (Prostigmin) remains the drug of choice in most cases. A typical dose is 15 mg 4 times daily. Pyridostigmine (Mestinon) is also widely used. Topical anticholinesterase drops, especially demecarium bromide (Humorsol), sometimes help with ocular signs, which are often particularly resistant to systemic therapy. Ptosis usually does respond to treatment, but extraocular muscle weakness often does not respond. Thymectomy appears to be of benefit for patients with generalized muscle weakness.

The course of this chronic disease is not steady, and remissions are frequent. During a severe exacerbation, the patient may die from paralysis of respiration.

The prognosis depends to a great extent upon the patients' response to medication and their ability to regulate medication. An intelligent patient, well oriented to his or her disease, can live a normal life span.

CEREBROMACULAR DEGENERATION

Genetically determined (autosomal recessive) neuronal lipid storage diseases of the brain may affect the neural elements of the retina as well. The clinical forms are classified mainly by the age at onset. The pathologic changes are present prenatally, with clinical manifestations occurring as a critical level of intraneuronal lipidosis is reached. A definite diagnosis can be established readily by rectal biopsy or appendectomy showing ganglioside accumulation even before clinical signs are present. Five forms of cerebromacular degeneration (ganglioside lipidosis) are recognized: congenital, infantile (Tay-Sachs), late infantile, juvenile (Spielmeyer-Vogt), and adult.

Severe mental and physical deterioration occurs, usually causing death within a few years. The later the onset, the milder the disease. The liver and spleen show increased gangliosides. The striking ocular finding of a cherry-red spot in the macula is seen in congenital and infantile cases (Fig 18–26). Optic atro-

Figure 18–26. Cherry-red spot of Tay-Sachs disease in an 18-month-old child.

phy and retinal pigmentary changes are frequently present in the juvenile and adult forms. Extraocular muscle dysfunction is a less frequent finding in all forms.

The exact enzymatic abnormalities are still not known, but a deficiency of serum fructose-1-phosphate aldolase is present in carriers as well as affected persons with Tay-Sachs disease.

NIEMANN-PICK DISEASE (Sphingomyelin-Sterol Lipidosis)

This entity is quite similar to the ganglioside lipidoses. There is a deposition of glycolipid in the ganglion cells of the brain and retina. The spleen, liver, and other reticuloendothelial organs are massively infiltrated with glycolipid. Inheritance is autosomal recessive, and 2 clinical forms are recognized. The infantile form is the most common and most severe, with death usually occurring in 2 or 3 years. A cherry-red spot in the macula may be present. The juvenile or adult form is much more benign and usually without eye findings.

REFERENCES

Asbury AK et al: Oculomotor palsy in diabetes mellitus: A clinicopathological study. *Brain* 1970;**93(Part 3):**555.

Balkan R, Hoyt CS: Associated neurologic abnormalities in congenital third nerve palsies. *Am J Ophthalmol* 1984;**97:**315.

Bever CT Jr et al: Prognosis of ocular myasthenia. *Ann Neurol* 1983;**14:**516.

Brown GC, Shields JA: Tumors of the optic nerve head. *Surv Ophthalmol* 1985;**29:**239.

Carroll FD: Nutritional amblyopia. *Arch Ophthalmol* 1966;**76:**406.

Chusid JG: *Correlative Neuroanatomy & Functional Neurology,* 18th ed. Lange, 1982.

Cogan DG: *Neurology of the Ocular Muscles,* 4th ed. Thomas, 1978.

Cogan DG, Lessell S: Neuro-ophthalmology and medical ophthalmology: A dialogue. *Arch Ophthalmol* 1976;**94:**393.

Currie J, Lubin JH, Lessell S: Chronic isolated abducens paresis from tumors at the base of the brain. *Arch Neurol* 1983;**40:**226.

Frisén L: Swelling of the optic nerve head: A staging scheme. *J Neurol Neurosurg Psychiatry* 1982;**45:**13.

Glaser JS: *Neuro-ophthalmology.* Harper & Row, 1978.

Halliday AM, McDonald WI: *Visual Evoked Potentials in Clinical Neurophysiology.* Stalberg E, Young RR (editors). Butterworth, 1981.

Halmagyi GM et al: Downbeating nystagmus: A review of 62 cases. *Arch Neurol* 1983;**40:**777.

Harrington DO: *The Visual Fields: A Textbook and Atlas of Clinical Perimetry,* 5th ed. Mosby, 1981.

Hayreh SS: Anterior ischemic optic neuropathy: Treatment, prophylaxis, and differential diagnosis. *Br J Ophthalmol* 1974;**58:**981.

Hayreh SS: Optic disc edema in raised intracranial pressure. 5. Pathogenesis. *Arch Ophthalmol* 1977;**95:**1553.

Hollenhorst RW: Vascular status of patients who have cholesterol emboli in the retina. *Am J Ophthalmol* 1966;**61:**1159.

Hotchkiss MG et al: Bilateral Duane's retraction syndrome: A clinical-pathologic case report. *Arch Ophthalmol* 1980;**98:**870.

Hoyt WF: Ophthalmoscopy of the retinal nerve fibre layer in neuro-ophthalmologic diagnosis. *Aust J Ophthalmol* 1976;**4:**14.

Huber A: *Eye Signs and Symptoms in Brain Tumors,* 3rd ed. Mosby, 1976.

Leonard TJK, Moseley IF, Sanders MD: Ophthalmoplegia in carotid cavernous sinus fistula. *Br J Ophthalmol* 1984;**68:**128.

Lessell S: Current concepts in ophthalmology: Optic neuropathies. *N Engl J Med* 1978;**299:**533.

Lindenberg R, Walsh FB, Sacks JG: *Neuropathology of Vision: An Atlas.* Lea & Febiger, 1973.

Lowenfeld ID: The Argyll Robertson pupil, 1869–1969: A critical survey of the literature. *Surv Ophthalmol* 1969;**14:**199.

McDonald WI: The significance of optic neuritis. *Trans Ophthalmol Soc UK* 1983;**103:**230.

Miller NR (editor): *Walsh & Hoyt's Clinical Neuro-ophthalmology,* 4th ed. Vol 1. Williams & Wilkins, 1982.

Moseley IF, Sanders MD: *Computerised Tomography in Neuroophthalmology.* Chapman & Hall, 1982.

Moses RA: *Adler's Physiology of the Eye: Clinical Application,* 7th ed. Mosby, 1981.

Moster ML et al: Isolated sixth-nerve palsies in younger adults. *Arch Ophthalmol* 1984;**102:**1328.

Nadeau SE, Trobe JD: Pupil sparing in oculomotor palsy: A brief review. *Ann Neurol* 1983;**13:**143.

O'Brien JF: The lysosomal storage diseases. *Mayo Clin Proc* 1982;**57:**192.

Page NGR, Sanders MD: Bilateral central scotomata due to intracranial tumour. *Br J Ophthalmol* 1984;**68:**449.

Parkin PJ, Hierons R, McDonald WI: Bilateral optic neuritis: A long-term follow-up. *Brain* 1984;**107:**951.

Paul TO, Hoyt WF: Funduscopic appearance of papilledema with optic tract atrophy. *Arch Ophthalmol* 1976;**94:**467.

Perkin GD, Rose FC: *Optic Neuritis and Its Differential Diagnosis.* Oxford Univ Press, 1979.

Quigley HA, Addicks EM: Quantitative studies of retinal nerve fiber layer defects. *Arch Ophthalmol* 1982;**100:**807.

Rush JA, Younge BR: Paralysis of cranial nerves III, IV, and VI: Cause and prognosis in 1,000 cases. *Arch Ophthalmol* 1981;**99:**76.

Spector RH, Troost BT: The ocular motor system. *Ann Neurol* 1981;**9:**517.

Stanbury JB et al (editors): Disorders of lysosomal enzymes. Pages 751–969 in: *The Metabolic Basis of Inherited Disease,* 5th ed. McGraw-Hill, 1983.

Thompson HS: Pupil in clinical diagnosis. (Symposium.) *Trans Am Acad Ophthalmol Otolaryngol* 1977;**83:**847.

Thompson HS: Pupillary signs in the diagnosis of optic nerve disease. *Trans Ophthalmol Soc UK* 1976;**96:**377.

Thompson HS et al (editors): *Topics in Neuro-ophthalmology.* Williams & Wilkins, 1979.

Womack LW, Liesegang TJ: Complications of herpes zoster ophthalmicus. *Arch Ophthalmol* 1983;**101:**42.

Young BR, Sulta F: Analysis of trochlear nerve palsies: Diagnosis, etiology and treatment. *Mayo Clin Proc* 1977;**52:**11.

19

Ocular Disorders Associated With Systemic Diseases

Michael D. Sanders, FRCP, FRCS, & Elizabeth M. Graham, MRCP, DO

Examination of the eye provides the ophthalmologist an opportunity to make a unique contribution to the diagnosis of systemic disease. Nowhere else in the body can a microcirculatory system be investigated with such precision, and nowhere else are the results of minute focal lesions so devastating. Most systemic diseases involve the eyes, and therapy demands some knowledge of the vascular, rheologic, and immunologic nature of these diseases.

VASCULAR DISEASE

NORMAL ANATOMY & PHYSIOLOGY

The blood supply to the eye is from the ophthalmic artery, which is the first branch of the internal carotid artery. The first branches of the ophthalmic artery are the central retinal artery and the long posterior ciliary arteries. The retina is therefore perfused by retinal and choroidal vessels that provide contrasting anatomic and physiologic circulations. The retinal arteries correspond to arterioles in the systemic circulation but are thin-walled, with several layers of medial muscle cells. They function as end arteries and feed a capillary bed consisting of small capillaries (7 μm) with tight endothelial junctions. Dependent on this anatomic arrangement is the maintenance of the blood-retina barrier, and this system is autoregulated, since there are no autonomic nerve fibers. Most of the blood within the eye, however, is in the choroidal circulation, which is characterized by a high flow rate, autonomic regulation, and an anatomic arrangement with collateral branching and large capillaries (30 μm), all of which have fenestrations in juxtaposition to Bruch's membrane. Clinical examination of the retinal vessels is facilitated by the use of red-free light, and fluorescein angiography enables us to obtain information about the dynamic and functional aspects of this circulation.

PATHOLOGIC APPEARANCES IN RETINAL VASCULAR DISEASE

Hemorrhages

Retinal hemorrhages result from diapedeses from veins or capillaries, and the morphologic appearances depend upon the size, site, and extent of damage to the vessel (Fig 19–1). Hemorrhages may be caused by any condition that alters the integrity of the endothelial cells. They usually indicate some abnormality of the retinal vascular system, and systemic factors should be considered in relation to (1) vessel wall disease (eg, hypertension, diabetes), (2) blood disorders (eg, leukemia, polycythemia), and (3) reduced perfusion (eg, carotid cavernous fistula, acute blood loss).

A. Preretinal Hemorrhages: These result from damage to the superficial disk or retinal vessels and are usually large, producing a gravity-dependent fluid level.

B. Linear Hemorrhages: These usually small hemorrhages lie in the superficial nerve fiber layers and hence have a characteristic linear appearance, conforming to the alignment of nerve fibers in any particular area of the fundus.

C. Punctate Hemorrhages: Hemorrhages situated deeper in the substance of the retina are punctate and derived from capillaries and smaller venules. The circular appearance is related to the anatomic arrangement of structures in the retina.

Figure 19–1. Flame-shaped retinal hemorrhages in the nerve fiber layer radiate out from the optic disk. Three days before the photograph was taken, the patient experienced sudden loss of vision, which left him with light perception only.

Figure 19–2. Cotton wool spots. *Left:* Numerous cotton wool spots are seen in the posterior pole in a patient with accelerated hypertension. *Right:* One month after hypotensive treatment. Note resolution of the infarcts.

D. Subretinal Hemorrhages: These hemorrhages are less common because normally there are no blood vessels between the retina and the choroid. Such hemorrhages are large and red, with a well-defined margin and no fluid level. They are seen in relation to the disk and in any condition where abnormal vessels pass from the choroidal circulation into the retina.

E. Hemorrhages Under the Pigment Epithelium: Hemorrhages situated under the pigment epithelium are usually dark and large, so that they must be differentiated from choroidal melanomas and hemangiomas.

F. White Central Hemorrhages (Roth's Spots): Superficial retinal hemorrhages with pale or white centers are not pathognomonic of any disease process but may arise in a variety of circumstances: (1) retinal infarction (cotton wool spot) with surrounding hemorrhage; (2) retinal hemorrhage in combination with extravasation of white corpuscles (eg, leukemia); and (3) retinal hemorrhage with central resolution.

Neuronal Effects of Focal Retinal Ischemia

The funduscopic appearance of arteriolar occlusion depends on the size of the vessel occluded, the duration of occlusion, and the time course. Occlusion of major arterioles produces a total, hemispheric, or segmental pallid swelling of the retina. Occlusion of a precapillary retinal arteriole produces the pathognomonic appearance of a cotton wool spot (Fig 19–2). This consists of a pale, slightly elevated swelling usually one-fourth to one-half the size of the optic disk. Pathologic examination shows distention of neurons, with cytoid bodies (Fig 19–3); electron microscopy shows the accumulation of axoplasm and organelles. Occlusion of arterioles, whether due to intrinsic vessel

wall disease or to intramural factors, may produce these pathognomonic signs.

A. Optic Disk Infarction (Ischemic Optic Neuropathy): Impairment of the blood supply to the optic disk produces sudden visual loss, usually with an altitudinal field defect and pallid swelling of the optic disk. The primary abnormality is complete or partial interruption of the choroidal blood supply to the disk, while the retinal capillaries on the surface of the disk appear dilated. Fluorescein angiography confirms the circulatory alterations (Fig 19–4). Optic disk infarction is often caused by giant cell arteritis in old age and by hypertension and arteriosclerotic disease in middle age.

Investigations should include serum lipids, blood

Figure 19–3. Cotton wool spot. Histologic examination shows cytoid bodies and distended neurons in the superficial retinal layers. Deeper retinal layers are normal. (Courtesy of Professor N Ashton.)

Figure 19–4. Ischemic optic neuropathy. Sudden visual loss in a 48-year-old man produced a complete inferior altitudinal field loss. *Left:* Fluorescein angiography shows impaired filling of the upper part of the disk with dilatation of retinal capillaries at the lower part of the disk. *Right:* Photograph 10 minutes after injection shows leakage of dye mainly at the lower part of the disk.

Figure 19–5. Cholesterol embolus (Hollenhorst plaque). *Left:* A cholesterol embolus at the optic disk, which is refractile and appears larger than the vessel that contains it. A collateral vessel is seen at the lower border of the disk. *Right:* Surgical specimen from a patient with a similar embolus shows an atheromatous ulcer at the bifurcation of the common carotid artery.

glucose, serologic tests for syphilis, and assessment of blood viscosity by hemoglobin, hematocrit, and fibrinogen determinations. Giant cell arteritis merits measurement of the erythrocyte sedimentation rate and temporal artery biopsy on an urgent basis. Corticosteroids are essential in the management of giant cell arteritis, but the results of use of these drugs are equivocal in nonarteritic disorders.

B. Choroidal Infarction: Though the connection has rarely been recognized, certain clinical appearances have been attributed to ciliary vessel occlusion. These include small pale areas in the equatorial region which resolve to leave mottled pigmentary areas (Elschnig's spots) due to necrosis of the pigment epithelium. Larger infarcts may occur, which may be triangular or linear.

C. Retinal Emboli: Transient episodes of monocular visual loss lasting 5–10 minutes are characteristic of amaurosis fugax. Patients often describe a curtain coming down from above or across their vision, usually with complete return of vision within seconds or minutes. Amaurosis fugax is most commonly due to retinal emboli.

Paresthesias in the contralateral limbs localize the disorder to the carotid artery and suggest involvement of the ophthalmic artery and middle cerebral artery. It is important for the ophthalmologist to auscultate the carotid for a systolic bruit and to search the fundus for emboli. Retinal emboli are of 3 main types:

1. Cholesterol emboli (Hollenhorst plaques)– These usually arise from an atheromatous plaque in the carotid artery and consist of cholesterol and fibrin. They lodge at the bifurcation of retinal arterioles, are refractile, and may appear larger than the vessel that contains them (Fig 19–5).

2. Calcific emboli–Originating from damaged cardiac valves, these emboli lodge within the arteriole, producing complete occlusion and infarction of the distal retina. Calcific emboli are solid and calcified and occur in younger patients with a variety of cardiac lesions.

3. Platelet/fibrin emboli–Most cases of amaurosis fugax are probably due to the transit of platelet aggregates through the retinal and choroidal circulations. The emboli are usually broken up as they traverse the retinal circulation and hence are rarely seen, though occasionally they produce retinal infarction. Arising from abnormalities of the heart or great vessels, they may be reduced by drugs that reduce platelet coagulability (eg, aspirin).

Patients with retinal emboli who are under 40 years of age should undergo cardiac studies (24-hour ECG, echocardiogram). In older patients, carotid disease should be suspected, and these patients should undergo digital subtraction angiography.

D. Other Causes: There are several other causes of amaurosis fugax, including factors that induce temporary reduction in ocular perfusion, eg, arterial disease, cardiac disorders, hematologic disorders, and, rarely, elevation of intraocular pressure (Table 19–1).

Table 19–1. Causes of amaurosis fugax.

Retinal emboli	(1) Cholesterol emboli
	(2) Calcific emboli
	(3) Platelet/fibrin emboli
Arterial disease	(1) Carotid artery stenosis
	(2) Carotid artery ulceration
	(a) Bifurcation
	(b) Carotid siphon
	(3) Ophthalmic artery stenosis
Cardiac disease	(1) Dysrhythmia
	(2) Valvular disease, eg, mitral leaflet prolapse
	(3) Left ventricular aneurysm or mural thrombus secondary to myocardial infarction
Hematologic disease	(1) Anemia
	(2) Polycythemia
	(3) Macroglobulinemia
	(4) Sickle cell disease
Other	(1) Mechanical compression of vertebral or carotid arteries
	(2) Hypertensive episode
	(3) Hypotensive episode
	(a) Drugs
	(b) Spontaneous (eg, diabetes mellitus, Addison's disease)
	(4) Arteritis
	(5) Raised intraocular pressure

Central Retinal Vein Occlusion (Fig 19–6)

Central retinal vein occlusion is an important cause of blindness in elderly people, particularly those with hypertension or glaucoma.

Fundus examination shows dilated tortuous veins with retinal and macular edema, hemorrhages all over the posterior pole, and soft exudates. The arterioles are usually attenuated, indicating generalized microvascular disease.

The prognosis for vision is poor. Fluorescein angiography demonstrates 2 types of response: a nonischemic type, with dilatation of retinal vessels and edema; and an ischemic type, which may be followed by the blinding complications of thrombotic glaucoma and retinal neovascularization.

Central retinal vein occlusion has an increased incidence in certain systemic conditions such as diabetes mellitus, hypertension, collagen vascular diseases, and hyperviscosity syndromes (eg, Waldenström's macroglobulinemia, angioimmunoblastic lymphadenopathy). Investigations include measurement of serum lipids, plasma proteins, a glucose load test, and assessment of blood viscosity by hemoglobin, hematocrit, and fibrinogen estimations. If hypertension is present, simple renal function tests, including urea and electrolytes, estimation of creatinine clearance, microscopic examination of the urine, and intravenous urography are indicated.

Treatment of retinal vein occlusion is unsatisfactory. Trials with anticoagulants and fibrinolytic agents have not been successful.

Figure 19–6. Central retinal vein occlusion. *Left:* Photograph shows linear hemorrhages in the nerve fiber layer and punctate hemorrhages in the deeper retinal layers. *Right:* Fluorescein angiogram shows dilatation of the veins.

Occasionally, central retinal vein occlusion occurs in young people and may be associated with cells in the vitreous, suggesting an inflammatory cause. Rheologic investigations are usually negative, and the prognosis for vision is good.

Retinal Branch Vein Occlusion (Fig 19–7)

Occlusion of a branch vein should be viewed as part of the spectrum of central retinal vein occlusion. Investigations are similar in the 2 conditions, but arterial disease—particularly hypertension—is found more commonly in patients with retinal branch vein occlusion than in those presenting with central retinal vein occlusion.

Figure 19–7. Retinal branch vein occlusion. The affected segment of retina shows changes of reduced perfusion. This results in irregularity of the arterioles and veins, areas of capillary closure, and dilated capillaries with microaneurysms.

ATHEROSCLEROSIS & ARTERIOSCLEROSIS

The process of atherosclerosis occurs in larger arteries and is due to fatty infiltration of a patchy nature occurring in the intima and associated with fibrosis. Involvement of smaller vessels (ie, less than 300 μm) by diffuse fibrosis and hyalinization is termed arteriosclerosis. The retinal vessels beyond the disk are less than 30 μm; therefore, involvement of the retinal arterioles should be termed arteriosclerosis, whereas involvement of the central retinal artery is properly termed atherosclerosis.

Atherosclerosis is a progressive change developing in the second decade, with lipid streaks in larger vessels, progressing to a fibrous plaque in the third decade. In the fourth and fifth decades, ulceration, hemorrhages, and thrombosis occur, and the lesion may be calcified. Destruction of the elastic and muscular elements of the media produces ectasia and rupture of the large vessels, though in smaller vessels obstruction is usually seen. The clinical results of atherosclerosis are seen several decades after the onset of the process. Contributing factors to atheroma include hyperlipidemia, hypertension, and obesity.

Arteriosclerosis is characterized by an enhanced light reflex, focal attenuation, and irregularity of caliber. These signs may also be seen in the arterioles of normotensive individuals in middle age. These findings are due to fibrosis and hyalinization as confirmed by fluorescein angiography and histologic examination. In elderly individuals with arteriosclerosis and associated mild hypertension, it is difficult to differentiate the changes of arteriosclerosis from those of hypertension.

Appearance of Retinal Vessels

A normal arteriolar wall is transparent, so that what is actually seen is the column of blood within the vessel. A thin, central light reflection in the center

Figure 19–8. Acute retinal infarction. Red-free photograph shows acute arterial occlusion in a congenitally anomalous vessel at the disk. The inferior retina is infarcted, but axoplasm has accumulated beneath the fovea in an irregular pattern owing to preserved neuronal function of the distal ganglion cells.

of the blood column appears as a yellow refractile line about one-fifth the width of the column. As the walls of the arterioles become infiltrated with lipids and cholesterol, the vessels become sclerotic. As this process continues, the vessel wall gradually loses its transparency and becomes visible; the blood column appears wider than normal, and the thin light reflex becomes broader. The grayish yellow fat products in the vessel wall blend with the red of the blood column to produce a typical "copper wire" appearance. This indicates moderate arteriosclerosis. As sclerosis proceeds, the blood column–vessel wall light reflection resembles "silver wire," which indicates severe arteriosclerosis; at times, even occlusion of an arteriolar branch may occur.

Red-free light (a white light with a green filter) allows details of hemorrhages, focal irregularity of blood vessels, and nerve fibers to be seen more clearly (Fig 19–8).

HYPERTENSIVE RETINOPATHY

A major contribution to the study of hypertensive retinopathy was made by Wagener and Keith in 1939. They placed patients with hypertensive retinopathy into 4 groups (Figs 19–9 to 19–12). Stages I and II were restricted to arteriolar changes with attenuation and an increased light reflex ("copper" or "silver" wiring). The changes are mild, and subsequent observers have experienced difficulty in differentiating between these 2 groups. More emphasis has been placed on stages III and IV, which include cotton wool spots, hard exudates, hemorrhages, and extensive microvascular changes.

Figure 19–10. Keith-Wagener retinopathy stage II. There is irregularity of caliber of the arterioles and focal attenuation. Signs of retinal vascular disease include hard exudates at the macula, a cotton wool patch below the macula, and grooves in the nerve fiber layer beneath the disk, suggesting previous microinfarcts.

Figure 19–9. Keith-Wagener retinopathy stage I. Minimal vascular changes; a nearly normal fundus.

Figure 19–11. Keith-Wagener retinopathy stage III. Marked attenuation of retinal arterioles is apparent, with numerous microinfarcts and a large retinal hemorrhage.

Figure 19–12. Keith-Wagener retinopathy stage IV. This may include the same retinal changes as stage III, but in addition there is disk swelling.

Stage IV is differentiated by the additional feature of edema of the optic disk. This was initially termed papilledema, but clinical and experimental evidence shows that the disk edema is due to infarction and hypoxia of the optic disk, resulting in axoplasmic accumulation and edema (the term papilledema being reserved for disk edema associated with elevated cerebrospinal fluid pressures).

The classification has been of particular value in assessing the prognosis of patients with hypertension. The 5-year survival rate of patients in group I is about 70%; in group IV it is about 1%.

The appearance of the fundus in hypertensive retinopathy is determined by the degree of elevation of the blood pressure and the state of the retinal arterioles. Thus, in young patients with accelerated hypertension, an extensive retinopathy is seen, with hemorrhages, retinal infarcts (cotton wool spots), choroidal infarcts (Elschnig's spots), and occasionally serous detachment of the retina (Fig 19–13). Experimental work on monkeys made hypertensive suggests that ateriolar spasm initially occurs as a response to the high blood pressure and that this is followed by degeneration of the muscle of the blood vessel, with subsequent breakdown of the endothelial cells lining the vessel lumen. Secondary closure of the vessels occurs as a result of infiltration of the wall by plasma and fibrinogen to produce fibrinoid necrosis. The vascular damage is often associated with fibrin degradation products in the plasma, and this may play a part in the vascular changes of accelerated hypertension.

In contrast, elderly patients with arteriosclerotic vessels are unable to respond in this manner, and their vessels are thus protected by the arteriosclerosis. It is for this reason that elderly patients seldom exhibit florid hypertensive retinopathy (Fig 19–14).

Fluorescein angiography has made possible accurate documentation of these microcirculatory changes. In young patients with hypertension, arteriolar attenuation and occlusion are seen, and capillary nonperfusion can be verified in relation to a cotton wool spot, which is surrounded by abnormal dilated capillaries and microaneurysms and demon-

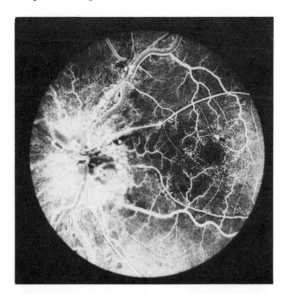

Figure 19–13. Accelerated hypertension. Fluorescein angiogram in a young man showing arteriolar constriction, dilatation of capillaries with microaneurysms, and areas of closure. Marked disk edema is present.

Figure 19–14. Accelerated hypertension. Fluorescein angiogram in an elderly woman showing marked arteriolar constriction and irregularity but few signs of florid retinopathy.

Figure 19–15. Pheochromocytoma. Marked circinate retinopathy with signs of recent retinal infarction and hemorrhages.

strates increased permeability on fluorescein angiography.

Resolution of the cotton wool spots and the arteriolar changes occurs with successful hypotensive therapy. In elderly patients, the underlying arteriosclerotic changes are irreversible.

Other Forms of Hypertensive Retinopathy

A severe retinopathy may be seen in advanced renal disease, in patients with pheochromocytoma, and in preeclampsia-eclampsia. All such patients should receive a complete medical workup to establish the nature of the hypertension, including measurement of 24-hour urinary vanillylmandelic acid excretion and occasionally measurement of blood levels of norepinephrine and selective adrenal angiography in cases of suspected pheochromocytoma (Fig 19–15).

BENIGN INTRACRANIAL HYPERTENSION

Benign intracranial hypertension is a term used to indicate raised intracranial pressure in the presence of normal radiologic studies and normal cerebrospinal fluid. Patients present with headache, tinnitus, and dizziness; obscurations, blurred vision, and diplopia are the ophthalmologic features. Etiologic factors include (1) drug therapy, particularly oral contraceptives, nalidixic acid, tetracyclines, sulfonamides, vitamin A, and prolonged steroid therapy or steroid withdrawal in children; (2) endocrine abnormalities (thyroid or parathyroid); (3) blood dyscrasia; (4) trauma; and (5) middle ear disease. Frequently, there is no obvious cause; in this (idiopathic) group, the

patients are usually young overweight women with irregular menstrual periods. Benign intracranial hypertension is very rare in men, and a thorough search for a precipitating cause is mandatory in these patients.

The cause of the intracranial pressure increase is unknown, although both diminished absorption of cerebrospinal fluid and cerebral edema secondary to abnormality of the cerebral vessels have been suggested.

On examination, visual fields are normal with enlarged blind spots due to gross papilledema. Cerebrospinal fluid pressure is raised and may be as high as 500 mm of water. The aims of treatment are to reduce spinal fluid pressure and prevent permanent visual loss and optic atrophy, which occurs in up to 50% of patients. Treatment includes strict diet, serial lumbar punctures, diuretics (eg, acetazolamide), and occasionally optic nerve sheath decompression or lumboperitoneal shunt procedures.

SUBACUTE INFECTIVE ENDOCARDITIS

Inflammatory changes on the cardiac valves may produce multiple embolization with frequent ocular manifestations. The emboli may arise from vegetations on the cardiac valves and may be composed of platelet and fibrinogen aggregates or calcified endocardial vegetations. Ocular changes therefore are related to transit or obstruction of emboli in the conjunctival, retinal, or choroidal circulatory systems (Fig 19–16). Focal vasculitis due to circulating immune complexes has been demonstrated in the kidney, and similar changes can presumably occur in the eye.

Figure 19–16. Subacute bacterial endocarditis. Calcific embolus impacted in arteriole below the disk, producing a distal area of retinal infarction.

HEMATOLOGIC & LYMPHATIC DISORDERS

PERNICIOUS ANEMIA

Pernicious anemia occurs when lack of intrinsic factor prevents absorption of vitamin B_{12}; the normal intake is 2 μg daily, and normal blood levels are 350 μg/L.

Macrocytic anemia with thrombocytopenia is the classic hematologic abnormality.

Ocular involvement is rare. Retinal and choroidal hemorrhages can occur as a result of platelet deficiency or if the red blood cell count is less than 2.5 million/μL. The paucity of red cells may produce characteristic pallor of the conjunctiva. Optic neuropathy is present in 5% of cases. Ophthalmoplegia occurs rarely.

Treatment is by intramuscular injection of hydroxocobalamin (vitamin B_{12}), 1000 μg weekly for 2 months and monthly thereafter for life.

ACUTE MASSIVE HEMORRHAGE

Complete and sudden permanent blindness occurs rarely following acute massive hemorrhage, most commonly if bleeding is from the gastrointestinal tract or uterus. Such loss of vision is usually due to ischemic optic neuropathy (infarction of the disk). Though common prior to the use of blood transfusion, this type of blindness is rarely seen today.

DISSEMINATED INTRAVASCULAR COAGULATION

Disseminated intravascular coagulation, an acquired coagulation disorder, is characterized by clotting in small blood vessels throughout the body, particularly the renal cortex, heart, and brain. Occlusion of the choroidal vessels occurs, producing hemorrhage, thinning of the pigment epithelium, and serous retinal detachments. The inner retina and its blood supply may be affected in neonates but not in adults.

LEUKEMIA

The ocular changes of leukemia occur primarily in those structures with a good blood supply, including the retina, the choroid, and the optic disk (Fig 19–17). Changes are most common in the acute leukemias, where hemorrhages are seen in the nerve fiber and preretinal layers. Visual loss may occur when the hemorrhage occurs at the macula, and some hemorrhages may have white centers. If the white blood cell count is excessively elevated, retinal evidence of hyperviscosity syndrome (see below) may occur, with dilatation of the retinal arteries and veins, microaneurysms, and deep punctate hemorrhages.

Infiltration by leukemic cells may also occur in the retina, producing irregular pale areas, or in the choroid, causing pigmentary mottling. Infiltration at the optic disk is characteristic of acute lymphoblastic leukemia of infancy, in which blindness usually results.

Figure 19–17. *Left:* Retinal changes in chronic myeloid leukemia, where dilated veins and hemorrhages may be seen. *Right:* In acute lymphoblastic leukemia, infiltration of the disk may be seen.

HYPERVISCOSITY SYNDROMES

Increased viscosity results in a reduced flow of blood through the eye. This produces a characteristic appearance in the fundus of dilatation of the arteries and veins, which appear darker than normal, and retinal hemorrhages, microaneurysms, and areas of capillary closure (Fig 19–18). The main factors that contribute to blood viscosity are the red blood cells and plasma constituents, notably fibrinogen and the immunoglobulins. Polycythemia (high red cell count), either primary or secondary, may produce a hyperviscosity syndrome; the other main causes are macroglobulinemia (high IgM concentration) and multiple myeloma. Reduction of the abnormalities producing hyperviscosity can reverse the retinal changes.

SICKLE CELL DISEASE

Sickle cell hemoglobinopathies are heritable disorders in which the normal adult hemoglobin is replaced by sickle hemoglobin in the red cell. This causes "sickle-shaped" deformity of the red cell on deoxygenation. Various types of sickling are described: sickle cell anemia (SS), sickle cell hemoglobin C (SC), and sickle cell thalassemia.

Ocular abnormalities include conjunctival changes, with "comma-shaped capillaries," and retinal changes, including arterial occlusions, neovascular patterns (sea fan), and extensive capillary closure (Fig 19–19). Vitreous hemorrhage may result from bleeding arising from neovascular membranes, and choroidal occlusive phenomena have also been reported.

MALIGNANT LYMPHOMA

Lymphocytes are now divided into T and B subsets. Lymphomas of T cell origin (eg, Hodgkin's disease) do not usually involve the eye or orbit. B cell lymphomas may be undifferentiated, histiocytic, mixed, or malignant. They characteristically affect the eye and orbit and may be associated with systemic involvement. Orbital involvement may be seen in the conjunctiva, the lacrimal gland, or within the muscle cone. Orbital lymphoma represents a common cause of proptosis in the elderly. Rarely, malignant lymphoma may present as posterior uveitis of the eye, progressing to multiple cerebral lymphomas. Diagnosis may be difficult to make, even with the use of vitreous biopsy, vitrectomy, and sophisticated monoclonal antibody diagnostic techniques.

NEOPLASTIC DISEASE
(Fig 19–20)

Increasing age is associated with an increasing incidence of malignant disease. Thus, the ophthalmologist encounters these diseases more frequently in elderly people and must be familiar with the broad spectrum of their manifestations.

Neoplastic disease may involve the eye and optic pathways by direct spread or by metastatic effects.

The effect of the metastases depends upon the size and site of the metastasis and the site of the primary lesion. The most frequent primary tumor metasta-

Figure 19–18. Hyperviscosity syndrome. Dilated arteries and veins, with hemorrhages and microaneurysms in a patient with hyperviscosity due to elevated IgM levels.

Figure 19–19. Sickle cell disease. Fluorescein angiogram of equatorial "sea fan," with extensive capillary closure peripheral to the fan.

Figure 19–20. Neoplastic disease. *Top left:* Normal fundus of a patient with rapid visual loss in his only eye. *Top right:* Chest x-ray showed left lower lobe consolidation and a hilar mass. *Bottom:* Carcinoma of the bronchus was confirmed at autopsy, and metastasis was found in the optic nerve in the region of the canal (arrows).

sizing to the eye is carcinoma of the breast in women and bronchial carcinoma in men, followed by neoplasms of the genitourinary and intestinal tracts and, less frequently, tumors of the kidney, thyroid, and prostate and malignant melanoma.

Metastatic Effects

A. Conjunctiva: Direct spread may occur from an iris or ciliary body melanoma. Subconjunctival hemorrhage occurs with bleeding disorders secondary to neoplasia (eg, liver failure, disseminated intravascular coagulation).

B. Sclera: Metastatic deposits are rare. Jaundice indicates biliary obstruction (eg, due to carcinoma of the head of the pancreas).

C. Iris, Ciliary Body, and Choroid: Melanoma deposits are common in all of these structures, and metastases from primary breast tumors are often seen in the choroid. These are often multiple, bilateral, and asymptomatic unless situated near the macula. Choroidal metastases probably represent the commonest choroidal neoplasm.

Uveitis sometimes occurs secondary to these metastases.

D. Vitreous: Neoplastic disease associated with immunologic disturbance (eg, reticulum cell sarcoma, carcinoma, lymphoma) may present in patients with posterior uveitis.

Vitreous hemorrhage may occur directly from choroidal or retinal neoplasm or secondary to retinal neovascularization.

Amyloidosis, which may follow slow-growing tumors, produces strands in the vitreous.

E. Retina: Retinal detachment is a complication of choroidal metastases. Retinal vascular occlusion occurs secondary to hematologic abnormalities resulting from distant carcinomas (eg, pancreas, renal cell carcinoma); more rarely, photoreceptor degeneration may occur.

F. Orbit: Direct invasion from lacrimal adenocarcinoma or from carcinoma of the paranasal sinuses and nasopharynx will produce proptosis and painful ophthalmoplegia (known as the orbital apex syndrome due to involvement at the orbital fissure of cranial nerves II, III, IV, and VI). Compression of the optic nerve may produce central scotomas with disk edema or optic atrophy.

G. Extraocular Muscles: Orbital apex syndrome is discussed above. Discrete metastases of the extraocular muscles are rare. Meningeal carcinomatosis may produce nuclear palsies of the extraocular muscles or sixth nerve palsy secondary to raised intracranial pressure.

H. Optic Nerve: Direct infiltration or compression of the optic nerve sheath from metastases or meningiomas results in progressive visual loss and optic atrophy. A carcinomatous optic neuropathy is reported in association with meningeal carcinomatosis when the visual loss is thought to have a vascular cause.

I. Optic Chiasm: Metastatic deposits characteristically present in patients with diabetes insipidus, because the highly vascular posterior pituitary is more susceptible to hematogenous spread of tumor cells. These patients therefore present with bitemporal field defects in addition to polyuria and polydipsia. Symptoms of dysfunction of the anterior pituitary or suprasellar extension to the chiasm may occur later.

J. Optic Tract, Optic Radiation, and Optic Cortex: Neoplasms in this area produce characteristic hemianopic field defects (see Chapter 18). These are associated with different symptoms (eg, temporal lobe epilepsy) according to the site of the neoplasm.

Nonmetastatic Effects

Uveitis occurs in patients with immunologic disturbances.

The myasthenic (Eaton-Lambert) syndrome occurs in patients with bronchial carcinoma and is characterized by fatigable weakness of skeletal muscles and, very rarely, ptosis and ophthalmoplegia. The electromyographic findings are diagnostic: The action potential of the motor unit is reduced in the resting muscle after a single maximal stimulus but increases after 4 seconds of tetanic stimulation.

Cerebellar degeneration occurs most commonly in women with ovarian carcinoma. The characteristic features include ataxia, dysarthria, and nystagmus.

METABOLIC DISORDERS

DIABETES MELLITUS

Diabetes mellitus is a complex metabolic disorder that also involves the small blood vessels, often causing widespread damage to many body tissues, including the eyes.

The ocular complications of diabetes are dependent not only upon impaired carbohydrate metabolism but also upon as yet undefined complexes of factors, and these may occur before the characteristic findings of glycosuria, hyperglycemia, polyuria, and polydipsia become manifest. The ocular complications occur approximately 20 years after onset despite apparently adequate diabetic control. Improved treatment measures (eg, improved insulins, antibiotics) that have lengthened the life span of diabetics have actually resulted in a marked increase in incidence of retinopathy and other ocular complications. Diabetes has become the most common cause of blindness in younger people throughout the world. The visual outlook for adult (maturity onset) diabetics is considerably better than for juvenile diabetics.

The possibility of diabetes should be considered in all patients with unexplained retinopathy, cataract, extraocular muscle palsy, optic neuropathy, or sudden changes in refractive error. Absence of glycosuria or a normal fasting blood glucose level does not exclude a diagnosis of diabetes. Postprandial blood glucose

Figure 19–21. Diabetic retinopathy stage I. Trypsin-digested whole mount showing microaneurysms of the retinal capillaries.

Figure 19–23. Diabetic retinopathy. Fluorescein angiogram shows florid retinopathy of diabetes with extensive areas of capillary closure, dilated capillaries with microaneurysms, and early new vessel formation at the optic disk.

Figure 19–22. Diabetic retinopathy. Fluorescein angiogram shows earliest stage with microaneurysm in the macular region.

Figure 19–24. Proliferative diabetic retinopathy. Fluorescein angiogram shows extensive growth of vessels into the vitreous with marked fluorescein leakage.

determinations and glucose tolerance tests may be required. Rarely, the diabetic ocular change may become evident before there is demonstrable evidence of impaired glucose tolerance.

Retinopathy (Figs 19–21 to 19–24)

Diabetic retinopathy is a common cause of blindness and now accounts for almost one-fourth of blind registrations in the western world.

Metabolic and hematologic factors are important in the development of diabetic retinopathy. Atheroma may be associated, and higher triglyceride and insulin levels are found in diabetics with atherosclerosis. Contributory rheologic factors include elevated blood viscosity and abnormal leukocyte and platelet function. The glycosylated hemoglobin HbA_{1c} increases the affinity of the blood for oxygen and is increased in diabetics to 12% from the normal level of 3.6% of total hemoglobin. The level of HbA_{1c} can be correlated with blood lipid concentrations and provides a measure of the efficacy of treatment.

HLA typing may be important in detecting diabetics who are vulnerable to severe diabetic retinopathy: (1) Increased incidence of HLA-A1 and HLA-B8 occurs in juvenile diabetes with microangiopathy; (2) HLA-B8, when occurring alone, is associated with severe diabetic retinopathy.

The presence and degree of retinopathy seem to be more closely related to the duration of the disease than to its severity. Control plays only a minor role (if any) in the onset, once the process is well under way.

The juvenile diabetic develops a severe form of retinopathy within 20 years in 60–75% of cases, even if under good control. The retinopathy often begins in stage IV and progresses to stage V. In older diabetic patients, retinopathy usually begins in stage I and seldom progresses beyond stage III. Macular degeneration may reduce the central visual acuity markedly in the later stages.

The details of characteristics and treatment of diabetic retinopathy are presented in Chapter 14.

Lens Changes

A. True Diabetic Cataract (Rare): Bilateral cataracts occasionally occur with a rapid onset in severe juvenile diabetes. The lens may become completely opaque in several weeks. The process starts as snow-white areas in the cortex—posterior subcapsular and some anterior subcapsular opacities that progressively involve more and more cortex—which finally become confluent to make the entire lens opaque.

B. Senile Cataract in the Diabetic (Common): Typical senile nuclear sclerosis, posterior subcapsular changes, and cortical opacities occur earlier and more frequently in diabetics.

C. Sudden Changes in the Refraction of the Lens: Especially when diabetes is not well controlled, changes in blood glucose levels cause changes in sugar alcohols of the lens that in turn cause changes in refractive power by as much as 3 or 4 diopters. This

results in blurred vision. Such changes do not occur when the disease is well controlled.

Iris Changes

Glycogen infiltration of the pigment epithelium and sphincter and dilator muscles of the iris may cause diminished pupillary responses. The reflexes may also be altered by the autonomic neuropathy of diabetes.

Rubeosis iridis is common in severe juvenile diabetes. Numerous small intertwining blood vessels develop on the anterior surface of the iris. Spontaneous hyphema may occur. The formation of peripheral anterior synechiae is aided by the vascularization of anterior chamber structures, eventually blocking aqueous outflow sufficiently to cause secondary glaucoma.

Extraocular Muscle Palsy (Fig 19–25)

This common occurrence in diabetes is manifested by a sudden onset of diplopia caused by paresis of an extraocular muscle. This may be the presenting sign and is due to infarction of the nerve. When the third nerve is involved, pain may be a prominent symptom. Differentiation from a posterior communicating aneurysm is important; in diabetic third nerve palsy, the pupil is usually spared. Recovery of ocular motor function usually occurs within a year and frequently within 6–8 weeks. The fourth and sixth nerves may be similarly involved.

Optic Neuropathy

Visual loss is usually due to infarction of the optic disk or nerve. A characteristic telangiectatic pattern is visible at the optic disk in some younger diabetics with sudden visual loss. There is also a form of optic neuropathy that is associated with diabetes insipidus, diabetes mellitus, and deafness.

Figure 19–25. Pupil-sparing third nerve palsy in diabetes mellitus. Sudden painful ophthalmoplegia, left ptosis, failure of adduction, and normal pupillary responses.

GOUT

Inflammatory changes in the eye, as in the joints, are due to the deposition of monosodium urate. This usually occurs in the conjunctiva and episclera, presenting as an acute and uncomfortable red eye. Less frequently, the sclera may be involved, and this can be associated with anterior uveitis, which is responsive to topical corticosteroid and cycloplegic therapy.

ENDOCRINE DISEASES

Disturbances of the endocrine glands have a number of important ocular manifestations. By far the most important of these are due to disturbances of the thyroid gland, although parathyroid and pituitary abnormalities also produce significant ocular changes.

THYROID GLAND DISORDERS

1. GRAVES' DISEASE

The general term Graves' disease has been used to describe patients with hyperthyroidism due to an autoimmune process. Patients with the eye signs of Graves' disease but without clinical evidence of hyperthyroidism are referred to as having ophthalmic Graves' disease. Apart from signs of hyperthyroidism, patients may have pretibial myxedema and clubbing of the fingers, and when these signs occur in combination with the ocular signs, the condition is termed thyroid acropachy.

Sophisticated diagnostic tests provide accurate diagnosis of thyroid disease (Table 19–2). These include the ability to recognize T_3 toxicosis and the ability to assess the hypothalamopituitary axis with the use of the TRH test.

Clinical Findings

Patients may present with nonspecific complaints such as dryness of the eyes, discomfort, or prominence of the eyes. The American Thyroid Association has graded the ocular signs in order of increasing severity:*

Class	Signs
0	No signs or symptoms
1	Only signs, which include upper lid retraction, with or without lid lag, or proptosis to 22 mm. No symptoms.
2	Soft tissue involvement
3	Proptosis > 22 mm
4	Extraocular muscle involvement
5	Corneal involvement
6	Sight loss due to optic nerve involvement

*Abridged classification of the eye signs of Graves' disease (after Werner).

Table 19–2. Thyroid function tests.

	Hyper-thyroid	Hypo-thyroid	Comments
Plasma T_4	+	−	
T_3 resin uptake	−	+	Thyopac technique. Other tests may vary.
Free thyroxine index	+	−	
Plasma TSH levels	−	+	In pituitary hypothyroidism, TSH is reduced.
Response to TRH	Absent	Exaggerated	Absent in pituitary hypothyroidism.
Autoantibodies	May be present	May be present (Hashimoto's)	

T_3 assay: A patient who is clinically hyperthyroid but with normal plasma T_4 may have T_3 thyrotoxicosis and raised plasma T_3 levels; the TRH test will show a hypothyroid response.

Lid retraction may be unilateral or bilateral and may be accompanied by impaired elevation of the eyes. Lid retraction appears to be pathognomonic of thyroid disease, particularly when associated with exophthalmos. The pathogenesis of lid retraction is not completely understood. Some features suggest overactivity of the sympathetic system, particularly the reversal of the retraction following administration of guanethidine eye drops. However, the absence of any pupillary dilatation has led to alternative explanations, and spasm of the striated levator palpebrae superioris muscle has been suggested.

A. Exophthalmos: (Fig 19–26.) The degree of exophthalmos may be extremely variable. Measurements using the Hertel or Krahn exophthalmometer range from minimal (20 mm) to excessive (28 mm or more). The condition is usually asymmetric and may be unilateral, and it is important clinically to assess the resistance to manual retropulsion of the globe. The increase in orbital contents that produces the exophthalmos is largely due to an increase in the bulk of the ocular muscles. Visualization of the ocular muscles is now possible with the advent of the CT scan (Fig 19–26), which can differentiate exophthalmos from an intraconal orbital tumor. In some cases, thickening of the ocular muscles may be restricted to certain muscles only (eg, medial or inferior rectus muscles).

B. Ophthalmoplegia: This is seen more commonly in ophthalmic Graves' disease, which usually affects older people and may be grossly asymmetric. Limitation of elevation is the most frequent finding, and this is mainly due to adhesions between the inferior rectus and inferior oblique muscles. Confirmation may be gained by measuring the intraocular pressure on elevation, when a substantial increase in the intraocular pressure suggests tethering. Often there is mild limitation of ocular movements in all positions of gaze. Patients complain of diplopia, which may be relieved by corticosteroid treatment, may sponta-

Figure 19–26. Thyroid ophthalmopathy. *Left:* Proptosis, visual loss, and ophthalmoplegia occurred in this elderly woman with a history of thyroid disease. *Right:* CT scans showed gross thickening of the ocular muscles, particularly in relation to the orbital apex. The increased intraorbital pressure is producing convexity of the medial orbital wall.

neously return to normal, or, if it remains static for 6–12 months, can frequently be relieved by surgical correction of one or more extraocular muscles.

C. Retinal and Optic Nerve Changes: Compression of the globe by the orbital contents may produce elevation of the intraocular pressure and retinal or choroidal striae. The optic disk may become swollen and progress to visual loss from optic atrophy. Optic neuropathy associated with Graves' disease occasionally occurs as a result of compression and ischemia of the optic nerve as it traverses the tense orbit.

D. Corneal Changes: In some patients, a superior limbic keratoconjunctivitis may be seen, though this is not specific for thyroid disease. In severe exophthalmos, corneal exposure and ulceration may occur.

Pathogenesis of the Ocular Signs

The main feature is gross distention of the ocular muscles due to the deposition of mucopolysaccharides. The mucopolysaccharides are strongly hygroscopic, which accounts for the increased water content of the orbits. There is an increase in the orbital connective tissue, with numerous fibroblasts, and the tissues are infiltrated by lymphocytes and plasma cells.

The pathogenesis of Graves' disease remains unknown, though an immunologic disorder involving both cellular and humoral elements has been implicated. Long-acting thyroid stimulator (LATS) is un-

likely to be of significance in humans, because it is not always found in patients with ocular signs. There has, however, been good correlation between hyperthyroidism and human-specific thyroid stimulator, previously known as LATS protector, although this correlation is not seen in patients with Graves' disease. Thyroid autoantibodies against thyroglobulin and the microsome fraction of thyroid cells are frequently found in Hashimoto's disease and less often in Graves' disease. There are now thought to be 2 pathogenetic components to Graves' disease: (1) immune complexes of thyroglobulin-antithyroglobulin bind to extraocular muscles and produce a myositis; and (2) exophthalmos-producing substance acts with ophthalmic immunoglobulins to displace thyroid-stimulating hormones from the retro-orbital membranes, which results in the increase of retro-orbital fat.

Cellular immunity is also abnormal in Graves' disease. Lymphocytes from patients show increased migration inhibition. The total T lymphocyte count in peripheral blood may be abnormal, and there may be differences in the subpopulations of T cells. Patients with reduced T lymphocyte counts respond well to treatment with corticosteroids, but those with increased counts failed to improve with steroids. The finding of thyroid autoantibodies in a number of patients adds further credence to the immunologic theory of pathogenesis of this disorder.

Treatment

A. Medical Treatment: Medical treatment includes adequate control of the hyperthyroidism as a primary measure. However, thyroid ophthalmopathy may occur in the euthyroid or hypothyroid states. Severe cases with visual loss, disk edema, or corneal ulceration merit urgent medical treatment with corticosteroids in high doses (eg, prednisolone, 100 mg); low doses are ineffective. Plasmapheresis is occasionally used with good results in the treatment of refractory cases of malignant exophthalmos, but full immunosuppression must follow plasmapheresis to prevent rebound increase of immunoglobulins and recurrence of disease. Immunosuppressive agents (eg, azathioprine) may play a supportive role and allow a lower maintenance dose of corticosteroids. In most cases, medical treatment produces adequate control, and surgical decompression is now performed less frequently. Guanethidine (Ismelin) eye drops, 10%, may produce temporary resolution of the lid retraction, which may be useful for cosmetic reasons.

B. Surgical Treatment: The lid retraction may be cosmetically improved by section of Müller's muscle (Henderson's operation) or by a lateral tarsorrhaphy. The latter may also provide some protection for the cornea. Decompression of the orbit may be performed from an intracranial approach (Krönlein's operation) with removal of the superior and lateral walls of the orbit. Currently in favor is antral decompression, in which the inferior and medial walls of the orbit are removed. Finally, if troublesome diplopia persists, ocular muscle surgery is often effective.

2. HYPOTHYROIDISM (Myxedema)

Significant ocular signs are not common in myxedema. Edema of the lids and periorbital tissue is commonly encountered. Thin superficial corneal opacities and small, flaky, white opacities in the lens cortex, neither of which seriously interferes with vision, may be present. Optic neuritis, with eventual optic atrophy and serious visual disability, occurs very rarely.

PARATHYROID GLAND DISORDERS

1. HYPOPARATHYROIDISM

Occasionally at thyroidectomy, the parathyroid glands are removed inadvertently, causing hypoparathyroidism. Spontaneous cases, although rare, should be suspected in young patients with cataracts. The blood calcium decreases, and serum phosphates are increased. Tetany may ensue and can be severe enough to cause generalized convulsions. The ocular manifestations consist of blepharospasm and twitching eyelids. Small, discrete, punctate opacities of the lens cortex develop that may eventually require lens extraction. Treatment with calcium salts, calciferol, and

dihydrotachysterol usually prevents further development of lens opacities, but any that have occurred prior to treatment remain.

2. HYPERPARATHYROIDISM

In hyperparathyroidism, deposition of calcium may rarely occur in soft tissue. "Metastatic" calcification of the cornea and conjunctiva may be an early sign of the hypercalcemia encountered in this disorder.

VITAMINS & EYE DISEASE

Vitamins are organic complexes that are essential for normal growth and maintenance of life. Vitamins A, D, and K are fat-soluble; vitamins B and E are water-soluble. Abnormal intake may produce systemic effects and ocular manifestations.

VITAMIN A

Vitamin A (retinol) is found in fish oil and liver, and its precursor (carotene) is found in plants, vegetables, and cream. The normal daily requirement is 5000–7000 IU, and the normal blood level is 50–70 IU/L.

1. VITAMIN A DEFICIENCY

Symptoms and signs of vitamin A deficiency do not occur until the blood level drops below 50 IU/L. Vitamin A is essential for the maintenance of epithelium throughout the body, and deficiency produces changes in (1) the corneal and conjunctival epithelia (**xerophthalmia**) (Fig 19–27) and (2) retinal function (**night blindness**). Deficiency is due to dietary factors in underdeveloped countries (eg, seasonal, pregnancy) and more commonly to malabsorption in developed

Figure 19–27. Keratomalacia. Case of xerophthalmia in a 5-month-old child.

Figure 19–28. Xerophthalmia. Bitot's spot is seen as a foamy, white, wedge-shaped area with the base at the limbus.

countries (eg, blind loop syndrome, massive gut resection).

Pathology

The conjunctival and corneal epithelia become dry and thickened; under the microscope, keratinized epithelium has replaced the normal columnar epithelium.

In the cornea, there is degeneration of Bowman's membrane and infiltration of the stroma with inflammatory cells and fluid. Yellow spots form in the cornea, and progression may result in hypopyon or perforation.

Clinical Findings

The damaged epithelium may produce dry, irritable eyes and blurred or distorted vision in severe cases. On examination, there are white foamy areas in the conjunctival tissue exposed by the palpebral apertures called Bitot's spots (Fig 19–28).

Xerosis of the corneal epithelium occurs in 2 stages: **prexerosis,** a loss of luster and reduction in corneal sensitivity; and **true xerosis,** an extension of conjunctival xerosis onto the cornea. Microscopic study of the scrapings from Bitot's spots shows large, keratinized epithelial cells with pale, indistinct cytoplasm and fragmented nuclei. The normal columnar conjunctival epithelium is keratinized and squamous. Xerosis bacilli (nonpathogenic diphtheroids originally thought to be the cause of xerosis) are numerous.

In severe cases, perforation of the cornea and subsequent loss of the eye can occur. Bilateral corneal scarring is common.

Night blindness is an early symptom and rarely severe. The fundi are normal, showing no pigmentary change, although yellow spots are occasionally seen in the retinal periphery.

The mechanism of any relationship between vitamin A deficiency and retinitis pigmentosa is not known.

Treatment

Both night blindness and xerophthalmia can be cured with adequate doses of vitamin A (eg, 20,000 IU/d). Recently, topical application of retinoic acid has been beneficial.

2. HYPERVITAMINOSIS A

Vitamin A intoxication has produced benign intracranial hypertension. These patients present with bilateral papilledema that may resolve months after ceasing ingestion.

VITAMIN B

The vitamin B complex is subdivided into 8 groups, but only vitamin B_1 and vitamin B_2 will be discussed here. Pernicious anemia (vitamin B_{12} deficiency) is discussed on p 271.

Vitamin B_1 Deficiency

Vitamin B_1 (thiamine) is found in animal and vegetable matter. The normal daily requirement is 1 mg, and the normal plasma levels are 21 $\mu g/L$.

Deficiency produces **beriberi,** characterized by high-output cardiac failure resulting in pleural and peritoneal effusions; in addition, peripheral neuritis is seen.

Seventy percent of patients have ocular abnormalities. Epithelial changes in the conjunctiva and cornea produce dry eyes and blurred vision. Visual loss with centrocecal scotomas may also be due to optic atrophy, and ocular motor palsies may be seen.

Treatment is by correction of dietary deficiency with liver, whole wheat bread, cereals, eggs, and yeast, or with parenteral injection of thiamine, 50 mg, or parenteral multivitamin preparation. **Wernicke's syndrome** of ophthalmoplegia, ptosis, and nystagmus is usually due to thiamine deficiency associated with alcoholism, although it can occur in other malnutrition states.

Vitamin B_2 Deficiency

Vitamin B_2 (nicotinic acid and riboflavin) is found in animals and vegetables, particularly liver, yeast, and wheat germ. The minimal daily requirement is 12–15 mg.

Nicotinic acid deficiency (pellagra) is quite common in alcoholics and is characterized by dermatitis, diarrhea, and dementia. Ocular involvement is rare, and optic neuritis or retinitis may develop.

Riboflavin deficiency has been said to cause a number of ocular changes. Rosacea keratitis, vascularization of the limbal cornea, seborrheic blepharitis, and secondary conjunctivitis have all been attributed to riboflavin deficiency, but these conditions seldom respond to riboflavin therapy. Optic atrophy is at times caused by ariboflavinosis. Definite riboflavin-deficient conditions respond well to dried (brewer's) yeast, 25–30 g 3 times daily.

VITAMIN C

Vitamin C (ascorbic acid) is found in fresh citrus fruits and green vegetables. The daily requirement is 50–100 mg, and the normal plasma level is 6.32 mg/L.

In vitamin C deficiency (scurvy), hemorrhages may develop in a variety of sites, eg, skin, mucous membranes, body cavities, the orbits, and subperiosteally in the joints. Hemorrhages may also occur into the lids, subconjunctival space, anterior chamber, vitreous cavity, and retina.

Treatment of vitamin C deficiency is with proper diet, particularly adequate amounts of citrus juice. Supplements of ascorbic acid, 200–300 mg/d orally, or sodium ascorbate injection, 0.5–1 g intravenously or intramuscularly daily in divided doses, will help correct vitamin C deficiency rapidly.

VITAMIN D

Vitamin D Deficiency

Children with rickets may develop zonular cataracts due to hypocalcemia.

Hypervitaminosis D

Calcium deposits in the cornea (forming band keratopathy) and in the conjunctiva are the most common ocular changes. Strabismus, epicanthal folds, osteosclerosis of orbital bones, nystagmus, papilledema, sluggish pupillary reaction, iritis, and cataract are less common ocular findings. The incidence of these changes has declined substantially since the content of vitamin D in milk and other foodstuffs has been subject to government regulation.

GRANULOMATOUS DISEASES

Many of the so-called granulomatous infectious diseases, including tuberculosis, sarcoidosis, brucellosis, leprosy, and toxoplasmosis, undergo a chronic course with frequent exacerbations and remissions. The eye is often involved, particularly by anterior uveitis. The following paragraphs deal with other ocular complications of these systemic diseases.

TUBERCULOSIS

Ocular tuberculosis results from endogenous spread from systemic foci. The incidence of eye involvement is less than 1% in known cases of pulmonary tuberculosis.

Tuberculosis of the Uveal Tract

A. Iritis (Anterior Uveitis): Many cases of granulomatous uveitis are said to be tuberculous, although very few cases have been established. At times only the anterior segment of the eye is involved. A few patients develop cells in the vitreous cavity with the picture of central retinal vein thrombosis. This may be associated with a high platelet count and may represent a hypersensitivity "erythema nodosum" reaction in the retina. Local treatment of iritis with mydriatics and corticosteroids is indicated. Systemic tuberculosis therapy is useful in the treatment of established cases of tuberculous uveitis.

B. Miliary Tuberculosis: In this usually fatal form of tuberculosis, many small discrete yellowish nodules are visible ophthalmoscopically in the posterior pole of the eye.

C. Solitary Tubercles: These occur as gray isolated masses about the size of the optic disk in the posterior fundus and usually cause minimal functional disturbance. The tubercles may be the first sign of an impending generalized uveitis. Solitary tubercles are occasionally seen in the iris or ciliary body.

Occasionally, orbital periostitis has occurred because of a tubercle.

Tuberculosis of the Retina

Acute retinal vasculitis may be seen in patients with a positive Mantoux test but without other signs of tuberculosis.

SARCOIDOSIS
(Fig 19–29)

Sarcoidosis is a multisystem disease, with pulmonary, ocular, cutaneous, and reticuloendothelial system manifestations. The pulmonary changes include hilar lymphadenopathy, although pulmonary fibrosis may occur in the later stages. Erythema nodosum is seen in some cases, and sarcoid infiltration of the skin also occurs. Hepatosplenomegaly and lymphadenopathy are important signs of generalized systemic involvement.

Clinical Findings

Enlargement of the parotid glands occurs and, when associated with uveitis, is called **Heerfordt's syndrome.** Enlargement of lacrimal and salivary glands (**Mikulicz's syndrome**) also occurs.

A granulomatous uveitis with large mutton fat keratic precipitates and posterior synechiae is the commonest ocular manifestation. Sarcoid follicles may also be seen in the conjunctiva. Recent reports have suggested that granulomatous involvement of the retina, choroid, and optic disk may be seen more frequently than heretofore recognized. There are also reports that vitreous inflammation and involvement of the pars plana may be due to sarcoidosis. Neurologic sarcoidosis may produce visual loss from optic nerve involvement, and ocular motor and other cranial nerve palsies may be seen.

Figure 19–29. Sarcoidosis. Focal periphlebitis is a feature of ocular sarcoid and responds dramatically to corticosteroids. *Left:* Before treatment. *Right:* After treatment.

Pathogenesis & Diagnosis

The immunologic basis of sarcoidosis is not fully understood, but there is a depression of cell-mediated immunity and hyperactivity of humoral immunity. Lymphopenia is common, and the distribution of T lymphocytes is abnormal. The T cell count in peripheral blood is reduced, although there is some evidence that it is raised in other organs (eg, lungs). There is no correlation between immunologic abnormalities and clinical status. The diagnosis depends on clinical suspicion and confirmation by biopsy. Tissue that has been biopsied includes the conjunctiva, liver, and scalene lymph node. Transbronchial biopsy is a useful technique that confirms the diagnosis in 85% of cases. If biopsy confirmation is not available, the Kveim test should be performed. This test consists of the intradermal injection of sarcoid material and then, after a period of 6 weeks, biopsy of the area, which, if positive, shows a granulomatous reaction with giant cells. Unfortunately, this test is less specific than transbronchial biopsy and is positive in only 20% of patients presenting with uveitis who later develop sarcoidosis. The Mantoux test should also be performed, although it is usually negative. Serum angiotensin-converting enzyme is produced by epithelioid cells, and raised levels may be found in sarcoidosis. This is an excellent test for assessing disease activity but not for diagnosis. Angiotensin-converting enzyme levels may also be high in tuberculosis, leprosy, primary biliary cirrhosis, experimental allergic alveolitis, and Hodgkin's disease.

Treatment

The uveitis is controlled by corticosteroids and mydriatics applied topically. The development of new vessels in the retina merits photocoagulation, in view of their propensity to cause vitreous hemorrhages. The systemic disease is controlled by the administration of oral corticosteroids.

EALES' DISEASE

This disease was originally reported to occur in young men in a poor general state of health who experienced recurrent vitreous hemorrhages from areas of retinal neovascularization. However, such symptoms are also known to occur in sarcoidosis, systemic lupus erythematosus, sickle cell disease, and diabetes. Extensive investigations are therefore indicated to exclude these conditions in patients with consistent clinical features. If test results are negative, Eales' disease is then appropriate as a diagnosis arrived at by exclusion. Photocoagulation of the new vessels can reduce the chance of further vitreous hemorrhage.

LEPROSY
(Hansen's Disease)

Leprosy is a chronic granulomatous disorder caused by *Mycobacterium leprae*, an acid-fast bacillus. It is estimated that 12–15 million people in the world have leprosy and that of this number, 20–50% (2.4 to 6 or 7 million) have ocular involvement. In tropical countries, the infection is endemic.

Three major types of leprosy are recognized: lepromatous, tuberculoid, and dimorphous. The type any given patient will develop depends upon the individual's immunity to the organism and the number of

Figure 19–30. Leprosy keratitis, left eye. (Courtesy of W Richards.)

invading organisms. Thus, a person with minimal or no cell-mediated immunity and in whom the organisms are numerous (multibacillary) develops lepromatous leprosy, whereas a person with strong resistance and few organisms (paucibacillary) develops tuberculoid leprosy. The eye may be affected in any type of leprosy, but ocular involvement is more common in the lepromatous type. Ocular lesions are due to direct invasion by *M leprae* of the ocular tissues or of the nerves supplying the eye and adnexa. Since the organism appears to grow better at lower temperatures, infection is more apt to involve the anterior segment of the eye than the posterior segment.

Clinical Findings

The early clinical signs of ocular leprosy are lagophthalmos, loss of the lateral portions of the eyebrows and eyelashes (madarosis), conjunctival hyperemia, and superficial keratitis (Fig 19–30), with interstitial keratitis—beginning typically in the superior temporal quadrant of the cornea—often supervening.

Scarring of the cornea from interstitial or exposure keratitis (or both) causes blurred vision and often blindness. Granulomatous iritis with lepromas (iris pearls) is common, and a low-grade iritis associated with iris atrophy and a pinpoint pupil may also occur. Hypertrophy of the eyebrows with deformities of the lids and trichiasis are late changes, and exposure keratitis, typically in the inferior and central cornea, can result from facial nerve palsy and absence of corneal sensation.

Ocular leprosy can be diagnosed on the basis of characteristic signs combined with a characteristic skin biopsy.

Treatment

The best drugs for treating leprosy are the sulfones, which are bacteriostatic, and clofazimine and rifampin, which are bactericidal. In multibacillary infections, it is now recommended that the 2 types of drugs be used together. Since the host may harbor the organisms for years, long-term therapy is necessary.

Drug reactions such as erythema nodosum leprosum may require corticosteroids or clofazimine for adequate control. Granulomatous iritis may be benefited by topical atropine and corticosteroids; low-grade iritis with iris atrophy is benefited by topical phenylephrine and epinephrine.

SYPHILIS

Congenital Syphilis

Manifestations of syphilis acquired in utero or at birth include mental deficiency, saddle nose, rhinitis, Hutchinson's teeth, alopecia, exanthemas, deafness, and bone lesions. The most common eye lesion is interstitial keratitis (see p 123). Chorioretinitis unassociated with interstitial keratitis occurs fairly often. There are many small yellow dots and pigment clumps in the peripheral fundus, giving the typical "salt and pepper" appearance. In other cases, the chorioretinitis occurs as larger isolated patches or may have the appearance of retinitis pigmentosa. Syphilitic conjunctivitis or dacryoadenitis is rare.

Congenital syphilis is treated with large doses of penicillin.

Acquired Syphilis

Ocular chancre (primary lesion) occurs rarely on the lid margins and follows the same course as a genital chancre.

Iritis and iridocyclitis occur in the secondary stage of syphilis along with the rash in about 5% of cases. The iritis is acute, with fibrous exudates in the anterior chamber.

Other less common ocular manifestations of acquired syphilis are interstitial keratitis and chorioretinitis, which occur much less frequently in acquired than in congenital syphilis; chorioretinitis usually is widespread and often involves the disk, producing posterior uveitis (Fig 19–31).

Most cases of syphilis can now be diagnosed by the Venereal Disease Research Laboratory (VDRL) or *Treponema pallidum* hemagglutination (TPHA) tests. Further tests include the *T pallidum* immobilization (TPI) test and the fluorescent treponemal antibody (FTA-ABS) test. The latter test can indicate whether a recent infection has occurred. The increasing incidence of syphilis requires the use of these tests in all patients with unexplained uveitis, vitritis, retinal vasculitis, ischemic optic neuropathy, or ocular motor nerve palsies. Treatment consists of systemic penicillin in very high dosage, with systemic corticosteroids.

Neuro-ophthalmologic Considerations

Neurosyphilis may be asymptomatic or may present as meningovascular syphilis, tabes dorsalis, or general paralysis of the insane. **Meningovascular syphilis** particularly involves the base of the brain and may produce cerebrovascular accidents (midbrain or pontine syndromes) or cranial nerve palsies. **Tabes**

Figure 19–31. Secondary syphilis. Bilateral visual loss occurred in a 24-year-old man. Late fluorescein photographs showed disk leakage with dilatation and leakage of peripapillary capillaries.

dorsalis occurs 20–30 years after the initial infection and typically is associated with lightning pains, ataxia, absent deep tendon reflexes, and loss of posterior columnar function. In 90% of cases, there are Argyll Robertson pupils, bilaterally small pupils that fail to constrict to light but constrict normally to accommodation. Optic atrophy is seen in 20% of cases. **General paralysis of the insane** is now an uncommon manifestation and represents progressive loss of cortical function due to chronic meningoencephalitis. Cranial nerve palsies, Argyll Robertson pupils, and optic atrophy are rare features.

When serologic tests and examination of cerebrospinal fluid suggest active treponemal infection, a 21-day course of penicillin should be given.

BRUCELLOSIS

During the chronic stage of this disease, ocular involvement by the endogenous route is fairly common. Iritis is the most frequent ocular complication. The uveitis is not always granulomatous; if nongranulomatous, the inflammation tends to subside in a short time. Less common complications include choroiditis, generalized uveitis, and nummular keratitis, which has the same clinical appearance as epidemic keratoconjunctivitis. These lesions usually heal well but occasionally ulcerate, and they can develop into chronic keratitis with periodic exacerbations and remissions.

Other ocular complications of brucellosis, including scleritis, are rarely seen. Cases of ocular brucel-

losis may respond to tetracycline and streptomycin, although the organism develops resistance easily. The iritis is treated locally by mydriatics. Corticosteroids are sometimes of value locally but are contraindicated systemically.

TOXOPLASMOSIS

This disease is of great ocular importance. The organism is a protozoal parasite that infects a great number of animals and birds and has worldwide distribution. Although there have not been a great many proved human cases, toxoplasmosis is probably the most common cause of posterior chorioretinitis.

Congenital Toxoplasmosis
(Fig 19–32)

Infection occurs in utero, and one-third of infants born to mothers who acquired toxoplasmosis during pregnancy—particularly during the third trimester—will be affected.

The disease is recognized after birth by the typical posterior polar chorioretinitis, which is usually seen in the inactive stage. A number of cases also show cerebral or cerebellar calcification by x-ray, although only a minority show signs of central nervous system disease such as convulsions, mental deficiency, hemiplegia, or paraplegia. The congenital form is nearly always arrested by the time it can be diagnosed.

Congenital toxoplasmosis is perhaps the most common cause of posterior uveitis. A focal choroiditis is seen, usually in the posterior pole, and an active lesion is often related to an old healed lesion. Episodes of posterior uveitis and chorioretinitis usually represent a reactivation of a congenital infection. Rarely, panuveitis may occur, or papillitis progressing to optic atrophy. Isolated anterior uveitis does not occur. Pe-

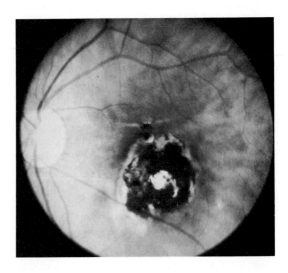

Figure 19–32. Healed toxoplasmic chorioretinitis. Note scarring in left macular area.

ripheral vision is preserved, but because the macula is involved in at least 50% of cases, central vision is reduced.

Treatment with systemic corticosteroids reduces inflammation but does not prevent scar formation. Subconjunctival or retrobulbar injection of corticosteroids is contraindicated, because it may cause severe exacerbation of disease. Clindamycin may be considered in acute cases, although pseudomembranous colitis is an infrequent complication of this treatment.

Acquired Toxoplasmosis

Acquired toxoplasmosis affects young adults and is characterized by general malaise, lymphadenopathy, sore throat, and hepatosplenomegaly similar to that seen in infectious mononucleosis. Uveitis or chorioretinitis does not occur in this disease. Acquired ocular toxoplasmosis may occur in immunosuppressed patients.

VIRAL DISEASES

HERPES SIMPLEX

The most common manifestation of herpes simplex is fever blisters on the lips. The most common and serious eye lesion is herpes simplex (dendritic) keratitis (see p 112). Vesicular skin lesions can also appear on the skin of the lids and the lid margins. Herpes simplex may cause iridocyclitis and may rarely cause severe encephalitis. (Corticosteroids should not be employed in early stages.)

There are 2 morphologic strains of the virus: type 1 and type 2. Ocular infections are usually produced by type 1, whereas genital infections are caused by type 2.

Retinitis due to herpes simplex virus type I occurs in adults suffering from herpes encephalitis or in immunosuppressed patients. Severe occlusive retinal vasculitis develops, followed by retinal necrosis and detachment. Type I antigens have been found in all layers of the retina, pigment epithelium, and choroid. Intravenous acyclovir prevents spread of the disease, and prophylactic retinal buckling may be useful.

Herpes simplex virus type 1, varicella-zoster virus, and cytomegalovirus have all been implicated in **acute retinal necrosis syndrome,** which produces a similar clinical picture but affects healthy young individuals.

HERPES ZOSTER
(See Chapter 18.)

POLIOMYELITIS

Bulbar poliomyelitis severe enough to cause lesions of the third, fourth, or sixth cranial nerve is usually fatal. Any type of internal or external ophthalmoplegia may result in survivors. Supranuclear abnormalities (''gaze'' palsies, paralysis of convergence or divergence) are rare residual defects. Optic neuritis is rarely present. Treatment is purely symptomatic, although occasionally a residual extraocular muscle imbalance can be greatly improved by strabismus surgery.

GERMAN MEASLES
(Rubella)

Maternal rubella during the first trimester of pregnancy causes congenital anomalies, including serious heart disease, genitourinary disorders, and many serious ocular diseases, in about 10% of infants. The most common eye complication is cataract, which is bilateral in 75% of cases. The embryonal and fetal nuclei of the lens are usually opaque, and visual acuity is often below 6/60 (20/200). Other congenital ocular anomalies are frequently associated with the cataracts, eg, uveal colobomas, searching nystagmus, microphthalmos, strabismus, retinopathy, and infantile glaucoma. Congenital cataract, especially if bilateral, may require surgical removal, but the prognosis is always guarded, since other ocular anomalies are often present that may not be recognized until the cataract is removed. Many physicians have felt that therapeutic abortion is advisable if rubella occurs during the first trimester of pregnancy, since the rate of serious congenital anomalies is so high.

Cataract surgery should be delayed until at least age 2, since the live virus is present in ocular tissues for many months after birth. The results of early surgery are unsatisfactory in a very high percentage of cases.

HEPATITIS B

The hepatitis B virus is transmitted primarily via blood transfusion or improperly sterilized syringes, needles, or scalpels. Infections produce a mild acute hepatitis; uveitis with disk edema is a rare complication. The virus has been implicated in the pathogenesis of glomerulonephritis and polyarteritis nodosa via immune complex formation, but there is no evidence for a similar association with idiopathic inflammatory eye disease.

MEASLES
(Rubeola)

Acute conjunctivitis is common early in the course of measles. Koplik's spots can occur on the conjunctiva. There may also be an associated epithelial keratitis.

Interest has recently been shown in the slow virus of measles, which produces an encephalitis (**subacute sclerosing panencephalitis**). Ocular signs include disk edema and macular changes due to neuroretinal involvement. The prognosis is extremely poor.

The treatment of the eye complications of measles is symptomatic unless there is secondary infection, in which case local antibiotic ointment is used.

MUMPS

The most common ocular complication of mumps is dacryoadenitis. A diffuse keratitis with corneal edema resembling the disciform keratitis of herpes simplex occurs rarely. It usually clears completely within 2–3 weeks. Other less common eye complications of mumps include episcleritis, iridocyclitis, choroiditis, and optic neuritis, all of which tend to heal with little or no residual damage. Mumps encephalitis can cause a wide variety of neuro-ophthalmologic abnormalities that may be permanent, including internal and external ophthalmoplegia, pupillary abnormalities, and gaze palsies. Convalescent serum and gamma globulin may help to modify the disease; otherwise, treatment is symptomatic.

CHICKENPOX
(Varicella)

Swollen lids, conjunctivitis, vesicular conjunctival lesions, and (rarely) optic neuritis may occur as part of the clinical picture of chickenpox.

INFECTIOUS MONONUCLEOSIS

Although this fairly common disease is often looked upon as benign and self-limited, there is increasing evidence that significant complications are not rare. The disease process can affect the eye directly, causing nongranulomatous uveitis, scleritis, conjunctivitis, retinitis, or papillitis. Complete recovery is usual, but residual visual loss can result. The central nervous system may also be involved, causing infranuclear muscle palsies, nystagmus, and pupillary abnormalities. No specific therapy is available, although gamma globulin has been used with questionable benefit.

CYTOMEGALIC INCLUSION DISEASE

Infection with cytomegalovirus, a member of the herpesvirus group, may range from a subclinical infection to classic manifestations of cytomegalic inclusion disease. The virus most frequently affects newborn infants and compromised hosts, and the disease can be acquired or congenital. The clinical findings in the newborn infant may include prematurity, hepatosplenomegaly, jaundice, and microcephaly. The ocular findings include focal necrotizing retinitis and choroiditis with perivascular infiltrates and retinal hemorrhages. Other reported ocular findings include microphthalmia, cataract, optic atrophy, and optic disk malformation.

Histopathologic examination of the retinal and choroidal lesion shows large inclusion-bearing cells characteristic of cytomegalovirus infections. There is disruption of the normal architecture of the retina and choroid, with evidence of necrosis and mononuclear and perivascular infiltration. Calcifications in the retina may be observed.

Laboratory studies include isolation of the virus from a fresh urine specimen, from a throat swab, or from a liver biopsy. Serologic tests, complement-fixing antibodies, and indirect FA tests may become positive. The evaluation of cord serum IgM and IgA in newborn infants is helpful as a nonspecific aid in the diagnosis of congenital cytomegalic inclusion disease.

The differential diagnosis in the congenital disease should include toxoplasmosis, rubella, herpesvirus hominis or herpes simplex infection, and syphilis.

No specific therapy has been shown to be effective against this virus. Some agents such as vidarabine and interferon-inducers (poly I:C) may induce a decrease in viruria but do not cure the disease.

FUNGAL DISEASE

CANDIDIASIS

The introduction of modern surgical and immunosuppressive methods of treatment to clinical medicine has resulted in a marked increase in the number of people with compromised immune systems and, therefore, an increase in the susceptibility of these patients to a large number of opportunistic pathogens that were previously considered saprophytes. *Candida albicans* is one of the most important opportunistic fungi.

Many factors are responsible for this apparent emergence of *Candida* as an important opportunistic organism. These factors include the increasing long-term use of corticosteroids and cytotoxic agents, widespread use of antibiotics, abdominal surgery, prolonged use of indwelling intravenous catheters and hyperalimentation, widespread abuse of intravenous narcotic drugs, infusion of glucose solutions, diabetes, debilitating diseases, malnutrition, and malignant diseases.

The ocular involvement accompanies systemic *Candida* infection and candidemia in approximately two-thirds of cases. The initial *Candida* lesion is a focal necrotizing granulomatous retinitis with or without choroiditis, characterized by fluffy white exudative lesions associated with cells in the vitreous overlying the lesion. Such lesions may spread to involve the optic nerve and other ocular structures. Endophthalmitis, panophthalmitis, Roth's spots, papillitis, and exudative retinal detachment may occur. Spread into the vitreous cavity may result in the formation of a vitreous abscess. Anterior uveitis occurs with cells and flare in the anterior chamber, and a hypopyon may form.

Treatment consists of vitrectomy and systemic administration of amphotericin B, flucytosine, and ketoconazole.

ACQUIRED IMMUNODEFICIENCY SYNDROME (AIDS)

Acquired immunodeficiency syndrome is caused by a retrovirus variously known as human T lymphotropic virus type III (HTLV-III), lymphadenopathy-associated virus (LAV), or AIDS-related retrovirus (ARV). The virus infects mature T helper cells, leading to immunosuppression, the severity of which depends on the balance between the rates of destruction and replacement of T cells. The persistent immunodeficiency leads to opportunistic infections. The virus has been recovered from various body fluids, including blood, semen, saliva, tears, and cerebrospinal fluid. It has also been isolated from brain tissue, suggesting potential neurotropism. The viral envelope undergoes continuous structural change, so that antibodies are rendered ineffective and the development of a vaccine is extremely difficult.

The virus is thought to have originated in the green monkey, native to central Africa, and then to have traversed the species barrier. The virus has spread from Africa to many other parts of the world, including Haiti and the USA. So far, 73% of adult cases have occurred in homosexual or bisexual men, 17% in intravenous drug abusers, 3% in recipients of blood or blood product transfusions (1% of these were patients with hemophilia or other blood coagulation disorders), and 1% in persons who have had heterosexual contact with an AIDS carrier or patient. Seventy-one percent of pediatric cases have occurred congenitally in children whose parents had AIDS or were at increased risk for AIDS.

Transmission of AIDS; Prevention

Transmission of the virus is by exchange of bodily fluids during sexual activity or by transfusion of contaminated whole blood or blood products. Use of screening tests for serum antibodies in donated blood and plasma is successfully preventing the virus from entering the blood supply. There is no evidence to suggest transmission by tears or saliva or via casual contact with an infected individual.

The virus can be inactivated readily in vitro by

Figure 19–33. Retinal changes in AIDS. Multiple cotton wool spots *(left)* and retinal necrosis with hemorrhage *(right)* due to opportunistic infection. (Courtesy of R Marsh.)

the use of a variety of common disinfectants, including isopropanol, ethanol, glutaraldehyde, and sodium hypochlorite, or by heat inactivation at 60 °C for relatively brief periods. The Centers for Disease Control has published specific guidelines for preventing possible transmission of the virus in tears.

Little is known as yet about the risk of transmission via corneal transplantation. If the virus is a neurotropic pathogen, this is a possibility; rabies and Jakob-Creutzfeldt disease have been transmitted in this way, presumably by involvement of corneal nerves. Patients may harbor the virus without being symptomatic or having serum antibodies. Thus, although a reliable screening test for serum antibodies is available, neither this nor careful clinical histories, nor even autopsy studies, will necessarily exclude all affected donors.

Clinical Findings

The spectrum of clinical disease is wide, presumably due to the degree of immunologic damage and the frequency and nature of opportunistic infections. Typically, an acute flulike illness occurs a few weeks after infection, followed by weight loss, fever, diarrhea, lymphadenopathy, and encephalopathy some months later. In third world countries, patients often develop tuberculosis, malaria, or bacterial pneumonia.

Ocular involvement occurs in 50–70% of cases. The commonest findings are retinal cotton wool spots and hemorrhages (Fig 19–33). The precise cause of these findings is unknown but may represent immune complex deposition. Opportunistic infections of the retina or choroid may be due to cytomegalovirus (which produces extensive retinal necrosis with severe visual loss), *Cryptococcus*, herpes simplex virus, or the *Mycobacterium avium-intracellulare* complex. In addition, Kaposi's sarcoma affects the conjunctiva.

Treatment

Treatments under study vary in different centers and include antiviral agents and immunomodulators.

MULTISYSTEM AUTOIMMUNE DISEASES

This ill-defined group of diseases is characterized by widespread inflammatory damage of connective tissue with deposition of fibrinoid tissue in the ground substance. There is evidence that an autoantibody reaction against normal tissue antigens produces tissue damage. Ocular involvement is frequent in most collagen diseases.

SYSTEMIC LUPUS ERYTHEMATOSUS

Discoid lupus erythematosus is localized to the skin region on either side of the nose, conforming to the characteristic "butterfly" distribution. There are no generalized features.

Systemic or disseminated lupus erythematosus is a multisystem disease including "butterfly skin lesions," pericarditis, Raynaud's phenomenon, renal involvement, arthritis, anemia, and central nervous system signs. Almost any ocular structure can be involved, but scleritis, conjunctivitis, and keratoconjunctivitis sicca (in 25% of cases) are predominant. Uveitis rarely occurs, and retinal involvement produces signs of arteriolar occlusion, probably a manifestation of arteritis. The fundus picture may be complicated by a hypertensive retinopathy, which in severe cases can cause capillary occlusion or even proliferative retinopathy.

Pathogenesis & Diagnosis

The disease is an immunologic disorder marked by the presence of circulating immune complexes. Diagnostic tests include anti-DNA antibodies and mitochondrial type V antibodies. Active disease is associated with raised circulating immune complexes and reduced fractions of complement.

Treatment

Systemic steroids and sometimes immunosuppressives may be very effective therapeutically.

DERMATOMYOSITIS

This rare disease occurs frequently in children. Characteristically there is a degenerative subacute inflammation of the muscles, sometimes including the extraocular muscles. The lids are commonly a part of the generalized dermal involvement and may show marked swelling and erythema. Retinopathy—consisting of multiple white, irregular opacities appearing much like cotton wool patches—as well as flame-shaped hemorrhages may occur. High doses of systemic corticosteroids will frequently effect a remission that continues even after cessation of therapy. The ultimate prognosis is poor, however.

SCLERODERMA

This rare chronic disease is characterized by widespread alterations in the collagenous tissues of the mucosa, bones, muscles, skin, and internal organs. Men and women between 15 and 45 years of age are affected. The skin in local areas becomes tense and "leathery," and the process may spread to involve large areas of the limbs, rendering them virtually immobile. The skin of the eyelids is often involved. Iritis and cataract occur less frequently. Retinopathy similar to lupus erythematosus and dermatomyositis may be

Figure 19–34. Polyarteritis nodosa. Bilateral sixth nerve palsies.

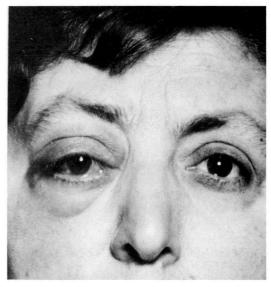

Figure 19–35. Classic Wegener's granulomatosis with proptosis, ptosis, and ophthalmoplegia. The condition has remained static for 10 years with use of corticosteroids and cyclophosphamide.

present. Systemic corticosteroid treatment has improved the prognosis substantially, and retinopathy usually improves or disappears.

POLYARTERITIS NODOSA

This collagen disease affects the medium-sized arteries, most commonly in men. There is intense inflammation of all the muscle layers of the arteries, with fibrinoid necrosis. The main clinical features are fever of unknown origin, weight loss, nephritis, hypertension, acute abdominal symptoms, pulmonary signs, peripheral neuropathy, and muscle pain with wasting. Cardiac involvement is common, although death is usually caused by renal dysfunction.

Ocular changes are seen in 20% of cases and consist of episcleritis and scleritis. When the limbal vessels are involved, guttering of the peripheral cornea may occur. The commonest ocular signs are seen in the retinal circulation, where cotton wool spots and hemorrhages reflect retinal arteritis. The central artery may be involved, and if the disk vessels are affected, disk edema results. Ophthalmoplegia may result from arteritis of the vasa nervorum (Fig 19–34). Systemic corticosteroids are of some value, but the long-term prognosis is uniformly bad.

WEGENER'S GRANULOMATOSIS

This granulomatous process shares certain clinical features with polyarteritis nodosa. The 3 diagnostic criteria are (1) necrotizing granulomatous lesions of the respiratory tract, (2) generalized necrotizing arteritis, and (3) renal involvement with necrotizing glomerulitis.

There is a spectrum of disease ranging from classic Wegener's granulomatosis, with the 3 features described above, to a more benign form, termed necrotizing sarcoidal granulomatosis.

Ocular complications occur in 50% of cases, and proptosis owing to orbital granulomatous involvement occurs with associated ocular muscle or optic nerve involvement (Fig 19–35). If the vasculitis affects the eye, conjunctivitis, episcleritis, scleritis, uveitis, and retinal vasculitis may occur. Nasolacrimal duct obstruction is a rare complication.

It has been suggested that there is a partial cell-mediated immunodeficiency, and therapy with combined corticosteroids and immunosuppressives (particularly cyclophosphamide) often produces a satisfactory response.

RHEUMATOID ARTHRITIS

Rheumatoid arthritis is a disease of middle and old age and is 3 times more common in women than in men. Uveitis is a rare complication, but scleritis and episcleritis are comparatively common. The scleritis may herald exacerbation of the systemic disease, tends to occur with widespread vasculitis, and may lead to scleromalacia perforans.

Corticosteroid drops are helpful in episcleritis or anterior uveitis, but systemic treatment (corticosteroids plus indomethacin or phenylbutazone) is necessary for scleritis. Operative procedures (subconjunctival injection, scleral biopsy) on the sclera are contraindicated, since risks are involved. Keratoconjunctivitis sicca is present in 15% of cases.

JUVENILE RHEUMATOID ARTHRITIS
(Still's Disease)

Ocular complications occur 3 times more frequently in girls, and particularly when few joints are affected, of which the knee is the most common. The systemic disease appears to be disproportionately mild in children with severe visual loss, and diagnosis and treatment may therefore be delayed. Ocular involvement may occur before joint involvement. A chronic insidious uveitis with a high incidence of anterior segment complications develops (eg, posterior synechiae, cataract, secondary glaucoma, band-shaped keratopathy). Antinuclear antibodies are positive in 88% of patients with juvenile rheumatoid arthritis who develop uveitis, whereas they are positive in only 30% of the group as a whole.

SJÖGREN'S SYNDROME

Sjögren's syndrome is a systemic disorder with diverse features. The disease is characterized by the clinical triad of keratoconjunctivitis sicca (see p 73), xerostomia or dryness of the mouth, and a connective tissue disease, usually rheumatoid arthritis. It is more common in females. The onset of ocular symptoms occurs most frequently during the fourth, fifth, and sixth decades. Lymphoid proliferation is a prominent feature of Sjögren's syndrome and may involve the kidneys, the lungs, or the liver, causing renal tubular acidosis, pulmonary fibrosis, or liver cirrhosis. Lymphoreticular malignant disease such as reticulum cell sarcoma may complicate the benign course of Sjögren's syndrome many years after the onset.

The histopathologic changes of the lacrimal glands consist of lymphocytic infiltration and occasional plasma cells leading to atrophy and destruction of the glandular structures. These changes are part of the generalized polyglandular affection in Sjögren's syndrome, resulting in dryness of the eyes, mouth, skin, and mucous membranes.

Because of the relative inaccessibility of the lacrimal gland, the labial salivary gland biopsy serves as an important diagnostic procedure in patients with suspected Sjögren's syndrome.

The tear lysozyme level is absent or reduced in over 90% of patients.

Tubuloreticular viruslike structures resembling the unenveloped nucleocapsids of paramyxovirus have been observed in the renal biopsy and in the capillary endothelial cells and infiltrating lymphocytes of the labial salivary glands in patients with Sjögren's syndrome. Although the pathogenesis is not yet clear, there is increasing evidence that immunologic and viral factors interact in a susceptible host to account for the disease process.

ANKYLOSING SPONDYLITIS

Ankylosing spondylitis is a disease occurring mainly in men 16–40 years of age. There is almost always uveitis occurring at some stage in the disease, which is intermittent, exudative, and may be accompanied by scleritis. There is a strong association with HLA-B27. There is an antigenic cross-reactivity between HLA-B27 and *Klebsiella pneumoniae*, and active uveitis in ankylosing spondylitis patients is associated with the presence of this organism in the feces.

REITER'S DISEASE

The diagnosis of Reiter's disease is based on a triad of signs that includes urethritis, conjunctivitis, and arthritis. Scleritis, keratitis, and uveitis may also be seen in addition to conjunctivitis. The disease has a high correlation with HLA-B27 antigen.

BEHÇET'S DISEASE

Behçet's disease consists of the clinical triad of relapsing iritis and aphthous and genital ulceration (Fig 19–36). Ocular signs occur in 75% of cases; the uveitis is severe, occasionally associated with hypopyon. Posterior uveitis is common, and retinal periphlebitis and papillitis may occur. Treatment is difficult, and the prognosis is poor. Systemic corticosteroids and azathioprine or chlorambucil constitute the most satisfactory regimen, but cyclosporine may also be beneficial.

Exacerbation of the disease coincides with a raised erythrocyte sedimentation rate, raised IgG (with fall in IgA in the acute phase and a later rise of IgA in the convalescent phase), and raised C9 levels with C-reactive protein. Fibrinolytic studies may also be abnormal, particularly in patients developing major vein thrombosis and retinal vein thrombosis.

Figure 19–36. Behçet's disease. Clinical features include oral and genital ulcers. Ocular features include increased capillary permeability and areas of retinal ischemia and infiltration. Marked leakage of capillaries is seen in the late stages of fluorescein angiography *(bottom right).*

UVEITIS WITH INFLAMMATORY BOWEL DISEASE

Scleral, episcleral, and uveal tract involvement may be seen in both ulcerative colitis and Crohn's disease. Conversely, bowel symptoms may be seen in patients with ankylosing spondylitis.

HUMAN LEUKOCYTE ANTIGENS

Histocompatability antigens are unique markers on the surfaces of all nucleated cells. The human leukocyte A system is the major group of such antigens.

The genes responsible for the formation of these antigens are found in 5 adjacent loci on each of the pair of chromosome 6. Therefore, each cell in a heterozygous individual can contain up to 10 different antigens.

The 5 loci are named A, B, C, D, and DR. Humoral antibodies that can be detected by serologic methods are bound to antigens at loci A, B, and C. Cross-reactivity occurs when an antiserum to one particular antigen reacts weakly with another antiserum. This may account for some of the associations of specific disorders with different HLA antigens. The antigen controlled by locus D can be detected by mixed lymphocyte culture when donor lymphocytes are incubated with lymphocytes of the proposed recipient and blastic transformation and division occur.

Some groups of HLA appear to be inherited together, eg, HLA-A8, HLA-B1, and HLA-Dw3, and are called haplotypes. This occurs because the different antigens are close together on a gene and therefore inherited "en bloc." This phenomenon is called linkage disequilibrium, because there is a reduction in the normal genetic transfer that occurs during meiosis.

The association between different HLA haplotypes (ie, different HLA groups inherited together) and specific diseases is well known. Ninety percent of people with ankylosing spondylitis have HLA-B27. A person with HLA-B27 is 100 times more likely to develop ankylosing spondylitis than a person without this haplotype. However, only 5% of people who do possess HLA-B27 actually develop ankylosing spondylitis.

Other associations are listed in Table 19–3.

The HLA-D–related (HLA-DR) locus is the most important in immunologically mediated conditions; it codes for class II cell surface antigens that are expressed on a restricted population of cells, including macrophages, activated T cells, B cells, and vascular endothelial cells and thymocytes.

The serum level of other immunoregulatory proteins is also genetically determined and may indicate disease susceptibility (eg, α_1-antitrypsin levels are increased in patients with retinal vasculitis).

HERITABLE CONNECTIVE TISSUE DISEASES

MARFAN'S SYNDROME (Arachnodactyly) (Fig 19–37)

The most striking feature of this rare syndrome is increased length of the long bones, particularly of the fingers and toes. Other characteristics include scanty subcutaneous fat, relaxed ligaments, and, less commonly, other associated developmental anomalies, including congenital heart disease and deformities of the spine and joints. Ocular complications are often seen—in particular, dislocation of the lenses, usually superiorly and nasally. Less common ocular anomalies include severe refractive errors, megalocornea, cataract, uveal colobomas, and secondary glaucoma. There is a high infant mortality rate. Removal of a dislocated lens may be necessary. The disease is genetically determined, nearly always as an autosomal dominant, often with incomplete expression, so that mild, incomplete forms of the syndrome are seen. Several reports have correlated cytogenetic changes with Marfan's syndrome.

MARCHESANI'S SYNDROME

This is a rare hereditary disorder characterized by multiple skeletal and ocular abnormalities, which is transmitted as an autosomal recessive trait. Patients are short and stocky, with well-developed muscles. The hands and feet are characteristically spade-shaped; in childhood, x-rays show delayed carpal and tarsal ossification. Ocular complications include spherophakia and ectopia lentis, which give rise to lenticular myopia, iridodonesis, and glaucoma. The prognosis for vision is usually poor because the glaucoma resists all forms of treatment.

Table 19–3. Association of HLA types with systemic diseases.

Behçet's disease	HLA-B5
Juvenile diabetic retinopathy	HLA-B8 (without A1)
Myasthenia gravis	HLA-DR3
	HLA-B8
Thyrotoxicosis	HLA-Dw3
	HLA-B8
Multiple sclerosis	HLA-DR3
	HLA-Dw2
Ankylosing spondylitis	HLA-B27
Reiter's disease	HLA-B27
Acute anterior uveitis	HLA-B27
Rheumatoid arthritis	HLA-DR4
	HLA-Dw4

Figure 19–37. Marfan's syndrome. Familial expression of arachnodactyly and upward dislocation of the lens.

OSTEOGENESIS IMPERFECTA
(Brittle Bones & Blue Scleras)

This rare autosomal dominant syndrome is characterized by multiple fractures, blue scleras, and, less commonly, deafness. The disease is usually manifest soon after birth. The long bones are very fragile, fracturing easily and often healing with fibrous bony union. The bones become more fragile with age. The very thin sclera allows the blue color imparted by the underlying uveal tract to show through. There is often no visual functional impairment. Occasionally, abnormalities such as keratoconus, megalocornea, and corneal or lenticular opacities are also present that do interfere with visual function.

Ophthalmologic treatment is seldom necessary.

HEREDITARY METABOLIC DISORDERS

MUCOPOLYSACCHARIDOSES

Mucopolysaccharides are long glycoside polymers consisting of a chain of 100 sugar residues attached to a protein core. The polymers are either dermatan or heparan sulfate, and in the mucopolysaccharidoses there is defective breakdown of those polymers due to enzyme deficiency, resulting in the deposition of mucopolysaccharide in the tissues and an elevated urinary excretion.

There are 6 clearly defined disorders of mucopolysaccharide metabolism (I–VI) that all used to be grouped together and called **gargoylism.**

Corneal clouding occurs in **Hurler's syndrome** (type I) (Fig 19–38), **Scheie's syndrome** (type I), **Morquio's disease** (type IV), and **Maroteaux-Lamy syndrome** (type V A+B) and noticeably not in **Hunter's syndrome** (type I), the only X-linked inherited variety; the others are all autosomal recessive. Other ocular features are megalocornea, buphthalmos, pigmentary retinopathy, and optic atrophy.

HEPATOLENTICULAR DEGENERATION
(Wilson's Disease)

This rare autosomal recessive disease of young adults, characterized by abnormal copper metabolism, causes changes in the basal nuclei, cirrhosis of the liver, and a pathognomonic corneal pigmentation called the Kayser-Fleischer ring. The ring appears as a green or brown band peripherally and deep in the stroma near Descemet's membrane and may only be visible with a slit lamp. The disease is progressive and often results in death by age 40.

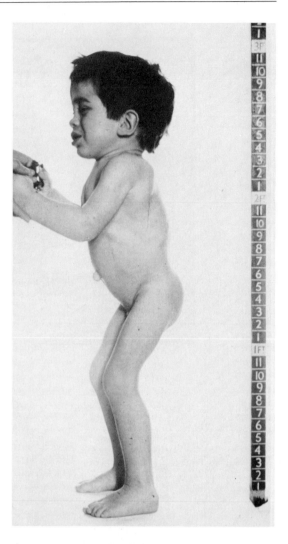

Figure 19–38. Clinical features of Hurler's syndrome include gargoylism, gibbus, and umbilical hernia.

Treatment with penicillamine has resulted in sustained clinical improvement in some cases.

CYSTINOSIS

This rare autosomal recessive derangement of amino acid metabolism causes widespread deposition of cystine crystals throughout the body. Dwarfism, nephropathy, and death in childhood from renal failure are the rule. Cystine crystals can be readily seen in the conjunctiva and cornea, where fine particles are seen predominantly in the outer third of the corneal stroma.

There is no treatment.

ALBINISM

Generalized albinism is a disease affecting the metabolism of melanin and is inherited as an autosomal recessive trait. The skin and hair are white, and there is a generalized lack of pigment throughout the body that is apparent from birth. The eyebrows and lashes are white. The irides appear reddish, and the pupil appears red. The fundus is red, with a prominent choroidal vessel pattern, since the pigment epithelium of the retina is deficient. Photophobia is prominent. The macula is often poorly developed, greatly impairing visual function, and this often causes an associated searching nystagmus that reduces visual acuity to about 6/60 (20/200).

HOMOCYSTINURIA

Homocystinuria is a rare autosomal recessive disorder of amino acid metabolism characterized clinically by mental retardation, downward dislocation of the lenses of the eyes, and genu valgum. The plasma homocystine and methionine levels are elevated. Urinary excretion of homocystine is increased, and the nitroprusside test of the urine is positive. Thrombosis of medium-sized arteries is common, often resulting in early death from cerebrovascular, coronary, or renal vascular occlusions. These are relatively common during general anesthesia and are due to excess platelet aggregation. Dietary therapy is possible with either a high-pyridoxine diet or a low-methionine diet with added cystine, or a combination of these two.

GALACTOSEMIA

Galactosemia is a rare autosomal recessive disorder of carbohydrate metabolism that becomes clinically manifest soon after birth by feeding problems, vomiting, diarrhea, abdominal distention, hepatomegaly, jaundice, ascites, cataracts, mental retardation, and elevated blood and urine galactose levels. Dietary exclusion of milk and all foods containing galactose and lactose for the first 3 years of life will prevent the clinical manifestations and will result in improvement of existing abnormalities. Even the cataract changes, which are characterized by vacuoles of the cortex, are reversible in the early stage.

Identification of the carrier state is possible by finding a 50% reduction of galactose-6-phosphatase.

MISCELLANEOUS SYSTEMIC DISEASES WITH OCULAR MANIFESTATIONS

VOGT-KOYANAGI-HARADA SYNDROME (Fig 19–39)

Bilateral uveitis associated with alopecia, poliosis, vitiligo, and hearing defects, usually in young adults, has been termed Vogt-Koyanagi disease. When the choroiditis is more exudative, serous retinal detachment occurs, and the complex is known as Harada's syndrome. Japanese and Italians are affected more commonly than other groups, but even among these

Figure 19–39. Vogt-Koyanagi-Harada syndrome. Acute pigment epithelial disease with disk swelling and cells in the vitreous *(left)*. Three months later, disk swelling has subsided and pigment epithelial damage is seen *(right)*.

the disease is rare. There is a tendency toward recovery of visual function, but this is not always complete. Corticosteroids have been reported to have a favorable effect upon the disease. Local corticosteroids and mydriatics are indicated. There have been a few reports of isolation of a virus from these cases, but a viral cause has not yet been definitely established.

ERYTHEMA MULTIFORME
(Stevens-Johnson Syndrome)

Erythema multiforme is a serious mucocutaneous disease that occurs as a hypersensitivity reaction to drugs or food. Children are most susceptible. The manifestations consist of generalized maculopapular rash, severe stomatitis, and purulent conjunctivitis, sometimes leading to symblepharon and occlusion of the lacrimal gland ducts (**dry eye syndrome).** In severe cases, corneal ulcers, perforations, panophthalmitis can destroy all visual function. Systemic corticosteroid treatment often favorably influences the course of the disease and usually preserves useful visual function. Secondary infection with *Staphylococcus aureus* is common and must be vigorously treated by local antibiotics instilled into the conjunctival sac. Frequently there is marked reduction of tear formation that can be helped by instillation of artificial tears.

GIANT CELL ARTERITIS
(Including Temporal or Cranial Arteritis)

This is a disease of elderly patients (over age 60). Medium-sized arteries are involved, particularly the intima of the vessels. Branches of the external carotid system are frequently involved, though pathologic studies have shown more diffuse arterial involvement. Polymyalgia rheumatica may precede or accompany the disease. Patients feel ill and have excruciating pain over the temporal or occipital arteries. Visual loss due to an ischemic optic neuropathy is frequent, and a few cases have a central retinal artery occlusion. Visual loss may also be due to cortical blindness. Other central nervous system signs include cranial nerve palsies and signs referable to brain stem lesions. The diagnosis is confirmed by a high erythrocyte sedimentation rate (ESR) and a positive temporal artery biopsy. In early stages of the disease, the ESR may be normal, but usually it is 80–100 mm in the first hour. It is important to make the diagnosis early, because immediate systemic corticosteroids produce dramatic improvement. The disease activity is monitored by the erythrocyte sedimentation rate and the clinical state. The corticosteroid dose may have to be maintained for several years and should be kept below 5 mg prednisolone daily if possible, since with higher doses the survival rate is markedly reduced.

IDIOPATHIC ARTERITIS OF TAKAYASU
(Pulseless Disease)

This disease, found most frequently in young women and occasionally in children, is a polyarteritis of unknown cause with increased predilection for the aorta and its branches. Manifestations may include evidence of cerebrovascular insufficiency, syncope, absence of pulsations in the upper extremities, and ophthalmologic changes compatible with chronic hypoxia of the ocular structures. Ophthalmodynamometry may be of value by demonstrating decreased carotid blood flow on one or both sides. The disease is sometimes associated with rheumatoid arthritis, which supports the idea that it is a collagen disease.

Thromboendarterectomy, prosthetic graft, and systemic corticosteroid therapy have been reported to be successful.

LAURENCE-MOON-BIEDL SYNDROME

Obesity, mental deficiency, polydactyly, hypogenitalism, and retinitis pigmentosa form the complete syndrome. The retinal changes are not always typical of retinitis pigmentosa and may be present soon after birth or develop during adolescence. This rare syndrome is genetically determined and follows an autosomal recessive pattern with a high rate of consanguinity. The heterozygous state may be identified by mild incomplete evidences of the disease. It is interesting that a single abnormal gene can account for such a multiplicity of clinical findings.

ROSACEA
(Acne Rosacea)

This disease of unknown cause is primarily dermatologic, beginning as a hyperemia of the face associated with acneiform lesions and eventually causing hypertrophy of tissues (such as rhinophyma). Chronic blepharitis due to staphylococcal infection or seborrhea is often present. Rosacea keratitis develops in about 5% of cases. Episcleritis, scleritis, and nongranulomatous iridocyclitis are rare ocular complications.

Topical corticosteroids help in controlling keratitis or iridocyclitis, but there is no specific therapy.

LOWE'S SYNDROME

This rare syndrome consists of cerebral defects, mental retardation, and ocular anomalies associated with dwarfism due to renal dysfunction (a congenital defect of reabsorption in the renal tubules, causing aminoaciduria). The eye findings include congenital cataract, infantile glaucoma, and nystagmus. All cases reported to date have occurred in males, suggesting X-linked inheritance. Early mortality rates are high.

Figure 19–40. Retinitis in an immunosuppressed patient. *Left:* This patient with myasthenia gravis underwent thymectomy and received long-term immunosuppression with cytotoxic agents. *Right:* He developed retinal necrosis and Ramsay Hunt syndrome following infection with herpes zoster.

IMMUNOSUPPRESSIVE AGENTS USED IN EYE DISEASE

Immunosuppressive agents are used to suppress inflammatory reactions within the eye, particularly those affecting the uveal tract but also the sclera, retina, and optic nerve. Frequently, the cause of inflammation is not known. and, hence, the use of these drugs is empirical. All patients must have a full medical examination before treatment is started. Special consideration must be given to patients with infections and blood diseases, and regular blood counts must be performed during the course of treatment.

Corticosteroids (eg, prednisolone) are the mainstay of immunosuppressive treatment in ophthalmology. High doses (eg, 60 mg of prednisolone daily) may be required to control inflammation, and there is a high incidence of side effects. Weight gain, acne, and hirsutism are common; peptic ulceration, myopathy, osteoporosis, and avascular necrosis are less frequently encountered. Alternate-day regimens pro-

Table 19—4. Cytotoxic agents used in the management of inflammatory eye disease.

Drug	Daily Dose (mg/kg)	Maximum Length of Treatment	Specific Indications	Side Effects
Azathioprine	2.5–3	18 months	Corticosteroid-sparing	Bone marrow depression (usually leukopenia, but may be anemia, thrombocytopenia, and bleeding) (irreversible in elderly patients). Skin rashes, drug fever, nausea and vomiting, sometimes diarrhea. Hepatic dysfunction (raised liver enzymes, mild jaundice). Lymphoma.
Chlorambucil	0.05–0.2	2½ years (4 g)	Behçet's disease	Moderate depression of peripheral blood count. Excessive doses produce severe bone marrow depression with leuko-
Cyclophosphamide	1.25–2.5	3 years	Wegener's granulomatosis	penia, thrombocytopenia, and bleeding. Lymphoma. Prevent cystitis with adequate hydration. Chlorambucil: Leukemia may occur. Large doses near puberty may cause infertility. Cyclophosphamide: Nausea and vomiting acutely. Alopecia and hemorrhagic cystitis occasionally. Infertility may occur.
Colchicine	0.01–0.03	5 years	Behçet's disease	Occasionally nausea, vomiting, abdominal pain, diarrhea. Rarely, hair loss, bone marrow depression, peripheral neuritis, myopathy.

duce fewer side effects in some patients. Azathioprine may be added as a corticosteroid-sparing drug. Ideally, the patient should be given only 40 mg/d for 3 consecutive months, and the dosage should then be reduced to 10 mg/d. The total course should not last for more than 3 years. Intravenous methylprednisolone (1 g/d given over 3 hours in dextrose saline for 3 days) is an effective method of controlling exacerbations in patients already taking high doses of corticosteroids.

Fortunately, cytotoxic agents are rarely indicated in the management of inflammatory eye disease, except in severe cases of Behçet's syndrome and Wegener's granulomatosis. These drugs and their important side effects are listed in Table 19–4. Cytotoxic agents are sometimes used in the treatment of myasthenia gravis (see Fig 19–40 and Chapter 18).

OCULAR COMPLICATIONS OF CERTAIN SYSTEMICALLY ADMINISTERED DRUGS
(See also Chapter 29.)

AMIODARONE

Amiodarone is a benzofuran derivative used to treat cardiac dysrhythmias, particularly Wolff-Parkinson-White syndrome, and angina pectoris. Most patients develop small punctate deposits in the basal cell layer of the corneal epithelium. The severity of keratopathy is related to the total daily dose and is mild at a dose of less than 200 mg daily. The deposits rarely interfere with vision, and although they progress with continued treatment, even in low dosage, they always resolve completely when treatment is stopped (Fig 19–41).

Figure 19–41. Amiodarone keratopathy. (Courtesy of DJ Spalton.)

ANTICHOLINERGICS
(Atropine & Related Synthetic Drugs)

All of these drugs, when given preoperatively or for gastrointestinal disorders, may cause blurred vision in presbyopic patients because of a direct action on accommodation. They also tend to dilate the pupils, so that in patients with narrow anterior chamber angles there is the added threat of angle-closure glaucoma. This is the cause of angle-closure glaucoma (frequently attributed to ''nervousness'') occasionally seen in patients hospitalized for general surgery.

ANTIDEPRESSANTS

Tricyclic antidepressants and monoamine oxidase inhibitors have an anticholinergic effect and theoretically may exacerbate open-angle glaucoma or provoke an attack of angle-closure glaucoma. However, this is rare in clinical practice, and if a patient is already receiving treatment for open-angle glaucoma, the medication will overcome any effect of the antidepressants.

CHLORAMPHENICOL

Chloramphenicol, in addition to the possibility of causing severe blood dyscrasias, hepatic and renal disease, and gastrointestinal disturbances, can sometimes cause optic neuritis. This is especially true in children. Bilateral blurred vision with central scotomas occurs. Stopping the drug does not always restore vision.

Despite the possibility of toxic optic neuropathy, chloramphenicol may still be required for the treatment of bacterial endophthalmitis. The drug is generally not administered for more than 1 week.

CHLOROQUINE

Originally employed as an antimalarial drug, chloroquine has also been widely used in the treatment of many collagen diseases, especially systemic lupus erythematosus and rheumatoid arthritis, and skin diseases, including discoid lupus erythematosus and sarcoidosis. With high dosage—often 250–750 mg daily administered for months or years—serious ocular toxicity has occurred. Corneal changes were described first and consisted of diffuse haziness of the epithelium and subepithelial area, occasionally sufficient to simulate an epithelial dystrophy. These changes cause only mild blurring of vision and are reversible upon drug withdrawal. Similar changes have been described in patients receiving quinacrine. Minimal corneal involvement is not necessarily an indication for discontinuance of chloroquine therapy. Corneal changes have been reported in about 30% of patients on long-term chloroquine treatment.

A less common but more serious ocular complication of long-term chloroquine therapy is retinal damage, causing loss of central vision as well as constriction of peripheral visual fields. Pigmentary changes and edema of the macula, marked alteration of the retinal vessels, and in some cases peripheral pigmentary changes can be seen ophthalmoscopically. Fluorescein fundus photography aids greatly in establishing early diagnosis or evaluating the extent of macular involvement. Visual field examination reveals central scotomas and peripheral field constriction. There are also changes in the electroretinogram, dark adaptation, and color vision. The damage is always bilateral and is usually equal in both eyes. The visual loss is irreversible and may even progress after cessation of therapy. No treatment is of any value.

Long-term chloroquine therapy must be undertaken only upon urgent indications. These patients should be examined by an ophthalmologist every 3–4 months. Between examinations, patients should make a rough test of visual acuity once weekly.

CHLOROTHIAZIDE

Xanthopsia (yellow vision) has been reported in patients taking this oral diuretic.

CONTRACEPTIVES, ORAL

Although numerous reports suggest that in predisposed individuals oral contraceptives can provoke or precipitate ophthalmic vascular occlusive disease or optic nerve damage, it is difficult to establish a definite cause and effect relationship. Optic neuritis, retinal arterial or venous thrombosis, and pseudotumor cerebri have been described in patients taking oral contraceptives. Since there is some uncertainty regarding the possibility of such ocular complications, oral contraceptives should be used only by healthy women with no history of vascular, neurologic, or ocular disease.

CORTICOSTEROIDS

It has been clearly demonstrated that long-term systemic corticosteroid therapy can cause chronic open-angle glaucoma and cataracts and can provoke and worsen attacks of herpes simplex keratitis. Locally administered corticosteroids are much more potent in this respect and have the added disadvantage of causing fungal overgrowth if the corneal epithelium is not intact. Steroid-induced subcapsular lens opacities cause some impairment of visual function but usually do not progress to advanced cataract. Cessation of therapy will arrest progression of the lenticular opacities, but the changes are irreversible.

Systemic corticosteroids may also cause papilledema associated with pseudotumor cerebri, both during administration and shortly after withdrawal.

DIGITALIS

Blurred vision and disturbed color vision are said to be the most common ocular complications of digitalis toxicity, although the actual incidence of such symptoms in patients receiving digitalis is extremely low. The purified glycosides of digitalis probably produce fewer of the toxic ocular symptoms than the whole leaf.

Visual acuity may be decreased. Objects may appear yellow (xanthopsia) or, less commonly, green, brown, red, "snowy," or white. The patient may complain of photophobia and flashes of light. Scotomas and, very rarely, transient and permanent amblyopia have been described. The toxic effects of digitalis may be due to direct effects on the retinal reception cells or retrobulbar neuritis, or they may be of central origin.

ETHAMBUTOL

Ocular complications are rare unless the daily dose is greater than 25 mg/kg, but they do occur because the drug is often used in resistant cases of tuberculosis. Optic neuropathy affecting the papillomacular bundle produces centrocecal scotoma and reduced color vision. A chiasmal pattern of involvement may also be seen. Visual loss is dose-dependent and may improve over 6 months after cessation of the drug.

OXYGEN

Premature infants who are given any concentration of oxygen in excess of that in air may develop retinopathy of prematurity (retrolental fibroplasia). These infants should receive only the amount of oxygen necessary for survival. The incidence of the condition was considerably reduced in the 1960s with rigid restriction of oxygen, but despite continued restriction, the incidence has recently risen again. This may be due to prematurity itself (with advanced medical techniques, smaller infants are surviving); the condition is found in 40–77% of infants weighing less than 1 kg. The clinical features are described in Chapter 14. Vitamin E given daily reduces the severity but not the incidence of retinopathy of prematurity.

In adults, administration of hyperbaric oxygen (3 atmospheres) can cause constriction of the retinal arterioles. In one reported case, a patient with an old inactive retrobulbar neuritis exposed to 100% oxygen at 2 atmospheres of pressure developed almost complete loss of visual field in 2 hours.

PHENOBARBITAL & PHENYTOIN

Ocular complications relate to oculomotor involvement, producing nystagmus and weakness of convergence and accommodation. The nystagmus may persist for many months after cessation of the drug, and the degree of oculomotor abnormality is related to drug dosage. Early abnormalities include disturbance of smooth pursuit.

PHENOTHIAZINES

The phenothiazines usually exert an atropinelike effect on the eye so that the pupils may be dilated, especially with large dosages. Of greater clinical significance, however, are the pigmentary ocular changes, which include pigmentary retinopathy and pigment deposits on the corneal endothelium and anterior lens capsule. The corneal and lens pigmentation may cause blurring of vision, but the pigment deposits usually disappear several months after the drug is discontinued. In pigmentary retinopathy, there is a diminution of central vision, night blindness, diffuse narrowing of the retinal arteries, and occasionally severe blindness.

The piperidine group (eg, thioridazine) has a higher risk of causing pigmentary retinopathy, and the maximum daily dose should not exceed 600 mg. The retinal changes are partly reversible under normal circumstances, but in some patients more severe irreversible changes occur at the "safe" dosage level.

The dimethylamine group (eg, chlorpromazine) rarely produces retinal pigmentary changes.

The piperazine group (eg, trifluoperazine) does not produce these retinal complications.

All of these drugs can produce an extrapyramidal syndrome that may involve eye movements. Large doses can provoke profound hypotension, which may produce ischemic optic neuropathy.

Patients receiving large dosages or prolonged treatment with phenothiazines should be questioned regarding visual disturbances and should have periodic ophthalmoscopic examinations.

QUININE & QUINACRINE

Quinine and quinacrine, when used in the treatment of malaria, may cause bilateral blurred vision, sometimes following a single dose. There is constriction of the visual field and, rarely, total blindness. The tendency is toward partial recovery, although usually there are permanent peripheral field defects. The ganglion cells of the retina are affected first, presumably as a result of vasoconstriction of the retinal arterioles. Varying degrees of retinal edema occur early. Optic atrophy is a late finding.

SALICYLATES

Hypersensitivity reactions are common with aspirin taken at therapeutic dosage levels, producing angioneurotic edema and conjunctivitis. Withdrawal of the drug usually results in improved visual function, but complete recovery is rare.

SEDATIVE TRANQUILIZERS

When taken regularly, the so-called minor tranquilizers can decrease tear production by the lacrimal gland, thus resulting in ocular irritation because of dry eyes. Tear production returns to normal when the tranquilizers are discontinued.

The principal drugs in this group are meprobamate, chlordiazepoxide, and diazepam.

FETAL EFFECTS OF DRUGS

The visual pathways of the fetus are occasionally affected by drugs taken by the mother during pregnancy.

Phenytoin may cause optic nerve hypoplasia.

Pigmentary retinopathy has been reported in a child of a mother taking **busulfan** for acute myeloid leukemia.

Warfarin is teratogenic and may produce a hypoplastic nose, stippled epiphyses, and skeletal abnormalities. Affected children may present with recurrent sticky eyes from obstruction of the nasolacrimal duct secondary to malformation of the nose. Other ocular abnormalities include optic atrophy, microphthalmia, and lens opacities. (**Heparin** does not produce these abnormalities, since it is a large molecule that does not cross the placenta.)

REFERENCES

Arruga J, Sanders MD: Ophthalmologic findings in 70 patients with evidence of retinal embolism. *Ophthalmology* 1982; **89:**1336.

Bergsma D, Bron AJ, Cotlier E (editors): *The Eye and Inborn Errors of Metabolism.* AR Liss, 1976.

Brewerton DA: The histocompatibility antigen (HLA 27) and acute anterior uveitis. *Trans Ophthalmol Soc UK* 1974; **94:**735.

Cant JS: *Vision and Circulation.* Mosby, 1976.

Centers for Disease Control: Acquired immunodeficiency syndrome (AIDS): Precautions for health care workers and allied professionals. *MMWR* 1983; **32:**450.

Centers for Disease Control: Recommendations for preventing possible transmission of human T-lymphotropic virus type III/lymphadenopathy-associated virus from tears. *MMWR* 1985; **34:**533.

Cogan DG: *Ophthalmic Manifestations of Systemic Vascular Disease.* Saunders, 1974.

Diabetic Retinopathy Study Group: Preliminary report on effects of photocoagulation therapy. *Am J Ophthalmol* 1976; **81:**383.

Dunlap EA (editor): *Gordon's Medical Management of Ocular Disease,* 2nd ed. Harper & Row, 1976.

Edwards JE Jr et al: Ocular manifestations of *Candida* septicemia: Review of seventy-six cases of hematogenous *Candida* endophthalmitis. *Medicine* 1974; **53:**47.

Eva PR, Pascoe PT, Vaughan DG: Refractive change in hyperglycaemia: Hyperopia, not myopia. *Br J Ophthalmol* 1982; **66:**500.

Ferry AP, Font RL: Carcinoma metastatic to the eye and orbit. *Arch Ophthalmol* 1975; **93:**472.

Fraunfelder FT: *Drug-Induced Ocular Side-Effects and Drug Interactions.* Lea & Febiger, 1976.

Fujikawa LS et al: Isolation of human T-cell leukemia/lymphotropic virus type III (HTLV-III) from the tears of a patient with acquired immunodeficiency syndrome (AIDS). *Lancet.* [In press.]

Garner LL, Wang RIH, Hieb E: Ocular effects of phenothiazines. *Med Lett Drugs Ther* (Dec) 1974; **4:**30.

Gass JDM, Olson CL: Sarcoidosis with optic nerve and retinal involvement. *Arch Ophthalmol* 1976; **94:**945.

Graham E et al: Prognosis in giant-cell arteritis. *Br Med J* 1981; **282:**269.

Griffin JR et al: Blood-borne *Candida* endophthalmitis. *Arch Ophthalmol* 1973; **89:**450.

Hanshaw JB: Congenital cytomegalovirus infection. *N Engl J Med* 1973; **288:**1406.

Hart PD, Russell E Jr, Remington JS: The compromised host and infection. 2. Deep fungal infections. *J Infect Dis* 1969; **120:**169.

James DG, Spiteri MA: Behçet's disease. *Ophthalmology* 1982; **89:**1279.

Jones IS, Jakobiec FA (editors): *Diseases of the Orbit.* Harper & Row, 1979.

Kaplan HJ, Waldrep JC: Immunologic insights into uveitis and retinitis: The immunoregulatory circuit. *Ophthalmology* 1984; **91:**655.

Keltner JL: Giant-cell arteritis: Signs and symptoms. *Ophthalmology* 1982; **89:**1101.

Martin LS, McDougal JS, Loskoski SL: Disinfection and inactivation of the human T lymphotropic virus type III/lymphadenopathy-associated virus. *J Infect Dis* 1985; **152:**400.

Mausolf FA: *The Eye and Systemic Disease.* Mosby, 1975.

O'Connor GR: Factors related to the initiation and recurrence of uveitis. *Am J Ophthalmol* 1983; **96:**577.

Orcutt JC, Page NGR, Sanders MD: Factors affecting visual loss in benign intracranial hypertension. *Ophthalmology* 1984; **92:**1303.

Pepose JS et al: Acquired immune deficiency syndrome: Pathogenic mechanisms of ocular disease. *Ophthalmology* 1985; **92:**472.

Rahi AHS, Barner A: *Immunopathology of the Eye.* Blackwell, 1976.

Rose FC (editor): *The Eye in General Medicine.* Chapman & Hall, 1983.

Spire B et al: Inactivation of lymphadenopathy associated virus by chemical disinfectants. *Lancet* 1984; **2:**899.

Walsh JB: Hypertensive retinopathy: Description, classification, and prognosis. *Ophthalmology* 1982; **89:**1127.

Watson PG, Hazleman BL (editors): *The Sclera and Systemic Disorders.* Saunders, 1976.

Wise GN, Dollery CT, Henkind P: *The Retinal Circulation.* Harper & Row, 1971.

20   Immunologic Diseases of the Eye

The eye is frequently considered to be a special target of immunologic disease processes, but proof of the causative role of these processes is lacking in all but a few disorders. In this sense, the immunopathology of the eye is much less clearly delineated than that of the kidney, the testis, or the thyroid gland. Because the eye is a highly vascularized organ and because the rather labile vessels of the conjunctiva are embedded in a nearly transparent medium, inflammatory eye disorders are more obvious (and often more painful) than those of other organs such as the thyroid or the kidney. The iris, ciliary body, and choroid are the most highly vascularized tissues of the eye. The similarity of the vascular supply of the uvea to that of the kidney and the choroid plexus of the brain has given rise to justified speculation concerning the selection of these 3 tissues, among others, as targets of immune complex diseases (eg, serum sickness).

Immunologic diseases of the eye can be grossly divided into 2 major categories: antibody-mediated and cell-mediated diseases. As is the case in other organs, there is ample opportunity for the interaction of these 2 systems in the eye.

ANTIBODY-DEPENDENT & ANTIBODY-MEDIATED DISEASES

Before it can be concluded that a disease of the eye is antibody-dependent, the following criteria must be satisfied: (1) There must be evidence of specific antibody in the patient's serum or plasma cells. (2) The antigen must be identified and, if feasible, characterized. (3) The same antigen must be shown to produce an immunologic response in the eye of an experimental animal, and the pathologic changes produced in the experimental animal must be similar to those observed in the human disease. (4) It must be possible to produce similar lesions in animals passively sensitized with serum from an affected animal upon challenge with the specific antigen.

Unless all of the above criteria are satisfied, the disease may be thought of as *possibly* antibody-dependent. In such circumstances, the disease can be regarded as antibody-mediated if only one of the following criteria is met: (1) if antibody to an antigen is present in higher quantities in the ocular fluids than in the serum (after adjustments have been made for the total amounts of immunoglobulins in each fluid); (2) if abnormal accumulations of plasma cells are present in the ocular lesion; (3) if abnormal accumulations of immunoglobulins are present at the site of the disease; (4) if complement is fixed by immunoglobulins at the site of the disease; (5) if an accumulation of eosinophils is present at the site of the disease; or (6) if the ocular disease is associated with an inflammatory disease elsewhere in the body for which antibody dependency has been proved or strongly suggested.

HAY FEVER CONJUNCTIVITIS

This disease is characterized by edema and hyperemia of the conjunctiva and lids (Fig 20–1) and by itching and watering of the eyes. There is often an associated itching sensation in the nose as well as rhinorrhea. The conjunctiva appears pale and boggy because of the intense edema, which is often rapid in onset. There is a distinct seasonal incidence, some patients being able to establish the onset of their symptoms at precisely the same time each year. These times usually correspond to the release of pollens by specific grasses, trees, or weeds.

Immunologic Pathogenesis

Hay fever conjunctivitis is one of the few inflammatory eye disorders for which antibody dependence has been definitely established. It is recognized as a form of atopic disease with an implied hereditary susceptibility. IgE (reaginic antibody) is believed to be attached to mast cells lying beneath the conjunctival epithelium. Contact of the offending antigen with IgE triggers the release of vasoactive amines, principally histamine, in this area, and this in turn results in vasodilatation and chemosis.

The role of circulating antibody to ragweed pollen in the pathogenesis of hay fever conjunctivitis has been demonstrated by passively transferring serum from a hypersensitive person to a nonsensitive one. When exposed to the offending pollen, the previously nonsensitive individual reacted with the typical signs of hay fever conjunctivitis.

Immunologic Diagnosis

Victims of hay fever conjunctivitis show many

Figure 20–1. Hay fever conjunctivitis. Note edema and hyperemia of the conjunctiva. (Courtesy of M Allansmith and B McClellan.)

eosinophils in Giemsa-stained scrapings of conjunctival epithelium. They show the **immediate** type of response, with wheal and flare, when tested by scratch tests of the skin with extracts of pollens or other offending antigens. Biopsies of the skin test sites have occasionally shown the full-blown picture of an **Arthus reaction,** with deposition of immune complexes in the walls of the dermal vessels. Passive cutaneous anaphylaxis can also be used to demonstrate the presence of circulating antibody.

Treatment

Systemically administered antihistaminics such as diphenhydramine or tripelennamine are effective, particularly when given prophylactically during the season of greatest exposure. Sustained-release capsules of antihistaminics such as Ornade (chlorpheniramine maleate) are preferred by some. Locally applied antihistaminics such as Prefrin-A drops contain both an antihistaminic agent (pyrilamine) and a vasosconstrictor (phenylephrine). Where conjunctival edema is severe and of sudden onset, epinephrine drops (1:100,000) instilled into the conjunctival sac may help to reduce the edema quickly. Corticosteroids applied locally offer some relief. Topical use of cromolyn (disodium cromoglycate; Opticrom), a stabilizer of the mast cell, appears to be a promising method of treatment for many allergic conditions.

Immunotherapy with gradually increasing doses of subcutaneously injected pollen extracts or other suspected allergens appears to reduce the severity of the disease in some individuals if started well in advance of the season. The mechanism is presumed to be production of blocking antibodies in response to the injection of small, graded doses of the antigen. This procedure cannot be recommended routinely, however, in view of the generally good results and relatively few complications of antihistamine therapy. Acute anaphylactoid reactions have occasionally resulted from overzealous immunotherapy.

VERNAL CONJUNCTIVITIS & ATOPIC KERATOCONJUNCTIVITIS

These 2 diseases also belong to the group of atopic disorders. Both are characterized by itching and lacrimation of the eyes but are more chronic than hay fever conjunctivitis. Furthermore, both ultimately result in structural modifications of the lids and conjunctiva.

Vernal conjunctivitis characteristically affects children and adolescents; the incidence decreases sharply after the second decade of life. Like hay fever conjunctivitis, vernal conjunctivitis occurs only in the warm months of the year. Most of its victims live in hot, dry climates. The disease characteristically produces giant ("cobblestone") papillae of the tarsal conjunctiva (Fig 20–2). The keratinized epithelium from these papillae may abrade the underlying cornea, giving rise to complaints of foreign body sensation.

Atopic keratoconjunctivitis affects individuals of all ages and has no specific seasonal incidence. The skin of the lids has a characteristic dry, scaly appearance. The conjunctiva is pale and boggy. Both the conjunctiva and the cornea may develop scarring in the later stages of the disease. Atopic cataract has also been described. Staphylococcal blepharitis, manifested by scales and crusts on the lids, commonly complicates this disease.

Immunologic Pathogenesis

Reaginic antibody (IgE) is fixed to subepithelial mast cells in both of these conditions. Contact between the offending antigen and IgE is thought to trigger degranulation of the mast cell, which in turn allows for the release of vasoactive amines in the tissues. It is unlikely, however, that antibody action alone is

Figure 20–2. Giant papillae ("cobblestones") in the tarsal conjunctiva of a patient with vernal conjunctivitis.

responsible, since—at least in the case of the papillae of vernal conjunctivitis—there is heavy papillary infiltration by mononuclear cells. Hay fever and asthma occur much more frequently in patients with vernal conjunctivitis and atopic keratoconjunctivitis than in the general population. Of the criteria outlined above (see p 302) for demonstration of *possibly* antibody-dependent diseases, (2), (5), and (6) have been met by atopic keratoconjunctivitis.

Immunologic Diagnosis

As in hay fever conjunctivitis, patients with atopic keratoconjunctivitis and vernal conjunctivitis regularly show large numbers of eosinophils in conjunctival scrapings. Skin testing with food extracts, pollens, and various other antigens reveals a wheal-and-flare type of reaction within 1 hour of testing, but the significance of these reactions is not established.

Treatment

Local instillations of corticosteroid drops or ointment relieve the symptoms. However, caution must be observed in the long-term use of these agents because of the possibility of steroid-induced glaucoma and cataract. Corticosteroids produce less dramatic relief in vernal conjunctivitis than in atopic keratoconjunctivitis, and the same can be said of the antihistamines. Cromolyn seems to be useful in treating both atopic and vernal conjunctivitis. It may also allow dosages of corticosteroids to be reduced.

Avoidance of known allergens is helpful; such objects as duck feathers, animal danders, and certain food proteins (egg albumin and others) are common offenders. Specific allergens have been much more difficult to demonstrate in the case of vernal disease, although some workers feel that such substances as rye grass pollens may play a causative role. Installation of air conditioning in the home or relocation to a cool, moist climate is useful in vernal conjunctivitis if economically feasible.

RHEUMATOID DISEASES AFFECTING THE EYE

The diseases in this category vary greatly in their clinical manifestations depending upon the specific disease entity and the age of the patient. Uveitis and scleritis are the principal ocular manifestations of the rheumatoid diseases. **Juvenile rheumatoid arthritis** affects females more frequently than males and is commonly accompanied by iridocyclitis of one or both eyes. The onset is often insidious, the patient having few or no complaints and the eye remaining white. Extensive synechia formation, cataract, and secondary glaucoma may be far-advanced before the parents notice that anything is wrong. The arthritis generally affects only one joint (eg, a knee) in cases with ocular involvement.

Ankylosing spondylitis affects males more frequently than females, and the onset is in the second to sixth decades. It may be accompanied by iridocyclitis of acute onset, often with fibrin in the anterior chamber (Fig 20–3). Pain, redness, and photophobia are the initial complaints, and synechia formation is common.

Rheumatoid arthritis of adult onset may be accompanied by acute scleritis or episcleritis (Fig 20–4). The ciliary body and choroid, lying adjacent to the sclera, are often involved secondarily with the inflammation. Rarely, serous detachment of the retina results. The onset is usually in the third to fifth decade, and women are affected more frequently than men.

Reiter's disease affects men more frequently than women. The first attack of ocular inflammation usually consists of a self-limited papillary conjunctivitis. It follows, at a highly variable interval, the onset of nonspecific urethritis and the appearance of inflammation in one or more of the weight-bearing joints. Subsequent attacks of ocular inflammation may consist of acute iridocyclitis of one or both eyes, occasionally with hypopyon (Fig 20–5).

Figure 20–3. Acute iridocyclitis in a patient with ankylosing spondylitis. Note fibrin clot in anterior chamber.

Figure 20–4. Scleral nodules in a patient with rheumatoid arthritis. (Courtesy of S Kimura.)

Figure 20–5. Acute iridocyclitis with hypopyon in a patient with Reiter's disease.

Figure 20–6. Scleral thinning in a patient with rheumatoid arthritis. Note dark color of the underlying uvea.

Immunologic Pathogenesis

Rheumatoid factor, an IgM autoantibody directed against the patient's own IgG, may play a major role in the pathogenesis of rheumatoid arthritis. The union of IgM antibody with IgG is followed by fixation of complement at the tissue site and the attraction of leukocytes and platelets to this area. An occlusive vasculitis, resulting from this train of events, is thought to be the cause of rheumatoid nodule formation in the sclera as well as elsewhere in the body. The occlusion of vessels supplying nutriments to the sclera is thought to be responsible for the "melting away" of the scleral collagen that is so characteristic of rheumatoid arthritis (Fig 20–6).

While this explanation may suffice for rheumatoid arthritis, patients with the ocular complications of juvenile rheumatoid arthritis, ankylosing spondylitis, and Reiter's syndrome usually have negative tests for rheumatoid factor, so other explanations must be sought.

Outside the eyeball itself, the lacrimal gland has been shown to be under attack by circulating antibodies. Destruction of acinar cells within the gland and invasion of the lacrimal gland (as well as the salivary glands) by mononuclear cells result in decreased tear secretion. The combination of dry eyes (keratoconjunctivitis sicca), dry mouth (xerostomia), and rheumatoid arthritis is known as Sjögren's syndrome (see Chapter 19).

A growing body of evidence indicates that the immunogenetic background of certain patients accounts for the expression of their ocular inflammatory disease in specific ways. Analysis of the HLA antigen system shows that the incidence of HLA-B27 is significantly greater in patients with ankylosing spondylitis and Reiter's syndrome than could be expected by chance alone. It is not known how this antigen controls specific inflammatory responses.

Immunologic Diagnosis

Rheumatoid factor can be detected in the serum by a number of standard tests involving the agglutination of IgG-coated erythrocytes or latex particles. Unfortunately, the test for rheumatoid factor is not positive in the majority of isolated rheumatoid afflictions of the eye.

The HLA types of individuals suspected of having ankylosing spondylitis and related diseases can be determined by standard cytotoxicity tests using highly specific antisera. This is generally done in tissue typing centers where work on organ transplantation necessitates such studies. X-ray of the sacroiliac area is a valuable screening procedure that may show evidence of spondylitis prior to the onset of low back pain in patients with the characteristic form of iridocyclitis.

Treatment

Patients with uveitis associated with rheumatoid disease respond well to local instillations of corticosteroid drops (eg, dexamethasone 0.1%) or ointments. Orally administered corticosteroids must occasionally be resorted to for brief periods. Salicylates given orally in divided doses with meals are thought to reduce the frequency and blunt the severity of recurrent attacks. Atropine drops (1%) are useful for the relief of photophobia during the acute attacks. Shorter-acting mydriatics such as phenylephrine 10% should be used in the subacute stages to prevent synechia formation. Corticosteroid-resistant cases, especially those causing progressive erosion of the sclera, have been treated successfully with immunosuppressive agents such as chlorambucil. Nonsteroidal anti-inflammatory agents such as piroxicam (Feldene) are useful in the symptomatic treatment of scleritis.

Figure 20–7. "Cotton wool" spots (cytoid bodies) in the retina of a patient with lupus erythematosus.

OTHER ANTIBODY-MEDIATED EYE DISEASES

The following antibody-mediated diseases are infrequently encountered by the practicing ophthalmologist.

Systemic lupus erythematosus, associated with the presence of circulating antibodies to DNA, produces an occlusive vasculitis of the nerve fiber layer of the retina. Such infarcts result in cytoid bodies or "cotton wool" spots in the retina (Fig 20–7).

Pemphigus vulgaris produces painful intraepithelial bullae of the conjunctiva. It is associated with the presence of circulating antibodies to an intercellular antigen located between the deeper cells of the conjunctival epithelium.

Cicatricial pemphigoid is characterized by subepithelial bullae of the conjunctiva. In the chronic stages of this disease, cicatricial contraction of the conjunctiva may result in severe scarring of the cornea, dryness of the eyes, and ultimate blindness. Pemphigoid is associated with local deposits of tissue antibodies directed against one or more antigens located in the basement membrane of the epithelium.

Lens-induced uveitis is a rare condition that may be associated with circulating antibodies to lens proteins. It is seen in individuals whose lens capsules have become permeable to these proteins as a result of trauma or other disease. Interest in this field dates back to Uhlenhuth (1903), who first demonstrated the organ-specific nature of antibodies to the lens. Witmer showed in 1962 that antibody to lens tissue may be produced by lymphoid cells of the ciliary body.

CELL-MEDIATED DISEASES

This group of diseases appears to be associated with cell-mediated immunity or delayed hypersensitivity. Various structures of the eye are invaded by mononuclear cells, principally lymphocytes and macrophages, in response to one or more chronic antigenic stimuli. In the case of chronic infections such as tuberculosis, leprosy, toxoplasmosis, and herpes simplex, the antigenic stimulus has clearly been identified as an infectious agent in the ocular tissue. Such infections are often associated with delayed skin test reactivity following the intradermal injection of an extract of the organism.

More intriguing but less well understood are the granulomatous diseases of the eye for which no infectious cause has been found. Such diseases are thought to represent cell-mediated, possibly autoimmune processes, but their origin remains obscure.

OCULAR SARCOIDOSIS

Ocular sarcoidosis is characterized by a panuveitis with occasional inflammatory involvement of the optic nerve and retinal blood vessels. It often presents as iridocyclitis of insidious onset. Less frequently, it occurs as acute iridocyclitis, with pain, photophobia, and redness of the eye. Large precipitates resembling drops of solidified "mutton fat" are seen on the corneal endothelium. The anterior chamber contains a good deal of protein and numerous cells, mostly lymphocytes. Nodules are often seen on the iris, both at the pupillary margin and in the substance of the iris stroma. The latter are often vascularized. Synechiae are commonly encountered, particularly in patients with dark skin. Severe cases ultimately involve the posterior segment of the eye. Coarse clumps of cells ("snowballs") are seen in the vitreous, and exudates resembling candle drippings may be seen along the course of retinal vessels. Patchy infiltrations of the choroid or optic nerve may also be seen.

Infiltrations of the lacrimal gland and of the conjunctiva have been noted on occasion. When the latter are present, the diagnosis can easily be confirmed by biopsy of the small opaque nodules.

Immunologic Pathogenesis

Although many infectious or allergic causes of sarcoidosis have been suggested, none has been confirmed. Noncaseating granulomas are seen in the uvea, optic nerve, and adnexal structures of the eye as well as elsewhere in the body. The presence of macrophages and giant cells suggests that particulate matter is being phagocytosed, but this material has not been identified.

Patients with sarcoidosis are usually anergic to extracts of the common microbial antigens such as those of mumps, *Trichophyton, Candida,* and *Mycobacterium tuberculosis.* As in other lymphoproliferative disorders such as Hodgkin's disease and chronic lymphocytic leukemia, this may represent suppression of T cell activity such that the normal delayed hypersensitivity responses to common antigens cannot take place. Meanwhile, circulating immunoglobulins are usually detectable in the serum at higher than normal levels.

Immunologic Diagnosis

The diagnosis is largely inferential. Negative skin tests to a battery of antigens to which the patient is known to have been exposed are highly suggestive, and the same is true of the elevation of serum immunoglobulins. Biopsy of a conjunctival nodule or scalene lymph node may provide positive histologic evidence of the disease. X-rays of the chest reveal hilar adenopathy in many cases. Elevated levels of serum lysozyme or serum angiotensin converting enzyme may be detected.

Treatment

Sarcoid lesions of the eye respond well to corticosteroid therapy. Frequent instillations of dexamethasone 0.1% eye drops generally bring the anterior uveitis under control. Atropine drops should be prescribed in the acute phase of the disease for the relief of pain and photophobia; short-acting pupillary dilators such as phenylephrine should be given later to prevent synechia formation. Systemic corticosteroids are sometimes necessary to control severe attacks of anterior uveitis and are always necessary for the control of retinal vasculitis and optic neuritis. The latter condition often accompanies cerebral involvement and carries a grave prognosis.

SYMPATHETIC OPHTHALMIA & VOGT-KOYANAGI-HARADA SYNDROME

These 2 disorders are discussed together because they have certain common clinical features. Both are thought to represent autoimmune phenomena affecting pigmented structures of the eye and skin, and both may give rise to meningeal symptoms.

Clinical Features

Sympathetic ophthalmia is an inflammation in the second eye after the other has been damaged by penetrating injury. In most cases, some portion of the uvea of the injured eye has been exposed to the atmosphere for at least 1 hour. The uninjured or "sympathizing" eye develops minor signs of anterior uveitis after a period ranging from 2 weeks to several years. Floating spots and loss of the power of accommodation are among the earliest symptoms. The disease may progress to severe iridocyclitis with pain and photophobia. Usually, however, the eye remains

relatively quiet and painless while the inflammatory disease spreads around the entire uvea. Despite the presence of panuveitis, the retina usually remains uninvolved except for perivascular cuffing of the retinal vessels with inflammatory cells. Papilledema and secondary glaucoma may occur. The disease may be accompanied by vitiligo (patchy depigmentation of the skin) and poliosis (whitening) of the eyelashes.

Vogt-Koyanagi-Harada syndrome consists of inflammation of the uvea of one or both eyes characterized by acute iridocyclitis, patchy choroiditis, and serous detachment of the retina. It usually begins with an acute febrile episode with headache, dysacusis, and occasionally vertigo. Patchy loss or whitening of the scalp hair is described in the first few months of the disease. Vitiligo and poliosis are commonly present but are not essential for the diagnosis. Although the initial iridocyclitis may subside quickly, the course of the posterior disease is often indolent, with long-standing serous detachment of the retina and significant visual impairment.

Immunologic Pathogenesis

In both sympathetic ophthalmia and Vogt-Koyanagi-Harada syndrome, delayed hypersensitivity to melanin-containing structures is thought to occur. Although a viral cause has been suggested for both of these disorders, there is no convincing evidence of an infectious origin. It is postulated that some insult, infectious or otherwise, alters the pigmented structures of the eye, skin, and hair in such a way as to provoke delayed hypersensitivity responses to them. Soluble materials from the outer segments of the photoreceptor layer of the retina have recently been incriminated as possible autoantigens. Patients with Vogt-Koyanagi-Harada syndrome are usually Orientals, which suggests an immunogenetic predisposition to the disease.

Histologic sections of the traumatized eye from a patient with sympathetic ophthalmia may show uniform infiltration of most of the uvea by lymphocytes, epithelioid cells, and giant cells. The overlying retina is characteristically intact, but nests of epithelioid cells may protrude through the pigment epithelium of the retina, giving rise to **Dalen-Fuchs nodules.** The inflammation may destroy the architecture of the entire uvea, leaving an atrophic, shrunken globe.

Immunologic Diagnosis

Skin tests with soluble extracts of human or bovine uveal tissue are said to elicit delayed hypersensitivity responses in these patients. Several investigators have recently shown that cultured lymphocytes from patients with these 2 diseases undergo transformation to lymphoblasts in vitro when extracts of uvea or rod outer segments are added to the culture medium. Circulating antibodies to uveal antigens have been found in patients with these diseases, but such antibodies are to be found in any patient with long-standing uveitis, including those suffering from several infectious entities. The spinal fluid of patients with Vogt-Koyanagi-Harada syndrome may show increased numbers of mononuclear cells and elevated protein in the early stages.

Treatment

Mild cases of sympathetic ophthalmia may be treated satisfactorily with locally applied corticosteroid drops and pupillary dilators. The more severe or progressive cases require systemic corticosteroids, often in high doses, for months or years. An alternate-day regimen of oral corticosteroids is recommended for such patients in order to avoid adrenal suppression. The same applies to the treatment of patients with Vogt-Koyanagi-Harada disease. Occasionally, patients with long-standing progressive disease become resistant to corticosteroids or cannot take additional corticosteroid medication because of pathologic fractures, mental changes, or other reasons. Such patients may become candidates for immunosuppressive therapy. Chlorambucil and cyclophosphamide have been used successfully for both conditions. More recently, cyclosporine has shown promise in the treatment of steroid-resistant uveitis.

OTHER DISEASES OF CELL-MEDIATED IMMUNITY

Giant cell arteritis (temporal arteritis) (see Chapter 19) may have disastrous effects on the eye, particularly in elderly individuals. The condition is manifested by pain in the temples and orbit, blurred vision, and scotomas. Examination of the fundus may reveal extensive occlusive retinal vasculitis and choroidal infarcts. Atrophy of the optic nerve head is a frequent complication. Such patients have an elevated sedimentation rate. Biopsy of the temporal artery reveals extensive infiltration of the vessel wall with giant cells and mononuclear cells.

Polyarteritis nodosa (see Chapter 19) can affect both the anterior and posterior segments of the eye. The corneas of such patients may show peripheral thinning and cellular infiltration. The retinal vessels reveal extensive necrotizing inflammation characterized by eosinophil, plasma cell, and lymphocyte infiltration.

Behçet's disease (see Chapter 19) has an uncertain place in the classification of immunologic disorders. It is characterized by recurrent iridocyclitis with hypopyon and occlusive vasculitis of the retinal vessels. Although it has many of the features of a delayed hypersensitivity disease, dramatic alterations of serum complement levels at the very beginning of an attack suggest an immune complex disorder. Furthermore, high levels of circulating immune complexes have recently been detected in patients with this disease. Most patients with eye symptoms are positive for HLA-B5.

Contact dermatitis of the eyelids represents a significant though minor disease caused by delayed hypersensitivity. Atropine, perfumed cosmetics, materials contained in plastic spectacle frames, and other

Figure 20–8. Phlyctenule (arrow) at the margin of the cornea. (Courtesy of P Thygeson.)

locally applied agents may act as the sensitizing hapten. The lower lid is more extensively involved than the upper lid when the sensitizing agent is applied in drop form. Periorbital involvement with erythematous, vesicular, pruritic lesions of the skin is characteristic.

Phlyctenular keratoconjunctivitis (Fig 20–8) represents a delayed hypersensitivity response to certain microbial antigens, principally those of *M tuberculosis*. It is characterized by acute pain and photophobia in the affected eye, and perforation of the peripheral cornea has been known to result from it. The disease responds rapidly to locally applied corticosteroids. Since the advent of chemotherapy for pulmonary tuberculosis, phlyctenulosis is much less of a problem than it was 30 years ago. It is still encountered occasionally, however, particularly among American Indians and Alaskan Eskimos. Other pathogens such as *Staphylococcus aureus* and *Coccidioides immitis* have also been implicated in phlyctenular disease.

CORNEAL GRAFT REACTIONS (Fig 20–9)

Blindness due to opacity or distortion of the central portion of the cornea is a remediable disease. If all other structures of the eye are intact, a patient whose vision is impaired solely by corneal opacity can expect great improvement from a graft of clear cornea into the diseased area. Trauma, including chemical burns, is one of the most common causes of central corneal opacity. Others include scars from herpetic keratitis, endothelial cell dysfunction with chronic corneal edema (including pseudophakic bullous keratopathy and Fuchs' dystrophy), keratoconus, and opacities from previous graft failures. All of these conditions represent indications for penetrating corneal grafts, provided the patient's eye is no longer inflamed and the opacity has been allowed maximal time to undergo spontaneous resolution (usually 6–12 months). It is estimated that approximately 10,000 corneal grafts are performed in the USA annually. Of these, about 90% can be expected to produce a beneficial result.

The cornea was one of the first human tissues to be successfully grafted. The fact that recipients of corneal grafts generally tolerate them well can be attributed to (1) the absence of blood vessels or lymphatics in the normal cornea and (2) the lack of pre-sensitization to tissue-specific antigens in most recipients. Reactions to corneal grafts do occur, however, particularly in individuals whose own corneas have been damaged by previous inflammatory disease. Such corneas may have developed both lymphatics and blood vessels, providing afferent and efferent channels for immunologic reactions in the engrafted cornea.

Although attempts have been made to transplant corneas from other species into human eyes (xenografts), particularly in countries where human material is not available for religious reasons, most corneal grafts have been taken from human eyes (allografts). Except in the case of identical twins, such grafts always represent the implantation of foreign tissue into a donor site; thus, the chance for a graft rejection due to an immune response to foreign antigens is virtually always present.

The cornea is a 3-layered structure composed of a surface epithelium, an oligocellular collagenous stroma, and a single-layered endothelium. Although the surface epithelium may be sloughed and later replaced by the recipient's epithelium, certain elements of the stroma and all of the donor's endothelium remain in place for the rest of the patient's life. This has been firmly established by sex chromosome markers in corneal cells when donor and recipient were of opposite sexes. The endothelium must remain healthy in order for the cornea to remain transparent, and an energy-dependent pump mechanism is required to keep the cornea from swelling with water. Since the recipient's endothelium is in most cases diseased, the central corneal endothelium must be replaced by healthy donor tissue.

A number of foreign elements exist in corneal grafts that might stimulate the immune system of the host to reject this tissue. In addition to those mentioned above, the corneal stroma is regularly perfused with IgG and serum albumin from the donor, although none—or only small amounts—of the other blood proteins are present. While these serum proteins of donor origin rapidly diffuse into the recipient stroma, these substances are theoretically immunogenic.

Although the ABO blood antigens have been shown to have no relationship to corneal graft rejection, the HLA antigen system probably plays a significant role in graft reactions. HLA incompatibility between donor and recipient has been shown by several authors to be significant in determining graft survival, particularly when the corneal bed is vascularized. It is known that most cells of the body possess these HLA antigens, including the endothelial cells of the corneal graft as well as certain stromal cells (keratocytes). The epithelium has been shown by Hall and others to possess a non-HLA antigen that diffuses into the anterior third of the stroma. Thus, while much foreign antigen may be eliminated by purposeful removal of the epithelium at the time of grafting, that amount of antigen which has already diffused into the stroma is automatically carried over into the recipient. Such antigens may be leached out by soaking the donor cornea in tissue culture for several weeks prior to engraftment.

Both humoral and cellular mechanisms have been implicated in corneal graft reactions. It is likely that early graft rejections (within 2 weeks) are cell-mediated reactions. Cytotoxic lymphocytes have been found in the limbal area and stroma of affected individuals, and phase microscopy in vivo has revealed an actual attack on the grafted endothelial cells by these lymphocytes. Such lymphocytes generally move inward from the periphery of the cornea, making what is known as a "rejection line" as they move centrally. The donor cornea becomes edematous as the endothelium becomes compromised by an accumulation of lymphoid cells.

Late rejection of a corneal graft may occur several weeks to many months after implantation of donor tissue into the recipient eye. Such reactions may be antibody-mediated, since cytotoxic antibodies have been isolated from the serum of patients with a history of multiple graft reactions in vascularized corneal beds. These antibody reactions are complement-dependent

Figure 20–9. A cornea severely scarred by chronic atopic keratoconjunctivitis into which a central graft of clear cornea has been placed. Note how distinctly the iris landmarks are seen through the transparent graft. (Reproduced, with permission, from Stites DP et al [editors]: *Basic & Clinical immunology,* 5th ed. Lange, 1984.)

and attract polymorphonuclear leukocytes, which may form dense rings in the cornea at the sites of maximum deposition of immune complexes. In experimental animals, similar reactions have been produced by corneal xenografts, but the intensity of the reaction can be markedly reduced either by decomplementing the animal or by reducing its leukocyte population through mechlorethamine therapy.

Treatment

The mainstay of the treatment of corneal graft reactions is corticosteroid therapy. This medication is generally given in the form of frequently applied eye drops (eg, prednisolone acetate, 1%, hourly) until the clinical signs abate. These clinical signs consist of conjunctival hyperemia in the perilimbal region, a cloudy cornea, cells and protein in the anterior chamber, and keratic precipitates on the corneal endothelium. The earlier treatment is applied, the more ef-

fective it is likely to be. Neglected cases may require systemic or periocular corticosteroids in addition to local eye drop therapy. Occasionally, vascularization and opacification of the cornea occur so rapidly as to make corticosteroid therapy useless, but even the most hopeless-appearing graft reactions have occasionally been reversed by corticosteroid therapy.

Patients known to have rejected many previous corneal grafts are managed somewhat differently, particularly if disease affects their only remaining eye. An attempt is made to find a close HLA match between donor and recipient. Pretreatment of the recipient with immunosuppressive agents such as azathioprine has also been resorted to in some cases. Although HLA testing of the recipient and the potential donor is indicated in cases of repeated corneal graft failure or in cases of severe corneal vascularization, such testing is not necessary or practicable in most cases requiring keratoplasty.

REFERENCES

Allansmith MR, O'Connor GR: Immunoglobulins: Structure, function, and relation to the eye. *Surv Ophthalmol* 1970; **14:**367.

Braude LS, Chandler JW: Corneal allograft rejection: The role of the major histocompatibility complex. *Surv Ophthalmol* 1983;**27:**290.

Chandler JW, Gillette TE: Immunologic defense mechanisms of the ocular surface. *Ophthalmology* 1983;**90:**585.

Cogan DG: Immunosuppression and eye disease. *Am J Ophthalmol* 1977;**83:**777.

Foulks GN et al: Histocompatibility testing for keratoplasty in high-risk patients. *Ophthalmology* 1983;**90:**239.

Friedlaender MH: *Allergy and Immunology of the Eye.* Harper & Row, 1979.

Friedlaender MH, Okumoto M, Kelley J: Diagnosis of allergic conjunctivitis. *Arch Ophthalmol* 1984;**102:**1198.

Gillette TE, Chandler JW, Greiner JV: Langerhans cells of the ocular surface. *Ophthalmology* 1982;**89:**700.

Godfrey WA et al: The use of chlorambucil in intractable idiopathic uveitis. *Am J Ophthalmol* 1974;**78:**415.

Jakobiec FA, Lefkowitch J, Knowles DM II: B- and T-lymphocytes in ocular disease. *Ophthalmology* 1984;**91:**635.

Kaplan HJ, Waldrep JC: Immunologic insights into uveitis and retinitis: The immunoregulatory circuit. *Ophthalmology* 1984;**91:**655.

McDevitt HO: Regulation of the immune response by the major histocompatibility system. *N Engl J Med* 1980;**303:**1514.

Mehra RM et al: Chlorambucil in the treatment of iridocyclitis in juvenile rheumatoid arthritis. *J Rheumatol* 1981;**8:**141.

Mondino BJ, Brown SI: Immunosuppressive therapy in ocular cicatricial pemphigoid. *Am J Ophthalmol* 1983;**96:**453.

Nichols CW et al: Conjunctival biopsy as an aid in evaluation of the patient with suspected sarcoidosis. *Ophthalmology* 1980;**87:**287.

Nussenblatt RB: HLA and ocular disease. Proceedings of the

Immunology of the Eye Workshop 1. Steinberg GM, Gery I, Nussenblatt RB (editors). *Immunology Abstracts* 1980;**Spr Suppl:**25.

O'Connor GR: Eye diseases. Chap 34, pp 673–681, in: *Basic & Clinical Immunology,* 5th ed. Stites DP et al (editors). Lange, 1984.

O'Connor GR (editor): *Immunologic Diseases of the Mucous Membranes: Pathology, Diagnosis, and Treatment.* Masson, 1980.

O'Connor GR, Chandler JW: *Advances in Immunology and Immunopathology of the Eye.* Masson, 1985.

Potts AM: The relation of immunology to the study of eye disease. Pages 335–338 in: *Year Book of Ophthalmology 1978.* Hughes WF (editor). Year Book, 1978.

Rahi AHS, Garner A: *Immunopathology of the Eye.* Blackwell, 1976.

Rao NA et al: The role of the penetrating wound in the development of sympathetic ophthalmia: Experimental observations. *Arch Ophthalmol* 1983;**101:**102.

Reed CE, Friedlaender MH: Immunologic aspects of diseases of the eye. *JAMA* 1982;**248:**2692. [Special issue.]

Rocklin RE et al: Generation of antigen-specific suppressor cells during allergy desensitization. *N Engl J Med* 1980;**302:**1213.

Salisbury JD, Gebhardt BM: Suppression of corneal allograft rejection by cyclosporin A. *Arch Ophthalmol* 1981;**99:**1640.

Silverstein AM, O'Connor GR (editors): *Immunology and Immunopathology of the Eye.* Masson, 1979.

Smolin G, O'Connor GR: *Ocular Immunology.* Lea & Febiger, 1981.

Theodore FH, Bloomfield SE, Mondino BJ: *Clinical Allergy and Immunology of the Eye.* Williams & Wilkins, 1983.

Wong VG, Anderson RR, McMaster PRB: Endogenous immune uveitis: The role of serum sickness. *Arch Ophthalmol* 1971;**85:**93.

Special Subjects of Pediatric Interest   21

The immediate examination of the newborn infant consists of a brief observation of color, responses, extremities, and digits, and a quick inspection of body surfaces. The more complete examination is done in the nursery.

Because the development of the eye often reflects organ and tissue development of the body as a whole, many congenital somatic defects are mirrored in the eye. A careful eye examination soon after birth may suggest the need for further investigative procedures. Subjective response is limited to the following response to a moving light. The only instruments required for the ocular examination of the newborn are a good hand light, an ophthalmoscope, and a loupe if necessary for magnification.

External Inspection

The eyelids are inspected for growths, deformities, lid notches, and symmetric movement with opening and closing of the eyes. The absolute and relative size of the eyeballs is noted, as well as position and alignment. Spontaneous and elicited conjugate eye movements may also be examined. The size and luster of the corneas are noted, and the anterior chambers are examined for clarity and iris configuration. The size, position, and light reaction of the pupils are also noted.

Ophthalmoscopic Examination

With undilated pupils, some information can be obtained by use of the ophthalmoscope in a dimly lighted room. Ideally, however, all newborns should be examined with an ophthalmoscope through dilated pupils. Ophthalmoscopic examination will demonstrate any corneal, lens, or vitreous opacities as well as abnormalities in the fundus. Preretinal hemorrhages have been reported in 30–45% of newborns, usually clearing completely within a few weeks and leaving no permanent visual dysfunction.

THE NORMAL EYE IN INFANTS & CHILDREN

Tests for Visual Acuity

In the early years, visual acuity should be appraised as part of each general "well child" examination. It is best not to wait until the child is old enough to respond to visual charts, since these may not furnish accurate information until school age. Estimations of vision should be made in the first few days by ascertaining the pupillary responses to light,

---

Pediatric Eye Examination Schedule

Hospital Nursery

External eye examination and ophthalmoscopic examination through dilated pupils as outlined in the text. Two drops of sterile 5% homatropine and 2.5% phenylephrine in each eye are instilled 1 hour prior to examination. Special emphasis should be placed on the optic disks and maculas; detailed examination of the peripheral retinas is not necessary.

Age 4

Visual acuity test with illiterate "E" chart and stereopsis by the random dot "E" test to rule out amblyopia. Visual acuity is normal (6/6–6/9) (20/20–20/30) by 4–5 years of age.

Age 5–16

Test visual acuity at age 5. If normal, test visual acuity with the Snellen chart every 2 years until age 16. Color vision should be tested at age 8–12. No other routine eye examination (eg, ophthalmoscopy) is necessary if visual acuity is normal and the eyes appear normal upon inspection.

---

which rules out complete dysfunction of the eyes. In later weeks, light fixation reflexes can be elicited—single and bilateral reflexes first, and then binocular following and converging reflexes. A good response consists of prompt fixation and following reflexes, equal in each eye, with the light reflex centered in the pupil when the source is near the examiner's eye.

These indirect inferences about the status of the developing sensory systems can now be augmented by the quantitative techniques of optokinetic nystagmus, forced-choice preferential looking methods, and visually evoked potentials (see Chapter 3). These tests have demonstrated that normal adult visual acuity is attained by about 2 years of age (Table 21–1).

During the growing years, the parents' observations of the child's clumsiness, awareness of surroundings, and apparent sharpness of vision are valuable aids. From about age 4 on, it becomes possible to elicit subjective responses by use of the illiterate "E" chart. Usually, at the first or second grade level, the regular Snellen chart may be employed.

Table 21–1. Development of visual
acuity (approximate).

Age	Visual Acuity
2 months	6/120 (20/400)
6 months	6/30 (20/100)
1 year	6/15 (20/50)
2 years	6/6 (20/20)

Eyeball

In the newborn, the eye is relatively larger in comparison with body size than in later life. However, the anteroposterior diameter, which determines the focusing of the eye, is relatively short (averaging about 17.3 mm). This would produce a marked hyperopia if it were not for the greater curvature of the lens at this time.

Cornea

The cornea of the newborn is also relatively large and reaches adult size by about 2 years of age. It is flatter than the adult cornea, however, and the curvature is greater at the periphery than in the center, whereas the opposite is true in the adult.

Lens

At birth the lens is more globular than in adulthood, and its greater refractive power compensates for the shortness of the eye. The lens grows throughout life as new fibers are added to the periphery, and this causes it to flatten. The consistency of the lens material changes throughout life from a soft plasticlike material to the glassy consistency seen in old age. This accounts for the gradual loss in power of accommodation with advancing age.

Refractive State

About 80% of children between the ages of 2 and 6 years are hyperopic, 5% myopic, and 15% emmetropic. About 10% have refractive errors that require correction before age 7 or 8. Hyperopia remains relatively static or gradually diminishes until 19 or 20 years of age. Myopia often develops between age 6–9 and increases throughout adolescence, with the greatest change at the time of puberty. Astigmatism is congenital and remains relatively constant throughout life. Transient refractive changes are well documented in the neonatal period.

Iris

At birth there is little or no pigment on the anterior surface of the iris. The posterior pigment layer shows through the translucent tissue, usually giving the effect of a bluish or slate-gray color. As the pigment begins to appear on the anterior surface, the iris assumes its definitive color. If considerable pigment is deposited, the eyes become brown. Less pigmentation results in blue, gray, hazel, or green eyes. It may take 1–2 years for the pigmentary deposits to occur; in the meantime it is impossible to ascertain the ultimate color of the eyes.

Pupil

In the newborn, the pupil is situated slightly to the nasal side of and below the center of the cornea. Because of the refractive power of the cornea in the neonatal period, the pupil appears larger than it actually is. The apparent diameter varies between 2.5 and 5.5 mm and averages about 4 mm. In infancy, the pupil is smaller than at birth. Congenital underdevelopment of the dilator muscle is common in children with congenital cataracts. The pupillary reflexes appear at about the fifth fetal month and are active by the sixth month. At about age 1 the pupil begins to widen, and it reaches its greatest diameter during adolescence. It again becomes smaller with advancing age. Myopes have larger pupils than hyperopes.

Normal pupils are round and regular and constantly move in response to changes in lighting and upon focusing. Anisocoria, a difference in the size of the 2 pupils, is often a normal finding; in the absence of neurologic abnormalities, it requires no further special diagnostic consideration.

Position

During the first month of life, eye movements may be poorly coordinated and there may be some doubt about the straightness of the eyes. By 3 months of age, however, the binocular reflexes are well developed; any deviation noted after that time should be investigated. Stereoacuity can be shown to develop in most infants beginning at 3 months of age. If strabismus is suspected after age 3 months, referral to an ophthalmologist is indicated.

Nasolacrimal System

The fetal development of the nasolacrimal passages begins as cords of cells that usually hollow out about the time of birth. Because there may normally be a few weeks' delay in duct formation, failure of tear production in the first few weeks does not necessarily indicate any difficulty; failure of the ducts to function by 6 months of age, however, needs attention.

Optic Nerve

By term, some fibers in the optic nerve near the globe begin to become myelinated, but the amount of myelin surrounding individual nerves increases dramatically during the ensuing months and may continue to increase up to the age of 2 years.

The Normal Ocular Fundus of Infants & Children

The ophthalmoscopic appearance of the normal fundus in an infant differs greatly from that of an adult. Most of the differences are due to the distribution of pigments.

In premature infants, remnants of the tunica vasculosa lentis are frequently visible with the ophthalmoscope, either in front of the lens, behind the lens, or in both positions. The remnants are usually absorbed by the time the infant has reached term, but rarely they remain permanently and appear as a complete or partial "cobweb" in the pupil. At other times remnants of the primitive hyaloid system fail to absorb completely, leaving a cone on the optic disk that projects into the vitreous and is called Bergmeister's papilla.

Physiologic cupping of the disk is usually not seen in premature infants and is rarely seen at term; if seen then, it is usually very slight. In such cases the optic disk will appear gray, resembling optic nerve atrophy. This relative pallor, however, gradually changes to the normal adult pink color at about 2 years of age.

The foveal light reflection is absent in infants. Instead, the macula has a bright "mother-of-pearl" appearance with a suggestion of elevation. This is more pronounced in black infants. At 3–4 months of age, the macula becomes slightly concave and the foveal light reflection appears.

The peripheral fundus in the infant is gray, in contrast to the orange-red fundus of the adult. In white infants the pigmentation is more pronounced near the posterior pole and gradually fades to almost white at the periphery. In black infants there is more pigment in the fundus and a gray-blue sheen is seen throughout the periphery. In white infants a white periphery is normal and should not be confused with retinoblastoma. During the next several months, pigment continues to be deposited in the retina, and usually at about 2 years of age the adult color is evident.

CONGENITAL EYE DEFECTS

Most congenital ocular defects are genetically determined. Examples include congenital ptosis, refractive errors, aniridia, strabismus, retinitis pigmentosa, and arachnodactyly (Marfan's syndrome). Absence of a positive family history is no proof that the defect is not in the germ plasm (see Chapter 22).

Other congenital defects may be caused by interference with the development of the embryo, such as the multiple defects associated with rubella infection of the mother during the first 3 months of pregnancy. In this instance the infant may suffer from any or all of the following: cataracts, heart disease, deafness, microcephaly, microphthalmos, and mental deficiency. Eye defects are common in cerebral palsy.

Anophthalmos

This is a rare condition in which one or both eyeballs are absent or rudimentary. There may be either a congenital absence of any ocular structure or an arrest of development to the point where only histologic evidence is present. The eyelids are usually present. They are often adherent at the margins but can be separated. Anophthalmos may be associated with a chromosomal variation and there may be associated intracranial anomalies.

Congenital Cystic Eye

This is a developmental abnormality resulting from complete or partial failure of invagination of the primary optic vesicle. The eye is variable in size and is usually associated with some degree of neuroglial proliferation. The malformation occurs at about the fourth week of embryonic life.

Cyclopia

Cyclopia, which is a rare midline fusion of developing eye structures together with generalized anterior brain and skull defects, is usually not compatible with life since it is transmitted by a recessive lethal gene.

Palpebral Colobomas

A unilateral cleft of one upper lid is the most common type of palpebral coloboma. Bilateral clefts or fissures can occur in lower as well as upper lids and may be associated with other malformations of the face or globe. No specific embryonic maldevelopment has been established as being causative. Large defects require early repair to avoid corneal ulceration due to exposure.

Microphthalmos

In microphthalmos, one or both eyes are markedly smaller than normal. Many other ocular abnormalities may be present also, eg, cataract, glaucoma, aniridia, and coloboma. Somatic abnormalities are also often present, eg, polydactyly, syndactyly, clubfoot, polycystic kidneys, cystic liver, cleft palate, and meningoencephalocele. Microphthalmos is nearly always genetically determined—most frequently as a recessive but occasionally as a dominant trait.

Corneal Defects

There may be partial or complete opacity of the corneas such as is found in congenital glaucoma, faulty development of the cornea with persistent corneal-lens attachments, birth injuries, intrauterine inflammation, interstitial keratitis, and mucopolysaccharide depositions of the cornea as in Hurler's syndrome. The most frequent cause of opaque corneas in infants and young children is congenital glaucoma. In most instances, the eye is larger than normal (macrophthalmos, hydrophthalmos, buphthalmos). Birth injuries may cause extensive corneal opacities with edema as a result of rupture of Descemet's membrane. These usually clear spontaneously.

Megalocornea is an enlarged cornea with normal function usually transmitted as an X-linked recessive trait. It must be differentiated from infantile glaucoma. There are usually no associated defects.

Iris & Pupillary Defects

Misplaced or ectopic pupils are frequently observed. The usual displacement is upward and laterally (temporally) from the center of the cornea. Such displacement is occasionally associated with ectopic lens, congenital glaucoma, or microcornea. Multiple pupils are known as **polycoria.** A true pupil must constrict on exposure to light, indicating a sphincter muscle. Congenital miosis is due to a poorly developed dilator muscle. Little change in pupillary size is noted after instillation of a mydriatic. Congenital mydriasis is characterized by large and inactive pupils and under-developed sphincter muscles and must be differen-tiated from mydriasis due to juvenile paresis and pineal tumor. **Coloboma of the iris** indicates incomplete closure of the fetal ocular cleft and usually occurs below and nasally. It may be associated with coloboma of the lens, choroid, and optic nerve. **Aniridia** (ab-sence of the iris) is a rare abnormality, frequently associated with secondary glaucoma (see p 195) and due to an autosomal dominant hereditary pattern. Var-ious abnormalities in the shape of the pupils have been described but are not necessarily significant. Persistent mesodermal remnants usually appear as threadlike bands running across the central pupillary space and attached to the lesser circle of the iris. They rarely have clinical significance or interfere with visual acu-ity.

The color of the iris is determined largely by he-redity. Abnormalities in color include **albinism** (see p 295), due to the absence of normal pigmentation of the ocular structures and frequently associated with poor visual acuity and nystagmus; and **hetero-chromia,** which is a difference in color in the 2 eyes that may be a primary developmental defect with no functional loss or may be secondary to an inflam-matory process.

Lens Abnormalities

The lens abnormalities most frequently noted are cataracts, although there may be faulty development, forming colobomas, or subluxation, as seen in Mar-fan's syndrome.

Any lens opacity that is present at birth is a con-genital cataract, regardless of whether or not it inter-feres with visual acuity. Congenital cataracts are often associated with other conditions. Maternal rubella during the first trimester of pregnancy is a common cause of congenital cataract. Other congenital cata-racts have a hereditary background.

If the opacity is small enough so that it does not occlude the pupil, adequate visual acuity is attained by focusing around the opacity. If the pupillary open-ing is entirely occluded, however, normal sight does not develop, and the poor fixation may lead to nys-tagmus and amblyopia. Good visual results have been reported with both monocular and binocular cataracts receiving early surgery and aphakic correction. Thus, early referral to an ophthalmologist is indicated.

Choroid & Retina

Gross defects of the choroid and retina are visible with the ophthalmoscope. The choroidal structures may show congenital colobomas, usually in the lower nasal region, which may also include the iris and all or part of the optic nerve. Posterior polar chorioretinal scarring is a pigmentary disturbance often caused by

intrauterine toxoplasmosis. Other congenital lesions of the choroid and retina include drusen, aneurysms, optic nerve malformations, medullated nerve fibers, hereditary macular degeneration, and those associated with intrauterine infections.

DEVELOPMENTAL BODY DEFECTS ASSOCIATED WITH OCULAR DEFECTS

Albinism

Congenital deficiency of pigment may involve the entire body (complete albinism) or a part of the body (incomplete albinism). When incomplete albinism in-volves only the eye, function may be normal or im-paired. In complete ocular albinism, there is usually an abnormal development of the macula, a significant refractive error, nystagmus, and severe photophobia. The eyebrows and eyelashes are white, the conjunctiva is hyperemic, the irides are gray or red, and the pupil appears red. Treatment consists of relieving photo-phobia with tinted glasses or opaque contact lenses with a clear central area 2–3 mm in diameter.

Marfan's Syndrome

A congenital disorder of mesodermal origin that is nearly always transmitted as an autosomal dominant trait; the major features are (1) long, thin fingers and toes (arachnodactyly), (2) generalized relaxation of ligaments, (3) generalized muscular underdevelop-ment, (4) bilateral dislocation of the lenses (ectopia lentis), (5) abnormalities of the heart and, occasion-ally, aortic aneurysm, (6) high-arched palate, and (7) other deformities of the sternum, thorax, and joints.

The lenses are usually dislocated and visual acuity suffers because the patient is not seeing through the lens centers. Cataracts frequently develop in the sub-luxated lenses. Cataract surgery may become neces-sary but has a less favorable prognosis than routine cataract surgery.

Osteogenesis Imperfecta

This rare affliction is characterized by increased fragility of the bones and laxity of the ligaments, with frequent fractures and dislocations, dental defects, deafness, and blue scleras. The blue color is darker in the anterior parts of the scleras over the ciliary bodies. It is thought to be due to abnormal thinness of the sclera and remains unchanged throughout life. Cataracts, megalocornea, and keratoconus may also be present. It nearly always occurs as an autosomal dominant trait.

Gargoylism (Hurler's Syndrome)

This is a rare condition due to autosomal recessive inheritance in which there is infiltration of mucopoly-saccharides into the tissues, especially the liver, spleen, lymph nodes, pituitary gland, and corneas. Other ocu-lar signs include slight ptosis, larger thickened eyelids, and strabismus (esotropia). The corneas show a diffuse haziness, which progresses to a milk-white opacity.

Glaucoma may eventually develop. There is no satisfactory treatment.

Oxycephaly (Acrocephaly, Tower Skull, Steeple Head)

This deformity is evident at birth but is often attributed to normal distortion during delivery and is seldom diagnosed at the time of delivery. It is characterized by a high, dome-shaped or pointed skull, high forehead, bulging temporal fossae, flattened cheekbones, shallow orbits, a high, narrow palatal arch, and synostosis of the cranial suture. Syndactyly may also be present. The ocular signs include exophthalmos (due to flatness of the orbits), wide separation of the eyes, and exotropia. Closure of the eyelids may be difficult or impossible. Loss of vision may follow increased intracranial pressure. Nystagmus is common. Various operative procedures have been devised for the relief of intracranial pressure. If vision is to be preserved, surgery must be performed before optic atrophy has progressed. The syndrome is due to an autosomal dominant gene of weak penetrance.

Acrobrachycephaly

In this abnormality the head is wide, whereas in oxycephaly it is narrow. Acrobrachycephaly is caused by premature closure of the coronal sutures. Growth occurs only laterally and vertically, and the anteroposterior diameter is short. The ocular signs are similar to those of oxycephaly.

Other abnormalities involving the development of the skull are scaphocephaly (increased anteroposterior diameter due to premature closure of the sagittal suture) and plagiocephaly (asymmetric flattening, usually due to premature closure of a single coronal suture).

Craniofacial Dysostosis (Crouzon's Disease)

This rare hereditary deformity, due to an autosomal dominant gene, is characterized by exophthalmos, atrophy of the maxilla, enlargement of the nasal bones, abnormal increase in the space between the eyes (ocular hypertelorism), optic atrophy, and bony abnormalities of the region of the perilongitudinal sinus. The palpebral fissures slant downward (in contrast to the upward slant of Down's syndrome). Strabismus and nystagmus are also present. The strabismus is secondary to both structural anomalies of the muscles and orbital angle anomalies.

Laurence-Moon-Biedl Syndrome

This syndrome includes retinitis pigmentosa, polydactyly, obesity, hypogenitalism, and mental retardation. It is inherited as an autosomal recessive.

POSTNATAL PROBLEMS

The most common ocular disorders of children are external infections of the conjunctiva and eyelids (bacterial conjunctivitis, sties, blepharitis), strabismus, ocular foreign bodies, allergic reactions of the conjunctiva and eyelids, refractive errors (particularly myopia), and congenital defects. Since it is more difficult to elicit an accurate history of causative factors and subjective complaints in children, it is not uncommon to overlook significant ocular disorders (especially in very young children). Aside from the altered frequency of occurrence of the types of ocular disorders, the causes, manifestations, and treatment of eye disorders are about the same for children as for adults. Certain special problems encountered more frequently in infants and children are discussed below.

Ophthalmia Neonatorum (Conjunctivitis of the Newborn)

Conjunctivitis in the newborn may be of chemical, bacterial, chlamydial, or viral origin. *Chlamydia* is now the commonest identifiable infectious cause of neonatal conjunctivitis in the USA. Differentiation is sometimes possible according to the timing of presentation, but appropriate smears and cultures are essential. Chemical conjunctivitis caused by the silver nitrate drops instilled into the conjunctival sac at birth is most apparent during the first or second day of life. Inclusion blennorrhea due to chlamydial infection has its onset between the fifth and 14th days; the presence of typical inclusion bodies in the epithelial cells of a conjunctival smear confirms this diagnosis. Bacterial conjunctivitis, usually due to *Staphylococcus aureus*, *Haemophilus* species, pneumococcus, enterococcus, *Neisseria gonorrhoeae*, or *Pseudomonas* species (the last 2 being the most serious because of potential corneal damage), presents between the second and fifth days after birth. Provisional identification of the causative organism may be made from conjunctival smears. Herpes simplex virus produces characteristic giant cells and viral inclusions on cytologic examination.

Silver nitrate conjunctivitis is usually self-limited. In inclusion blennorrhea, systemic therapy with erythromycin is more effective than topical therapy and aids in the eradication of concurrent nasopharyngeal carriage, which may predispose to the development of pneumonitis. Gonococcal conjunctivitis necessitates parenteral therapy with aqueous crystalline benzylpenicillin given intravenously for penicillin-sensitive strains, and cefotaxime given intravenously with topical erythromycin for penicillinase-producing strains. In all cases due to *Chlamydia* or gonococci, both parents should also be given systemic treatment. Other types of bacterial conjunctivitis require topical instillation of antibacterial agents, such as sodium sulfacetamide, bacitracin, or tetracycline, as soon as results of smears are known. Herpetic keratoconjunctivitis usually resolves spontaneously but may require antiviral therapy, particularly when associated with disseminated infection.

Silver nitrate solution (1%) should be contained in sealed single-use disposable containers. Because of the possibility of chemical conjunctivitis and the lack of effectiveness of silver nitrate against *Chlamydia*, some authorities advocate use of topical erythromycin or tetracycline instead for prophylaxis. Instillation of silver nitrate or an antibiotic is still required in most states in the USA.

Antenatal diagnosis and treatment of maternal genital infections should prevent many cases of neonatal conjunctivitis. The presence of active maternal genital herpes at the time of delivery is an indication for elective cesarean section.

Retinopathy of Prematurity (Retrolental Fibroplasia)

In the early stages of retinopathy of prematurity, demarcated areas of avascularity develop in the peripheral retina. These are followed by extraretinal fibrovascular proliferation and retinal detachment. Supplemental oxygen therapy in neonatal intensive care units was strongly implicated as a causative factor in the original epidemic of 1943–1953. There was a marked reduction in the incidence of disease once oxygen therapy was more carefully controlled. A recent resurgence has been noted by many ophthalmologists, particularly in premature infants of very low birth weight (< 1000 g). The causative factors in these cases are as yet unclear. (See also Chapter 14 and discussion of oxygen in Chapter 19.)

Congenital Glaucoma

Congenital glaucoma (see Chapter 15) may occur alone or in association with many other congenital lesions. Early recognition is essential to prevent permanent blindness. Involvement is often bilateral. The most striking symptom is extreme photophobia. Early signs are corneal haze or opacity, increased corneal diameter, and increased intraocular pressure. Since the outer coats of the eyeball are not as rigid in the child, the increased intraocular pressure expands the corneal and scleral tissues. Useful vision may be preserved by early diagnosis and medical and surgical treatment by an ophthalmologist.

Leukocoria (White Pupil)

Parents will occasionally see a white spot through the infant's pupil (leukocoria). Although retinoblastoma must be ruled out, the opacity is more often due to cataract, retrolental fibroplasia, persistence of the tunica vasculosa lentis, or corneal scarring.

Retinoblastoma

This rare malignant tumor of childhood is fatal if untreated. Two-thirds of cases occur before the end of the third year; rarely, cases have been reported in later childhood, adolescence, and even (very rarely) in adults. In about 30% of cases, retinoblastoma is bilateral. Development of the tumor is thought to occur because of the loss, from both members of the chromosome pair, of the normally protective dominant allele at a single locus within chromosomal band 13q14. This is caused by mutations, either in the somatic retinal cells alone (nonheritable retinoblastoma) or in the germ line cells as well (heritable retinoblastoma). In heritable retinoblastoma, children of survivors have a nearly 50% chance of having the disease, and it is more apt to be bilateral in succeeding generations. Parents who have produced one child with retinoblastoma run a 4–7% risk of producing the disease in each subsequently born child. Retinoblastoma is usually not discovered until it has advanced far enough to produce an opaque pupil. Infants and children with presenting symptoms of strabismus should be examined carefully to rule out retinoblastoma, since a deviating eye may be the first sign of the tumor.

Enucleation is the treatment of choice in nearly all unilateral cases of retinoblastoma. Additional discussion, including other possible methods for treatment, is presented on p 331.

Strabismus

Strabismus is present in about 2% of children. Its early recognition is often the responsibility of the pediatrician or the family physician. Occasionally, childhood strabismus has neurologic significance. Treatment of strabismus is best started at the age of 6 months to ensure development of the best possible visual acuity and a good cosmetic and functional result (binocular vision). The idea that a child may outgrow crossed eyes should be discouraged. Neglect in the treatment of strabismus may lead to undesirable cosmetic effects, psychic trauma, and amblyopia (see below) in the deviating eye. Strabismus is covered in depth in Chapter 16.

Amblyopia

Amblyopia is decreased visual acuity of one eye (uncorrectable with lenses) in the absence of organic eye disease.

Normal development of the physiologic mechanisms of the retina and visual cortex is determined by postnatal visual experience. Monocular deprivation due to any cause, congenital or acquired, during a critical period of development (probably lasting up to age 10 in humans) prevents the establishment of normal vision in the involved eye. Reversal of this effect is possible only within a much more limited time period, which decreases with increasing age from a few months to only a few weeks. Early suspicion and prompt referral for treatment of the underlying condition are important in preventing amblyopia.

The most common causes of amblyopia are strabismus, in which the image from the deviated eye is suppressed to prevent diplopia, and anisometropia, in which an inability to focus the eyes simultaneously causes suppression of the image of one eye. Both of these conditions are treatable. (See Chapter 16.)

Since poor visual function in a young child may go unnoticed, routine testing of visual acuity at age 4 is essential in reducing the number of cases of amblyopia.

REFERENCES

Atkinson J et al: Screening for refractive errors in 6–9 month old infants by photorefraction. *Br J Ophthalmol* 1984;**68:**105.

Balkan R, Hoyt CS: Associated neurologic abnormalities in congenital third nerve palsies. *Am J Ophthalmol* 1984;**97:**315.

Banks MS: Infant refraction and accommodation. *Int Ophthalmol Clin* 1980;**20:**205.

Beller R et al: Good visual function after neonatal surgery for congenital monocular cataracts. *Am J Ophthalmol* 1981; **91:**559.

Cameron JH, Cameron M: Visual screening of pre-school children. *Br Med J* 1978;**2:**1693.

Campbell PB et al: Incidence of retinopathy of prematurity in a tertiary newborn intensive care unit. *Arch Ophthalmol* 1983; **101:**1686.

Fulton AB, Hansen RM, Manning KA: Measuring visual acuity in infants. *Surv Ophthalmol* 1981;**25:**325.

Gallie BL, Phillips RA: Retinoblastoma: A model of oncogenesis. *Ophthalmology* 1984;**91:**667.

Garner A: An international classification of retinopathy of prematurity. *Br J Ophthalmol* 1984;**68:**690.

Hall SM, Pugh AG, Hall DMB: Vision screening in the under-5s. *Br Med J* 1982;**285:**1096.

Halloran SL et al: Accuracy of detection of the retinoblastoma gene by esterase D linkage. *Arch Ophthalmol* 1985;**103:**1329.

Hammerschlag MR et al: Erythromycin ointment for ocular prophylaxis of neonatal chlamydial infection. *JAMA* 1980; **244:**2291.

Harley RD (editor): *Pediatric Ophthalmology,* 2nd ed. Saunders, 1983.

Hoskins HD, Shaffer RN, Hetherington J: Anatomical classification of the developmental glaucomas. *Arch Ophthalmol* 1984;**102:**1331.

Hoyt CS, Nickel BL, Billson FA: Ophthalmological examination of the infant. *Surv Ophthalmol* 1982;**26:**177.

Kalina RE: Examination of the premature infant. *Ophthalmology* 1979;**86:**1690.

Mayer DL, Fulton AB, Rodier D: Grating and recognition acuities of pediatric patients. *Ophthalmology* 1984;**91:**947.

Mukai S et al: Linkage of genes for human esterase D and hereditary retinoblastoma. *Am J Ophthalmol* 1984;**97:**681.

Nelson LB: *Pediatric Ophthalmology: Major Problems in Clincal Pediatrics.* Vol 25. Saunders, 1984.

Nelson LB (editor): *Symposium on Pediatric Ophthalmology: The Pediatric Clinics of North America.* Vol 30. Saunders, 1983.

Ophthalmia neonatorum today. (Editorial.) *Lancet* 1984;**2:**1375.

Pierce JM, Ward ME, Seal DV: Ophthalmia neonatorum in the 1980s: Incidence, aetiology and treatment. *Br J Ophthalmol* 1982;**66:**728.

Reinecke RD, Feman SS: *Handbook of Pediatric Ophthalmology.* Grune & Stratton, 1978.

Rice NSC, Taylor D: Congenital cataract: A cause of preventable blindness in children. (Editorial.) *Br Med J* 1982;**285:**581.

Skarf B, Hoyt CS: Optic nerve hypoplasia in children: Association with anomalies of the endocrine and CNS. *Arch Ophthalmol* 1984;**102:**62.

Taylor D: The assessment of visual function in young children: An overview. Regrettably there are no rapid and infallible methods. *Clin Pediatr* 1978;**17:**226.

Wybar K, Taylor D (editors): *Paediatric Ophthalmology: Current Aspects.* Marcel Dekker, 1983.

22

Genetic Aspects

Genetic influences are being described in an increasing number of diseases, and a primary causative role for genetic defects is being more clearly defined in many instances. Thus, it becomes increasingly important to understand the principles of genetic transmission. Much of the background work in clinical genetics has been done in ophthalmology. The eye seems to be unusually prone to genetically determined disease, and an accurate diagnosis of ocular disease can usually be arrived at on the basis of careful clinical examination.

Clinicians can estimate the risk of occurrence of many genetically determined diseases (usually the rare but severe ones), but the familial incidence of many other diseases also known to be genetically determined still cannot be accurately predicted.

Mechanisms of Inheritance

An individual's genetic identity (**genotype**) is carried by **chromosomes,** which are composed of DNA. There are 23 pairs of chromosomes in the nucleus of the normal human somatic cell. Twenty-two of these pairs are somewhat similar (homologous) and are therefore termed **autosomal.** The 23rd pair is composed of the **sex chromosomes** (X and Y). In the female this pair is homologous (XX), whereas in the male it is heterologous (XY). A number of agents (quinacrine mustard, trypsin, Giemsa's stain) produce morphologic banding of human chromosomes that permits their identification and classification into a number of groups.

Each chromosome is composed of many small functional units termed **genes,** which are situated at specific sites (**loci**) along the length of the chromosome. Genes are thus also arranged in pairs. The alternate forms of a gene at a locus controlling a particular characteristic are known as **alleles.** There are commonly 2 alternate forms, but there may be more. When the alleles at a particular locus are the same, the individual is said to be homozygous, and when they are different, heterozygous.

Genes exert their effects by controlling the production of proteins within the cell cytoplasm. Complementary copies of the DNA constituting specific genes are formed with RNA, and these are used to direct protein synthesis. The mechanisms regulating gene expression are complex.

DNA recombinant technology using isolated human DNA fragments inserted into bacterial cells has led to the identification of the DNA sequences and protein products of specific genes. Linkage studies and DNA probes have identified the position of specific gene loci and carriers for certain mutant genes.

The **gametes** (spermatozoon and ovum) are produced by a special type of cell division called **reduction-division meiosis,** in which the 23 pairs of chromosomes dissociate, each daughter cell receiving one chromosome of each pair. One of each pair passes into each daughter cell as a random occurrence. Exchange of chromosomal material (**translocation**) between the members of each pair also occurs. At fertilization, each chromosome of the spermatozoon joins its corresponding chromosome of the ovum to produce a cell with 46 chromosomes of unique genetic constitution. All cell divisions after fertilization (**mitosis**) involve duplication and separation of all the chromosomes to produce cells with the constant number of 46 chromosomes and identical genetic constitution.

The expression of the genotype in physical characteristics is known as the **phenotype.** The inheritance of certain characteristics of the human phenotype, such as eye color, can be explained on the basis of interaction between the 2 alleles at a single chromosomal locus. Each allele determines the development of one form of the particular characteristic. In the homozygous individual, this form is correspondingly expressed. In the heterozygous individual, one allele is said to be **dominant** because it determines the phenotype, while the other is **recessive** (not expressed). This is the basis of **mendelian inheritance,** from which are derived many of the terms used to describe patterns of inheritance. The inheritance of many phenotypic characteristics, however, cannot easily be classified in this way. This has led to modifications of the original mendelian concepts, including variable expression and variable penetration of genes. Recent improvements in the understanding of gene regulation and expression, as well as recognition of the role of environmental factors, have demonstrated why this model breaks down. Nevertheless, the framework of mendelian inheritance is still of immense value in clinical genetics as a means of describing modes of inheritance and estimating the risk of transmission of certain genetically determined abnormalities. The major alternative patterns of inheritance are those due to chromosomal abnormalities and those described as multifactorial, involving multiple genes or major environmental influences.

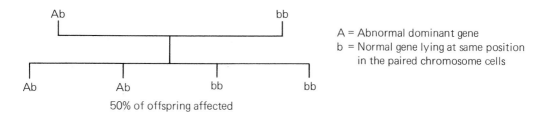

A = Abnormal dominant gene
b = Normal gene lying at same position in the paired chromosome cells

50% of offspring affected

Figure 22–1. Autosomal dominant inheritance.

MENDELIAN INHERITANCE

Mendelian inheritance can be divided into 3 main groups: autosomal dominant, autosomal recessive, and X-linked recessive.

Autosomal Dominant Inheritance

An abnormal dominant gene produces its specific abnormality even though its paired gene (allele) is normal. Males and females are affected alike and, being heterozygous, have a theoretical 50% chance of passing along the affected gene (and therefore the abnormality) to each of their offspring, even when mated to genotypically normal individuals (Fig 22– 1).

Given a particular group of pedigrees, autosomal dominant inheritance is established if the following conditions are met: (1) Males and females are equally affected. (2) Direct transmission has occurred over 2 or more generations. (3) About 50% of individuals in the pedigrees are affected.

Quite a large number of uncommon but serious diseases with ocular manifestations are transmitted in this way: forms of juvenile glaucoma, Marfan's syndrome, congenital stationary night blindness (Fig 22– 2), osteogenesis imperfecta, and all the phakomatoses, which include neurofibromatosis, Lindau-Von Hippel disease, tuberous sclerosis, and Sturge-Weber syndrome. The process of natural selection tends to keep most of these serious diseases at a low incidence in the general population, since many of these people are unable to produce children even if they do manage to live to the age of reproduction.

Dominant disease may be more or less severe from generation to generation depending upon its **expression;** a disease with ''variable expression'' is one that can occur in a mild or severe form. An example is neurofibromatosis, in which genotypically affected individuals may have merely café au lait spots or may have many serious manifestations. One cannot predict if or when the disease will be more serious (with central nervous system tumors or optic nerve gliomas) in a succeeding generation. If the genetic pattern is present but there is no evidence of the disease, one says that its **penetrance** is reduced. It may be quite difficult to differentiate dominant inheritance with reduced penetrance from recessive inheritance (see below). To quote Duke-Elder, ''It may well be said that dominance and recessiveness are not two distinct antitheses but represent the two extremes of a continuous series of variable types of hereditary transmission, all of which are fundamentally the same.'' Those pedigrees which demonstrate neither a definite autosomal dominant nor a definite recessive pattern are properly classified as irregular dominants (dominant inheritance with variable expression) or incomplete recessives (carrier state identifiable clinically).

In certain diseases such as hemoglobin S disease, there is a clearly defined intermediate phenotype that corresponds to the heterozygous individual. This is known as **codominant inheritance.**

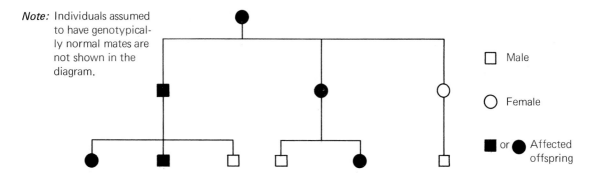

Note: Individuals assumed to have genotypically normal mates are not shown in the diagram.

☐ Male

○ Female

■ or ● Affected offspring

Figure 22–2. Pedigree of congenital stationary night blindness (abnormal dominant gene).

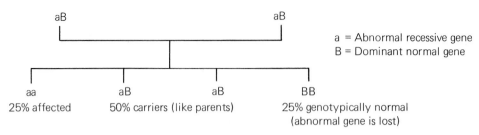

a = Abnormal recessive gene
B = Dominant normal gene

Figure 22–3. Mating of 2 carriers.

Autosomal Recessive Inheritance

Abnormal recessive genes must lie in pairs (duplex state) to produce manifest abnormality. Thus, each parent must contribute one recessive abnormal gene. Each parent is clinically unaffected (genotypically affected but phenotypically normal), since a normal dominant gene makes the abnormal gene recessive (Fig 22– 3).

It is difficult to establish that a given disease results from autosomal recessive inheritance. Some of the criteria used to establish recessive inheritance are the following:

(1) Occurrence of the same disease in collateral branches of the family.

(2) History of consanguinity. The higher the rate of consanguinity in the pedigrees of a given disease, the more likely the disease is to be recessive and the rarer the occurrence of the disease in the general population. Consanguinity creates greater opportunities for the genes to lie in the duplex state, inasmuch as an individual with 2 related parents can receive the same affected gene from each, a common ancestor having originally passed on the affected gene.

(3) The occurrence of the disease in about 25% of siblings. This only holds for groups of pedigrees. There is a 25% chance that the 2 abnormal genes will be passed on to one individual. There is a 50% chance that a normal gene will modify the affected gene. In this case, the individual is a carrier of the disease (just like the parents) but is not affected with the disease (ie, genotypically affected but phenotypically normal). In the remaining 25% of siblings, 2 normal genes lie together and the abnormal gene is completely lost (ie, the individual is genotypically normal). Although a number of pedigrees are required to definitely establish recessive inheritance, even a single pedigree is suggestive if more than one sibling is similarly affected without antecedent history.

Many disease processes have been definitely established as resulting from autosomal recessive inheritance, and many others are suspected of having such a genetic background. Included among the definite cases are Laurence-Moon-Biedl syndrome and inborn errors of metabolism such as oculocutaneous albinism (Fig 22– 4), galactokinase deficiency, and Tay-Sachs disease.

X-Linked (Sex-Linked) Recessive Inheritance

The sex chromosomes are one of the 23 pairs of human chromosomes. Identical chromosomes appear in females; these have been labeled with X chromosomes. One such chromosome appears with a dissimilar mate in the male; this smaller chromosome has been labeled the Y chromosome. Therefore, XX is female and XY is male.

The criteria for X-linked inheritance are (1) that only males are affected, (2) that the disease is transmitted through carrier females to half of the sons, and (3) that there is no father-to-son transmission.

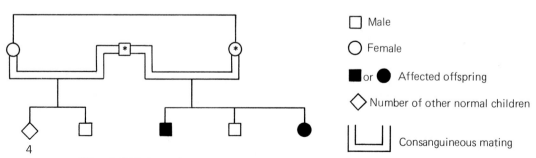

☐ Male

◯ Female

■ or ● Affected offspring

◇ Number of other normal children

Consanguineous mating

*These individuals must be carriers, although there may be no clinical method of detection.

Figure 22–4. Pedigree of oculocutaneous albinism. In this case a man married successively 2 sisters, his first cousins.

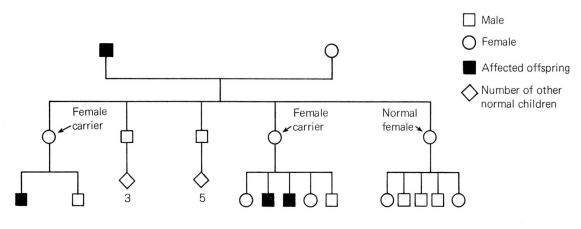

Figure 22–5. Pedigree of red-green color blindness.

Many of the genes of the X chromosome are unopposed by a gene of the Y chromosome. Abnormalities of these genes cause disease in the male, whereas in the female an abnormal recessive gene of the sex chromosome is masked by its normal allele. Therefore, nearly all of the X-linked diseases are manifested in males, whereas the disease is passed through the female. A male and his maternal grandfather are affected, and the intervening female is the carrier.

Among the important eye diseases with an X-linked genetic pattern are color blindness (Fig 22–5), ocular albinism, and one type of retinitis pigmentosa.

Females have a mosaic of somatic cells consisting of cell groups with one X chromosome functioning and cell groups with the other X chromosome functioning (Lyon hypothesis). When the female is a carrier of an X-linked disease, this mosaicism is occasionally detectable. Such is the case in female carriers of ocular albinism, in whom groups of pigmented and albino retinal pigment epithelial cells are visible ophthalmoscopically.

CHROMOSOMAL ABNORMALITIES

When mitosis is interrupted in metaphase, the chromosomes can be spread on a slide, counted, and photographed. These cytogenetic studies have made possible the classification of chromosomes into 7 groups based upon characteristics such as size and the position of the centromere. The groups contain as few as 2 or as many as 7 chromosomes, with the chromosomes of any group being indistinguishable from each other. The study of cytogenetics has also established that some clinical states can be correlated with an abnormal number of chromosomes, most frequently one more (trisomy) or occasionally one less (monosomy) than the normal number of 46. A few of the more common syndromes are summarized briefly below. Since the addition or subtraction of an entire gene is obviously a major genetic abnormality, these syndromes are characterized by many and extensive deformities. Many such abnormal fertilizations result in early abortions and stillbirths.

1. SYNDROMES ASSOCIATED WITH AN ABNORMAL NUMBER OF CHROMOSOMES

Trisomy 13 (Patau's Syndrome)

Anophthalmos, microphthalmos, retinal dysplasia, optic atrophy, coloboma of the uvea, and cataracts are the major eye anomalies; cerebral defects, cleft palate, heart lesions, polydactyly, and hemangiomas are the more severe nonophthalmic changes. Cytogenetically, there is an extra chromosome indistinguishable from group 13–15. Death by age 6 months is the rule.

Trisomy 18 (Edward's Syndrome)

The main features of this rare syndrome are mental and physical retardation, congenital heart defects, and renal abnormalities. Corneal and lenticular opacities, unilateral ptosis, and optic atrophy have been described.

Trisomy 21 (Down's Syndrome)

Although Down's syndrome is a fairly common and well-known entity, the hereditary pattern was long ill-defined. Waardenburg originally suggested that Down's syndrome was a chromosomal problem in 1932. Cytogenetic studies in 1958 revealed an extra chromosome indistinguishable from chromosome 21. The principal manifestations are small stature, a flattened, round, mongoloid facies, saddle nose, thick lower lip, large tongue, soft, seborrheic skin, smooth hair, obesity, small genitalia, short fingers, a simian fold, congenital heart anomalies, mental retardation, and frequent psychic disturbances. The ocular signs include hyperplasia of the iris, narrow palpebral fissures with Oriental slant, frequent strabismus, epicanthus, frequent cataract, high myopia (33%), and Brushfield (silver-gray) spots on the iris.

The incidence of Down's syndrome is significantly increased in children born to older women, particularly those past age 35.

2. ABNORMALITIES INVOLVING SEX CHROMOSOMES

Turner's syndrome is a monosomy (45 chromosomes). For some reason, the affected female receives only one X chromosome. Clinically, growth retardation, rudimentary ovaries and female genitalia, amenorrhea, pterygium colli, epicanthus, cubitus valgus, and ptosis occur. Of particular ophthalmic interest is the high incidence of color blindness (8%). This is the same frequency as for males (female incidence, 0.4%) and is readily explained by the fact that the normally recessive gene is unopposed and is expressed just as in the male.

Klinefelter's syndrome is a trisomy involving the X chromosomes. These phenotypical males have 47 chromosomes: the normal 44 autosomes and 3 sex chromosomes, XXY. These individuals are sterile, with small testes, have a eunuchoid physique, and frequently gynecomastia. The ocular finding of interest is the very rare occurrence of color blindness, since the recessive X chromosome is masked by a normal dominant (as in the normal female).

OTHER GENETIC CONSIDERATIONS

Genetic Counseling

Valuable advice can often be given to families concerned with the possibilities of transmitting serious disease to future generations. This entails a working knowledge of basic genetic principles and sensitive counseling skills. A careful history of the pedigree in question is very important, as a single disease may have more than one mode of transmission (eg, retinitis pigmentosa has 3 or more basic patterns). On the other hand, careful inquiries about maternal health during pregnancy may suggest that the anomaly is developmental and therefore unrelated to the genes. The recognition of the genetic carrier state may enable the physician to give intelligent advice.

Consanguineous mating increases the risk of birth defects, since it is estimated that the average individual carries several undesirable recessive genes.

In some cases it is possible to offer families at risk for a specific hereditary disease the option of prenatal diagnosis. This may involve searching for chromosomal abnormalities or specific structural protein defects such as enzyme deficiencies. Currently, techniques are being devised to identify abnormalities at the gene level using DNA linkage studies (eg, in X-linked retinitis pigmentosa) or DNA probes. Prenatal diagnosis by testing amniotic fluid cells obtained by amniocentesis at 14–16 gestational weeks has become a safe and practical procedure. The list of he-

reditary diseases that can be diagnosed with this method is rapidly increasing. There is, however, a 3-week delay before results of cytogenetic analysis become available. Chorionic villus sampling has certain advantages: It can be undertaken at 8–12 gestational weeks, and results are known within 24 hours. Its overall safety is still being determined.

Genetic Carrier State

Recognition of the genetic carrier state is most important. Detection is possible in many diseases. There are 3 types:

(1) Autosomal dominant diseases in which the disease appears in a mild or subclinical form (low expression). Because the offspring of such individuals still have the theoretical 50% chance of passing on the disease process, the recognition of this carrier state is important in genetic counseling.

(2) Autosomal recessive diseases with heterozygous manifestations. Affected genes that are normally balanced by a normal allele may cause minor subclinical abnormalities which disclose the presence of the abnormal gene. One can predict the 25% possibility of occurrence of some autosomal recessive diseases if the carrier state can be recognized in both potential mates.

(3) Female carrier in X-linked recessive disease. Subclinical evidence of the disease in daughters of affected fathers differentiates carriers from noncarriers in a number of X-linked recessive diseases (often quite obvious in tapetoretinal degenerative conditions).

Mutation

Mutation occurs when a gene undergoes alteration in the germ cell as a result of spontaneous chemical change within the gene and the change is manifested by a new characteristic. The causes of the change are not well understood, but such extrinsic environmental factors as heat, x-rays, and exposure to radioactive materials may induce it. Most often the new characteristic is unfavorable (ie, disease-producing), but some mutations are favorable and account for the evolution of species (Darwin).

Certain mutations occur repeatedly in specific genes and cause specific disease. Hemophilia, which follows an X-linked pattern, and retinoblastoma, in which a single locus on chromosome 13 q is involved, are examples of disease occurring as a result of mutation. Very few individuals with severe abnormalities reproduce, so that the incidence of such diseases is dependent almost entirely upon mutation. Mutations causing less severe diseases are inherited as dominant, recessive, or X-linked traits depending upon the type of mutated gene.

GLOSSARY OF GENETIC TERMS*

Abiotrophic disease: Genetically determined disease which is not evident at birth but which becomes manifest later in life.

Acquired: Not hereditary; contracted after birth or in utero.

Alleles: Paired genes or partner genes; genes occupying the same locus on homologous (paired) chromosomes and which, therefore, normally segregate from each other during the reduction-division of mitosis.

Autosomes: The chromosomes (22 pairs of autosomes in humans) other than the sex chromosomes.

Chromosome: A small threadlike or rodlike structure into which the nuclear chromatin separates during mitosis. The number of chromosomes is constant for any given species (23 pairs in humans: 22 pairs of autosomes and one pair of sex chromosomes).

Congenital: Existing at or before birth; not necessarily hereditary.

Dominant: Designating a gene whose phenotypic effect largely or entirely obscures that of its allele.

Familial: Pertaining to traits, either hereditary or acquired, which tend to occur in families.

Gamete (germ cell): A cell that is capable of uniting with another cell in sexual reproduction (ie, the ovum and spermatozoon).

Gene: A unit of heredity which occupies a specific locus in the chromosome which, either alone or in combination, produces a single characteristic. It is usually a single unit that is capable of self-duplication or mutation.

Genetic carrier state: A condition wherein a given hereditary characteristic is not manifest in one individual but may be genetically transmitted to the offspring of that individual.

Genotype: The hereditary constitution, or combination of genes, that characterizes a given individual or a group of genetically identical organisms.

Germ cell: See Gamete, above.

*Modified from Krupp MA et al: *Physician's Handbook,* 21st ed. Lange, 1985.

Hereditary: Transmitted from ancestor to offspring through the germ plasm.

Heterozygous: Having 2 members of a given hereditary factor pair that are dissimilar, ie, the 2 genes of an allelic pair are not the same.

Homozygous: Having 2 members of a given hereditary factor pair that are similar, ie, the 2 genes of an allelic pair are identical.

Meiosis: A special type of cell division occurring during the maturation of sex cells, by which the normal diploid set of chromosomes is reduced to a single (haploid) set, 2 successive nuclear divisions occurring, while the chromosomes divide only once.

Mitosis: Cell division in which daughter nuclei receive identical components of the number of chromosomes characteristic of the species.

Mutation: A transformation of a gene, often sudden and dramatic, with or without known cause, into a different gene occupying the same locus as the original gene on a particular chromosome; the new gene is allelic to the normal gene from which it has arisen.

Penetrance: The likelihood or probability that a gene will become morphologically (phenotypically) expressed. The degree of penetrance may depend upon acquired as well as genetic factors.

Phenotype: The visible characteristics of an individual or those which are common to a group of apparently identical individuals.

Recessive: Designating a gene whose phenotypic effect is largely or entirely obscured by the effect of its allele.

Sex chromosome: The chromosome or pair of chromosomes that determines the sex of the individual. (In the human female, the sex chromosome pair is homologous, XX; in the male, heterologous, XY.)

Sex linkage: See X linkage, below.

Somatic cells: Cells incapable of reproducing the organism.

Trisomy: The existence of 3 chromosomes of one variety, rather than the normal pair of chromosomes.

X linkage: The pattern of inheritance of genes located on the X chromosome.

Zygote: The cell formed by the union of 2 gametes in sexual reproduction.

REFERENCES

Bergsma D (editor): *Birth Defects Compendium,* 2nd ed. AR Liss, 1979.

Deutman AF: Genetically determined retinal and choroidal disease. *Trans Ophthalmol Soc UK* 1974;**94**:1014.

Duke-Elder S: *System of Ophthalmology.* Vol 7. Mosby, 1962.

Edlin G: *Genetic Principles: Human and Social Consequences.* Jones & Bartlett, 1984.

François J: "Counseling" in ophthalmology. *Ann Ophthalmol* 1976;**8**:265.

François J: *Heredity in Ophthalmology.* Mosby, 1961.

Gallie BL, Phillips RA: Retinoblastoma: A model of oncogenesis. *Ophthalmology* 1984;**91**:666.

Goldberg MF (editor): *Genetic and Metabolic Eye Disease.* Little, Brown, 1974.

Gorlin RJ, Pindborg JJ, Cohen MM Jr: *Syndromes of the Head and Neck,* 2nd ed. McGraw-Hill, 1976.

Green JS, Johnson GJ: Hereditary diseases as causes of blindness in Newfoundland: Preliminary report. *Can J Ophthalmol* 1983;**18**:281.

Keith CG: *Genetics and Ophthalmology.* Churchill Livingstone, 1978.

Kinnear PE, Jay B, Witkop CJ Jr: Albinism. *Surv Ophthalmol* 1985;**30**:75.

McKusick VA: *Human Genetics,* 2nd ed. Prentice-Hall, 1969.

McKusick VA: *Mendelian Inheritance in Man,* 6th ed. Johns Hopkins Univ Press, 1983.

Mets MB, Maumenee IH: The eye and the chromosome. *Surv Ophthalmol* 1983;**28**:20.

Miller M: Fetal alcohol syndrome. *J Pediatr Ophthalmol Strabismus* 1981;**18**:5.

Mukai S et al: Linkage between the X-linked retinitis pigmentosa locus and the L1.28 locus. *Am J Ophthalmol* 1985;**100**:225.

Newell F: *Hereditary Disorders of the Eye and Ocular Adnexa.* Ophthalmic Publishers, 1981.

Stanbury JB et al: *The Metabolic Basis of Inherited Disease,* 5th ed. McGraw-Hill, 1983.

Tabbara KF, Badr IA: Changing pattern of childhood blindness in Saudi Arabia. *Br J Ophthalmol* 1985;**69**:312.

Ullman S, Nelson LB, Jackson LG: Prenatal diagnostic techniques: Chorionic villus sampling. *Surv Ophthalmol* 1985;**30**:33.

Waardenburg PJ, Franceschetti A, Klein D: *Genetics and Ophthalmology.* 2 vols. Thomas, 1961, 1963.

Tumors

23

J. Brooks Crawford, MD

Both benign and malignant tumors are encountered in the eye and its related structures. Most can be diagnosed early since they are visible, interfere with vision, or displace the eyeball. Care must be taken not to overlook the possibility of malignancy. Ultrasonography may be very useful in detecting orbital and intraocular masses, especially when visibility with an ophthalmoscope is poor, as occurs when cataract is present. Delay in diagnosis may make curative surgery technically more difficult and may result in loss of useful vision. As far as possible, biopsies should be taken of all accessible suspicious lesions, with complete excision of smaller lesions, since a positive diagnosis of malignancy can only be made by histologic examination.

Secondary (metastatic) ocular malignant tumors are probably more common than primary intraocular ones. The most frequent site of metastasis is the choroid. The ophthalmoscopic appearance may be difficult to differentiate from that of primary tumors of the choroid; therefore, the finding of a primary elsewhere may be of diagnostic importance. Ultrasonography may help in differentiating primary from metastatic intraocular tumors. Radiotherapy or other treatment may relieve ocular symptoms, but enucleation is sometimes necessary to relieve pain.

Physiology of Symptoms

Small tumors of the lids are asymptomatic except in the case of verrucae and molluscum contagiosum, which occasionally cause conjunctivitis. Tumors of the conjunctiva are usually painless unless they have a rough, keratinized surface. A central corneal lesion causes decrease in vision. An intraocular lesion involving the macula causes blurring of vision as a presenting symptom. Extramacular tumors are not manifested until they become large enough to obstruct vision or produce secondary changes in the eye such as retinal detachment, a rise in intraocular pressure, or anterior uveitis. Retrobulbar tumors may be relatively asymptomatic until they are well-developed, at which time diplopia, displacement, or exophthalmos is likely to occur.

A history of recent change in size or appearance of an external ocular growth calls for careful observation, including photographs. If there is any suspicion of malignancy, biopsy or total removal is indicated for microscopic examination.

LID TUMORS

BENIGN TUMORS OF THE LIDS

Nevus

Melanocytic nevi of the eyelids are common benign tumors with the same pathologic structure as nevi found elsewhere. They are usually congenital but may be relatively unpigmented at birth, enlarging and darkening during adolescence. Many never acquire visible pigment, and many resemble benign papillomas. Nevi rarely become malignant.

Nevi may be removed by shave excision if desired for cosmetic reasons.

Verrucae (Warts)

Warts commonly appear along the margins of the lids as fleshy, multilobulated, flat-based to pedunculated lesions. They are thought to be caused by viruses.

If treatment is indicated for cosmetic reasons, verrucae may be removed by excision with cauterization at the base of the lesion. Care must be exercised to avoid producing a marginal notch in the eyelid.

Molluscum Contagiosum (Fig 23–1)

The typical lesion of this unusual disorder is a small, flat, symmetric, centrally umbilicated growth along the lid margin. It is caused by a large virus and

Figure 23–1. Molluscum contagiosum. Note central umbilication.

Figure 23–2. Xanthelasma. (Courtesy of M Quickert.)

may produce conjunctivitis and even keratitis if the lesion sheds into the conjunctival space.

Cure can usually be obtained by incision, cautery, or excision.

Xanthelasma (Fig 23–2)

Xanthelasma is a common disorder that occurs on the anterior surface of the eyelid, usually bilaterally near the inner angle of the eye. The lesions appear as yellow, wrinkled patches on the skin and occur more often in elderly people. Xanthelasma represents lipid deposits in histiocytes in the dermis of the lid. Clinical evaluation of serum cholesterol levels is indicated, but only rarely is a direct relationship found.

Treatment is indicated for cosmetic reasons. Surgical removal is simple. Cauterization of the smaller lesions is sometimes effective. Recurrence following removal is not unusual.

Hemangioma (Fig 23–3)

Two main types of congenital vascular tumors occur in the lids: cavernous hemangiomas and capillary hemangiomas. **Cavernous hemangiomas** are composed of large venous channels lying in the subcutaneous tissue; they are bluish in color and change in size according to their distention with blood. **Capillary hemangiomas,** when superficial, are bright red (strawberry) spots. These and the more invasive type are composed of proliferating capillaries and endothelial cells. They may grow rapidly in the first few

Figure 23–3. Cavernous hemangioma of left upper lid.

months of life. Both types frequently undergo spontaneous involution, usually by age 5.

Treatment is usually not indicated in infancy or childhood unless the defect is extensive enough to cause occlusion amblyopia. Refractive amblyopia can also occur owing to astigmatism or anisometropia produced by the tumor. It is important to detect this and treat it as it develops. If the hemangioma blocks the pupil or does not spontaneously involute, surgical excision may be necessary. Some of these hemangiomas respond to the injection of steroids.

PRIMARY MALIGNANT TUMORS OF THE LIDS

Carcinoma
(Figs 23–4 and 23–5)

Basal cell and squamous cell carcinomas of the lids are the most common malignant ocular tumors. These tumors occur most frequently in fair-complexioned individuals who have had chronic exposure to the sun. Ninety-five percent of lid carcinomas are of the basal cell type. The remaining 5% consist of squamous cell carcinomas and meibomian gland carcinomas. Keratoacanthomas and inverted follicular keratoses are benign lesions that resemble squamous cell carcinomas. In the past this was not recognized, and the incidence of squamous cell carcinomas was thought to be higher than it actually is. Diagnosis is based upon clinical appearance and biopsy.

Squamous cell carcinoma may spread via the lymphatic system to the preauricular and submaxillary lymph nodes. Most do not spread if they are recognized and treated. Basal cell tumors grow very slowly, are locally invasive, and do not spread to the regional lymph nodes.

Squamous cell carcinoma grows slowly and painlessly, and it may be present for many months before it is noted. It usually begins as a small warty growth

Figure 23–4. Squamous cell carcinoma of upper lid. (Courtesy of A Rosenberg.)

Figure 23–5. Basal cell carcinoma of left lower lid. (Courtesy of S Mettier, Jr.)

with a keratotic covering, gradually eroding and fissuring until an ulcer develops. The base of the ulcer is indurated and hyperemic and the edges hard. Unless the tumor is excised early it grows through the skin, connective tissue, cartilage, and bone until large areas are destroyed in a fungating crater that may eventually reach the cranial cavity. Pain then becomes severe and constant. When sensory nerves are involved, the pain may be excruciating. The patient may die of hemorrhage, meningitis, or general debility.

Basal cell carcinoma begins in a similar manner, eventually forming the typical rodent ulcer with a raised nodular border and indurated base. It eventually erodes the surrounding tissue in somewhat the same way as squamous cell carcinoma but much more slowly. Biopsy of the tumor itself is a simple office procedure and is the only sure method of diagnosis.

Basal cell tumors of the lower lid near the inner canthus tend to invade the structures of the inner canthus and the orbit. Complete eradication of these tumors is important.

The sclerosing or morphealike basal cell carcinoma, an unusually aggressive variety of basal cell carcinoma, may lie beneath the skin surface and manifest its presence by subtle signs such as alopecia, lid notching, ectropion, or entropion.

Sebaceous gland carcinomas of the eyelid, most of which arise from the meibomian glands and the glands of Zeis, are potentially fatal neoplasms; about half of them may resemble benign inflammatory diseases such as chalazions and chronic blepharitis.

Any suspicious growths on the lids should be submitted for pathologic examination.

The objective of treatment is complete destruction of the tumor. Surgery is an effective method, particularly if frozen sections are used to ensure complete excision. Radiotherapy can also be effective for basal cell carcinomas and squamous cell carcinomas; cryotherapy has been successful in the treatment of some basal cell carcinomas.

Carcinoma Associated With Xeroderma Pigmentosum

This rare disease is characterized by the appearance of a large number of freckles in the areas of the skin exposed to the sun. These are followed by telangiectases, atrophic patches, and eventually a warty growth that may undergo carcinomatous degeneration. The eyelids are frequently affected and may be the first area to show degenerative changes, causing atrophy and ectropion with secondary inflammatory changes of the conjunctiva, symblepharon, corneal ulceration, and carcinoma of the lids. Malignant tumors include basal cell carcinomas, squamous cell carcinomas, and malignant melanomas. This condition is inherited as an autosomal recessive trait. Carriers can often be identified by excessive freckling.

The disease appears early in life and in most cases is fatal by adolescence as a result of metastasis. Life may be prolonged by carefully protecting the skin from actinic rays and treating carcinomatous tumors as rapidly as they appear.

Sarcoma

Sarcoma of the lids is rare and usually represents an anterior extension of an orbital sarcoma. Rhabdomyosarcomas involving the orbit and lids represent the most common malignant tumor in these tissues in the first decade of life. Other sarcomas (usually named after the predominant type of cell) also occur. Most are radiosensitive, but a combination of surgery and radiation is often required. They may be associated with similar lesions elsewhere in the body.

Malignant Melanoma

Malignant melanomas of the eyelids are similar to those elsewhere in the skin and include 3 distinct varieties: superficial spreading melanoma, lentigo maligna melanoma, and nodular melanoma. Not all malignant melanomas are pigmented. Most pigmented lesions on the eyelid skin are not melanomas. Therefore, biopsy should be used to establish the diagnosis. The prognosis for melanomas of the skin depends upon the depth of invasion or the thickness of the lesion.

CONJUNCTIVAL TUMORS

PRIMARY BENIGN TUMORS OF THE CONJUNCTIVA

Nevus (Fig 23–6)

One-third of melanocytic nevi of the conjunctiva lack pigment. Over half have cystic epithelial inclusions that can be seen clinically.

Histologically, conjunctival nevi are composed of nests or sheets of typical nevus cells. Conjunctival nevi, like other nevi, rarely become malignant. Many are excised because they are disfiguring.

Figure 23–6. Conjunctival nevus. (Courtesy of A Irvine, Jr.)

Papilloma

Conjunctival papillomas are not rare, occurring most frequently near the limbus, on the caruncle, or at the lid margins. Those on the caruncle and lid margin are usually soft and pedunculated, with irregular surfaces. They frequently recur after removal.

Granuloma

Pyogenic granulomas are a variety of capillary hemangiomas. They frequently occur on the palpebral conjunctiva over chalazions or in an area of recent surgical incision.

Granulomatous inflammation occurs around foreign bodies and in association with diseases such as coccidioidomycosis and sarcoidosis. These inflammatory foci may form elevated plaques or nodules in the skin or the conjunctiva of the eyelids.

Dermoid Tumor
(Fig 23–7)

This rare congenital tumor appears as a smooth, rounded, yellow elevated mass, frequently with hairs protruding. A dermoid tumor may remain quiescent,

Figure 23–7. Dermoid tumor at the inferior limbus. (Courtesy of A Irvine, Jr.)

although it often increases in size during puberty. Removal is indicated only if cosmetic deformity is significant or if vision is impaired or threatened.

Dermolipoma

Dermolipoma is a common congenital tumor that usually appears as a smoothly rounded growth in the upper temporal quadrant of the bulbar conjunctiva near the lateral canthus. Treatment is usually not indicated, but at least partial removal may be indicated if the growth is enlarging or is cosmetically disfiguring. Posterior dissection must be undertaken with extreme care (if at all) since this lesion is frequently continuous with orbital fat; orbital derangement may cause scarring and complications far more serious than the original lesion.

Lymphoma & Lymphoid Hyperplasia

These are uncommon conjunctival lesions that may appear in adults without evidence of systemic disease or as part of the clinical picture of lymphosarcoma, lymphocytic leukemia, Hodgkin's disease, or other related conditions. Benign lymphoid hyperplasia can sometimes be distinguished by a pebbly appearance corresponding to follicle formation. However, the clinical appearance of benign lymphoid hyperplasia and malignant lymphoma can be similar; therefore, biopsy is essential to establish a diagnosis.

Treatment of both benign and malignant lesions is best accomplished with radiotherapy.

Fibroma

Fibromas are rare small, smooth, pedunculated, transparent growths that may appear anywhere in the conjunctival tissues but are most often seen in the lower fornix. Histologically, they consist of fibrous overgrowths covered by epithelium. Treatment is by excision.

Angioma

Conjunctival angiomas may occur as isolated, circumscribed capillary hemangiomas or as more diffuse vascular tumors, often associated with a more extensive lid or orbital capillary or cavernous hemangioma. Hemangiomas should be distinguished from telangiectases involving conjunctival capillaries. Telangiectases of the conjunctival vessels are not always associated with inflammatory disease; they occasionally occur over an underlying melanoma of the ciliary body.

PRIMARY MALIGNANT TUMORS OF THE BULBAR CONJUNCTIVA

Carcinoma

Carcinoma of the conjunctiva (Fig 23– 8) arises most frequently at the limbus in the area of the palpebral fissure and less often in nonexposed areas of the conjunctiva. Some of these tumors may resemble pterygiums. Most have a gelatinous surface; some-

Figure 23–8. Intraepithelial epithelioma. (Courtesy of A Irvine, Jr.)

CORNEAL TUMORS

PRIMARY MALIGNANT TUMORS OF THE CORNEA

Carcinomas of the corneal epithelium are rare; extension of conjunctival carcinoma (especially at the limbus) onto the cornea is not uncommon. The same is true for melanomas in the corneal epithelium.

INTRAOCULAR TUMORS

PRIMARY BENIGN INTRAOCULAR TUMORS

Nevus

Nevi may occur on any of the 3 portions of the uvea: the iris, ciliary body, or choroid (Figs 23– 9 and 23– 10). They are usually flat pigmented lesions lying in the stroma of the tissue. On the anterior surface of the iris they may be noted as iris "freckles." Posteriorly in the choroid one may see flat pigmented areas. Large choroidal nevi are difficult to differentiate from malignant melanomas. Their unchanging slate-gray color and flat appearance and the lack of extension are important in the differential diagnosis from malignant melanoma.

Because of the difficulties in differentiation from malignant melanomas, fundus photographs or careful line drawings should be made of all suspicious lesions. Observations should be made periodically for changes.

Retinal Angioma*

Angioma of the retina is a rare congenital disorder. Blurring of vision may result if bleeding occurs or if the retina is secondarily detached. Occasionally, angioma is associated with angioma in the cerebral cortex (Lindau's disease) (Fig 23– 11). It is globular in outline and may be located near one of the pairs of enlarged retinal vessels. Angiomas may enlarge. Photocoagulation therapy (xenon or argon laser) and cryotherapy are currently utilized to eradicate these lesions.

Tuberous Sclerosis (Bourneville's Disease) (Fig 23–12)

The rare intraocular tumor (glial hamartoma) associated with tuberous sclerosis in about half of cases varies in size and color but is most often a yellow or white nodular swelling, frequently mulberry in appearance, located in any portion of the posterior fundus but with a predilection for the area near the optic

times, abnormal keratinization of the epithelium produces leukoplakia. Growth is slow, and deep invasion and metastases are extremely rare; therefore, complete excision is effective treatment. Recurrences are common if the lesion is incompletely excised; treatment consists of reexcision.

Conjunctival dysplasia, a benign condition that occurs as an isolated lesion or sometimes over pterygiums and pingueculas, can resemble carcinoma in situ clinically and even histologically. Excisional biopsy will establish a diagnosis and result in cure of most of these lesions. The use of cryotherapy may help to prevent recurrences.

Malignant Melanoma

Malignant melanoma of the conjunctiva is rare. It may arise from a preexisting nevus, from an area of acquired melanosis, or de novo from formerly normal-appearing conjunctiva. Pigmentation may vary greatly, and the clinical course is often unpredictable.

Many tumors can be locally excised. More radical surgery (eg, exenteration of the orbit) does not usually improve the prognosis. The use of cryotherapy after excision of melanotic tumors may help to prevent recurrences.

Lymphosarcoma

Malignant lymphomas of the conjunctiva are much rarer than benign lymphoid hyperplasia. Many also involve the orbit, and a few are associated with systemic lymphoma. However, the conjunctival lesion may be the initial sign of a systemic problem.

*See also Angiomatosis Retinae in Chapter 18.

Figure 23–9. Nevus of the iris. (Courtesy of A Rosenberg.)

Figure 23–11. Angiomatosis retinae of Von Hippel-Lindau disease (drawing). (Courtesy of F Cordes.)

nerve. Other manifestations of tuberous sclerosis include skin changes (adenoma sebaceum), intracranial changes causing epilepsy and mental retardation, and other neurologic symptoms (see p 256).

Hemangioma of the Choroid

Choroidal hemangioma occurs in most cases of Sturge-Weber syndrome associated with unilateral infantile glaucoma (see p 256). Cases occurring with no other signs of Sturge-Weber syndrome are frequently mistaken for malignant melanoma of the choroid (see below), and the mistaken diagnosis has often led to unnecessary removal of the affected eye. The tumor involves the posterior pole, usually near the optic disk and sometimes extending out to the equator, most often on the temporal side. It may produce a solid elevation or a serous detachment of the retina. The borders are irregular, and the tumor is never

pigmented. Hemangiomas can produce arcuate field defects or localized scotomas.

Histologically, the tumor consists of endothelium-lined spaces engorged with blood separated by sparse connective tissue. Retinal degeneration over the tumor is common.

Secondary glaucoma, usually severe and refractory to any treatment, is associated with larger choroidal hemangiomas.

The differentiation from malignant melanoma is most important and frequently difficult.

Occasionally, choroidal hemangiomas can be treated with photocoagulation to limit the extent and

Figure 23–10. Nevus of the choroid. (Photo by Diane Beeston.)

Figure 23–12. Tuberous sclerosis.

degree of associated serous detachment of the retina. Enucleation may be necessary for those tumors associated with intractable, painful glaucoma.

PRIMARY MALIGNANT TUMORS OF THE INTRAOCULAR STRUCTURES

Malignant Melanoma

It has been estimated that intraocular malignant melanoma occurs in 0.02–0.06% of the total eye patient population in the USA. It is seen only in the uveal tract and is the most common intraocular malignant tumor in the white population. The average age of patients with this disorder is 50 years. It is almost always unilateral. Eighty-five percent appear in the choroid, 9% in the ciliary body, and 6% in the iris. Most of the choroidal tumors are in the posterior portion of the eye, especially on the temporal side. In the iris, the lower half is most often affected. Intraocular malignant melanoma is rare in blacks, although uveal nevi are common (Fig 23– 13).

This tumor may be seen in its early stages only accidentally during routine ophthalmoscopic examination or because of blurring due to macular invasion. Blood-borne metastases may occur at any time, and death may occur before local spread or ocular symptoms appear. Glaucoma may be a late manifestation.

Histologically, these tumors are composed of spindle-shaped cells, with or without prominent nucleoli, and large epithelioid tumor cells. Tumors composed of the former have a good prognosis; tumors with the latter, a poor prognosis.

Intraocular malignant melanomas may spread directly through the sclera, by local invasion of intraocular structures, or by metastasis.

Clinical manifestations are usually absent unless the macula is involved. In the later stages, growth of the tumor may lead to retinal detachment with loss of a large amount of visual field. A tumor located in the iris may be large enough to change the color of the iris or deform the pupil. Pain does not occur in the absence of glaucoma.

The first step in diagnosis is to suspect the lesion. Most intraocular malignant melanomas can be seen ophthalmoscopically. Transillumination is of some value in differentiation from serous retinal detachment.

A high incidence of intraocular tumors has been found in the study of blind, painful, phthisic (atrophic) eyes, one writer reporting that 10% of such eyes contained previously unsuspected malignant melanomas.

Enucleation of an eye with a choroidal melanoma has been the traditional treatment. Recently, other forms of therapy, particularly radiotherapy with charged particles such as helium ions and protons or with plaques of radioactive isotopes sutured to the sclera, have been used for eyes with small tumors and useful vision. Very small melanomas (< 10 mm in diameter) have an excellent prognosis and are often impossible to differentiate from benign nevi; therefore, many authorities advocate not treating these tumors until unequivocal growth can be documented (usually with serial photographs or ultrasound measurements).

Small melanomas of the iris that have not invaded the iris root can be safely observed until growth is documented; then they can be removed by iridectomy. Lesions that invade the iris root and ciliary body can sometimes be treated with iridocyclectomy. Iris melanomas have an excellent prognosis; the mortality rate is less than 1%. Many pigmented iris tumors are actually large nevi rather than malignant melanomas.

Retinoblastoma (Fig 23–14)

Retinoblastoma is a rare but life-endangering tumor of childhood. Two-thirds of cases appear before the end of the third year; rare cases have been reported at almost every age. The tumor is bilateral in about 30% of cases. Retinoblastoma was formerly thought to result from mutation of an autosomal dominant gene, but it is now thought that an allele at a single

Figure 23–13. Malignant melanoma of the choroid, macular area, left eye (drawing). (Courtesy of F Cordes.)

Figure 23–14. Retinoblastoma visible through pupil.

locus within chromosomal band 13q14 controls both the heritable and nonheritable forms of the tumor. (See Chapter 22 for further discussion of genetic aspects of ocular disease.) About 94% of retinoblastomas arise by mutation; therefore, only about 6% are familial. When the inheritance is familial or the mutation involves germinal tissue, a retinoblastoma survivor has approximately a 50% chance of producing an affected child.

Retinoblastomas usually arise from the posterior retina. Growth tends to be nodular, with numerous satellite or seeding nodules that may produce multiple secondary tumors (Fig 23–15). They gradually fill the eye and extend through the optic nerve to the brain and along the emissary vessels and nerves in the sclera to the orbital tissues. Microscopically, most retinoblastomas are composed of small, closely packed, round or polygonal cells with large, darkly staining nuclei and scanty cytoplasm. They sometimes form characteristic Flexner-Wintersteiner rosettes, which are indicative of photoreceptor differentiation. Degenerative changes are frequent, with necrosis and calcification. A few spontaneous cures have been reported.

Retinoblastoma usually remains unnoticed until it has advanced far enough to produce a white pupil—unless strabismus has occurred, leading to earlier diagnosis. Otherwise, the tumor is usually seen in the early stages only when sought for, as in children having a hereditary background or where the other eye has been affected. In the early stages small, yellowish-white nodular masses may be seen protruding into the vitreous from the retina. Infants and children with esotropia should be examined to rule out retinoblastoma, since blind eyes of children will often turn inward.

Retrolental fibroplasia, persistence of the primary vitreous, retinal dysplasia, Coats' disease, and nematode endophthalmitis may simulate retinoblastoma.

In general, the earlier the discovery and treatment of the tumor, the better the chance to prevent spread through the optic nerve and orbital tissues.

Enucleation is the treatment of choice for large retinoblastomas; smaller ones in eyes with potentially useful vision can be effectively treated with radiotherapy, sometimes augmented by chemotherapy, cryotherapy, or photocoagulation (Fig 23–16).

Medulloepitheliomas ("Diktyoma") of the Ciliary Body

Benign and malignant medulloepitheliomas are rare tumors that may arise from the ciliary body epithelium. Those with one or more heteroplastic elements, such as hyaline cartilage, brain tissue, or rhabdomyoblasts, are called teratoid medulloepitheliomas. Those that arise soon after birth may infiltrate the area around the lens and produce a white pupillary reflex similar to that seen in eyes with retinoblastoma.

ORBITAL TUMORS

Gradually enlarging orbital tumors may attain a diameter of 1 cm before any displacement of the eyeball is noted (Fig 23–17). The direction of displacement offers a clue to the location of the tumor—eg, posterior tumors tend to displace the eyeball anteriorly, whereas tumors between the eyeball and one of the walls of the orbit will cause lateral displacement. These observations indicate the site of exploration when biopsy is indicated.

With displacement of the eyeball, diplopia is a common symptom. Pressure resulting from marked exophthalmos may interfere with blood supply to the optic nerve and retina, causing blurred vision. Ex-

Figure 23 –15. Retinoblastoma with multiple seedings and optic nerve invasion. (Courtesy of B Crawford and W Spencer.)

Figure 23 –16. Retinoblastoma after x-ray radiation.

Figure 23–17. Orbital tumor displacing left eye.

4. Upper respiratory tract–Carcinoma of the upper respiratory epithelium, sarcoma, mucocele.
5. Cranial–Meningioma, other intracranial tumors.

C. Metastatic From Distant Sites: Carcinoma, sarcoma, neuroblastoma.

D. Other Types:
1. Reticuloendothelioses–Juvenile xanthogranuloma, eosinophilic granuloma, other rare entities.
2. Metabolic disorders–Thyroid exophthalmos (see p 277).
3. Phakomatoses–Neurofibromatosis (Recklinghausen's disease) (see p 255).

posure of the eye due to inability to close the lids causes corneal epithelial damage with resultant pain and irritation.

The use of CT scan, MRI (magnetic resonance imaging), and ultrasonography has helped resolve the diagnostic dilemma presented by many orbital tumors. These techniques can also aid the surgeon in determining when and where to explore the orbit for these masses.

The common or otherwise important tumors from the following classification will be discussed below. References are given to discussions elsewhere in the text. The uncommon orbital tumors are briefly described or only listed.

Classification*
A. Primary in Orbit:
1. Choristomas–Dermoid cyst, epidermal cyst, teratoma.
2. Hamartomas–Hemangioma, neurofibroma.
3. Mesenchymal–
   a. Adipose–ipoma, liposarcoma.
   b. Fibrous–Fibroma, fibrosarcoma.
   c. Myomatous–Rhabdomyosarcoma.
   d. Cartilaginous–Chondroma, chondrosarcoma.
   e. Osseous–Osteoma, osteosarcoma.
4. Neural–Neurofibroma, neurilemmoma, other rare tumors.
5. Epithelial–Lacrimal gland tumors.
6. Lymphoid tumors–Lymphomas, lymphoid hyperplasia, and other inflammatory infiltrates (granulomas, sarcoid, and others).

B. Secondary in Orbit From Adjacent Structures:
1. Intraocular–Malignant melanoma, retinoblastoma.
2. Cornea and conjunctiva–Malignant melanoma, epidermoid carcinoma.
3. Eyelids and face–Basal cell carcinoma, other rare malignant tumors.

*Modified from Spencer WH (editor): *Ophthalmic Pathology,* 3nd ed. 3 vols. Saunders, 1962.

PRIMARY ORBITAL TUMORS

Choristomas
A choristoma is defined as a tumor composed of tissue elements not normally present in the area. For the orbit this includes dermoid cyst, epidermal cyst, and teratoma.

Dermoid cysts are most often found in the superior temporal portion of the orbit, usually anterior to the lacrimal gland. They are benign. They frequently contain particles of hair. Rupture of these cysts, either spontaneously or after trauma, may produce a granulomatous inflammatory reaction that is often the first sign of the tumor.

Hamartomas
A. Hemangiomas: Capillary hemangiomas usually become apparent before the age of 6 months and tend to enlarge before finally involuting by age 5 years. Approximately one-third have a superficial component. Orbital enlargement, detectable by radiography, is apparent in approximately 70%. Amblyopia secondary to astigmatism or anisometropia affects up to 50% of children with this tumor and must be recognized and treated.

Cavernous hemangiomas tend to occur later in life than capillary hemangiomas (usually in the second or fourth decades) and show slowly progressive enlargement without a tendency to spontaneously involute. Most occur within the muscle cone and produce slowly progressive exophthalmos. These are usually well encapsulated and are composed of large, relatively uniform, endothelium-lined channels surrounded by multilaminar smooth muscle cells.

B. Neurofibroma: There is doubt that this tumor ever occurs as an isolated orbital tumor without other evidence of neurofibromatosis (Recklinghausen's disease) (see p 255).

Mesenchymal Tumors
A. Lipoma: Rare. Usually minor or no clinical signs.

B. Liposarcoma: Very rare malignant orbital tumor.

C. Fibroma: Simple fibromas are rare, but they are more common in the upper and inner portions of the orbit than elsewhere. They are usually evident by the third decade. Exophthalmos, diplopia, and displacement of the eyeball are the first symptoms.

Fibromatous tumors are usually encapsulated, firm, and have a meager blood supply. Simple excision to relieve symptoms is feasible in many cases.

D. Rhabdomyosarcoma: This is the most common primary malignant orbital tumor in children. It usually occurs prior to age 15, and there is a slight male preponderance. Rhabdomyosarcoma usually causes proptosis downward and temporally and grows rapidly. Metastases to the brain and lung are common. The prognosis for complete cure is excellent with the use of irradiation and chemotherapy.

E. Cartilaginous: Chondromas and chondrosarcomas are very rare in the orbit. Chondrosarcoma is associated with osteosarcoma following radiation therapy for retinoblastoma.

F. Osseous: Osteoma and osteosarcoma are very rare.

Neural

Neurofibroma (see above) and other rare tumors.

Epithelial (Lacrimal Gland) Tumors

There are 3 main types of tumors of the lacrimal fossa: (1) epithelial tumors of the lacrimal gland (50%), (2) inflammatory pseudotumors (30%), and (3) lymphomas and lymphoid hyperplasias (20%). The latter 2 are classified below under inflammatory tumors (pseudotumors) of the orbit.

Lacrimal gland tumors are classified as benign and malignant mixed tumors and carcinomas unrelated to mixed tumors.

Most mixed tumors are benign but locally invasive. Complete surgical removal is indicated; recurrence is common if excision has not been complete.

Carcinomas not associated with mixed tumor (adenoid cystic carcinoma and adenocarcinoma) are more apt to produce pain than benign mixed tumors and have an extremely poor prognosis. Standard x-rays and CT scan can often help in distinguishing mixed tumors from the more malignant carcinomas.

Lymphoid Tumors

Benign lymphoid hyperplasia, sometimes erroneously called a pseudotumor, is a common orbital tumor of unknown cause composed of proliferating benign lymphoreticular elements. The clinical course may be quite varied, and inflammatory signs are often not evident. Proptosis may be marked, and ocular muscle abnormalities are common. High doses of systemic corticosteroids may effectively treat some of these lesions. However, the absence of a response to steroid therapy does not rule out an inflammatory tumor, and the presence of a response to steroid therapy does not prove that the tumor is a benign process. (Some malignant tumors, particularly those with an inflammatory component, can show an apparent temporary resolution with corticosteroid therapy.)

Malignant lymphomas of the orbit can occur as isolated tumors or can be part of a systemic malignant lymphoma. When confronted with these tumors, it is important to search for a malignant process elsewhere in the body.

Radiotherapy is usually the best treatment for malignant lymphomas and may be useful for treating benign lymphoid hyperplasia that does not respond satisfactorily to corticosteroid therapy.

SECONDARY ORBITAL TUMORS & METASTATIC TUMORS FROM DISTANT SITES

These are listed in the orbital tumor classification (see above).

All tumors from adjacent structures invade the orbit by direct extension and usually call for a radical surgical approach, including exenteration, unless the prognosis is already hopeless because of malignant tumor spread.

Metastatic orbital tumor masses are rarely removed surgically. Radiation is occasionally used in the orbit as a palliative measure. The orbit is a relatively uncommon site for blood-borne metastases.

REFERENCES

Abramson DH et al: The management of unilateral retinoblastoma without primary enucleation. *Arch Ophthalmol* 1982;**100**:1249.

Beard C: Observations on treatment of basal cell carcinoma of eyelids. *Trans Am Acad Ophthalmol Otolaryngol* 1975; **79**:O664.

Bedford MA: *Color Atlas of Ocular Tumors.* Year Book, 1979.

Bedford MA, Bedotto C, Macfaul PA: Retinoblastoma. *Br J Ophthalmol* 1971;**55**:19.

Blodi FC: Ocular melanocytosis and melanoma. *Am J Ophthalmol* 1975;**80**:389.

Boniuk M, Zimmerman LE: Sebaceous carcinoma of the eyelid, eyebrow, caruncle and orbit. *Trans Am Acad Ophthalmol Otolaryngol* 1968;**72**:619.

Bullock JD, Beard C, Sullivan JH: Cryotherapy of basal cell carcinoma in oculoplastic surgery. *Am J Ophthalmol* 1976; **82**:841.

Char DH: The management of small choroidal melanomas. *Surv Ophthalmol* 1978;**22**:377.

Char DH: Therapeutic options in uveal melanoma. (Editorial.) *Am J Ophthalmol* 1984;**98**:796.

Collin JRO: Basal cell carcinoma in the eyelid region. *Br J Ophthalmol* 1976;**60**:806.

Davidorf FH: Conservative management of malignant melanoma. 2. Transscleral diathermy as a method of treatment for malignant melanomas of the choroid. *Arch Ophthalmol* 1970; **82**:273.

Davidorf FH, Lang JR: The natural history of malignant melanoma of the choroid: Small vs large tumors. *Trans Am Acad Ophthalmol Otolaryngol* 1975;**79**:310.

Duane TD (editor): *Clinical Ophthalmology.* Harper & Row, 1985.

Ellis JH et al: Lymphoid tumors of the ocular adnexa: Clinical correlation with the working formulation classification and immunoperoxidase staining of paraffin sections. *Ophthalmology* 1985;**92**:1311.

Fraunfelder FT et al: The role of cryosurgery in external ocular and periocular disease. *Trans Am Acad Ophthalmol Otolaryngol* 1977;**83**:713.

Gallie BL, Phillips RA: Retinoblastoma: A model of oncogenesis. *Ophthalmology* 1984;**91**:667.

Gass JDM: Problems in the differential diagnosis of choroidal nevi and malignant melanomas: The 33rd Edward Jackson memorial lecture. *Trans Am Acad Ophthalmol Otolaryngol* 1977;**83**:19.

Geisse LJ, Robertson DM: Iris melanomas. *Am J Ophthalmol* 1985;**99**:638.

Halloran SL et al: Accuracy of detection of the retinoblastoma gene by esterase D linkage. *Arch Ophthalmol* 1985;**103**:1329.

Henderson JW: *Orbital Tumors.* Thieme-Stratton, 1980.

Jakobiec FA (editor): *Ocular and Adnexal Tumors.* Aesculapius Publishing Co, 1978.

Jensen RD, Miller RW: Retinoblastoma: Epidemiologic characteristics. *N Engl J Med* 1971;**285**:307.

Jones IS, Jakobiec FA: *Diseases of the Orbit.* Harper & Row. 1979.

Knowles DM II, Jakobiec FA: Orbital lymphoid neoplasms: A clinicopathologic study of 60 cases. *Cancer* 1980;**46**:576.

Knowles DM II, Jakobiec FA, Halper JP: Immunologic characterization of ocular adnexal lymphoid neoplasms. *Am J Ophthalmol* 1979;**87**:603.

Kopf AW, Bart RS, Rodriguez-Sains BA: Malignant melanoma: A review. *J Dermatol Surg Oncol* 1977;**3**:43.

Lee DA et al: A clinicopathologic study of primary adenoid cystic carcinoma of the lacrimal gland. *Ophthalmology* 1985;**92**:128.

McLean IW, Foster WD, Zimmerman LE: Prognostic factors in small malignant melanomas of choroid and ciliary body. *Arch Ophthalmol* 1977;**95**:48.

Messmer EP, Font RL: Applications of immunohistochemistry to ophthalmic pathology. *Ophthalmology* 1984;**91**:701.

Reese AB: *Tumors of the Eye,* 3rd ed. Harper & Row, 1976.

Robins JH et al: Xeroderma pigmentosum. *Ann Intern Med* 1974;**80**:221.

Seddon JM et al: Comparison of survival rates for patients with uveal melanoma after treatment with proton beam irradiation or enucleation. *Am J Ophthalmol* 1985;**99**:282.

Shields JA: *The Diagnosis and Management of Intraocular Tumors.* Mosby, 1982.

Sigelman J, Jakobiec FA: Lymphoid lesions of the conjunctiva: Relation of histopathology to clinical outcome. *Trans Am Acad Ophthalmol Otolaryngol* 1978;**85**:818.

Spencer WH: Optic nerve extension of intraocular neoplasms. *Am J Ophthalmol* 1975;**80**:465.

Spencer WH (editor): *Ophthalmic Pathology,* 3rd ed. 3 vols. Saunders, 1985.

Thompson RW et al: Treatment of retinoblastoma. *Ophthalmol Digest* 1972;**34**:17.

Yanoff M, Fine BS: *Ocular Pathology,* 2nd ed. Harper & Row, 1982.

Ocular trauma is a common cause of unilateral blindness in children and young adults; persons in these age groups sustain the majority of severe ocular injuries. In adults, work- and alcohol-related ocular injuries frequently result in litigation.

Eye injuries incurred during athletic activity are becoming more common with the increasing popularity of indoor court games. A recent survey found racquetball to exceed other sports in generating ocular injuries, followed by tennis, baseball, basketball, and soccer. Hyphemas and corneal abrasions were the most common injuries sustained, and over 14% of patients had permanent partial or total visual loss.

Initial Examination of Ocular Trauma

Examination begins with the history, which should include an estimate of visual acuity prior to and immediately following the injury. It should be noted whether any visual loss was progressive or sudden. An intraocular foreign body must be suspected if the patient was hammering metal on metal. Injuries in a child that are said to have occurred late at night or several days earlier or a history that is not appropriate for the injury sustained may indicate child abuse. In all cases of ocular trauma, the "uninjured" eye should also be carefully examined.

Visual acuity must be measured and recorded before the injured eye is examined. (The eye should be tested again upon recovery from injury and a refraction performed if vision is below normal. This record may have legal significance.) If visual loss is severe, check for light projection, 2-point discrimination, and the presence of an afferent pupillary defect. Test ocular motility and periorbital skin sensation, and palpate for defects in the bony orbital rim. At the bedside, the presence of enophthalmos can be determined by viewing the profiles of the corneas from over the brow. If a slit lamp is not available in the emergency room, a penlight, loupe, or direct ophthalmoscope set on +10 (black numbers) can be used to examine the inner surfaces of the lids and the anterior segment.

The anterior surface of the cornea is examined for foreign materials or wounds, regularity, and luster. The bulbar conjunctiva is inspected for hemorrhage, foreign material, or tears. The depth and clarity of the anterior chamber are noted. The size, shape, and light reaction of the pupil should be compared with those of the pupil of the uninjured eye. If the eyeball is intact, the lids, palpebral conjunctiva, and fornices are carefully inspected, the upper lid being everted. A moist cotton-tipped applicator is used to sweep away foreign material from the conjunctival fornices. The direct and indirect ophthalmoscopes are used to view the lens, vitreous, optic disk, and posterior retina. Photographic documentation may be appropriate with external trauma.

Immediate Management of Ocular Trauma

If there is obvious rupture of the globe, avoid further manipulation until the patient has been given general anesthesia. No cycloplegic agents or topical antibiotics should be applied prior to surgery. A Fox shield (or the bottom third of a paper cup) is taped over the eye, and parenteral broad-spectrum antibiotics are started. Analgesics, antiemetics, and tetanus antitoxin are given as needed, with restriction of food and fluids. Induction of general anesthesia should not include the use of depolarizing neuromuscular blocking agents, because these transiently increase pressure on the globe, thus increasing any tendency to extrusion of intraocular contents. Small children may also be better examined with the aid of a short-acting general anesthetic.

In severe injuries it is important for the nonspecialist to bear in mind the possibility of causing further damage by unnecessary manipulation.

Caution: Topical anesthetics, dyes, and other medications placed in an injured eye *must be sterile.* Both tetracaine and fluorescein can be autoclaved repeatedly without impairment of their pharmacologic properties. Most ophthalmic solutions are now available in individual disposable sterile units.

ABRASIONS & LACERATIONS OF THE LIDS

Particulate matter should be removed from abrasions of the lids to reduce skin tattooing. The wound is then irrigated with saline and covered with an antibiotic ointment and sterile dressing. Avulsed tissue is cleaned and reattached. Because of the excellent vascularity of the lids, there is a good chance that such tissues will heal.

Many lacerations of the lid do not involve the margins and may be sutured in the same way as other lacerations of the skin. If the margin of the lid is involved, however, precautions must be taken to prevent marginal notching. The most effective technique is to freshen the lacerated edges by vertical incisions perpendicular to the lid margins through the full height of the tarsus. The incisions are then joined by a "V," thus forming a pentagonal wedge. The conjunctiva and tarsus are closed by interrupted gut sutures, anatomically reapproximating the layers, with conjunctiva and tarsus posteriorly and skin and orbicularis muscle anteriorly. The tarsal edges are kept straight and perpendicular to the lid margin. Several partial-thickness sutures are passed through the exposed tarsal edges. The sutures should not be exposed to the conjunctival surfaces. The edges of the skin are closed with interrupted 6-0 silk or monofilament suture. The lid margin is carefully aligned with two 7-0 silk sutures: one in the posterior margin through the orifices of the meibomian glands and the other in the anterior lid margin through the lash line. The sutures are allowed to remain about 5 mm long and are tied over the skin closure sutures to prevent their abrading the cornea. Skin grafting can be delayed 1–2 days by keeping exposed tissues moist and covered with antibiotics and a sterile dressing.

If primary repair is not effected within 24 hours, edema may necessitate delayed closure. The wound should be cleansed well and antibiotics administered. After swelling has subsided, repair may be performed. Debridement should be minimized, especially if the skin is not lax.

Lacerations near the inner canthus frequently involve the canaliculi. Early repair is desirable, since the tissue becomes more difficult to identify with swelling. The upper canaliculus is rarely essential to lacrimal drainage but can often serve as the sole excretory path when the lower one has been destroyed. Nonetheless, it is preferable to repair lacerations of the canaliculi to prevent stricture.

Sharp lacerations through the distal canaliculus can be repaired with a Veirs rod stent. Avulsions or proximal canalicular lacerations require silicone nasocanalicular intubation with Quickert probes (Fig 24–1). Use of a pigtail probe can create false passages and should be avoided by the inexperienced. Note that crepitus indicates a sinus fracture, usually ethmoidal, and swelling can signal orbital or preseptal cellulitis.

Figure 24–1. Laceration of upper and lower canaliculi and medial canthal region. Silicone tube encircling puncta. (Courtesy of J Sullivan.)

Figure 24–2. Metallic corneal foreign body. (Courtesy of A Rosenberg.)

FOREIGN BODIES IN THE EYE & CORNEAL ABRASIONS

Foreign bodies in the eye can be felt during eye and lid movement, and corneal epithelial defects may cause a similar sensation. Fluorescein will stain the exposed basement membrane of an epithelial defect and can highlight aqueous leakage from penetrating wounds (Seidel's test). A pattern of vertical scratch marks on the cornea indicates particles embedded on the conjunctival surface of the upper lid. Contact lens overwear produces edema of the central corneal epithelium.

Simple corneal epithelial defects are treated with antibiotics, a cycloplegic agent of intermediate duration (scopolamine, 0.25%), and a pressure patch to immobilize the lids. For removal of foreign material, a topical anesthetic can be given and a moist cotton-tipped applicator, spud, or fine-gauge needle used to remove the material during slit lamp examination. Metallic rings surrounding copper or iron fragments (Fig 24–2) can be removed with a battery-operated drill with a burr tip. Deeply embedded inert materials (eg, glass, carbon) may be allowed to remain in the cornea. If removal of deeply embedded fragments is necessary or if there is an aqueous leak requiring sutures or cyanoacrylate glue, the procedure should be undertaken in an operating room, where the anterior chamber can be re-formed (if necessary) under sterile conditions.

Following removal of a foreign body, an antibiotic ointment such as polymyxin B–bacitracin or gentamicin should be instilled 3 times a day into the conjunctival sac to prevent infection. If the wound is extensive, an eye bandage can be used to minimize movement of the lid over the injured area. The wound should be inspected daily for evidence of infection until it is completely healed.

Never give a topical anesthetic solution to the

patient for repeated use after a corneal injury, as this delays healing and masks further damage. Steroids should be avoided while an epithelial defect exists. Recurrent epithelial erosions sometimes follow corneal injuries and are treated with patching or a bandage contact lens.

PENETRATING INJURIES & CONTUSIONS OF THE EYEBALL

Rupture of the eyeball can occur with sharp penetrating injuries or a blunt contusive force. A blunt object produces a rise in orbital and intraocular pressure, with deformation of the globe. Decompression occurs when the eye wall ruptures or the orbital contents herniate into adjacent sinuses (blowout fracture). The superonasal limbus is the most common site of rupture.

While most penetrating injuries cause a marked loss of vision, injuries due to small high-velocity particles generated by grinding or hammering might present with only mild pain and blurring. Other signs include hemorrhagic chemosis, conjunctival laceration, a shallow anterior chamber with an eccentrically placed pupil, hyphema, and vitreous hemorrhage. The intraocular pressure can be low, normal, or even slightly elevated.

In addition to rupture of the wall, contusive forces to the eyeball can result in motility disorders, subconjunctival hemorrhage, corneal edema, aqueous cell and flare, hyphema and angle-recession glaucoma, traumatic mydriasis, rupture of the iris sphincter, iridodialysis, paralysis of accommodation, lens dislocation, and cataract. Injuries sustained by posterior structures include vitreal and retinal hemorrhages, retinal edema (commotio retinae, or Berlin's edema),

retinal holes, vitreous base avulsions, retinal detachment, choroidal rupture, and optic nerve contusion (Figs 24–3 and 24–4).

Many of these injuries cannot be seen on external observation. Some, such as cataract, may not develop for many days or weeks following the injury.

Treatment

Except for injuries involving rupture of the eyeball itself, most of the effects of contusion of the eye do not require immediate definitive treatment. However, any injury severe enough to cause intraocular hemorrhage involves the danger of delayed secondary hemorrhage from a damaged uveal vessel, which may cause intractable glaucoma and permanent damage to the eyeball. The further management of these cases is described in the section below on hyphema.

In the closure of anterior segment wounds, corneal tissue is accurately realigned to form a watertight closure. To minimize astigmatism, centrally placed corneal sutures should be 10-0 nylon, of short length, and more closely spaced than those positioned near the limbus. An incarcerated iris or ciliary body exposed for less than 24 hours can be reposited in the globe by introducing a cyclodialysis spatula through a limbal stab incision and sweeping the tissue into position. If this cannot be achieved or if the tissue has been exposed for more than 24 hours, then the prolapsing tissue should be excised at the level of the wound lip. Any excised tissue should be sent for pathologic examination. Bacterial cultures are taken intraoperatively. Lens remnants and blood are removed by anterior vitrectomy. Viscoelastic materials (sodium hyaluronate), air, or saline injected into the anterior chamber will help realign the edges and prevent incarceration by providing support during wound closure.

Figure 24–3. Hole in retina, macular area, posttraumatic.

Figure 24–4. Choroidal tears. (Photo by Diane Beeston.)

Scleral wounds are closed with an interrupted 7-0 or 8-0 nonabsorbable suture. The rectus muscles may be temporarily disinserted to provide better exposure. Posterior scleral exit wounds in a double penetrating injury are self-sealing, and generally no attempt is made at closure.

The prognosis for traumatic retinal detachments is poor because of the macular injury, giant retinal tears, and formation of intravitreal fibrocellular membranes that occur with penetrating injury. Such intravitreal membranes generate sufficient contractile force to detach the retina. Vitrectomy is effective in their treatment, but the timing of this procedure remains controversial. Early vitrectomy is indicated for endophthalmitis. In noninfected cases, delaying surgery for 10–14 days may decrease the risk of intraoperative hemorrhage and permit a posterior vitreous detachment to develop, making surgery technically easier.

Vitreoretinal surgery in the presence of large corneal wounds can be done through a temporary Landers-Foulks keratoprosthesis, to avoid damaging a corneal graft. Primary enucleation or evisceration should only be considered when the globe is completely disorganized. The remaining eye is susceptible to sympathetic ophthalmia whenever penetrating ocular trauma occurs, particularly if there has been damage to the uveal tissues.

INTRAOCULAR FOREIGN BODIES (Fig 24–5)

Foreign bodies that have become lodged within the eye should be identified and localized as soon as possible. Particles of iron or copper must be removed to prevent later disorganization of ocular tissues by degenerative changes (siderosis from iron and chalcosis from copper). Some of the newer alloys are more inert and may be tolerated. Other kinds of particles, such as glass or porcelain, may be tolerated indefinitely and are usually better left alone.

Figure 24–5. Ophthalmoscopic view of intraocular metallic (iron) foreign body in vitreous.

A complaint of discomfort in the eye with blurred vision and a history of striking steel upon steel should arouse a strong suspicion of an intraocular foreign body. The anterior portion of the eye, including the cornea, iris, lens, and sclera, should be inspected with a loupe or slit lamp in an attempt to localize the wound of entry. Direct ophthalmoscopic visualization of an intraocular foreign body may be possible. An orbital soft tissue x-ray must be taken to verify the presence of a radiopaque foreign body as well as for medicolegal reasons.

Various radiologic methods can be used to localize intraocular foreign bodies, including the geometric method of Sweet or the Comberg contact lens (containing a post and ring). Ultrasonography and coronal CT scan of the orbits can precisely locate fragments relative to orbital structures. The Berman metal locator, an electronic instrument, is useful in pinpointing an intraocular foreign body located near one of the accessible areas of the eyeball. The wand of the instrument can be sterilized and passed posteriorly over the exposed field at surgery.

Treatment

If the foreign body is anterior to the lens zonules, it should be removed through an incision into the anterior chamber at the limbus. If it is located behind the lens and anterior to the equator, it should be removed through the area of the pars plana that is nearest to the foreign body because less retinal damage is caused in that manner. If the foreign body is posterior to the equator, it should be removed directly through that point on the wall of the eyeball which is nearest to it, unless that area is at the macula.

If the foreign body has magnetic properties, the sterilized tip of a hand magnet (or giant magnet) near the area of exit can be used to facilitate its removal. If it is nonmagnetic and removal is essential, small forceps are available for introduction into the posterior portion of the eye with minimal displacement and trauma. A special instrument has been devised to grasp a spherical air rifle or shotgun pellet.

Any damaged area of the retina must be treated with diathermy or photocoagulation to prevent retinal detachment.

HYPHEMA

Contusive forces will frequently tear the iris vessels and damage the anterior chamber angle. Blood in the aqueous may settle out in a visible layer. Acute glaucoma occurs when the filtration meshwork is blocked by fibrin and cells or when clot formation produces pupillary block.

Treatment

Patients with visible hyphemas filling more than 5% of the anterior chamber should be hospitalized for 5 days of bed rest, cycloplegia to prevent movement of damaged iris vessels, and patching of the affected eye. The eye is examined daily for secondary bleeding, glaucoma, or corneal blood staining from iron pigment. Glaucoma management includes the use of ocular timolol 0.5% applied twice a day; acetazolamide, 250 mg orally 4 times a day, and hyperosmotic agents (mannitol, glycerol, or sorbitol).

Rebleeding occurs in 16–20% of cases within 2–3 days. This complication carries a high risk of glaucoma and corneal staining. The use of oral aminocaproic acid to stabilize clot formation may reduce the risk of rebleeding.

The hyphema must be surgically evacuated if the intraocular pressure remains elevated (> 35 mm Hg for 7 days or 50 mm Hg for 5 days) to avoid optic nerve damage or if corneal staining occurs. If the patient has hemoglobinopathy, optic atrophy is likely to develop much more readily and operation should be considered much earlier. Vitrectomy instruments are used to excise the central clot and lavage the anterior chamber. The mechanized probe and irrigation port are introduced anterior to the limbus through clear cornea, to avoid damage to the iris and lens. No attempt is made to extract the clot from the anterior chamber angle or from iris tissue. A peripheral iridectomy is then performed.

Late-onset glaucoma may follow several months to years later, as a result of trabecular meshwork damage. Corneal blood staining will clear slowly over a period of months.

BURNS OF THE EYE

Chemical Burns

All chemical burns must be treated as ophthalmic emergencies. If possible, a tap-water lavage should be started at the site of injury before the patient is transported. In the emergency room, obtain a brief history and perform a brief examination; then begin copious irrigation of the ocular surfaces, including the conjunctival fornices. Sterile isotonic saline (several liters per injured eye) can be conveniently instilled with standard intravenous tubing. A lid speculum and even local anesthetic infiltration of the lids may be necessary to overcome blepharospasm. Give analgesics and topical anesthetic and cycloplegic agents. Use a moist cotton-tipped applicator to remove particulate matter from the fornices. Watch for respiratory distress due to soft tissue swelling of the upper airways. The pH can be checked by placing a strip of indicator paper in the fornix; resume irrigation if it is not between 7.3 and 7.7. After lavage, apply an antibiotic ointment and a pressure dressing.

Alkali rapidly penetrates into deep tissues and will continue to cause damage long after the injury is sustained; therefore, prolonged lavage and repeated pH checks are needed. Acids form a barrier of precipitated tissue that tends to limit further damage. Alkali burns cause an immediate rise in the intraocular pressure owing to contraction of the sclera. A secondary rise occurs 2–4 hours later owing to release of prostaglandin; this increases blood flow to the iris, ciliary processes, and choroid. An intense uveitis develops, which is difficult to monitor through the opaque cornea. Treatment is with topical steroids, antiglaucoma agents, and pupillary dilation during the first 2 weeks. Beyond 2 weeks, steroids are used with caution because they can enhance corneal melting by the collagenases present in the inflammatory response. A trial with collagenase inhibitors (acetylcysteine) may prove beneficial.

Corneal exposure and persistent epithelial defects are treated with artificial lubricants, tarsorrhaphy, and a bandage contact lens. Long-term complications include angle-closure glaucoma, corneal scarring, symblepharon, entropion, and keratitis sicca. Competency of the conjunctival and scleral vasculature has been shown to be of prognostic value. A greater loss of perilimbal epithelium and increased scleral blanching correspond to a poorer prognosis.

Thermal Burns

Thermal burns of the lids are treated with topical antibiotics and sterile dressings. If corneal damage is sustained, the extensive lid swelling initially makes pressure patching unnecessary. At 2–3 days, ectropion and lid retraction begin. Tarsorrhaphies and moisture chambers fashioned from plastic wrap then protect the cornea. Full-thickness skin grafts are delayed until skin contraction is no longer progressing.

Ultraviolet irradiation, even in moderate doses, often produces a superficial keratitis that is quite painful, although recovery occurs within 12–36 hours without complications. Pain often comes on 6–12 hours after exposure. This type of injury occurs following exposure to an electric welding arc without the protection of a filter. Many "flash burns" are caused by careless exposure in the mistaken belief that the eyes can be burned in this way only when looking directly at the arc. A short circuit in a high-voltage line may cause the same type of injury.

In severe cases of "flash burn," instillation of a sterile topical anesthetic may be necessary for examination. A mydriatic (eg, homatropine hydrobromide, 2–5%) should be used. Systemic sedation or narcotics are preferable to topical anesthetics, which interfere with corneal healing. Patching and cold compresses are indicated to relieve discomfort.

Infrared exposure rarely produces an ocular reaction. ("Glassblower's cataract" is rare today but once was common among workers who were required to watch the color changes in molten glass in furnaces without proper filters.) Radiant energy from viewing the sun or an eclipse of the sun without an adequate filter, however, may produce a serious burn of the macula, resulting in permanent impairment of vision. Persons using hallucinogenic drugs such as LSD have been particularly prone to solar macular burns.

Excessive exposure to radiation (x-ray) produces cataractous changes that may not appear for many months after the exposure. The same risk is inherent in exposure to nuclear radiation.

INJURIES INVOLVING THE ORBIT & ITS CONTENTS

Orbital Fractures

Orbital fractures can have concurrent facial trauma, and the appropriate consulting services should be notified. Fractures of the maxilla are classified by the Le Fort system: type I is below the orbital floor; type II passes through the nasal and lacrimal bones in addition to the maxilla forming the medial orbital floor; and type III involves the medial and lateral walls and the orbital floor in the presence of separation of the facial skeleton from the cranium. Orbital roof fractures are rare and are generally caused by penetrating injuries. If visual loss is progressing in the presence of an optic canal fracture, steroids and surgical decompression may be necessary. When visual loss is sudden and complete, however, recovery is less likely. Carotid–cavernous sinus fistulas are associated with orbital apex fractures, and the orbit should therefore be auscultated for bruits.

Tripod fractures of the zygoma involve the orbital floor but in the absence of dislocation may not need surgical repair. Zygomatic arch fractures do not involve the orbit. Telescoping fractures of the frontal process of the maxilla and the lacrimal and ethmoid bones produce a saddle-nose deformity with telecanthus and lacrimal system obstruction.

When the orbital entrance receives a blow, the compressive forces can fracture the thin medial and inferior walls, with prolapse and entrapment of soft tissues. This force may be transmitted by the soft tissues or directly through the bone without producing an orbital rim fracture. If the blowout is large, enophthalmos of the globe may develop immediately. Alternatively, this may occur at a later time, when the swelling subsides and atrophy or scarring of the soft tissues develops.

Diplopia can be caused by direct neuromuscular damage or swelling of orbital contents. It must be differentiated from entrapment within the fracture of the inferior oblique and rectus muscles or adjacent tissues. This is done by testing forced ductions and noting the presence of pain on attempted upgaze or downgaze. When entrapment is present, passive movement of the eye with forceps is restricted. Sufficient time should pass to allow for spontaneous improvement in eye movements with the resolution of swelling. Sensation is tested in the distribution of the infraorbital nerve. A series of plain x-ray films of the bony orbit should include a Waters view x-ray to show the maxillary sinus (antral) roof. These x-rays may reveal bony defects, an air-fluid level in the sinus, or herniated soft tissues. Only when interpretation of these films is equivocal should CT scan be performed.

The indications for surgical repair of the blowout fracture are (1) persistent diplopia within 30 degrees of the primary position of gaze in the presence of entrapment; (2) enophthalmos of 2 mm or more; or (3) a large fracture (half the orbital floor), which is likely to develop late enophthalmos. Delaying surgery for 1–2 weeks helps the surgeon to assess whether the diplopia will resolve without intervention. Longer delays decrease the likelihood of successful repair of enophthalmos and strabismus.

Surgical repair is usually accomplished via an infraciliary or transconjunctival route, although transantral and infraorbital approaches are also done. The periorbita is incised and elevated to expose the fracture site in the floor and medial walls. Herniated tissue is pulled back into the orbit, and the defect is covered by an alloplastic implant, with care being taken not to damage the infraorbital neurovascular bundle. Complications include blindness, diplopia, extruded implant, hemorrhage, infection, lower eyelid retraction, and infraorbital anesthesia. Subsequent procedures for strabismus and ptosis may be needed.

Penetrating Injury of the Orbit

Penetrating injuries of the orbital tissue may be produced by flying missiles or sharp instruments. Radiopaque foreign bodies can be localized by x-ray methods similar to those used in locating foreign bodies within the eye. Most orbital foreign bodies are best left alone.

Contusions of the Orbit

Contusion injuries to the orbital contents may result in hemorrhage or subsequent atrophy of the tissue, with enophthalmos. Traumatic paresis of the extraocular muscles occasionally occurs in this way but is usually transient.

Pulsating Exophthalmos Following Orbital Injury

Pulsating exophthalmos occasionally follows a penetrating or contusion injury to the orbital contents that has caused a shunt between the arterial and venous channels, so that the pulse is transmitted into the orbital tissues. (This condition may develop spontaneously but is more frequently traumatic in origin.) A common site of involvement is a fracture through the cavernous sinus.

Pulsating exophthalmos occasionally requires ligation of the carotid artery on the side of the fistula.

PREVENTION OF INJURIES TO THE EYE DURING ATHLETIC ACTIVITY

Persons who engage in athletic activities while wearing prescription lenses made of glass or plastic are at increased risk from shattered lens fragments. The eyewear most effective in preventing injuries consists of polycarbonate lenses in polyamide frames with a posterior retention rim. Solid wraparound frames should be used (rather than hinged frames) because they better withstand lateral blows. Eye guards without lenses do not always prevent a ball from compressing itself between the upper and lower rims and striking the eye.

REFERENCES

Bhimani S, Virapongse C, Sarwar M: Computed tomography in penetrating injury to the eye. *Am J Ophthalmol* 1984;**97**:583.

Brown SI, Tragakis MP, Pearce DB: Treatment of the alkali-burned cornea. *Am J Ophthalmol* 1972;**74**:316.

Cleary PE, Ryan SJ: Method of production and natural history of experimental posterior penetrating eye injury in the rhesus monkey. *Am J Ophthalmol* 1979;**88**:212.

Coleman DJ: Early vitrectomy in the management of the severely traumatized eye. *Am J Ophthalmol* 1982;**93**:543.

de Juan E Jr, Sternberg P Jr, Michels RG: Timing of vitrectomy after penetrating ocular injuries. *Am J Ophthalmol* 1984;**91**:1072.

de Juan E Jr et al: Evaluation of vitrectomy in penetrating ocular trauma. *Arch Ophthalmol* 1984;**102**:1160.

Deutsch TA, Feller DB: *Paton and Goldberg's Management of Ocular Injuries,* 2nd ed. Saunders, 1985.

Eagling EM: Ocular damage after blunt trauma to the eye. *Br J Ophthalmol* 1974;**58**:126.

Eagling EM: Perforating injuries of the eye. *Br J Ophthalmol* 1976;**60**:732.

Green K, Paterson CA, Siddiqui A: Ocular blood flow after experimental alkali burns and prostaglandin administration. *Arch Ophthalmol* 1985;**103**:569.

Grove AS: Computerized tomography in the management of orbital trauma. *Ophthalmology* 1982;**89**:433.

Hawes MJ, Dortzbach RK: Surgery on orbital floor fractures. *Ophthalmology* 1983;**90**:1066.

Landers MB III et al: Temporary keratoprosthesis for use during pars plana vitrectomy. *Am J Ophthalmol* 1981;**91**:615.

Lemp MA: Cornea and sclera. *Arch Ophthalmol* 1974;**92**:158.

McCuen BW, Fung WE: The role of vitrectomy instrumentation in the treatment of severe traumatic hyphema. *Am J Ophthalmol* 1979;**88**:930.

McGetrick JJ et al: Aminocaproic acid decreases secondary hemorrhage after traumatic hyphema. *Arch Ophthalmol* 1983;**101**:1031.

Parrish R, Bernardine V Jr: Iridectomy in the surgical management of eight-ball hyphema. *Arch Ophthalmol* 1982;**100**:435.

Read J, Goldberg MF: Comparison of medical treatment for traumatic hyphema. *Ophthalmology* 1974;**78**:799.

Ryan SJ, Allen AW: Pars plana vitrectomy in ocular trauma. *Am J Ophthalmol* 1979;**88**:483.

Shock JP, Adams D: Long-term visual acuity results after penetrating and perforating ocular injuries. *Am J Ophthalmol* 1985;**100**:714.

Sternberg P Jr et al: Ocular BB injuries. *Ophthalmology* 1984;**91**:1269.

Optics & Refraction

25

Orson W. White, MD

The correct interpretation of visual information depends on the eye's ability to focus incoming rays of light on the retina. An understanding of this process and how it can be influenced by normal variations or ocular disease is essential to the successful use of any optical aids: glasses, contact lenses, intraocular lenses, or low vision aids. To achieve this understanding, it is necessary to master the concepts of geometric optics, which define the effect on light rays as they pass through different surfaces and media.

The first part of this chapter will outline the principles of geometric optics and provide some definitions of terms used in specification of lenses. Mathematical schemes for calculating the effects of individual and compound lens systems will then be described. It will be emphasized that the popular algebraic method cannot be applied to the problems of modern ophthalmic optics, particularly the selection of intraocular lenses. Thus, it is absolutely necessary to understand trigonometric ray tracing.

A discussion of the normal human eye, outlining concepts used to reduce it to optically simpler component parts, will be followed by a description of refractive errors and ways of correcting them. Throughout the chapter, attention will be called to a number of misconceptions current in the teaching of ophthalmic optics.

GEOMETRIC OPTICS

Speed, Frequency, & Wavelength of Light

Speed, frequency, and wavelength of light are related by the expression

$$\text{Frequency} = \frac{\text{Speed}}{\text{Wavelength}}$$

In different optical media, speed and wavelength of light change, but frequency is constant. Color depends on frequency, so that the color of a ray of light is not altered as it passes through optical media except by selective nontransmittance or fluorescence. The optical characteristics of a substance can only be defined with respect to clearly specified frequencies of light. A substance to be used for lenses to refract visible light is usually tested with the yellow sodium light (D line) and the blue (F line) and the red (C line) of a rarefied hydrogen discharge tube.

In a vacuum, the speed of all frequencies of light is the same, ie, 299,792.46 kilometers per second (186,282.40 statute miles per second). Since the frequency of the yellow D line is approximately 5.085×10^{14} Hz, the wavelength of this line in a vacuum is 0.5896 μm. Similarly, the wavelengths in a vacuum of the blue F and red C lines are 0.4861 μm and 0.6563 μm, respectively.

Index of Refraction

If the speed of a light ray is altered by a change in the optical medium, refraction of the ray will also occur. The effect of an optical substance on the speed of light is expressed as its index of refraction, n. The higher the index, the slower the speed and the greater the effect on refraction.

In a vacuum, n has the value of 1.00000. The **absolute index of refraction** of a substance is the ratio of the speed of light in a vacuum to the speed of light in the substance. The **relative index of refraction** of a substance is calculated with reference to the speed of light in air. The absolute index of refraction of air varies with the temperature, pressure, and humidity of the air and the frequency of the light, but it is about 1.00032. In optics, n is assumed to be relative to air unless specified as absolute.

Thermal Coefficient of Index of Refraction

The index of refraction changes with the temperature of the medium—it is higher when the substance is colder. This lability of n to temperature is different for different substances. The change in n per degree Celsius for the following substances (all to be multiplied by 10^{-7}) is as follows: glass, 1; fluorite, 10; plastic, 140; water, aqueous, and vitreous, 185. This makes plastic undesirable for precision optical devices. (Plastic also has 8 times the thermal expansion of glass.) Water lenses date back to antiquity but are not practical, because of problems with thermal instability, evaporation, freezing, and susceptibility to contamination. It is interesting that in the eye, these objections all but disappear, making the fluid lenses of the eye acceptable.

Dispersion of Light

In a vacuum, the speed of all frequencies of light is the same; thus, the index of refraction is also the same for all colors (1.00000). In all substances, n is different for each color or frequency, being larger at the blue end and smaller at the red end of the spectrum.

This difference can be quantified as the dispersion value, V:

$$V = \frac{n_D - 1}{n_F - n_C}$$

where n_D, n_F, and n_C are the indices of refraction for the yellow sodium light and the blue and the red hydrogen lines.

The higher the value of V, the less the dispersion of colors. Table 25–1 gives the indices of refraction and some dispersion values for substances of ophthalmologic interest.

Transmittance of Light

Optical materials vary in their transmittance or transparency to different frequencies. Some "transparent" materials such as glass are almost opaque to ultraviolet light. Red glass would be almost opaque to the green frequency. Optical media must be selected according to the specific wavelength of light with which they are to be used.

Laws of Reflection & Refraction

The laws of reflection and refraction were formulated in 1621 by the Dutch astronomer and mathematician Willebrod Snell at the University of Leyden. These laws, together with Fermat's principle, form the basis of applied geometric optics. They can all be stated as follows (Fig 25–1):

(1) Incident, reflected, and refracted rays all reside in a plane known as the plane of incidence, which is normal (at a right angle) to the interface.

(2) The angle of incidence equals the angle of reflection but has the opposite sign: $I = -I'$.

(3) The product of the index of refraction of the

Table 25–1. Indices of refraction and dispersion values of some substances of ophthalmologic interest.

Substance (20 °C unless noted)	Indices of Refraction (n_D)	Dispersion Values (V)
Water	1.33299	
Water 37 °C	1.33093	55.6
Sea water	1.344	
Sea water, 11,000 meters' depth	1.361	
Polymethylmethacrylate	1.49166	57.37
Polymethylmethacrylate 37 °C	1.48928	
Acrylonitrile styrene copolymer	1.56735	34.87
Polystyrene	1.59027	30.92
Fluorite	1.4338	95.2
Spectacle crown glass	1.523	58.8
Flint glass	1.617	36.6
Aqueous and vitreous 37 °C	1.3337	55.6
Hydroxyethylmethacrylate (HEMA)	1.43	
Cellulose acetate butyrate (CAB)	1.47	
Silicone	1.439	

medium of the incident ray and the sine of the angle of incidence of the incident ray is equal to the product of the same terms of the refracted ray. The refracted ray is denoted by a prime: $n \sin I = n' \sin I'$ (**Snell's law**).

(4) A ray of light passing from one point to another follows the path that takes the least time to negotiate (**Fermat's principle**). Optical path length is the index of refraction times the actual path length.

Critical Angle & Total Reflection

In Fig 25–1, consider the ray in the more dense medium as the arriving ray. We see that it is refracted into the less dense medium away from the normal. If

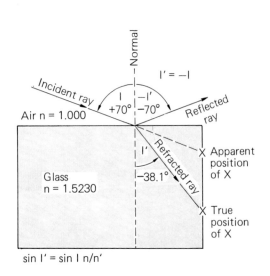

$\sin I' = \sin I \, n/n'$

Figure 25–1. Example of the laws of reflection and refraction.

Figure 25–2. Example of the critical angle.

we gradually increase the angle of incidence (Fig 25–2) in the denser medium until we reach the critical angle, a startling event takes place: None of the light escapes, but all is suddenly, totally, and perfectly reflected (total internal reflection). This angle is reached as the sine of the incident ray in the denser medium reaches the value $-n'/n$. This is one method used to determine the index of refraction. For water with an index of refraction of 1.330, the critical angle has the sine of $-1/1.330$, or -48.75 degrees.

Total reflection obeys the laws of regular reflection, ie, $I = -I'$. This allows perfect reflection without coatings and is used extensively in prisms and fiberoptics.

In Fig 25–2, the shaded area is not visible from the surface. This is why the angle of the eye cannot be inspected except with the gonioscopic lens (see Chapter 3). The index of refraction of the *aqueous*—and not the index of refraction of the tears or cornea, as is frequently stated—is the determining factor in this context.

CALCULATIONS USED IN OPTICS

There are 2 approaches to the application of the principles of geometric optics to single lenses or to compound lens systems. **Trigonometric ray tracing** is the more valid and exact approach, as it makes no other assumptions than those already determined by the laws of refraction. The **algebraic method** involves many hypothetical limitations. The lenses are assumed to be very thin, with minimal distances between them, and the beams of light are restricted in size by very small apertures. These limitations greatly reduce the accuracy and usefulness of the algebraic method when applied to actual lens systems, including those in the eye.

Unfortunately, the trigonometric method, although firmly established as the absolute reference system among scientists working in the field of geometric optics, has been largely ignored by ophthalmologists because of its supposed complexity. Most books on physiologic optics or refraction, most ophthalmology residency programs, most postgraduate "continuing education" courses, and even most courses in general physics stress only the algebraic method. The trigonometric method, if mentioned at all, is usually dismissed as being too complicated for practical purposes. However, it must be emphasized here that *the optical problems currently confronting the practicing ophthalmologist*—contact lenses, intraocular lenses, surgery that changes the shape of the eye, etc—*cannot be dealt with using the algebraic method*. The practice of ophthalmology has undergone a dramatic change with the introduction of the intraocular lens. Previously, when refractive problems after cataract surgery were dealt with solely by aphakic spectacles or contact lenses, mistakes in lens prescriptions because of difficult refractions, changes in refractive state, or incorrect calculation of the nec-

essary lens specifications were simple to put right, since one could always adjust the contact lenses or glasses. Now every ophthalmologist must realize that when undertaking an irreversible procedure such as insertion of an intraocular lens, the rough approximations of the algebraic method are intolerable. This becomes particularly apparent when it is realized that many of the problems caused by selecting the wrong intraocular lens are not amenable to correction by postoperative refraction. Reliance must be placed on an accurate, logical system: trigonometric ray tracing.

This chapter will demonstrate both the logic and the feasibility of trigonometric ray tracing. The supposed difficulties arise from the necessity for calculating the path of a number of rays through each refracting medium in turn. Fortunately, this task can now be easily performed with programmable calculators or computers.

Trigonometric Ray Tracing

Not every ophthalmologist who does refractions will choose to acquire facility with trigonometric ray tracing. However, every reader of this book should know of its existence and should know that *trigonometric ray tracing is the correct method for calculating complex lens systems*. Those who become familiar with the technique will be rewarded with a powerful tool in optics. Complex lens systems can be "made" mathematically and tested without the expense of actual production, and many controversial questions can be resolved with modest effort.

Graphic ray tracing is a comparable system that uses scale drawings to determine the optical properties of lens systems; it should not be confused with the method of "ray tracing" described in several books, in which tracings of an image are based on nodal points and focal planes (a derivation of the thin lens algebraic system).

A. Technique of Trigonometric Ray Tracing: The trigonometric method of ray tracing requires no higher

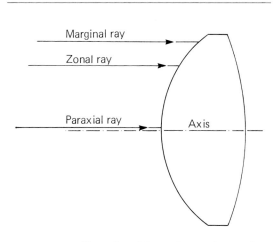

Figure 25–3. Illustration of 3 rays frequently traced.

mathematical skills other than elementary trigonometry. It consists of mathematically plotting the course of certain specified representative rays through the lens systems, calculating the change in direction produced at each refracting surface by using the principles of Snell's law.

The 3 rays most frequently traced are shown in Fig 25–3. They are named according to their positions relative to the first refracting surface. The marginal ray enters at the margin of the lens, the paraxial ray very near the optical axis (center of the lens), and the zonal ray in the portion of the lens where the average luminous flux of light passes. In this discussion, the paraxial ray will be placed at a distance of 0.01 times the semidiameter of the lens from the optical axis and the zonal ray at a distance from the optical axis that equals the semidiameter of the lens times the square root of 0.5. At each refracting surface, it is also necessary to know the radius of curvature of the surface, the index of refraction of the medium on each side, and the distance to the next surface.

Figure 25–4A shows the simplest situation, in which there is a single refracting surface and the light source is at infinity, such that the rays to be traced are all parallel to the optical axis. The points at which the particular ray under consideration and the optical axis intersect the refracting surface are designated P and A, respectively. Y is the distance of P from the optical axis along the perpendicular. For the marginal ray, this will equal the semidiameter of the lens; for the zonal ray, the semidiameter times the square root of 0.5; and for the paraxial ray, 0.01 times the semidiameter. The angles of incidence of the incident and refracted rays are I and I', both measured relative to the normal to the refracting surface. U' is the angle of the refracted ray relative to the optical axis. I and I' are positive if a ruler must be turned counterclockwise from the normal to reach the ray. Conversely, U' is positive if a ruler moves clockwise from the optical axis to the ray. L' is the distance between A and the intersection of the refracted ray and the optical axis. As with all measurements along the optical axis, those distances to the right of A are positive. When referring to the paraxial ray, small letters are commonly substituted for the capitals (eg, y for Y).

The radius of curvature of the refracting surface is r. It is positive if the center of curvature is to the right of the surface. n and n' are the indices of refraction before and after the refracting surface.

For infinite rays, Fig 25–4A:

$$\sin I = \frac{Y}{r} \qquad (1)$$

$$\sin I' = \frac{n}{n'} \sin I \qquad (2)$$

$$U' = I - I' \qquad (3)$$

$$PA = \frac{Y}{\cos \frac{I}{2}} \qquad (4)$$

$$L' = \frac{PA \cos \frac{I' - U'}{2}}{\sin U'} \qquad (5)$$

This produces an exact determination of the distance L'.

When the light source is situated at a finite distance from the refracting surface (Fig 25–4B), the distance between them along the optical axis is L, bearing in mind that the distances to the left of A are negative and the angle to the optical axis of the ray to be traced is U (with the same sign convention as U'). Equations 1, 3, and 4 are now modified to 1', 3', and 4'.

$$\sin I = \sin U \frac{L - r}{r} \qquad (1')$$

$$U' = U + I - I' \qquad (3')$$

$$PA = \frac{L \sin U}{\cos \frac{I - U}{2}} \qquad (4')$$

Equations 2 and 5 remain the same.

As shown in the diagram, unprimed letters are used before refraction and primed letters after refraction. With multiple surfaces, a numerical subscript, consecutively identifying each of the surfaces, is added to all of the relevant letters (Fig 25–4C). Moving from one surface to the next causes all of the primed letters to lose their prime as the refracted ray becomes the incident ray, and the numerical subscript is increased by 1.

Once a ray has entered the system, the above equations will automatically generate the value of U for the next surface. Furthermore, if the distance between the consecutive surfaces is d, the value of L for the second surface, denoted here as L_{x+1}, is related to L' of the first surface (L_x') by the equation

$$L_{x+1} = L_x' - d \qquad (6)$$

Thus, at each refracting surface subsequent to the very first, it is necessary only to additionally provide values for r, n, n', and d in order to derive the value of L for the last surface.

It is imperative to obey the stipulated sign conventions at all times. If during the calculation $\sin I$ becomes greater than 1, it means that the ray has missed the lens surface. A value of $\sin I'$ greater than 1 indicates total internal reflection. All of the equations can be adapted to fit a computer program.

Whenever a flat surface is encountered, such as the back surface of a convex-plano intraocular lens, the radius of curvature is infinite. Separate equations

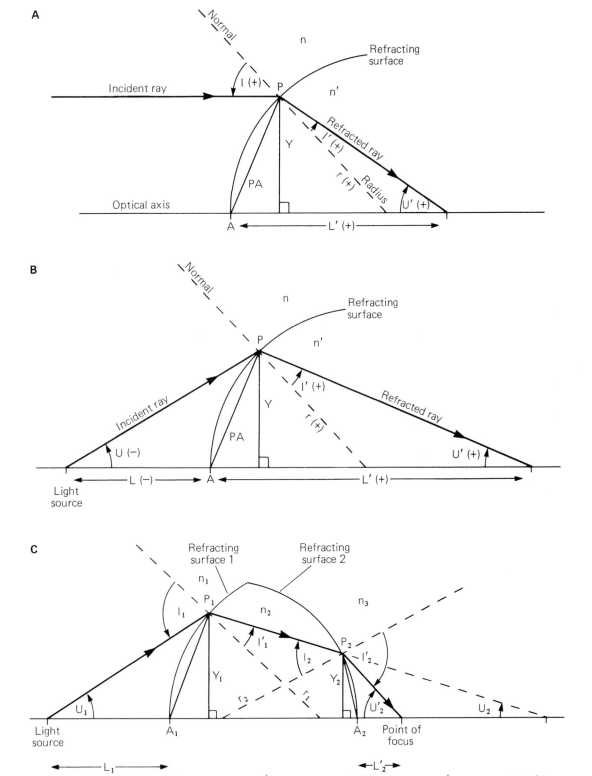

Figure 25–4. Trigonometric ray tracing notation. *A:* Single refracting surface with light source at infinity. *B:* Single refracting surface with light source at finite distance. *C:* Multiple refracting surfaces. Abbreviations are explained in the text.

may be used to avoid the division by zero that this introduces. However, the above equations may be used if a flat surface is assigned a very large radius of curvature, such as 10^9. **Optical flats (spacers)** are lenses with parallel flat surfaces. They are frequently used in optical devices to increase the focal length without a corresponding increase in magnification.

B. Use of Trigonometric Ray Tracing Determinations: Once the parameters of the final surface have been used in the calculations, L', the final back focal length, is determined and is the distance along the optical axis from the last surface to the point of focus of the ray in question. This point of focus is an exact location. The algebraic method will provide only an approximate location of the point of focus, with the tolerance degrading more and more as the system becomes more complex. Algebraic methods are unacceptably inaccurate when used with such determinations as the proper power of an intraocular lens. The trigonometric method will provide accurate determinations of the point of focus and information on the quality of the image formed.

Trigonometric ray tracing demonstrates that the back focal lengths for each of the different rays are almost never the same. The difference between the back focal lengths of the marginal and paraxial rays is a measure of the "spread of focus," thus indicating the degree of **spherical aberration.** Similarly, if rays of different color (frequency), with their different indices of refraction in each medium, are traced through the system, the degree of **chromatic aberration** will be determined. The optical pathway is the sum of the actual distances a ray passes through the substances multiplied by the index of refraction in the various substances through which it passes. How closely the optical pathways of the marginal and paraxial rays match predicts the brightness and contrast of the final image.

By using trigonometric ray tracing, one may determine the performance of each surface relative to the contribution to the final image. For example, it is easily shown that an intraocular lens gives a better image with the convex surface forward and the flat surface closer to the retina. The point of focus often requires—and is easily adjusted by—postoperative refraction. *However, the distorted image caused by selecting an intraocular lens of improper shape cannot be repaired by refraction. Suitability in this respect must be achieved by proper lens design preoperatively, and this can only be calculated using the trigonometric method of ray tracing.* Such calculations are not always undertaken by manufacturers of intraocular lenses. For best results, they should also be applied to each individual patient in turn. Since the optical quality of any lens cannot be judged in isolation, it must be assessed with respect to its place in a complete system.

Proportionality Principle

Optics, unlike mechanics but like geometry and mathematics, follows the laws of proportionality. Thus, a well-designed lens will function just as well if all components are made many times larger or smaller. If a model eye could be constructed the size of a swimming pool, with all structures correctly proportioned and the quality of the image—eg, in aphakia with glasses, with contact lenses, or with intraocular lenses—studied, the results would be valid.

Magnification

Linear magnification is the ratio of the height of the image to the height of the object. For an infinitely thin lens in air, this ratio is equal to the ratio of the distance of the image to the distance of the object. However, as usual, these relations are not valid for the eye. For real lens systems such as those of the eye, one must make use of the **LaGrange invariant.** Joseph Louis LaGrange (1736–1813) found that the height, H, times the index of refraction, n, times the sine of the angle of the ray, $\sin U$, results in a constant for any ray as it is traced through the system. The initial conditions at the object are noted by subscript 1, and subscript k represents the final conditions at the image. The final magnification of the system is then derived by the following equation:

$$M = \frac{n_1 \, \sin \, U_1}{n_k \, \sin \, U_k}$$

Note that the index of refraction of the vitreous, n_k of 1.3337, is involved.

In any system, only the initial U_1 and the final U_k (which are obtained from the ray tracing equations) and the initial and final n are required. Longitudinal magnification $\overline{M}$, which we are not as concerned with, has a different equation:

$$\overline{M} = \frac{n_1 \, (\sin \, U_1)^2}{n_k \, (\sin \, U_k)^2}$$

This explains the difference in perspective with a wide-angle lens and a telephoto lens. Portraits taken with a wide-angle lens are usually not flattering. The claim in the literature, that "$\overline{M} = M^2$," is warranted only when the object and the image are in the same medium, which is not the case in the eye.

A lens placed at the anterior focal plane of a lens system is often said to have no effect on the size of the image. This location has no less influence on the size of the image than any other location.

Algebraic Method

Correct trigonometric optical methods were well known in the time of the mathematician Karl Friedrich Gauss (1777–1855). The calculations were very time-consuming, as they involved multiple use of logarithm and trigonometry tables for each calculation. Gauss refined a method that in the beginning was far more simple and gave reasonable results if applied to thin lenses with small diameters placed close together. In fact, the restrictions are for "infinitely thin lenses," etc. By assuming these mythical conditions, we rid

$$\text{Diopters} \cong \frac{1}{\text{Focal length}} \cong \frac{1}{\text{Distance of image}} - \frac{1}{\text{Distance of object}}$$

$$\text{Diopters} \cong (n-1) \; \frac{1}{\text{Radius}_1} - \frac{1}{\text{Radius}_2}$$

$$\frac{\text{Size of image}}{\text{Distance of image}} \cong \frac{\text{Size of object}}{\text{Distance of object}}$$

$$\text{Magnification} = \frac{\text{Size of image}}{\text{Size of object}} \cong \frac{\text{Distance of image}}{\text{Distance of object}}$$

Power for Several Lenses Combined

$$\text{Diopters total} \cong \text{Dio}_1 + \text{Dio}_2 + \text{Dio}_3, \text{etc}$$

Figure 25–5. Algebraic thin lens approximations. All lengths in meters. $\cong$ indicates approximations. Diopters = power in diopters.

the equations of sines and cosines and no longer must use the tables. The restraints allow one to assume that any angle involved will be so small, measured in radians, that it will have the same value as the sine of the angle. Also, the sine and the tangent of the angle will be close enough to be assumed to be the same. From this, Gauss derived the general **thin lens equations** used by opticians to calculate curves for lenses. "Fudge factors" will be found at the bench of the optician and the "lathe man" for contact lenses to enter corrections shown by experience to help correct inaccuracies in the equations. These equations must not be used to calculate complicated thick lens systems such as those of the eye.

Fig 25–5 shows some of the important thin lens algebraic equations.

Diopter

The diopter is a measure of lens power. It was first introduced in 1872 by Felix Monoyer, a French ophthalmologist. It is defined as the reciprocal of the focal length measured in air in meters. It is, however, an algebraic approximation concept and not acceptable when calculating complex lens systems such as those that make up the eye.

Diopters are supposedly additive, such that a +2 diopter lens combined with a +1 diopter lens results in almost a +3 diopter lens. If these 2 lenses are combined with a −1 diopter lens, the result is nearly +2 diopters, and so on. This formula breaks down for lenses of high power (eg, a "+20 diopter" lens combined with a "+40 diopter" lens does not nearly equal a "+60 diopter" lens). The result varies greatly with the separation distance and with thickness. The phrase "60 diopter lens" has almost no meaning, because the powers at the edge, middle, and center portions are vastly different. *Strong lenses must be described by 3 values:* (1) radii of curvature, (2) index of refraction, and (3) thickness.

Curvature

Curvature *(c)* is a term used by optical engineers to express a function similar to diopters in that it

increases with lens power and is approximately additive. It is the reciprocal of the radius of curvature. It is useful in "bending" lenses, which is frequently done to achieve a better image. "Bending" a lens changes both curves, keeping the effective power the same. The effective power of the lens will remain about the same if the result of the front curvature minus the back curvature is kept constant.

Further Applications of the Algebraic Method

If a lens of given power at a given distance from the eye is moved to a different distance from the eye **(vertex distance)**, it will have a different effect. To calculate a new lens that will have the same effect at the new distance, we may use the following equation:

(Dio = power in diopters)

$$\text{Dio}_2 \approx \frac{1}{\frac{1}{\text{Dio}_1} - (\text{Dist}_1 - \text{Dist}_2)}$$

Example 1: A +13 diopter lens at 11 mm (0.011 m) is to be replaced by a lens at 9 mm (0.009 m)

$$\text{Dio}_2 \cong \frac{1}{\frac{1}{13} - (0.011 - 0.009)} \cong 13.347 \text{ diopters}$$

Example 2: Same lens to be replaced by a contact lens

$$\text{Dist}_2 = 0$$

$$\text{Dio}_2 \cong \frac{1}{\frac{1}{13} - (0.011)} \cong 15.169 \text{ diopters}$$

Remember that the vertex equation is also an approximate equation. It is used incorrectly for intraocular lens calculations; this partially explains why different authors using the equation arrive at different results.

In an attempt to make the thin lens equations more accurate for thicker lenses, a "thick lens equation" (below) has been derived. It is still an algebraic approximation but will give more accurate results for making high plus contacts or thick spectacle lenses.

$$\text{Dio} \cong \frac{1}{F} \cong (n - 1)\left[\frac{1}{r_1} - \frac{1}{r_2} - \frac{(n - 1)d}{nr_1r_2}\right]$$

where F = focal length, r = radius, and d = thickness of lens, all measured in meters.

The sign convention for the radius of curvature varies from author to author. The above formulas agree with the sign convention used in our discussion of trigonometric ray tracing. Another equation that may be of interest to the practicing ophthalmologist is the conversion of "diopters" to radius of curvature with contact lenses, since it is based on the above equations.

$$\text{Dio} \approx \frac{(n - 1)}{r} \approx \frac{1.3375 - 1}{r} \approx \frac{337.5}{\text{rmm}} \text{ and rmm} \approx \frac{337.5}{\text{Dio}}$$

n of "cornea" is for this purpose assumed to be 1.3375. Rmm = radius in millimeters.

The algebraic equations of Gauss do not all remain simple (as above) but may become very complex. This may lead one to the erroneous conclusion that because of their complexity they are accurate. One may not want to spend hours of study on these complex methods if one is aware of their limitations. These are the equations that involve principal planes, principal points, nodal points, etc. When these terms are mentioned in works on optics, one knows that the algebraic method was employed and that the results are not reliable. Magnification by these equations also results in incorrect answers when the results are applied to ophthalmologic optics. Again, this can save hours of study. Sylvanus P. Thompson (1851–1916), an En-

glish physicist, called these calculations "examination optics," involving mathematical acrobatics, as opposed to "real optics." A caution is required at this point. Nearly all examinations given today in ophthalmology are based on thin lens algebraic methods. The student should be prepared to use algebraic equations for examinations (at present) but should learn how to use trigonometric methods when seeking "real answers" in the spirit of the quotation of Thompson more than 70 years ago.

Prisms

In ophthalmology, prisms are used with the nearer face normal to the visual axis; this is not the classic minimal deviation angle of a symmetric prism usually given in texts on optics. Thus, prism equations are slightly different for ophthalmology. Fig 25–6 represents a prism as used in ophthalmology. The eye is to the left of the prism. This solution demonstrates an important point in optics; one may trace rays forward or backward with no change in the results. In the example, it is easier to trace the ray as if it emanated from the eye to the object (as was once popularly believed to happen). The ray strikes the prism and is not refracted by the first surface, as the ray is normal to this surface. At the second surface, the angle of incidence is seen to be the same as A, the apex angle. From Snell's law, $\sin I' = n/n' \sin A$. For example, if the prism is of glass with $n = 1.523$ and $A = 30$ degrees, then $\sin I'$ is 1.523×0.5, or 0.7615. I' is 49.6 degrees. The angle of deviation is $I' - A$, or 19.6 degrees. An object seen through the prism appears deviated toward the apex A, or away from the base. The power of a prism is measured in prism diopters (Δ). One prism diopter deviates an image 1 cm at 1 m. The arc tangent of 1/100 is 0.57 degrees. So 1 Δ is almost one-half degree. The "rule of thumb" is that 2 Δ = 1 degree.

Prisms are used in ophthalmology both to measure

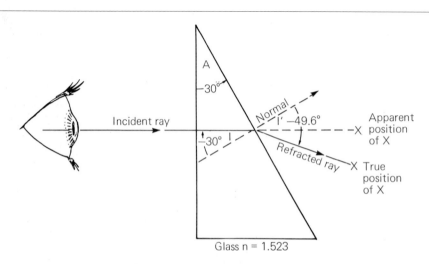

Figure 25–6. Example of the prism as used in ophthalmology.

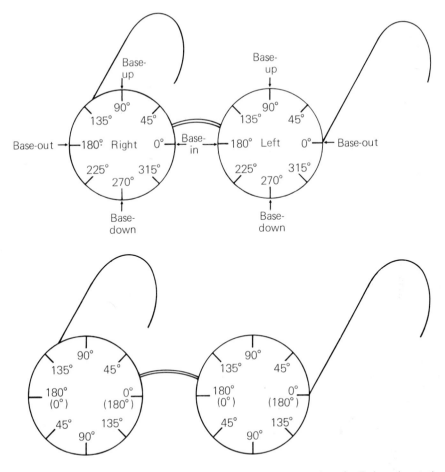

Figure 25–7. *Top:* Illustration of prism base notation. *Bottom:* Illustration of cylinder axis notation.

and to treat heterotropia and heterophoria (see Chapter 16). The prism is prescribed as magnitude in prism diopters and direction of the base, ie, "base-up right eye," "base-down left eye," "base-in," or "base-out." Prisms may be prescribed by the direction of the base in the usual mathematical way (Fig 25–7 top). Prisms obey vector laws. Vector addition is explained in the manual of any calculator capable of polar to rectangular and rectangular to polar operations.

OPTICS & THE EYE

Euclid (ca 300 BC) taught that some sort of sensory rays emanated from the eye and detected objects in a manner similar to the sensation of touch. Later, before the time of Johannes Kepler (1571–1630), the eye was thought of as a miniature camera obscura. The camera obscura was usually a darkroom or box with a small hole at one end that cast an inverted image of the scene against the opposite wall or side without the use of lenses. Kepler suggested that the cornea and lens together refracted the rays and formed the

image on the retina. Christopher Scheiner (1579–1650) made the first measurement of corneal curvature. He also demonstrated the small image of objects formed on the posterior surface of enucleated animal eyes.

Many models have been devised to represent the optical properties of the human eye, the most prominent of which is the **schematic eye of Gullstrand.** For each of these models, numerical values for the refractive index of each of the component parts are derived mathematically. Unfortunately, these numbers have become accepted by many as the true physiologic values. This has led to a compounding of errors in the practice of ophthalmic optics. It is only very recently that the true value of the refractive index of aqueous was found to be 1.3337 (for the sodium D line at 37 °C), as compared to the value of 1.336 used in Gullstrand's model.

Lenses of the Eye

The concept that the image of the retina is focused by 2 lens elements, the cornea contributing about 43 diopters and the lens the remaining 19 diopters, is still widely entertained today. Study of Fig 25–8 will show that a 3-lens system is a more realistic concept. All

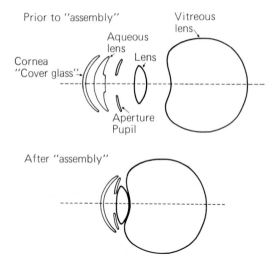

Prior to "assembly"

Cornea "Cover glass"

Aqueous lens

Lens

Aperture Pupil

Vitreous lens

After "assembly"

Figure 25–8. The optical system of the eye, illustrating the 3-lens concept.

3 lenses satisfy the thick lens definition: the aqueous lens, the lens lens, and the vitreous lens. In Fig 25–8, these 3 lenses are illustrated "prior to assembly" and then "assembled." The assembly is similar to a cemented system of lenses in cameras.

A. Cornea: Contrary to popular belief, the cornea has almost no power of refraction in the optical system of the eye. Since the cornea has been regarded as the most important "lens" of the eye for over 300 years, some explanation and proof are in order. The cornea is important optically only in shaping the anterior curve of the aqueous lens. Using trigonometric ray tracing, the possible refractive effect of the corneal substance can be removed mathematically. As long as the aqueous is kept in its former shape, image location and quality are for all practical purposes the same. Further proof of this concept can be obtained by considering 3 glass flasks of almost spherical shape (Fig 25–9). All the flasks are identical. The "empty" flask of air has almost no refractive power. The flask filled with water is a strong convex lens. The flask

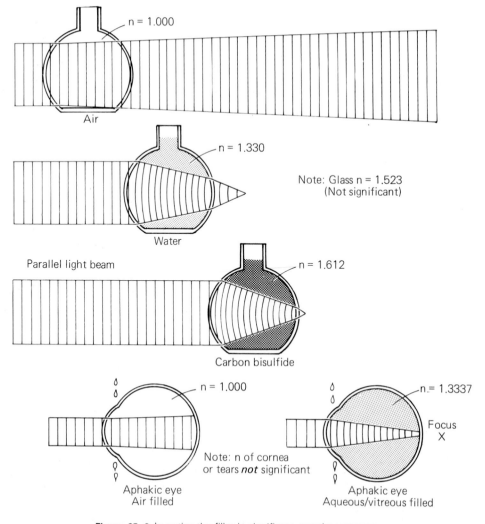

$n = 1.000$

Air

$n = 1.330$

Water

Note: Glass $n = 1.523$
(Not significant)

Parallel light beam

$n = 1.612$

Carbon bisulfide

$n = 1.000$

Aphakic eye
Air filled

Note: n of cornea or tears *not* significant

$n = 1.3337$

Focus
X

Aphakic eye
Aqueous/vitreous filled

Figure 25–9. In optics the filler is significant, not the wrapper.

filled with carbon bisulfide is a very strong convex lens. The actual values calculated by ray tracing are illustrated. The index of refraction of the glass container has almost no effect, whereas the index of refraction of the fluid content of the flask accounts almost entirely for the lens power of the flasks. In an analogous manner, the eye without the lens has almost no refractive power if filled with air. Its refractive power is then dependent on the filling fluid—just like the flasks. The index of refraction of the tears is of *no* importance to the refraction system of the eye; that of the cornea is of *almost no* importance.

B. Aqueous Lens: The first lens system of the eye, the aqueous, is a very powerful thick lens. If it is removed (replaced by air), the effect on refraction is striking. This also may be calculated by ray tracing techniques.

C. Lens Lens: The lens lens (**crystalline lens**), the second lens of the ocular system, is the most baffling component of the ocular refracting system. The equations used in optical calculations depend on a constant index of refraction for any one element. They also assume either spherical surfaces or surfaces with stable configurations and optical properties. The crystalline lens does not satisfy any of these requirements. The index of refraction of the lens changes like that of a syrup and water mixture, since the lens is more dense near the center. Various approximations have been made in an effort to create a hypothetical lens that might be used in ray tracing calculations. In the aphakic eye, conventional optical equations may be used. Thus, aphakic correction by glasses, contact lenses, and intraocular lenses may be studied as to quality of image, magnification, and focus.

D. Vitreous Lens: The third lens of the eye system is the vitreous lens. In a camera system, this would be the largest, heaviest, most expensive, and most important lens. When this vitreous lens is removed (replaced by air), there is a profound change in the refraction system of the eye. This too, of course, may be calculated by ray tracing. The vitreous lens has a major effect on magnification that is frequently ignored.

It should be noted that the aqueous lens, lens lens, and vitreous lens each have an optical spacer effect, ie, they alter the focal length of the system without a corresponding change in magnification.

The reader must be cautioned again that the present testing system in ophthalmology courses assumes the validity of the 2-lens theory, ie, that the cornea is the main lens and the crystalline lens the secondary lens.

Accommodation

The eye changes refractive power to focus on near objects by a process called accommodation. Thomas Young helped explain the principles of accommodation in 1801. Young himself had very prominent eyes. He was able to place one blade of a pair of calipers on his cornea and the other blade on the posterior pole of his eye. He claimed that he noted no increase in the size of the retinal scotoma from the caliper pressure when he accommodated. This discredited the theory that the eye accommodated by lengthening. Purkinje in 1823 described the various images reflected from the optical surfaces in the eye. Many observers have shown that the images from the lens change during accommodation. Contraction of the ciliary muscle results in thickening and increased curvature of the lens. This is probably due to relaxation of the elastic lens capsule. In the 3-lens concept, this causes a decrease in thickness and an increase in posterior curvature of the aqueous lens; an increase in thickness and both curvatures of the lens lens; and a slight decrease in thickness and an increase in anterior curvature of the vitreous lens. These peculiar changing fluid lenses are unfamiliar to optical engineers.

Visual Acuity

Visual field testing of peripheral retinal function is described briefly in Chapter 3. Foveal vision is assessed by testing the ability to distinguish small objects. By tradition, Alcor, the second star in the handle of the Big Dipper, and its optical double, Mizar, have been used to determine "good vision." Since these stars are separated by 11.8 minutes of arc, they do not make a very demanding test of visual acuity. (This angle has not changed significantly during the history of the human race, as the 2 stars travel together.) Euclid suggested that the average resolving power of the normal eye was 1 minute of arc. This is still the value used for 6/6 (20/20) vision. Robert Hooke (1635–1703) stated that the sharpest vision was about 30 seconds of arc, or 6/3 (20/10). Hermann Snellen (1834–1908), a Dutch ophthalmologist, devised the type of chart still in use (see Chapter 3). The Snellen "block E" letters (Fig 25–10) are made from squares of 5-by-5 units. For "normal" vision, the eye should discriminate a letter with a total block size of 5 minutes of angle, or 1 minute of angle per square of information. Thus, a person with "normal vision" could perceive a double star of 1 minute separation or could determine, for example, that an *F* is

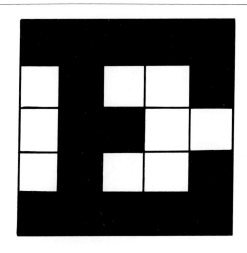

Figure 25–10. Snellen block E.

an *F* and not a *P* if the whole letter is 5 minutes high and 5 minutes wide. Acuity is noted as a fraction: 6/6 (20/20), 6/12 (20/40), etc. Distance visual acuity is usually measured at 6 meters (or 20 feet, which is approximately the same); this is the numerator of the fraction. The denominator represents the distance at which a letter that size would make a visual angle of 5 minutes. Thus a 6/6 (20/20) size letter has a visual angle of 5 minutes at 6 meters (or 20 feet). A 6/12 (20/40) size letter has a visual angle of 5 minutes at 12 meters (40 feet). Another approach would be to say that a person with 6/12 (20/40) visual acuity can discriminate a size of letter at 6 meters (20 feet) that a person with 6/6 (20/20) vision could discriminate at 12 meters (40 feet). The letters must have good contrast and be illuminated by sufficient light (800–1000 lux, or about 80–100 footcandles).

The 6/6 (20/20) letter at 6 meters (20 feet) is about 8.7 mm (0.35 in) high and wide. To calibrate a projector chart, one adjusts the height of the 6/60 letter to be 87.3 mm times the distance to the patient's eye in meters divided by 6. Similarly, the 20/200 letter should be 3.49 in times the distance to the patient's eye in feet divided by 20. (These heights are equal to the tangent of 50 minutes times either 6000 [6 meters in mm] or 240 [20 feet in inches].) By ray tracing, one finds that the eye minifies an image at 6 meters (20 feet) by about 350 times. Therefore, the size of the 6/6 (20/20) letter on the retina is 0.025 mm high and wide. Photographic films are often rated for resolution capacity by lines per millimeter. Vision of 6/6 (20/20) is 100 lines per millimeter, and 6/3 (20/10) is 200 lines per millimeter. For a 6-mm pupil and light of wavelength 0.560 μm (in air), the absolute theoretic limit would be 345 lines per millimeter.

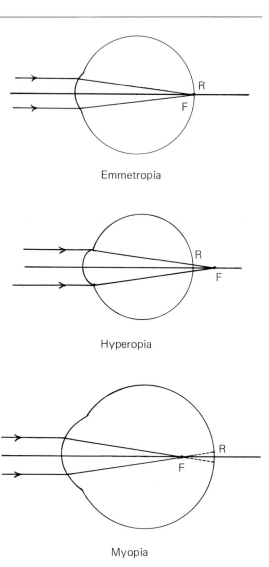

Figure 25–11. Emmetropia, hyperopia, and myopia. F = focal point; R = retina.

REFRACTIVE ERRORS

The terms **emmetropia,** having no refractive error, and **ametropia,** having a refractive error, are used infrequently at present. Refractive errors are illustrated in Figs 25–11 and 25–12.

Presbyopia

The loss of accommodation that comes to all people is called presbyopia (Table 25–2). A person with emmetropic eyes (no refractive error) will begin to notice inability to read small print or discriminate fine close objects at about age 44–46. This is worse in dim light and usually worse early in the morning or when the subject is fatigued. Many people complain of a feeling of sleepiness when reading. These symptoms increase until about age 55, when they stabilize but persist. This is a major annoyance, but no more than that, whereas before glasses became available, presbyopia had a devastating effect on the performance and well-being of the race.

Presbyopia is corrected by use of a plus lens to make up for the lost automatic focusing power of the lens. This is analogous to the close-up lens of a camera. The plus lens may be used in several ways. Reading glasses have the near correction in the entire aperture of the glasses, making them fine for reading but blurred for distant objects. Half-glasses can be worn to abate this nuisance by leaving the top open and uncorrected for distance vision. Bifocals do the same but allow correction of other refractive errors. Trifocals correct the distance vision by the top segment, the middle distance by the middle section, and the near distance by the lower segment.

Myopia

When the image of distant objects focuses in front of the retina in the unaccommodated eye, the eye is myopic or nearsighted. If the eye is longer than average, the error is called axial myopia. If the refractive elements are more refractive than average, the error

Table 25–2. Table of accommodation.

Age (Years)	Mean Accommodation (Diopters)
8	13.8
25	9.9
35	7.3
40	5.8
45	3.6
50	1.9
55	1.3

is called curvature myopia or refractive myopia. As the object is brought closer than 6 meters, the image moves closer to the retina and comes into sharper focus. The point reached where the image is most sharply focused on the retina is called the ''far point.'' One may estimate the extent of myopia by calculating the reciprocal of the far point. Thus, a far point of 0.25 m would suggest a 4-diopter minus lens correction for distance. The myopic person has the advantage of being able to read at the far point without glasses even at the age of presbyopia.

Concave spherical (minus) lenses are used to correct the image in myopia. These lenses move the image back to the retina. One may detect a minus lens by looking through it 0.5 m (19 inches) or so from the eye and moving the lens at right angles to the visual axis. The image seen through the lens will tend to move *with* the minus lens. The same test with a convex or plus lens causes the image to tend to move *away from* the direction of motion. An astigmatic (cylindric) lens shows changing distortion of the image when the lens is rotated about the visual axis. Spherical lenses cause no change in the image when rotated about the visual axis.

A high degree of myopia results in greater susceptibility to degenerative retinal changes, including retinal detachment.

Hyperopia

Hyperopia (hypermetropia, farsightedness) is the state in which the unaccommodated eye would focus the image behind the retina. Hyperopia is a more difficult concept to explain than myopia. The term ''farsighted'' contributes to the difficulty, as does the prevalent misconception among laymen that presbyopia is farsightedness and that one who sees well far away is farsighted. If hyperopia is not too great, a young person may obtain a sharp distant image by accommodating, as a normal eye would to read. The young hyperopic person may also make a sharp near image by accommodating more—or much more than one without hyperopia. This extra effort may result in eye fatigue and is more so for near work. The degree of hyperopia a person may have without symptoms is—like most clinical conditions—variable. However, the amount decreases with age as presbyopia (decrease in ability to accommodate) increases.

Three diopters of hyperopia might be tolerated in a teenager but will require glasses later, even though the hyperopia has not increased. If the hyperopia is too high, the eye may be unable to correct the image by accommodation. The hyperopia that cannot be corrected by accommodation is termed manifest hyperopia. This is one of the common causes of deprivation amblyopia in children and can be bilateral. There is a reflex correlation between accommodation and convergence of the 2 eyes. Hyperopia is therefore a frequent cause of esotropia (crossed eyes) and monocular amblyopia (see Chapter 16).

Latent Hyperopia

As explained above, a prepresbyopic person with hyperopia may obtain a clear retinal image by accommodation. This may become a ''set condition.'' If one carries a heavy backpack all day, when the pack is removed the ''set condition'' remains for some time, and one has a peculiar feeling of lightness or jumping about, since muscular responses are still modified by the discarded extra weight. The ciliary muscle is no different. It is not unusual for an uncorrected hyperope to observe that any plus lens blurs the image. The diagnosis may thus be missed or the hyperopia greatly underestimated. When cycloplegic drops are instilled to extinguish accommodation, the full extent of the hyperopia may be found. This is ''latent'' (hidden) hyperopia, ie, hyperopia that is not demonstrated until cycloplegic refraction is done. Refraction with a cycloplegic is very important in young patients who complain of eyestrain when reading and is vital in esotropia, where full correction of hyperopia may achieve a cure.

Remember that a moderately ''farsighted'' person may see well for near or far when young. However, as presbyopia comes on, the hyperope first has trouble with close work and at an earlier age than the non-hyperope. Finally, the hyperope has blurred vision for near *and far* and requires glasses for both near and far.

Astigmatism

Astigmatism is a type of refractive error that occurs when some of the refractive components of the eye are ''out of round'' or ''off center'' or ''tilted.'' Any of the refractive components may be defective in this way, but the cornea shaping the aqueous lens is the usual major cause of astigmatism. The lens may also contribute to astigmatic error. In contact lens terminology, lenticular astigmatism is called residual astigmatism, for it is not corrected by the usual spherical hard contact lens, which does correct ''corneal astigmatism.'' Astigmatism can be at any angle from 0 to 180 degrees. The nature and extent of image distortion depend on the magnitude of the astigmatism and its angle (Fig 25–12).

Astigmatism can make level objects appear slanted. All sorts of slanting may occur with the image of eyes being interpreted by the brain. The brain is very ingenious at correcting this ''out of plumb'' condition.

Figure 25–12. *A:* Emmetropia. *B:* Myopia or manifest hyperopia. *C, D, E, F:* Astigmatism.

Figure 25–12 (cont'd). *G, H, I:* Astigmatism.

(The brain cannot correct for the diminished visual acuity astigmatism causes.) When a patient has adapted to an uncorrected astigmatic error or if the correction has changed, the patient wearing new glasses that correct the error will still receive "aid" from the brain and for a week or so will have the impression of tilting. Finally, the "gyro" adjusts and levels are again correct. This is not always easy to explain to patients who are sure their glasses are incorrect because of slanting of the image.

Astigmatic errors can be corrected with cylindric lenses. Cylindric lenses may be positive or negative. They are frequently combined with spherical lenses. A typical prescription for nearsighted astigmatism might read as follows:

$$-3.00 +2.25 \times 175$$
$$-2.50 +1.75 \times 160$$

The top line refers to the right eye correction and the second line to the left eye. In the top line, -3.00 specifies the power of the spherical correction and

$+2.25$ specifies diopters of magnitude of the cylindric correction to be combined with the sphere for the total correction. Most ophthalmologists use only plus or only minus cylinders; however, the same prescription may be written in either form. To change the form is called transposing. To transpose a prescription for glasses, one algebraically adds the sphere and cylinder magnitudes to obtain the new sphere. Then one changes the sign of the cylinder and finally the axis by 90 degrees, keeping it between 0 and 180 degrees. For example, the former prescription transposed would read as follows:

$$-0.75 -2.25 \times 85$$
$$-0.75 -1.75 \times 70$$

The 2 prescriptions have the same meaning. The axis of the cylinder lens is the line of no refractive effect. Looking at the patient, zero degrees begins nasally in the right lens and temporally in the left lens and proceeds in a counterclockwise direction to 180 degrees (see Fig 25–7B). Further turning is a repetition. A cyclindric lens combined with one of the same magnitude at right angles to the first has the effect of a spherical lens of the same magnitude as either of the cylinders. The refractive power of a cylindric lens is 0 on axis and the nominal amount at 90 degrees from the axis. At other angles, the power is given by the sine squared of the angle off axis times the nominal value. The addition of 2 cylinders at oblique angles is a form of vector addition but is somewhat complex. Programmable calculators make this a simple task. Thus, overrefraction using spectacle addition and spectacle subtraction is now a practical aid to refraction, especially with strong lenses.

GRIN (Gradient-Index) Lenses

Having discussed the important 3-lens concept of the eye system, we must amplify the discussion of the unique and peculiar lens lens, or crystalline lens. As previously mentioned, the index of refraction within the crystalline lens is not constant but is maximal at the center of the lens and decreases outwardly along the X, Y, and Z axes as a spherical gradient. James Clerk Maxwell over a century ago developed the theoretic mathematical properties of such lenses using the partial derivative and vector equations. Such a lens, a gradient-index lens, is called a GRIN lens. In classic optics, a ray of light travels in straight lines until it meets an interface between 2 media with different indices of refraction, where it abruptly changes course along a new straight line until the next interface. Within a GRIN lens, the ray of light is bent along a gradient relative to the changing index of refraction and is therefore a curved line. A GRIN lens with parallel surfaces may function as a lens (Fig 25–13). A GRIN lens with curved surfaces such as the crystalline lens will be an even more effective lens (Fig 25–14). Earth's atmosphere is also a GRIN lens, and this may be the principal cause of sunset colors.

The optics of the eye submerged in seawater is of great importance in the phylogenesis of the eye. In submersion, the arriving incident ray is in water. This for all practical purposes cancels the effect of the aqueous lens and vitreous lens. The fish eye therefore has essentially one lens element—the crystalline lens, which is a GRIN lens. The full properties of GRIN lenses await further study. They should permit better transmission because there is less reflection from the surface. The lens may have the same n at the surface as the medium of the arriving ray. The effect on spherical aberration and chromatic aberration is unknown. To the author's knowledge, no investigator has yet produced a spherical gradient GRIN lens so that its properties could be investigated. This type of GRIN lens could be easily made in zero gravity outer space.

As a nuclear cataract develops, it is common for the patient to develop myopia, which may be of high degree. At first, this may again allow reading without glasses and for that reason is called "second sight." The myopia is due to an increase in the gradient of the GRIN lens. High elevations of blood glucose may also cause profound hyperopia, which is usually reversible. The mechanism is not clearly established. (The increased index of refraction of the aqueous lens and the vitreous lens owing to the increased glucose level is not of sufficient magnitude to explain the change.)

History of Spectacles

The history of the correction of refractive errors and presbyopia with spectacles is somewhat complex and vague, partly as a result of confusion about the definition of "spectacle." Spherical glass flasks found in many Egyptian tombs become functional presbyopic reading glasses when filled with water. However, conventional plus lenses did not come into use until the 13th century. Minus lenses probably date from the 15th or 16th century. The astronomer Sir George Biddell Airy corrected his own astigmatism in 1827, introducing this advance to humankind. Benjamin Franklin made the first bifocal spectacle lens in about 1775. It is a startling fact and unappreciated

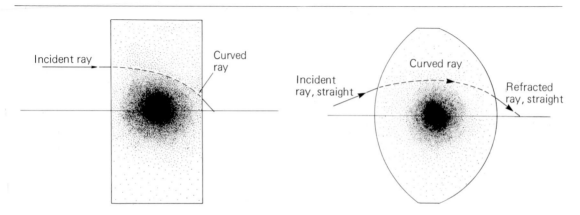

Figure 25–13. A noncurved GRIN lens simulating a convex lens.

Figure 25–14. GRIN crystalline lens of the eye.

by most that *until very recently, the most common cause of functional blindness was refractive error, including presbyopia.*

Natural History of Refractive Status

Most babies are slightly hyperopic at birth. The hyperopia slowly decreases, with a slight acceleration in the teens, to approach emmetropia. The corneal curvature is much steeper (6.59 mm radius) at birth and flattens to nearly the adult curvature (7.71 mm) by about 1 year. The lens is much more spherical at birth and reaches adult conformation at about 6 years. The axial length is short at birth (6.2 mm), lengthens rapidly in the first 2 or 3 years (to 24.1 mm), then moderately (0.4 mm/yr) until age 6, and then slowly (about 1 mm total) to stability at about 10 or 15 years. Presbyopia becomes manifest in the fifth decade.

Refractive errors are inherited. The mode of inheritance is complex, as it involves so many variables. The final result is the sum of the variables. Refractive errors, though inherited, need not be present at birth any more than tallness, which is also inherited, need be present at birth. For example, a child who reaches emmetropia at age 10 years will probably soon become myopic. Myopia usually increases during the teens. This should be expected, just as the need for larger shoes is expected, and not looked on with alarm by the patient and his or her parents. In a similar way, hyperopia usually decreases slightly during the teens. Myopia does not generally decrease with age, as is popularly believed, nor does farsightedness come with aging.

REFRACTION

Detailed discussion of refraction is better left to more specialized texts. However, some points are of general interest.

Patients over about 6 years of age can usually be refracted by eliciting subjective responses. Thus, the patient tells whether various steps are better or worse or the same until an end point is reached. One frequently begins with the correction of the patient's present glasses or with the correction indicated by the previous record and progresses from there to the new prescription. The retinoscope can be used to make a preliminary reading. With patients unable to give subjective replies, the retinoscope is the key to refraction. Cycloplegic drops are used to place the eye in an unaccommodated rested state. The large pupil that results makes retinoscopy and ophthalmoscopy easier, but arrested accommodation is the main advantage of cycloplegia. Performing a refraction by retinoscopy in a young person without using cycloplegic drops has been likened to measuring a man for a suit of clothes while he is running down the street. The retinoscope casts a light through the pupil. The examiner moves the light back and forth and observes the direction of the light reflection from the retina (often called the shadow). One adds plus or minus lenses

depending on the character of the motion until a reversal occurs. This is the end point. The magnitude and axis of the cylindric correction may also be determined using this technique. Thus, even day-old infants may be refracted. Early refraction is vital in strabismus. Opacity of the media of course makes retinoscopy impossible. Most ophthalmologists agree that subjective refraction, if possible, is more precise than retinoscopy alone.

Contact Lenses

A major stimulus to development of contact lenses was the problem of keratoconus, discussed in Chapter 9. In this condition, the cornea bulges forward progressively and irregularly, making the aqueous fluid lens cone-shaped. This creates an irregular astigmatism and, usually, increasing myopia that cannot be fully corrected by ordinary sphere-cylinder corrections. Before contact lenses became available, the next step was corneal transplant. It has long been known that if the cornea could be covered by a more perfectly curved substance, vision could be corrected. Leonardo da Vinci used a large bowl filled with water in which the eye was immersed. This in 1508 theoretically corrected the distorted vision. Thomas Young in 1801 immersed his prominent eye in a tube of water and, by adding lenses to the end of the tube, obtained a sharp image. Adolph Eugen Fick, a Zurich physician, first used glass contact lenses to correct irregular astigmatism in 1887. The Carl Zeiss Company of Jena manufactured a wide selection of glass fluid-filled scleral contact lenses. These were difficult to wear for extended periods and caused corneal edema and much ocular discomfort. Great efforts were made to perfect the fluid, without much success. In 1948, Kevin Tuohy made plastic corneal lenses that rested on the cornea with no added fluid. His lenses used the tears to fill the spaces between the lens and the cornea. These lenses have been made smaller and thinner, with various bevels and rounding and finishing of the edges, but they are basically the same today. This type of lens was so successful that it gained wide use for cosmetic replacement of glasses as well as its first use as an optical aid for keratoconus. In aphakia, the contact lens gave a wider field than glasses and much less magnification of the image. This allowed most patients with monocular aphakia to fuse with the nonaphakic eye and achieve stereopsis—a major breakthrough in the treatment of aphakia.

A hard contact lens corrects refractive errors in 2 ways. The *first* way may be explained by considering a contact lens as a shell with no refracting power per se. Assume that the cornea shapes the aqueous lens to a radius of 7.5 mm. Placing a shell contact lens on this eye with a steeper curvature of radius of 7.34 mm will increase the power of the aqueous lens by about 1 diopter. The vault or void under the contact is filled with tears, and there is some molding of the cornea to partially fill the void. This effect will be much the same no matter what the index of refraction of the cornea, tears, or contact lens. These substances are like cement in a cemented lens and largely cancel out. This you may prove if you have become familiar with ray tracing. Clinical experience proves the same point. The effect also rids the cornea of any astigmatic errors. There is much confusion about tear lenses, water lenses, or whether the index of refraction of the plastic suddenly makes the first lens system much stronger. These are all false concepts. In any event, *the back curvature of this shell lens, called the base curve, makes the new curve of the aqueous lens.*

The *second* way in which plastic contact lenses correct refractive error is inherent in the **refractive power** that exists when the front curvature is different from the back curvature. The algebraic equations may be used for these calculations without causing too great an error, especially if the thick lens modification is used. The index of refraction of the plastic is important here. This equation will tell the lathe man the radius of the front curve (knowing the base curve) so that the so-called power of the contact will be known. The actual power may be called the **total power** and is the sum of this power (that may be measured by the lensometer) and the power of the base curve converted into diopters. (The base curve may be measured by the radiuscope.) Remember that by convention, 337.5 divided by the base curve in millimeters gives power in diopters and, conversely, divided by diopters gives the base curve in millimeters. Thus, a 44-diopter base curve lens with no added refractive power (a shell) produces the same clinical effect as a 40-diopter base curve lens with +4 diopters of refractive power. The sum is 44 for both lenses. A lens of 46-diopter base curve with −2.00 refractive power is another twin.

A reliable method of fitting contact lenses is to select a trial contact near the base curve desired with a refractive power near that estimated. Overrefraction is performed with spheres. *These 3 values are added*, ie, the base curve in diopters of the trial contact, the refractive power of the contact, and the power of the overrefraction, and called the **total required power**. The base curve of the lens to be ordered is then determined. The sum of this base curve in diopters and its refractive power in diopters should equal the above total required power found by the trial lens.

The selection of the base curve depends on the philosophy and training of the clinician. A significant clue is the keratometer reading of the corneal curve.

During overrefraction, one may determine the astigmatic correction along with the sphere used for the best power correction. This astigmatic correction represents the "residual astigmatism" (mostly in the lens of the eye). If a great deal of residual astigmatism is present, a clear image cannot be achieved with spherical contact lenses. Fewer than 10% of patients have this problem.

A contact lens should have the proper thickness, considering the front curve, the back curve, and the diameter, to ensure proper integrity of the center, the edge, and enough material on the edge to permit proper beveling and edging. These may all be programmed for the computer so that each lens can be designed to perfection. Those who boast about making "ultrathin lenses" apparently are not aware of the mathematics involved, for it takes little skill to make a lens too thin.

Soft Contact Lenses

Otto Wichterle of Czechoslovakia introduced a soft hydrophilic plastic and made the first soft contact lenses. Several companies make various types of soft lenses, and the field is in a state of flux. The lens has been declared a medical device and is therefore controlled by the Food and Drug Administration in the USA. Some of these lenses have a very high water content and can be worn for extended periods. They tend to follow the astigmatism of the cornea to some extent and are not as effective with high astigmatism.

Other plastic materials are being used and have virtues, the total value of which must still be determined. Cellulose acetate butyrate is like a hard lens with increased gas permeability. Silicone lenses have superior oxygen and carbon dioxide permeability.

Intraocular Lenses

The principle of replacing a removed cataractous lens with a clear prosthesis of similar refracting power in or near the original position has obvious appeal. Harold Ridley of England observed that RAF pilots during World War II did rather well with retained intraocular foreign bodies of plexiglass windshields (polymethylmethacrylate). About 1949, he began using PMMA intraocular lens prostheses placed in the former lens position, ie, the posterior chamber. Many patients developed corneal edema, some several years later. Some of the patients had a remaining refractive error that was rather alarming. Cornelius Binkhorst of the Netherlands has for over 20 years used various types of lenses of his own design. At present, the intraocular lens has wide popularity. There are many styles, all with their devotees. The method has not been without severe complications. The hope is always that "this modification will prevent the complications." The lenses have been placed in the anterior chamber, at the iris plane, and in the posterior chamber. They have been supported by the iris, the angle, the ciliary sulcus, and the capsular bag of cataract removed extracapsularly (the method that leaves the posterior capsule of the lens in the eye). Posts in the pupil (especially metal ones) caused some glare, and some iris-supported lenses may "jiggle," but most of the present lenses give an excellent optical result. The long-term safety of the lenses is still not fully known and is a worry to many ophthalmologists.

Many equations have been proposed in the effort to determine the proper power of an intraocular lens for a given eye length as determined by ultrasonographic measurements and a given corneal curvature as measured by keratometry. The calculated powers are significantly different depending upon which equation is used. Algebraic thin lens equations are not appropriate for these calculations and should not be used.

At present, the most popular method for determining intraocular lens power is the **regression method**, which involves accumulating experience with lenses of one style and then by "hindsight" determining which would have been the best linear (straight line) fit that would have given the best correction for all of the cases. A constant is then derived, and the keratometer readings and axial lengths are given weighted values. An example is the **SRK (Sanders-Retzlaff-Kraff) equation,**

$$\text{Power IOL} = A - 2.5\,L - 0.9\,K$$

where A is the constant determined for an intraocular lens of one particular type and brand name, L is the axial length in millimeters, and K is the keratometer reading in diopters. This procedure gives clinically satisfactory results in most cases. When the eye is not of "average" dimensions, the results are less good. The reason is obvious: A linear equation cannot reliably determine a value from a nonlinear function.

Ray tracing does accurately predict the power of intraocular lenses. The parameters of a representative intraocular lens—radius of curvature, thickness, and index of refraction, as provided by the manufacturer—are entered into the ray tracing equations in the computer, along with the dimensions of the patient's eye—the length of the eye, the anterior chamber depth, and the radius of the corneal curvature. The point of focus of this intraocular lens if placed in the patient's eye can now be determined. The error is then calculated, and by automatic iteration, other lenses of this style from this manufacturer can be substituted until the best choice for the power of the intraocular lens is arrived at. This rigorous method of determining the correct power of intraocular lenses for an individual patient was impractical before computers became available and impossible before the manufacturers of intraocular lenses published the data required to perform the computations.

REFERENCES

*Conrady AE: *Applied Optics and Optical Design*. Vol 1. Oxford Univ Press, 1929. Dover Publications, Inc, 1957. Vol 2. (Edited and completed by Kingslake R.) Dover Publications, Inc, 1960.

Duke-Elder S (editor): *System of Ophthalmology*. Vol 5. *Ophthalmic Optics and Refraction*. Mosby, 1970.

Eva PR, Pascoe PT, Vaughan DG: Refractive change in hyperglycaemia: Hyperopia, not myopia. *Br J Ophthalmol* 1982; **66**:500.

Gordon RA, Donzis PB: Refractive development of the human eye. *Arch Ophthalmol* 1985;**103**:785.

Hales RH: *Contact Lenses: A Clinical Approach to Fitting*, 2nd ed. Williams & Wilkins, 1983.

Helmholtz H: *Helmholtz' Treatise on Physiological Optics, 1910*. Optical Society of America, 1925. [English edition.]

*Kingslake R: *Lens Design Fundamentals*. Academic Press, 1978.

Meyer-Arendt JR: *Introduction to Classical and Modern Optics*, 2nd ed. Prentice-Hall, 1984.

Michaels DD: *Visual Optics and Refraction: A Clinical Approach*. Mosby, 1980.

Smith WJ: *Modern Optical Engineering*. McGraw-Hill, 1966.

White O: Spectacle addition and spectacle subtraction. *Trans Pac Coast Otoophthalmol Soc* 1980;**61**:7.

*Wyld J: The design of refractor objectives by ray tracing. In: *Amateur Telescope Making*. Ingalls AG (editor). Vol 3. Kingsport Press/Scientific American, 1974.

*Ray tracing references.

26 Preventive Ophthalmology

The decade of the 1980s might be called the decade of preventive medicine. General medicine and all of the specialties have participated in this movement, and ophthalmology has been no exception. Prevention of ocular injuries in industry, in the schools, and in the home has had a long and successful history, but much remains to be done in the fields of infection, genetic disorders, iatrogenic disease, and other special areas.

Much of the responsibility for prevention of nontraumatic ocular disease rests with the pediatrician, the general practitioner, and the internist, but the ophthalmologist has a major role as disseminator of necessary information. Meanwhile, the nonophthalmologist practitioner must be aware of the eye problems that can be treated before visual loss has occurred if detected at an early stage.

Important problems fitting into this category are glaucoma, strabismus, and the complications of such systemic diseases as diabetes, tuberculosis, sarcoidosis, syphilis, and leprosy. It is indeed a tragedy to find hitherto undetected advanced ocular disease in a patient who has been receiving regular medical treatment for another illness. It is hoped that this chapter will give medical students, pediatricians, and general physicians—as well as young ophthalmology residents-in-training—a survey of preventive ophthalmology and that it will alert them to the huge opportunities available to them in sight conservation.

PREVENTION OF THE SEVERE CONSEQUENCES OF UNDIAGNOSED GLAUCOMA

About 1–2% of all people over age 35 have glaucoma. In the USA alone it is estimated that there are at least 300,000 people with undetected glaucoma. About 90% of them have chronic open-angle glaucoma, which does not cause symptoms in the early stages but can ultimately lead to blindness. Patients often do not seek treatment until late in the disease, because there is no pain and the visual acuity (central vision) remains good even when the peripheral fields constrict.

The best way to detect glaucoma is to examine tonometrically all people over 20 every 3 years (or every year if there is a family history of glaucoma). The next most important diagnostic steps are the visual field examination and the ophthalmoscopic examination for pathologic cupping of the optic disk. The visual field examination is normally done on the tangent screen; confrontation field testing in which the examiner's fingers are used as a target will pick up only gross visual field defects.

Tonometry and ophthalmoscopy should be part of every physical examination in the age group over 20. Unfortunately, the overdiagnosis of glaucoma is also a problem. It is also unfortunate that once a patient has been placed on miotics or other antiglaucomatous drugs, it is very difficult to establish the diagnosis of "nondisease."

PREVENTION OF AMBLYOPIA ("Lazy Eye")

Amblyopia can be defined for the purposes of this discussion as diminished visual acuity in one eye in the absence of organic eye disease. Central vision develops from birth to age 6 or 7; if vision has not developed by then, there is little or no chance that it will develop later. In the absence of eye disease, the 2 main abnormalities that will prevent a child from acquiring binocular vision are strabismus and anisometropia.

Strabismus

Esotropia or exotropia in a young child causes double vision. The child quickly learns to suppress the image in the deviating eye and learns to see normally with one eye. Unfortunately, vision does not develop in the unused eye; unless the good eye is patched, thus forcing the child to use the deviating eye, sight will never develop in that eye. The child will grow up with one perfectly normal eye that is essentially blind, since it has never developed a functional connection with the visual centers of the brain. This is more likely to occur with esotropia than with exotropia.

Anisometropia

Young children are more concerned with perception of near objects than with those at a distance. If one eye is nearsighted (myopic) and the other farsighted (hyperopic), the child will favor the nearsighted eye. Thus, the farsighted eye will not be used even though it is straight. The result will be the same as in untreated strabismus, ie, monocular blindness due to failure of visual development in an unused eye. The incidence of anisometropia is about 0.75–1%.

Early Diagnosis

The best way to prevent amblyopia is to test the visual acuity of all preschool children. By the time a child reaches school, it is usually too late for occlusion therapy. The parents can perform the test at home with the illiterate "E" chart. This is sometimes known as the "Home Eye Test." Pediatricians and others responsible for the care of small children should test visual acuity no later than age 4.

PREVENTION OF OCULAR INFECTION

In view of its exposure to the environment, the intact eye is remarkably resistant to infection; but once the epithelium of the cornea is breached, microorganisms find susceptible tissues, and even such opportunistic pathogens as *Pseudomonas aeruginosa* may proliferate. Protection of the corneal epithelium thus becomes all-important in the prevention of ocular infection. There are a few bacteria, particularly *Neisseria gonorrhoeae* and *Neisseria meningitidis*, that can proliferate on an intact epithelium, and it is of historical interest that Credé silver nitrate prophylaxis, introduced in 1881, has been responsible for saving thousands of eyes from total visual loss. Even viral infection such as herpes simplex virus infection (a cause of much ocular disability) is in large part dependent on corneal epithelial damage. It is safe to say that the majority of ocular infections, whether bacterial, fungal, chlamydial, or viral in origin, are preventable.

Ophthalmia neonatorum, especially inclusion blennorrhea, is still a problem despite the worldwide use of silver nitrate and other antimicrobial agents at birth. But recent research suggests that the antibiotic erythromycin, instilled in the eye of the newborn, may be effective in controlling not only gonococcal infection but chlamydial infection (inclusion blennorrhea) as well. In view of the high prevalence of gonococcal genital infection in this country and elsewhere, prophylaxis cannot be abandoned, but many state laws concerned with it are currently undergoing revision.

Corneal infections in general, particularly hypopyon ulcer, are a major cause of visual loss. It is therefore of first importance to realize that they are in large part preventable. Once the epithelial barrier is breached, the cornea is subject to infection with many pathogens, especially the pneumococcus, and with many opportunistic bacteria and fungi, especially *P aeruginosa, Candida* species, and *Fusarium* species.

The prevention of damage to the corneal epithelium is indisputably the key to the prevention of corneal infection. Fortunately, although direct trauma often occurs, minor abrasions heal so rapidly that infection can only follow a massive inoculation of bacteria or fungi. Such massive inoculations can come from (1) contaminated solutions, (2) dacryocystitis, (3) severe staphylococcal blepharitis, (4) a contami-

nated contact lens, etc, and all of these can be prevented or treated satisfactorily as called for.

Contact lenses can be contaminated by their carrying cases and can themselves cause epithelial damage by abrasion or oxygen deprivation. All contact lens wearers should be cautioned to report for examination at the first sign of inflammation. Pain, a helpful warning sign, may be absent, since partial corneal anesthesia develops characteristically in contact lens wearers.

Accidental epithelial injury incurred while participating in various sports is also common, and severe epithelial damage may be caused by (1) exposure during coma; (2) ultraviolet light while welding or skiing; or (3) desiccation associated with exophthalmos, facial nerve paralysis, or ectropion of the lower lid, eg, after a severe burn. Many of these damaged eyes have been lost as a result of infection when simple methods of protection have been omitted.

Temporary protection pending definitive therapy can be achieved by patching, tarsorrhaphy, or frequent instillations of ointment or artificial tears; exceptionally, the brief applications of soft contact lenses can be effective.

Intraocular infection is a common sequela to **penetrating injuries** to the eye, particularly those involving a retained foreign body. Prevention of such injuries requires use of protective lenses on a regular basis, not only in industry but also in daily activities. Every individual should be encouraged to have a pair of protective lenses on hand for use around the house to prevent injuries caused by corks from champagne and other bottles, fireworks, power mowers, power drills and other machines, and hazardous chemicals such as those used for opening drains or fertilizing crops (eg, liquids containing ammonia).

Prevention of intraocular infection after **cataract extraction** or other intraocular surgery deserves much attention, since such infections are almost always avoidable. They should in fact never occur in a modern hospital, where committees on infections have the responsibility for preventing them. Fortunately, eye surgery requires such a brief stay in the hospital that colonization of an eye with so-called hospital bacteria is rare indeed.

Most intraocular infections come from (1) contaminated solutions; (2) chronic conjunctival or lid margin infections or chronic dacryocystitis; (3) rarely, aerosols from the noses and throats of surgeons and their assistants; and (4) prolonged surgery, vitreous loss, or ocular implants. All of these complications can be prevented or minimized. At the time of surgery, the susceptible tissues are exposed for only a short time, and the surgical wound seals rapidly. The eye's local defense mechanisms seem to be able to handle small numbers of microorganisms without difficulty unless compromised by topical corticosteroids or other immunosuppressive drugs.

Since most intraocular surgery is elective, the surgeon has time to assess the patient's immunologic status and to correct any immunodepression due to malnutrition, alcoholism, narcotic addiction, stress, etc. There is also time to make sure that the external eye is not compromised by blepharoconjunctivitis, overt or intermittent dacryocystitis and stenosis, or tear deficiency. Most of these conditions are correctable—or can at least be ameliorated—before surgery.

The bacterial flora of the lids and conjunctiva should be assessed prior to elective intraocular surgery, although not necessarily by means of preoperative cultures. If clinical examination shows normal lid margins and conjunctivas and if there is no history of exudate or gumming of the lids on waking, further examination is unnecessary. But if the external eye is *not* normal, the bacterial flora should be studied for potential pathogens, particularly gram-negative opportunistic pathogens such as *P aeruginosa* and *Proteus* species.

Elimination of such potential pathogens by suitable treatment is mandatory. Antibiotics or antibiotic mixtures used preoperatively cannot be relied upon, and the prolonged use of such agents before surgery tends to inhibit the growth of the normally harmless gram-positive flora. This unfortunately encourages the colonization of both gram-negative bacteria and fungi. There is no substitute for a careful preoperative clinical examination combined with a careful history of previous infection, particularly of intermittent dacryocystitis during the common cold.

If emergency intraocular surgery must be performed in the presence of external eye disease, careful irrigation of the conjunctiva to remove exudate and bacteria-containing mucous threads is indicated. If there is dacryocystitis to deal with, the puncta can be temporarily sealed by cautery.

PREVENTION OF IATROGENIC OCULAR INFECTION

Ophthalmologists have been clearly implicated in the transmission of infectious eye disease. Outbreaks of **epidemic keratoconjunctivitis** have been traced to contamination in the ophthalmologist's office. The adenovirus is transmitted via the ophthalmologist's hands, a tonometer, or solutions contaminated by droppers accidentally rubbed against the infected conjunctiva or lid margin of a patient. Contaminated ophthalmic solutions have also been the source of infection in bacterial corneal ulcers and endophthalmitis following intraocular surgery. *Pseudomonas aeruginosa* used to be a common contaminant of ophthalmic solutions, particularly fluorescein. Instillation of contaminated fluorescein solution to delineate corneal epithelial defects (eg, after removal of a corneal foreign body) may result in severe pseudomonal keratitis and, frequently, loss of the eye.

Other infections can be similarly spread, but their occurrence is not generally recognized. The ophthalmologist should be alert to the possibility that if ophthalmic instruments are improperly sterilized (as by cold sterilization), they may be contaminated with hepatitis B virus. Recent identification of the AIDS virus in tears has suggested a small possibility of transmission by ophthalmologists (see p 287). To date, no such incident has occurred.

Ophthalmologists and their staffs must maintain the highest level of personal hygiene at all times and must use standard sterile technique when appropriate, keeping in mind the possibility of contamination of any solution brought into contact with the eye.

Hands play a major role in the transmission of infection. They should be washed or disinfected (eg, with isopropyl alcohol) before and after the examination of every patient, regardless of whether an ocular infection is thought to be present. Applanation tonometer heads should be wiped clean with a sterile solution after each use and should be thoroughly disinfected at least twice a day and after use on an infected eye. Schiotz tonometers require frequent disinfection because they may harbor organisms within the barrel of the plunger.

Intraocular procedures and injuries to the eye interfere with many of the natural barriers to infection, rendering the eye particularly susceptible. Any surgical ophthalmic procedure or treatment of an injured eye must be performed with strict sterile technique.

Use of contaminated eye solutions should be avoided at all costs. Sterility of solutions is the responsibility of physicians, pharmacists, and pharmaceutical companies, as well as of nurses and even patients.

Single-use disposable vials containing sterile ophthalmic solutions are an absolute requirement in ophthalmic surgery and in treating an injured eye; all operating and emergency rooms should be equipped accordingly. Single-use vials are also the preferred means of administering topical agents to patients in the ophthalmologist's office. The use of multiple-dose containers should be limited to the intact eye. These containers should never be used for other patients after use on an infected eye. The sterility of any ophthalmic solution should be confirmed prior to use. At the time of surgery, the type of solution, its correct formulation, and its sterility should be verified by the surgeon and at least one other person. A useful safeguard is to filter all solutions to be used in intraocular surgery through a membrane (Millipore-type) filter.

PREVENTION OF RADIATION INJURY

Ultraviolet irradiation may cause superficial epithelial keratitis accompanied by pain, redness, and photophobia. The symptoms appear 6–12 hours after exposure to ultraviolet light, eg, while skiing or using an electric welding device. Prevention consists of avoidance of exposure or the wearing of appropriate protective sunglasses or goggles.

Solar retinitis (eclipse retinopathy) is a specific type of radiation injury that usually occurs after solar eclipses as a result of direct observation of the sun without an adequate filter. Under normal circumstances, sun-gazing is difficult because of the glare, but cases have been reported in young people who have suffered self-inflicted macular damage by deliberate sun-gazing, perhaps while under the influence of drugs.

The optical system of the eye behaves as a strong magnifying lens, focusing the light onto a small spot on the macula, usually in one eye only, and producing a thermal burn. The resulting edema of the retinal tissue may clear with minimal loss of function, or it may cause significant atrophy of the tissue and produce a defect that is visible ophthalmoscopically as a macular hole. In the latter event, a permanent central scotoma results.

Eclipse retinopathy can easily be prevented by the use of adequate filters when observing eclipses, but the surest way to prevent it is to watch the eclipse on television.

Workers with improperly screened nuclear materials face an increasingly important problem because of the frequent formation of cataracts.

Pterygium is an occupational disease of farmers, sheepherders, and others who live largely outdoors. It is presumably due to exposure (ultraviolet light, desiccation by wind, etc) and can be prevented by wearing protective lenses. This applies also to **basal cell carcinoma** and probably also to **melanoma** of the lids and lid margins. In patients with xeroderma pigmentosum, the eyelids and bulbar conjunctiva frequently develop carcinomas and melanomas, and their development can be minimized, if not prevented entirely, by protective lenses.

PREVENTION OF EXPOSURE KERATITIS

Patients in coma or under prolonged anesthesia who have lid retraction (eg, exophthalmos) or facial nerve paralysis may develop exposure keratitis. This condition can be prevented by patching the eyes, suturing the lids together (tarsorrhaphy), instilling artificial tears, or applying a soft contact lens.

PREVENTION OF XEROPHTHALMIA

Even in the USA, where it should now be all but unknown, occasional cases of xerophthalmia still occur, and in the underdeveloped areas the world over, where nutrition is often poor, it is still common. Vitamin A deficiency disease, in which the eye changes (xerophthalmia and keratomalacia) are the most damaging and often cause blindness (see Chapter 27), is usually the result of a deficient diet associated with poverty. It should be borne in mind, however, that it may also be associated with chronic alcoholism, weight-reducing diets, dietary management of food allergy, or poor absorption from the gastrointestinal tract due to the use of mineral oil or gastrointestinal disease such as chronic diarrhea.

In vitamin A–deficient children, measles may result in severe corneal disease. Because of the eye signs (ie, night blindness, Bitot's spots, or a lackluster corneal epithelium), the ophthalmologist may be the first to recognize vitamin A deficiency. Early recognition and treatment can prevent loss of vision or blindness due to secondary infection and corneal perforation. Treatment of the acute condition may require large intramuscular doses of vitamin A followed by corrective diet and careful analysis of all possible causes.

PREVENTION OF VISUAL LOSS DUE TO DRUGS

All drugs can cause adverse reactions. It is the ophthalmologist's responsibility to prevent visual loss or major ocular disability from drugs used to treat eye diseases.

Ophthalmic drugs should be packaged and labeled so that mistakes are not made by elderly or poorly sighted patients. Atropine and other strong medications may call for color-labeling. On the first visit to a new ophthalmologist, the patient should be asked to bring along any previously prescribed medications in order to avoid duplication and possible overdosage.

Certain ophthalmic drugs have such frequently occurring and damaging side effects that their use requires special monitoring and special warnings to the patient. Atropine and scopolamine, used to dilate the pupil in iridocyclitis, may precipitate acute glaucoma in certain patients with narrow anterior chamber angles. After prolonged use, they can also lead to conjunctivitis and allergic eczema of the eyelids. Many antiglaucoma drugs can produce stenosis of the puncta and shrinkage of the conjunctiva.

Corticosteroids used locally in drop or ointment forms may depress the local defense mechanisms and precipitate corneal ulceration, often fungal. They may also worsen herpetic keratitis and other corneal infections, and on prolonged use may lead to open-angle glaucoma and to posterior polar cataract. Much of the severity of both herpes simplex virus and varicella-zoster virus corneal infections can be blamed on the unwise use of topical corticosteroids. In this situation, short-term improvement has been traded for long-term disaster. Fungal endophthalmitis after cataract surgery is usually the result of the unnecessary use of corticosteroids at the time of the operation and is therefore preventable.

Many drugs used **systemically** have serious ocular side effects, eg, keratopathy, retrobulbar neuritis, retinopathy, and Stevens-Johnson syndrome (erythema multiforme). For this reason, the ophthalmologist must take a careful history of the patient's use of drugs as part of the initial examination. Of special interest are the keratopathy and retinopathy that often follow the use of chloroquine in discoid lupus erythematosus. It is the function of the consulting ophthalmologist to detect any early ocular changes and to inform the dermatologist of them so that he can substitute another medication.

PREVENTION OF METABOLIC & GENETIC DISEASES

Until recently, the prevention of metabolic and genetic disorders received little attention. Now, however, there are genetic counseling centers in many medical centers, and the genetic nature of the transmissibility of many genetic and metabolic traits that affect the eye is recognized and their transmission better understood than formerly. In conference with internists and pediatricians, it is up to the ophthalmologist to recommend genetic counseling for patients contemplating marriage and children. Patients with histories of childhood diabetes, retinitis pigmentosa, consanguineous mating, hemophilia, etc, need genetic counseling to prevent disaster for their offspring.

Some clinical conditions, eg, Down's syndrome (trisomy 21), are associated with an abnormal number of chromosomes or with abnormalities of the sex chromosomes. Prenatal diagnosis can now be made by testing amniotic fluid cells obtained by amniocentesis (a safe and practical procedure), and a positive diagnosis gives the patient the option of abortion.

Viral disease of the mother with resultant embryopathy may lead to such ocular anomalies in the offspring as retinopathy, infantile glaucoma, cataract, uveal tract coloboma, etc, and prevention may in some cases be possible. Two viruses, rubella and cytomegalovirus, can be extremely damaging to the infant, and one of them—rubella virus—can be prevented by vaccinations. Once a common childhood disease, rubella led to lifelong immunity, but vaccination is now indicated for susceptible young women approaching childbearing age. Susceptibility can be determined by assessing the antibody content of the young woman's blood. If a mother contracts rubella during early pregnancy, she should be informed of the likelihood of ocular and other abnormalities in her baby, and the arguments for and against abortion should be presented.

Unfortunately, cytomegalovirus (the other virus causing a high incidence of congenital anomalies) continues to be a serious and unsolved threat. No protective vaccine is currently available, though one is currently under study.

PREVENTION OF HERPES SIMPLEX & HERPES ZOSTER

Some progress has been made in the prevention of herpetic disease. The epidemiology of herpes simplex virus type 1 is such that protection of highly susceptible young children (under 5 years of age) from salivary exposure to relatives with labial herpes could conceivably prevent many cases of primary infection, labial or ocular. As for the recurrent disease, many cases can be prevented by modifying the trigger mechanisms—stress, fever, overexposure to sunlight, trauma, etc. Fever, the most frequent trigger, can be reduced by aspirin used at the onset of coryza or other upper respiratory infection, and stress can be minimized by office psychotherapy and, if necessary, by a tranquilizer. The patient with recurrent ocular herpes can be taught to recognize his own trigger mechanisms and to modify them.

Primary infection of the newborn with herpesvirus type 2 can be prevented only by a change in the sexual mores of the population and by the cesarean delivery of mothers with vaginal or cervical herpetic infection.

Zoster ophthalmicus can be prevented by any means effective in preventing childhood varicella. There is as yet no effective vaccine, but varicella-zoster (VZ) immune globulin is available for immunosuppressed children (eg, with leukemia) who have been exposed to VZ virus. Recurrent infection (zoster) is known to have occurred only in patients immunosuppressed by Hodgkin's disease and other tumors, surgical shock, immunosuppressive drugs (eg, corticosteroids), extreme fatigue, advanced age, etc. Some of these trigger mechanisms, such as stress, may be preventable. Ways of measuring and reducing the immunosuppression of old age—the principal trigger for ophthalmic zoster—are currently under study.

Blindness

In this chapter we shall discuss blindness as a worldwide health problem, with emphasis on avoidable forms of this dread human affliction. The World Health Organization defines visual impairment as shown in Table 27–1. WHO officials encourage investigators and reporting agencies in all countries to report blindness and near blindness according to the categories defined in this table. WHO estimates that there are 28 million blind people in the world today. This figure rises to about 42 million if the criterion is extended to visual acuity of 6/60 or worse.

In the USA, the most widely used definition of partial blindness is that used by the Internal Revenue Service for the purpose of determining who is eligible for tax deductions on that basis: *Central visual acuity of 6/60 (20/200) or less in the better eye with best correction, or widest diameter of visual field subtending an angle of no greater than 20 degrees.* An alternative functional definition favored by the authors is *loss of vision sufficient to prevent one from being self-supporting in an occupation, making the individual dependent on other persons, agencies, or devices in order to live.*

Table 27–1. Categories of visual impairment. (Adapted from the International Classification of Diseases, World Health Organization, 1977.)

Category of Visual Impairment		Visual Acuity (Best Corrected)
Low vision	1	6/18 3/10 (0.3) 20/70
	2	6/60 1/10 (0.1) 20/200
Blindness	3	3/60 (finger counting at 3 m) 1/20 (0.05) 20/400
	4	1/60 (finger counting at 1 m) 1/50 (0.02) 5/300
	5	No light perception

Visual Field

Patients with a visual field radius no greater than 10 degrees but greater than 5 degrees around central fixation should be placed in category 3 and patients with a field no greater than 5 degrees around central fixation in category 4—even if the central acuity is not impaired.

"Industrial blindness" is said to be present when a worker can no longer pursue an occupation because of poor vision; "automobile blindness" when vision is so poor that the responsible licensing agency in that state will not issue a driver's license. The term color blindness is a misnomer since this genetically transmitted disorder is not blindness as that term is generally understood and is only a minor handicap to a few people. Loss of vision may affect only the central fields, only the peripheral fields, or only specific portions of the peripheral fields in one or both eyes. Total loss of vision in one eye is said to reduce visual capacity by only 10%, though it makes the other eye infinitely more valuable.

All of the disorders that may cause blindness are discussed more fully in other parts of this book. This chapter is an attempt to summarize some pertinent information about the epidemiology of blindness as a worldwide health problem with emphasis on those categories of blindness that are preventable by the combined efforts of physicians and health agencies.

PREVALENCE OF BLINDNESS THROUGHOUT THE WORLD

Table 27–2 lists some countries where fairly reliable data are available about the prevalence of blindness. Even where health statistics are most reliable, the methods of counting the blind are often crude and may be applied according to different criteria in different places and at different times within any extensive geographic area. Furthermore, extrapolations are often made from small sample studies to large populations.

The kind of effort it would take to make a substantial reduction in the prevalence of blindness is almost too vast to contemplate. The same was true years ago when the public health profession set out to eradicate smallpox as one of the scourges of humanity. Smallpox formerly caused much blindness, but it is most unlikely that anyone will ever again be blinded, disfigured, or killed by what was an almost universal public health concern only a few decades ago. Fortunately, it is not necessary in the health professions that success be unqualified and total to earn the label of "success." Eliminating one cause of blindness would be a magnificent victory even if the other causes were unaffected. It is precisely because the numbers are so great that partial success in the effort to treat and prevent blindness must be sought by all available means. WHO estimates that 75% of cases of blindness in developing countries are avoidable.

CAUSES OF BLINDNESS

The leading causes of preventable blindness in the world are trachoma, leprosy, onchocerciasis, and xerophthalmia. Between 6 and 9 million people are blind from trachoma, at least 1 million from leprosy, and 1 million from onchocerciasis. Xerophthalmia is estimated to affect 5 million children each year; 500,000 develop active corneal involvement, and half of these go blind. Although curable, cataract is still responsible for an estimated 17 million cases of blindness worldwide. Glaucoma, retinal detachment, and diabetic retinopathy have not been separately identified in WHO's statistical compilations, but many ophthalmologists believe that each of these disorders would rank ahead of onchocerciasis and xerophthalmia as a cause of blindness. Since some form of treatment is available for all 3 disorders, there is no reason why they should not be included among the avoidable causes of blindness.

Table 27–3 lists areas of the eye afflicted by major blinding diseases.

Trachoma

Trachoma is an infectious disease caused by *Chlamydia trachomatis*. It causes bilateral keratoconjunctivitis that leads to corneal scarring, which, when severe, causes blindness. About 500 million people have trachoma, most of them in Africa, the Middle East, and Asia. It can be prevented by adequate diet, proper sanitary facilities, and education and can be cured by sulfonamides or tetracycline drugs.

Leprosy

Leprosy (Hansen's disease) affects 15– 16 million people in the world and has a higher percentage of ocular involvement than any other systemic disease. The type and frequency of ocular involvement differ in different parts of the world, and surveys of leprosy hospitals reveal that 6– 90% of patients have ocular involvement. Many investigators feel that all leprosy patients will have ocular manifestations if the disease persists long enough. Reports on the prevalence of blindness among such patients indicate that up to 10% of leprosy patients may be blind from the disease, which means that over 1 million people are blind from leprosy worldwide. Such figures would place leprosy as the second leading cause of blindness resulting from an infectious disease and therefore a greater visual threat than onchocerciasis.

Onchocerciasis

Onchocerciasis (due to *Onchocerca volvulus*, a roundworm) is transmitted by bites of the blackfly *Simulium damnosum* in Africa and other species of *Simulium* in Central and South America. The larvae of the blackfly develop in clear running streams (hence the name river blindness). The adult female harbors the larvae of *O volvulus* and transmits the infection between humans by biting. The parasite larvae develop into mature worms in subcutaneous nodules, and the female produces large numbers of microfilariae, which invade other tissues, including the eye. The major blinding lesion in onchocerchiasis is sclerosing keratitis.

Onchocerciasis is endemic in the greater part of tropical Africa and Central and South America. The most heavily infested zone is the Volta River basin, which extends over parts of Dahomey, Ghana, Ivory Coast, Mali, Niger, Togo, and Upper Volta. Drug treatment (diethylcarbamazine [Hetrazan*]) is not very effective and may result in a harmful hypersensitivity reaction to the killed parasites. The best hope for control of the disease is insect eradication and personal protection by screening.

*Available in the USA only from Lederle Laboratories.

Table 27–2. Approximate prevalence of blindness (%). (Estimates based on WHO surveys.)*

Chad	3.2–5	Malawi	1
Liberia	3.2	Brazil	0.3
Egypt	2.6	Mexico	0.3
Phillipines	2.1	Australia	0.2
Afghanistan	2	Japan	0.2
Bangladesh	2	USA	0.2
Pakistan	2	UK	0.18
Saudi Arabia	2	Canada	0.15
India	1.5	USSR	0.12
Indonesia	1.3	China	0.1
Chile	1	Germany	0.1

*Based on available data, 1969–1980. Some data were only rough estimates when obtained and may have changed markedly since then. In some cases, the survey criteria used did not correspond to WHO definitions. Data taken from Maitchouk IF: Data on blindness: Prevalence and causes throughout the world. In: Lim ASM, Jones BR (editors): World's major blinding conditions. *Vision* 1982;1:99. (International Agency for the Prevention of Blindness.)

Table 27–3. Areas of eye afflicted by major blinding diseases.

Anterior segment diseases
Trachoma
Leprosy
Onchocerciasis
Xerophthalmia
Cataract
Herpes simplex keratitis
Posterior segment diseases
Glaucoma
Retinal degeneration
Retinal detachment
Diabetic retinopathy

Note: In general, the anterior segment diseases are more preventable than the posterior segment diseases.

Xerophthalmia

Xerophthalmia is due to hypovitaminosis A. Clinically, there is xerosis of the conjunctiva with characteristic Bitot's spots and softening of the cornea (keratomalacia), which may lead to corneal perforation. Protein malnutrition exacerbates the condition and renders it refractory to treatment. Xerophthalmia is a common cause of blindness in infants, particularly in India, Bangladesh, Indonesia, and the Philippines. Affected infants often do not reach adulthood, dying from malnutrition, pneumonia, or diarrhea.

Xerophthalmia can be prevented by general dietary improvement or vitamin A supplementation. If the problems of distribution and administration were solved, the cost of a quantity of the vitamin sufficient to prevent blindness in 1000 infants would be only about $25.

Cataract

Cataract accounts for 40–80% of cases of blindness in developing countries. As life expectancy increases, there is a continuing rise in the total number of people affected. It is not known why the frequency of cataract in different geographic areas varies so much. Mobile eye camps have aided in management, but there are too few to control the disorder. Many more cataract surgeons are needed in countries such as India and Pakistan.

In most Western countries, the relative prevalence of cataract is low; there is an oversupply of cataract surgeons; and patients at all economic levels have easy access to surgery, which has a 90–95% success rate. Many ophthalmologists, especially in the USA, do not consider cataract to be a cause of blindness in their countries.

Other Causes

Glaucoma, retinal detachment, and diabetic retinopathy are discussed in greater detail elsewhere in this text. The incidence of blindness due to glaucoma has decreased in recent years as a result of earlier detection, improved medical and surgical treatment, and a greater awareness and understanding of the disorder by the lay population.

Diabetic retinopathy is an increasingly more common cause of blindness everywhere in the world. Recent advances in surgical treatment (vitrectomy, laser therapy) are of some help, but many patients still suffer from progressive retinal hemorrhages, proliferative retinopathy, and eventual bilateral blindness. A vast research effort directed at all aspects of diabetes is in progress, and there is justification for hoping that the next generation of diabetics will benefit greatly from what is being done now.

Hereditary conditions are important causes of blindness but should gradually decrease in incidence in response to the efforts of genetic counselors to increase public awareness of the preventable nature of these disorders.

As is true also in other countries where medical care and social services are widely available, blindness in the USA is to a great extent related to the aging process, and about half of the legally blind people in this country are over age 65. The leading causes of blindness in this age group are degenerative retinal disorders, glaucoma, diabetes, and vascular diseases.

Amblyopia ("lazy eye") is decreased visual acuity in one eye in the absence of any organic eye disease responsible for the visual impairment. The function of vision develops from birth to age 7. If vision has not developed (because of disuse of the eye) by age 7, there is no chance that it will develop later.

PREVENTION OF BLINDNESS

It should be obvious from the foregoing discussion of the prevalence and causes of blindness that the solution to the problem of blindness lies in prevention rather than treatment. Little has been done where much could be done, particularly in the developing countries, and there, most especially, in children. If a choice must be made, it would be a simple one between (a) spending millions on organ transplant research to keep a few people alive a few years longer and (b) using that money to solve some of the truly desperate problems of the earth's people. In some cases simple remedies are available and are not being used.

Some examples of what can be achieved for modest outlays of scarce funds are as follows:

(1) To cure one person of trachoma in Saudi Arabia: $1.25.

(2) To restore vision to one person in Pakistan blinded by cataracts: $25.

(3) To prevent blindness due to xerophthalmia in one infant in Java: 27 cents.

Recently, on the advice of WHO experts, the World Council for the Welfare of the Blind and several international professional ophthalmic societies and agencies agreed to take the initiative, which led to the establishment in 1974 of the International Agency for Prevention of Blindness (Vision International), with Sir John Wilson, a blind barrister, as president. The aim of this agency is to work with groups formed for the purpose of preventing blindness. Its theme, Foresight Prevents Blindness, was brought into prominent display when WHO celebrated the first World Health Day on April 7, 1976. Its goal was stated as follows: "In every donor country during 1976, every family should be asked—in thanksgiving for sight—to give $10 to save the sight of its fellow countrymen or of the millions in the third world. If we can raise this campaign to that degree of universal appeal, the result could be spectacular."

REHABILITATION OF THE BLIND

Technologic developments in recent years have created new opportunities for richer and more productive lives for blind people. In assessing these advances it is necessary to be aware of the blind population one is dealing with. Different categories of the blind have different needs, and some blind people simply cannot benefit from some of the more glamorous technical achievements. It has been said that over half of the blind people in the USA are over age 65. The elderly widowed housewife may need or want no more than mobility training in home care and a steady supply of Talking Books. A young person facing blindness in later life due to retinitis pigmentosa requires the full range of social services, including educational assessment, job rehabilitation, and psychologic counseling. The physician's role is to know what referral sources are available and how to use them skillfully. This means personally investigating the quality of services offered. Medical social workers, public health nurses, and counseling services and agencies serving the blind and visually handicapped are common sources of reliable information.

Low Vision Aid Clinics

Persons characterized as visually handicapped or partially sighted probably exceed in numbers those defined as legally blind by at least 3:1. Because these people have the potential for improved vision, low vision clinics have been established in many large medical centers and in special centers for the blind and visually handicapped. These clinics offer better refraction techniques and a wider range of optical aids, particularly for improved near vision, than would be available in the office of the practicing ophthalmologist. It should always be assumed that refraction will benefit such patients until proved otherwise.

A number of eye problems require nothing more than simple magnification, either by using aids such as large-print books, periodicals, or newspapers or by using lenses. A hand magnifier for use when needed may be the best and most practical optical aid for many people. This is especially true of central field losses and macular lesions and disorders characterized by dimness of vision. Magnification is less useful for extensive peripheral field losses. Fresnel prisms or mirrors may be helpful in hemianopias. Patients with constricted visual fields often do not benefit from optical aids and may have to rely on nonvisual aids.

Patients rarely accept telescopic eyewear for long periods. Spectacle magnifiers for near vision up to +10 diopter sphere for both eyes and +40 diopter sphere for one eye are fairly well accepted.

The importance of adequate illumination should not be underestimated, since older patients even with vision normal for age need at least twice as much light for reading as younger persons. Pupillary dilation may be useful when light transmission through the eye is reduced. Excessive light, particularly glare, may present problems.

Braille

This remarkably effective system of reading for the blind was introduced in 1825. The Braille characters consist of raised dots arranged in 2 columns of three. The system is so simple that a blind child can quickly learn to read Braille, and proficient readers can learn to read Braille as fast as they can talk. The system has been adapted to musical notation and technical and scientific uses also. An international Braille code was introduced in 1951.

Braille is used less commonly now than formerly, since many blind people prefer auditory aids both for informational and recreational purposes. For the partially sighted, large-print editions may be easier to use and are more readily available. Braille continues to be essential on tags attached to items in common personal use even for people who do not wish to use it for reading.

All paper money in the Netherlands and Switzerland is Braille-printed to show the denomination.

Mobility Training

Many state commissions for the blind offer a wide variety of mobility training courses, either directly or in cooperation with private agencies. The courses are offered on an outpatient and residential basis and have varied objectives according to the special needs of the people who apply for help. The curriculum commonly includes self-care, home functions, and mobility within the community.

Guide Dogs

The popular concept of the guide dog is somewhat unrealistic and no doubt colored by the natural affection most people have for these handsome animals. The guide dog is not trained to think and thus help its master function better in a strange and hostile world; its major function is to obey commands, and its usefulness is therefore directly related to the competence of its master. It may be said that a cane is not much of a companion, but neither does it have to be fed or housed or taken to the veterinarian when it gets sick. Older patients have trouble with the dogs because considerable physical strength is required to hold them in check. Guide dogs are most useful for students and professional men and women in good health who lead fairly well organized lives. At this time less than 2% of blind people in the USA use guide dogs. Sonar sensor canes may ultimately be a better answer to the mobility problem even for those who are now using a dog successfully.

Electronic Devices

Optacon is an electronic device that converts visual images of letters into tactile forms. It is easily portable and can be used with almost any kind of reading matter. Auditory aids are becoming increasingly important (eg, talking calculators, clocks, paper money identifiers). There are a variety of optical enlargers, some of them based upon closed television circuitry. The Apollo electronic visual aid includes a camera with zoom lens, scanning table, and illuminator. Many of these systems are gradually becoming cheaper, but at current prices (about $1500) they are beyond the means of all but a few who could use them.

FINANCIAL ASSISTANCE PROGRAMS

It is unfortunate that over half of the blind people in the USA are essentially dependent upon Social Security and whatever local supplemental aid may be available to them. For the younger blind population, rehabilitation programs are commonly administered at the state level by a division of the department of education specifically set up to serve blind people in the state. Some of these programs are better than others, and all physicians should support efforts to increase the effectiveness of such programs in their geographic area of influence. The programs are of wide scope and offer preliminary counseling followed by academic or vocational training as the circumstances warrant. Once a realistic vocational objective has been established, full financial support is commonly available. This single resource is probably the most crucial referral available to the ophthalmologist, particularly in the case of young patients. Counseling services are available as early as the junior high school years to assure compliance with a curriculum consistent with measured aptitudes and interests. In many states, such rehabilitation programs as mobility training are administered under state auspices but contracted to private agencies for operational purposes.

In many countries of the world, the blind receive no financial or other support from their governments and are either cared for by their families or left to manage by themselves in any way they can.

REFERENCES

General

Baghdassarian SA, Tabbara KF: Childhood blindness in Lebanon. *Am J Ophthalmol* 1975;**79**:827.

Belfort R Jr, Moraes MAP: Oncocercose ocular no Brasil. *Rev Assoc Med Brasil* 1979;**25**:123.

Brand M: The care of the eye. In: *The Star.* National Hansen's Disease Center, 1980.

Choyce DP: Blindness in leprosy. *Trop Doct* (Jan) 1973;**3**:16.

Dawson CR, Jones BR, Tarizzo ML: *Guide to Trachoma Control in Programmes for the Prevention of Blindness.* World Health Organization, 1981.

Faye EE (editor): *Clinical Low Vision,* 2nd ed. Little, Brown, 1984.

Ffytche TJ: Role of iris changes as a cause of blindness in lepromatous leprosy. *Br J Ophthalmol* 1981;**65**:231.

Ghafour IM, Allan D, Foulds WS: Common causes of blindness and visual handicap in the west of Scotland. *Br J Ophthalmol* 1983;**67**:209.

Hobbs HE, Choyce DP: The blinding lesions of leprosy. *Lepr Rev* 1971;**42**:131.

Jones BR: General obstacles to the prevention of blindness. *Trans Ophthalmol Soc UK* 1978;**98**:316.

Jones BR: The prevention of blindness from trachoma. *Trans Ophthalmol Soc UK* 1975;**95**:16.

Law FW: World Health Day: 7 April 1976. *Br J Ophthalmol* 1976;**60**:231.

Lim ASM, Jones BR (editors): World's major blinding conditions. *Vision* 1982;**1**:1. [Entire issue.]

MacKay DM: The psychology of seeing. *Trans Ophthalmol Soc UK* 1973;**93**:391.

Marron JA, Bailey IL: Visual factors and orientation-mobility performance. *Am J Optom Physiol Opt* 1982;**59**:413.

Nizetić B: Prevention of "blindness": Potentialities of a systems analysis approach. *Acta Ophthalmol (Copenh)* 1974;**52**:134.

Onchocerciasis. (Editorial.) *Br J Ophthalmol* 1976;**60**:1.

Pirie A: Vitamin A deficiency and child blindness in the developing world. *Proc Nutr Soc* 1983;**42**:53.

The Prevention of Blindness: Report of a WHO Study Group. World Health Organization Technical Report Series 518, 1973. [Entire issue.]

Roper-Hall MJ: Prevention of blindness from trauma. *Trans Ophthalmol Soc UK* 1978;**98**(Part 2):313.

Roy FH: World blindness: Definition, incidence and major treatable causes. *Ann Ophthalmol* 1974;**6**:1049.

Sloan LL, Habel A, Feiock K: High illumination as an auxiliary reading aid in diseases of the macula. *Am J Ophthalmol* 1973;**76**:745.

Sommer A: *Nutritional Blindness: Xerophthalmia and Keratomalacia.* Oxford Univ Press, 1982.

Sommer A et al: Xerophthalmia and anterior segment blindness among preschool-age children in El Salvador. *Am J Ophthalmol* 1976;**80**:1066.

Stetten D Jr: Coping with blindness. *N Engl J Med* 1981;**305**:458.

Strategies for the Prevention of Blindness in National Programmes: A Primary Health Care Approach. World Health Organization, 1984.

Tabbara KF, Badr IA: Changing pattern of childhood blindness in Saudi Arabia. *Br J Ophthalmol* 1985;**69**:312.

Additional References & Sources

Division for the Blind and Physically Handicapped, Library of Congress.

Recording for the Blind, New York.

World Health Magazine (Jan) 1983.

28   Commonly Used Eye Medications

Philip P. Ellis, MD

The following is intended to serve as a brief formulary of commonly used ophthalmic drugs. Standard pharmacology and physiology texts should be consulted for more detailed information.

TOPICAL ANESTHETICS

Topical anesthetics are useful for several diagnostic and therapeutic procedures, including tonometry, removal of foreign bodies or sutures, gonioscopy, conjunctival scraping, and minor surgical operations on the cornea and conjunctiva. One or 2 instillations are usually sufficient, but the dosage may be repeated during the procedure.

Tetracaine, proparacaine, and benoxinate are the most commonly used topical anesthetics. For practical purposes, they can be said to have equivalent anesthetic potency.

Other available topical anesthetic solutions include piperocaine (Metycaine), 2%, and cocaine, 1–4%.

Tetracaine Hydrochloride (Pontocaine)
Preparations: Solution, 0.5–1%.
Dosage: 1 drop and repeat as necessary.
Onset and duration of action: Anesthesia occurs within 1 minute and lasts for 15–20 minutes.
Comment: Stings considerably on instillation.

Proparacaine Hydrochloride (Ak-Taine, Alcaine, Ophthaine, Ophthetic)
Preparation: Solution, 0.5%.
Dosage: 1 drop and repeat as necessary.
Onset and duration of action: Anesthesia begins within 20 seconds and lasts 10–15 minutes.
Comment: Least irritating of the topical anesthetics.

Benoxinate Hydrochloride
Preparation: Solution, 0.4%.
Dosage: 1 drop and repeat as necessary.
Onset and duration of action: Anesthesia begins within 1 or 2 minutes and lasts for 10–15 minutes.
Comment: Activity and duration of action are approximately equivalent to those of proparacaine. Benoxinate is the only anesthetic compatible with fluorescein. These 2 agents are available in a combined solution (Fluress) for use prior to applanation tonometry.

LOCAL ANESTHETICS FOR INJECTION

Lidocaine, procaine, and mepivacaine are commonly used local anesthetics for eye surgery. Longer-acting agents such as bupivacaine and etidocaine are often mixed with other local anesthetics to prolong the duration of effect. Local anesthetics are extremely safe when used with discretion, but the physician must be aware of the potential systemic toxic action when rapid absorption occurs from the site of the injection, with excessive dosage, or following inadvertent intravascular injection.

The addition of hyaluronidase encourages spreading of the anesthetic and shortens the onset to as little as 1 minute. For these reasons, hyaluronidase is commonly used in retrobulbar injections prior to cataract extraction. Up to 4 mL may be injected behind the globe with relative safety. Injectable anesthetics are used by ophthalmologists most commonly in older patients, who may be susceptible to cardiac arrhythmias; therefore, epinephrine should not be used in concentrations greater than 1:200,000.

Lidocaine Hydrochloride (Xylocaine)
Owing to its rapid onset and longer action (1–2 hours), lidocaine has become the most commonly used local anesthetic. It is approximately twice as potent as procaine. Thirty mL of 1% solution, without epinephrine, may be used safely. In cataract surgery, 20 mL is more than adequate. The maximum safe dose is 4.5 mg/kg without epinephrine and 7 mg/kg with epinephrine.

Procaine Hydrochloride
Preparations: Solution, 1 and 2%.
Dosage: Approximately 50 mL of a 1% solution can be safely injected without systemic effects. The maximum safe dose is 10 mg/kg.
Duration of action: 45–60 minutes.

Mepivacaine Hydrochloride (Carbocaine)
Preparations: Solution, 1 and 2%.
Dosage: Infiltration and nerve block, up to 20 mL of 1 or 2% solution.
Duration of action: Approximately 2 hours.
Comment: Carbocaine is similar to lidocaine in potency. It is usually used in patients who are allergic to lidocaine. The maximum safe dose is 7 mg/kg.

Bupivacaine Hydrochloride (Marcaine, Sensorcaine)

Preparations: Solution, 0.25%, 0.5%, and 0.75%.

Dosage: The 0.75% solution has been used most frequently in ophthalmology. The maximum safe dose in an adult is 250 mg with epinephrine and 200 mg without epinephrine. Bupivacaine is frequently mixed with an equal amount of lidocaine.

Onset and duration of action: The onset of action is slower than that of lidocaine, but it persists much longer (up to 4–6 hours).

Etidocaine Hydrochloride (Duranest)

Preparations: Solution, 0.5% and 1%.

Dosage: The maximum safe dose of etidocaine is 4 mg/kg without epinephrine and 5.5 mg/kg with epinephrine. This agent is frequently mixed with lidocaine for local anesthesia in ophthalmic surgery.

Onset and duration of action: The onset of action is slower than that of lidocaine but more rapid than that of bupivacaine. The duration of action is approximately twice as long as that of lidocaine.

MYDRIATICS & CYCLOPLEGICS

Mydriatics and cycloplegics both dilate the pupil. In addition, cycloplegics cause paralysis of accommodation (patient unable to see near objects, eg, printed words). They are commonly used drugs in ophthalmology, singly and in combination. Their prime uses are (1) for dilating the pupils to facilitate ophthalmoscopy; (2) for paralyzing the muscles of accommodation, particularly in young patients, as an aid in refraction; and (3) for dilating the pupil and paralyzing the muscles of accommodation in uveitis to prevent synechia formation and relieve pain and photophobia. Since mydriatics and cycloplegics both dilate the pupil, they should not be used in eyes with narrow anterior chamber angles since either a mydriatic or a cycloplegic can cause angle-closure glaucoma in such eyes.

1. MYDRIATICS (Sympathomimetics)

Phenylephrine is a mydriatic with no cycloplegic effect.

Phenylephrine Hydrochloride (Ak-Dilate, Efricel, Mydfrin, Neo-Synephrine)

Preparations: Solution, 2.5–10%.

Dosage: 1 drop and repeat in 5–10 minutes.

Onset and duration of action: The effect usually occurs within 30 minutes after instillation and lasts 2–3 hours.

Comment: Phenylephrine is used both singly and with cycloplegics to facilitate ophthalmoscopy, in treatment of uveitis, and to dilate the pupil prior to cataract surgery. It is used almost to the exclusion of all other mydriatics. If a patient is allergic to phenylephrine, hydroxyamphetamine hydrobromide (Paredrine) may be substituted. The 10% solution should not be used in newborn infants, in cardiac patients, or in patients receiving reserpine, guanethidine, or tricyclic antidepressants, because of increased susceptibility to the vasopressor effects.

2. CYCLOPLEGICS (Parasympatholytics)

Atropine Sulfate

Preparations: Solution, 0.25–2%; ointment, 0.5 and 1%.

Dosage: For refraction in children, instill 1 drop of 0.25–0.5% solution in each eye twice a day for 1 or 2 days before the examination and then 1 drop 1 hour before the examination.

Onset and duration of action: The onset of action is within 30–40 minutes. A maximum effect is reached in about 2 hours. The effect lasts for up to 2 weeks in a normal eye, but in the presence of acute inflammation the drug must be instilled 2–3 times daily to maintain its effect.

Toxicity: Atropine drops must be used with caution to avoid toxic reactions resulting from systemic absorption. Restlessness and excited behavior with dryness and flushing of the skin of the face, dry mouth, fever, inhibition of sweating, and tachycardia are prominent toxic symptoms, particularly in young children.

Comment: Atropine is an effective and long-acting cycloplegic. In addition to its use for cycloplegia in children, atropine is applied topically 2–3 times daily in the treatment of iritis. Atropine is used by many eye surgeons to dilate the pupil for a few weeks after cataract surgery.

Scopolamine Hydrobromide

Preparation: Solution, 0.25%.

Dosage: 1 drop 2 or 3 times daily.

Onset and duration of action: Cycloplegia occurs in about 40 minutes and lasts for 3–5 days when scopolamine is used as an aid to refraction in normal eyes. The duration of action is much shorter in inflamed eyes.

Toxicity: Scopolamine occasionally causes dizziness and disorientation, mainly in older people.

Comment: Scopolamine is an effective cycloplegic. It is used in the treatment of uveitis, in refraction of children, and in postoperative cataract patients.

Homatropine Hydrobromide

Preparations: Solution, 1, 2, and 5%.

Dosage: For refraction, 1 drop in each eye and repeat 2 or 3 times at intervals of 10– 15 minutes.

Onset and duration of action: Maximal cycloplegic effect lasts for about 3 hours, but complete recovery time is about 36– 48 hours. In certain cases, the shorter action is an advantage over scopolamine and atropine.

Toxicity: Sensitivity and side effects associated with the topical instillation of homatropine are rare.

Cyclopentolate Hydrochloride
(Ak-Pentolate, Cyclogyl)

Preparations: Solution, 0.5 and 1%.

Dosage: For refraction, 1 drop in each eye and repeat after 10 minutes.

Onset and duration of action: The onset of dilatation and cycloplegia is within 30– 60 minutes. The duration of action is less than 24 hours.

Comment: Cyclopentolate is more popular than homatropine and scopolamine in refraction because of its shorter duration of action. Occasionally, neurotoxicity may occur, manifested by incoherence, visual hallucinations, slurred speech, and ataxia.

Tropicamide
(Mydriacyl, Mydriafair, Tropicacyl)

Preparations: Solution, 0.5 and 1%.

Dosage: 1 drop of 1% solution 2 or 3 times at 5-minute intervals.

Onset and duration of action: The time required to reach the maximum cycloplegic effect is usually 20– 25 minutes, and the duration of this effect is only 15– 20 minutes; therefore, the timing of the examination after instilling tropicamide is important. Complete recovery requires 5– 6 hours.

Comment: Tropicamide is an effective mydriatic with weak cycloplegic action and is therefore most useful for ophthalmoscopy.

DRUGS USED IN THE TREATMENT OF GLAUCOMA

The concentration used and the frequency of instillation should be individualized on the basis of tonometric measurements. Use the smallest dosage that effectively controls the intraocular pressure and prevents optic nerve damage.

1. DIRECT-ACTING CHOLINERGIC (PARASYMPATHOMIMETIC) DRUGS

Pilocarpine Hydrochloride

Preparations: Solution, 0.5– 6%; gel, 4%.

Dosage: 1 drop up to 6 times a day; a ½-inch strip of gel in lower conjunctival cul-de-sac at bedtime.

Comment: Pilocarpine was introduced in 1876 and is still a commonly used antiglaucoma drug.

Carbachol

Preparations: Solution, 0.75– 3%.

Dosage: 1 drop in each eye 3– 4 times a day.

Comment: Carbachol is poorly absorbed through the cornea and usually is used if pilocarpine is ineffective. Its duration of action is 4– 6 hours. If benzalkonium chloride is used as the vehicle, the penetration of carbachol is significantly increased.

2. INDIRECT-ACTING REVERSIBLE ANTICHOLINESTERASE DRUGS

Physostigmine Salicylate
(Eserine)

Preparations: Solution, 0.25– 0.5%.

Dosage: 1 drop 3 or 4 times a day.

Comment: A high incidence of allergic reactions has limited the use of this old but effective antiglaucoma drug. It can be combined in the same solution with pilocarpine.

Neostigmine Bromide

Preparations: Solution, 2.5– 5%.

Dosage: 1 or 2 drops in each eye 2– 6 times a day.

3. INDIRECT-ACTING IRREVERSIBLE ANTICHOLINESTERASE DRUGS

These drugs are strong and long-lasting and are used when pilocarpine, carbachol, and epinephrine fail to control the intraocular pressure. The miosis produced is extreme. Local irritation is common, and phospholine iodide is believed to be cataractogenic in some patients. Pupillary block may occur. (See p 191.)

Isoflurophate (Floropryl)

Preparation: Ointment, 0.025%.

Dosage: A ¼-inch strip of ointment inside lower eyelid once or twice daily.

Echothiophate Iodide
(Phospholine Iodide)

Preparations: Solution, 0.03– 0.25%.

Dosage: 1 drop once or twice daily or less often, depending upon the response.

Comment: Echothiophate iodide is a long-acting drug similar to isoflurophate that has the advantages of being water-soluble and causing less local irritation. Systemic toxicity may occur in the form of cholinergic stimulation, including salivation, nausea, vomiting, and diarrhea.

Demecarium Bromide (Humorsol)

Preparations: Solution, 0.12 and 0.25%.

Dosage: 1 drop once or twice a day.

Comment: Systemic toxicity similar to that associated with echothiophate iodide may occur.

4. ADRENERGIC (SYMPATHOMIMETIC) DRUGS

In the treatment of glaucoma, epinephrine has the advantages of long duration of action (12– 72 hours) and no miosis, which is especially important in patients with incipient cataracts (effect on vision not accentuated). At least 25% of patients develop local allergies; others complain of headache and heart palpitation (less common with dipivefrin).

Epinephrine acts by increasing outflow of aqueous humor.

Some of the preparations available for use in open-angle glaucoma are listed below. The dosage is the same for all, ie, 1 drop once or twice daily:

Epinephryl borate (Epinal, Eppy/N), 0.5 and 1%.
Epinephrine bitartrate (Epitrate, Murocoll), 1% and 2%.
Epinephrine hydrochloride (Epifrin, Glaucon), 0.25, 0.5, 1, and 2%.
Dipivefrin (Propine), 0.1%.

5. BETA-ADRENERGIC BLOCKING DRUGS

Timolol Maleate (Timoptic)

Preparations: Solution, 0.25 and 0.5%.

Dosage: 1 drop of 0.25% solution twice daily. Increase to 1 drop of 0.5% solution in each eye twice daily if needed.

Comment: Timolol maleate is a beta-adrenergic blocking agent applied topically for treatment of open-angle glaucoma, aphakic glaucoma, and some types of secondary glaucoma. A single application can lower the intraocular pressure for 12– 24 hours. Timolol has been found to be effective in some patients with severe glaucoma inadequately controlled by maximum tolerated antiglaucoma therapy with other drugs. The drug does not affect pupillary size or visual acuity. Although timolol is usually well tolerated, it should be prescribed cautiously for patients with known contraindications to systemic use of beta-adrenergic blocking drugs (eg, asthma, heart failure). (See discussion of side effects, below.)

Betaxolol Hydrochloride (Betoptic)

Preparation: Solution, 0.5%.

Dosage: 1 drop twice daily.

Comment: Betaxolol has comparable efficacy to timolol in the treatment of glaucoma. Its relative beta-1 receptor selectivity reduces the risk of pulmonary side effects, particularly in patients with reactive airway disease.

Levobunolol Hydrochloride (Betagan)

Preparation: Solution, 0.5%.

Dosage: 1 drop twice daily.

Comment: Levobunolol is a nonselective beta-1 and beta-2 blocker. It has comparable effects to timolol in the treatment of glaucoma.

6. CARBONIC ANHYDRASE INHIBITORS

Inhibition of carbonic anhydrase in the ciliary body reduces the secretion of aqueous. The oral administration of carbonic anhydrase is especially useful in reducing the intraocular pressure in selected cases of open-angle glaucoma and can be used with some effect in angle-closure glaucoma.

The carbonic anhydrase inhibitors in use are sulfonamide derivatives. Oral administration produces the maximum effect in approximately 2 hours; intravenous administration, in 20 minutes. The duration of maximal effect is 4– 6 hours following oral administration.

The carbonic anhydrase inhibitors are used in patients whose intraocular pressure cannot be controlled with eye drops. They are valuable for this purpose but have many undesirable side effects, including potassium depletion, gastric distress, diarrhea, exfoliative dermatitis, renal stone formation, shortness of breath, fatigue, acidosis, and tingling of the extremities. Since the advent of timolol and laser therapy, carbonic anhydrase inhibitors are being used less frequently.

Acetazolamide (Diamox)

Preparations and dosages:

Oral: Tablets, 125 and 250 mg; give 125– 250 mg 2– 4 times a day (dosage not to exceed 1 g in 24 hours). Sustained-release capsules, 500 mg; give 1 capsule once or twice a day.

Parenteral: May give 500-mg ampules intramuscularly or intravenously for short periods in patients who cannot tolerate the drug orally.

Dichlorphenamide (Daranide)

Preparation: Tablets, 50 mg.

Dosage: Give a priming dose of 100– 200 mg followed by 100 mg every 12 hours until the desired response is obtained. The usual maintenance dosage for glaucoma is 25– 50 mg 3– 4 times daily. The total daily dosage should not exceed 300 mg daily.

Ethoxzolamide

Preparation: Tablets, 125 mg.
Dosage: 125 mg 2– 4 times daily.

Methazolamide (Neptazane)

Preparation: Tablets, 50 mg.
Dosage: 50– 100 mg 2 or 3 times daily (total not to exceed 600 mg/d).

7. OSMOTIC AGENTS

Hyperosmotic agents such as urea, mannitol, and glycerin are used to reduce intraocular pressure by making the plasma hypertonic to aqueous humor. These agents are generally used in the management of acute (angle-closure) glaucoma and occasionally in pre- or postoperative surgery when reduction of intraocular pressure is indicated. The dosage for all is approximately 1.5 g/kg.

Urea (Ureaphil)

Preparation: 30% solution of lyophilized urea in invert sugar.
Dosage: 1– 1.5 g/kg intravenously.
Onset and duration of action: Maximum hypotensive effect occurs in about 1 hour and lasts 5– 6 hours.
Toxicity: Accidental extravasation at the injection site may cause local reactions ranging from mild irritation to tissue necrosis.

Mannitol (Osmitrol)

Preparation: 20% solution in water.
Dosage: 1.5– 2 g/kg intravenously.
Onset and duration of action: Maximum hypotensive effect occurs in about 1 hour and lasts 5– 6 hours.

Glycerin (Glyrol, Osmoglyn)

Preparations and dosage: Glycerin is usually given orally as 50% solution with water, orange juice, or flavored normal saline solution over ice (1 mL of glycerin weighs 1.25 g). Dose is 1– 1.5 g/kg.
Onset and duration of action: Maximum hypotensive effect occurs in 1 hour and lasts 4– 5 hours.
Toxicity: Nausea, vomiting, and headache occasionally occur.
Comment: Oral administration and the absence of diuretic effect are significant advantages of glycerin over the other hyperosmotic agents.

TOPICAL CORTICOSTEROIDS

Indications

Topical corticosteroid therapy is indicated for inflammatory conditions of the anterior segment of the globe. Some examples are allergic conjunctivitis, uveitis, episcleritis, scleritis, phlyctenulosis, superficial punctate keratitis, interstitial keratitis, and vernal conjunctivitis.

Administration & Dosage

The corticosteroids and certain derivatives vary in their anti-inflammatory activity. The relative potency of prednisolone to hydrocortisone is 4 times; of dexamethasone and betamethasone, 25 times. The side effects are not decreased with the higher-potency drugs even though the therapeutic dosage is lower.

The duration of treatment will vary with the type of lesion and may extend from a few days to several months.

Initial therapy for a severely inflamed eye consists of instilling drops every 1 or 2 hours during waking hours. When a favorable response is observed, gradually reduce the dosage and discontinue as soon as possible.

Caution: The steroids enhance the activity of the herpes simplex virus, as shown by the fact that perforation of the cornea occasionally occurs when they are used in the eye for treatment of herpes simplex keratitis. Corneal perforation was an extremely rare complication of herpes simplex keratitis before the steroids came into general use. Other side effects of local steroid therapy are fungal overgrowth, cataract formation (unusual), and open-angle glaucoma (common). These effects are produced to a lesser degree with systemic steroid therapy. Any patient receiving local ocular corticosteroid therapy or long-term systemic corticosteroid therapy should be under the care of an ophthalmologist.

A partial list of the available topical corticosteroids for ophthalmologic use is as follows:

Hydrocortisone acetate suspension, 2.5%.
Prednisolone acetate suspension, 0.125% and 1%.
Prednisolone sodium phosphate solution, 0.125 and 1%.
Dexamethasone sodium phosphate suspension, 0.1%.
Medrysone suspension, 1%.
Fluorometholone suspension, 0.1%.

OTHER DRUGS USED IN THE TREATMENT OF ALLERGIC CONJUNCTIVITIS

Cromolyn Sodium (Opticrom)

Preparation: Solution, 4%.
Dosage: 1 drop 4– 6 times a day.
Comment: Cromolyn has a prophylactic effect in allergic conjunctivitis. Symptomatic improvement may not occur until 1– 2 weeks after initiation of therapy. Cromolyn is not useful in the treatment of acute symptoms. Soft contact lenses should not be worn during treatment.

ANTI-INFECTIVE OPHTHALMIC DRUGS

1. TOPICAL ANTIBIOTIC SOLUTIONS & OINTMENTS

Antibiotics are commonly used in the treatment of external ocular infection, including bacterial conjunctivitis, sties, marginal blepharitis, and bacterial corneal ulcers. The frequency of use is related to the severity of the condition. Antibiotic treatment of intraocular infection is discussed in Table 28–1.

Bacitracin, neomycin, polymyxin, erythromycin, tetracycline, gentamicin, and tobramycin are the most commonly used topical antibiotics. They are used separately and in combination as solutions and as ointments.

Bacitracin

Preparation: Ointment, 500 units/g. Commercially available in combinations with bacitracin and polymyxin B.

Comment: Most gram-positive organisms are sensitive to bacitracin. It is not used systemically because of nephrotoxicity.

Erythromycin

Erythromycin, 0.5% ointment, is an effective agent, particularly in staphylococcal conjunctivitis. May be used instead of silver nitrate in prophylaxis of ophthalmia neonatorum.

Table 28–1. A method of treating postoperative bacterial endophthalmitis.

---

(1) Aspiration of aqueous and vitreous:
    (a) Giemsa's stain.
    (b) Gram's stain.
    (c) Cultures (blood agar, thioglycolate, Sabouraud's) and antibiotic sensitivity tests.
(2) Intravitreal injection of antibiotics after diagnostic tap: Gentamicin, 0.1 mg, and cephaloridine, 2.25 mg, in 0.1 mL volume. Inject into central part of vitreous cavity.
(3) Intravenous antibiotics: Cefazolin, 1000 mg every 6 hours, and gentamicin, 1 mg/kg every 8 hours.
(4) Subconjunctival antibiotics:
    (a) Cefazolin, 50–100 mg.
    (b) Gentamicin, 20–30 mg.
(5) Topical agents: Gentamicin, 9–14 mg/mL, 1–2 drops every hour; prednisolone acetate 1%, 1–2 drops 4–6 times daily; and atropine 1%, 1–2 drops 3 times daily.
(6) Specific antibiotic treatment in maximum doses should be started as soon as causative organisms are identified and sensitivity studies completed.
(7) Diagnostic and therapeutic vitrectomy may be indicated initially, particularly in severe cases or if fungal endophthalmitis is present.
(8) Vitreous aspiration and intravitreal injection of antibiotics may be repeated in 48–72 hours if improvement has not occurred.

Neomycin

Preparations: Solution, 2.5– 5 mg/mL; ointment, 3.5– 5 mg/g. Commerically available in combinations with bacitracin and polymyxin B.

Dosage: Apply ointment or drops 3 or 4 times daily. Solutions containing 50– 100 mg/mL have been used for corneal ulcers.

Comment: Effective against gram-negative and gram-positive organisms. Neomycin is usually combined with some other drug to widen its spectrum of activity. It is best known in ophthalmologic practice as Neosporin, both in ointment and solution form, in which it is combined with polymyxin and bacitracin. Contact skin sensitivity develops in 5% of patients if the drug is continued for longer than a week.

2. TOPICAL PREPARATIONS OF SYSTEMIC ANTIBIOTICS

Topical use of the antibiotics commonly used systemically should be avoided if possible, because sensitization of the patient may interfere with future systemic use. However, in certain instances clinical judgment overrides this principle if the drug is particularly effective locally and the disorder is serious. A prime example of this is tetracycline in the treatment of trachoma, the commonest eye infection in the world.

Tetracyclines

Preparations: Solution, 10 mg/mL; ointment, 10 mg/g.

Comment: Tetracycline, oxytetracycline, and chlortetracycline have limited uses in ophthalmology because their effectiveness is so often impaired by the development of resistant strains. Solutions of these compounds are unstable with the exception of Achromycin in sesame oil, which is widely used in the treatment of trachoma. Ointment may be used for prophylaxis of ophthalmia neonatorum.

Gentamicin (Garamycin, Genoptic, Gentacidin)

Preparations: Solution, 3 mg/mL; ointment, 3 mg/g.

Comment: Gentamicin is widely accepted for use in serious ocular infections, especially corneal ulcers caused by gram-negative organisms. It is also effective against many gram-positive staphylococci but is not effective against streptococci.

Tobramycin (Tobrex)

Preparations: Solution, 3 mg/mL; ointment, 3 mg/g.

Comment: Similar antimicrobial activity to gentamicin but more effective against streptococci. Best reserved for treatment of *Pseudomonas* keratitis, for which it is more effective.

Chloramphenicol

Preparations: Solution, 5–10 mg/mL; ointment, 10 mg/g.

Comment: Chloramphenicol is effective against a wide variety of gram-positive and gram-negative organisms. It rarely causes local sensitization, but cases of aplastic anemia have occurred with long-term therapy.

3. SULFONAMIDES

The sulfonamides are the most commonly used drugs in the treatment of bacterial conjunctivitis. Their advantages include (1) activity against both gram-positive and gram-negative organisms, (2) relatively low cost, (3) low allergenicity, and (4) the fact that their use is not complicated by secondary fungal infections, as sometimes occurs following prolonged use of antibiotics.

The commonest sulfonamides employed are sulfisoxazole and sulfacetamide sodium.

Sulfacetamide Sodium (Sulamyd)

Preparations: Ophthalmic solution, 10 and 30%; ointment, 10%.

Dosage: Instill 1 drop frequently, depending upon the severity of the conjunctivitis.

Sulfisoxazole (Gantrisin)

Preparations: Ophthalmic solution, 4%; ointment, 4%.

Dosage: As for sulfacetamide sodium (above).

4. TOPICAL ANTIFUNGAL AGENTS

Natamycin (Natacyn)

Preparation: 5% suspension.

Dosage: Instill 1 drop every 1–2 hours.

Comment: Effective against filamentary and yeast forms. Initial drug of choice for most mycotic corneal ulcers.

Nystatin (Mycostatin)

Not available in ophthalmic ointment form, but the dermatologic preparation (100,000 units/g) is not irritating to ocular tissues and can be used in the treatment of fungal infection of the eye.

Amphotericin B (Fungizone)

More effective than nystatin but not available in ophthalmic ointment form. The dermatologic preparation is highly irritating. A solution (0.5–1.5 mg/mL of distilled water in 5% dextrose) must be made up in the pharmacy from the powdered drug. Many patients have extreme ocular discomfort following application of this drug.

Miconazole (Monistat)

A 1% solution is available in the form of an in-travenous preparation that may be applied directly into the eye. The drug is not available in an ophthalmologic form.

5. ANTIVIRAL AGENTS

Idoxuridine (Dendrid, Herplex, Stoxil)

Preparations: Ophthalmic solution, 0.1%; ointment, 0.5%.

Dosage: 1 drop every hour during the day and every 2 hours at night. With improvement (as determined by fluorescein staining), the frequency of instillation is gradually reduced. The ointment may be used 4–6 times daily, or the solution may be used during the day and the ointment at bedtime.

Comment: Used in the treatment of herpes simplex keratitis. Epithelial infection usually improves within a few days. Therapy should be continued for 3 or 4 days after apparent healing. Many ophthalmologists still prefer to denude the affected corneal epithelium and not use idoxuridine.

Vidarabine (Adenine Arabinoside, Ara-A, Vira-A)

Preparation: Ophthalmic ointment, 3%.

Dosage: In herpetic epithelial keratitis, apply 4 times daily for 7–10 days.

Comment: Ara-A is effective against herpes simplex virus but not other RNA or DNA viruses. It is effective in some patients unresponsive to idoxuridine. Ara-A interferes with viral DNA synthesis. The principal metabolite is arabinosylhypoxanthine (Ara-Hx). The drug is effective against herpetic corneal epithelial disease and has limited efficacy in stromal keratitis or uveitis. It may cause cellular toxicity and delay corneal regeneration. The cellular toxicity is less than that of idoxuridine.

Trifluridine (Viroptic)

Preparation: 1% solution.

Dosage: One drop every 2 hours (maximum total, 9 drops daily).

Comment: Acts by interfering with viral DNA synthesis. More soluble than either idoxuridine or vidarabine and probably more effective in stromal disease.

Acyclovir (Investigational)

Acyclovir (acycloguanosine) is a new antiviral agent, still investigational for ophthalmologic use, which shows great promise in the treatment of herpes simplex and herpes zoster infections. It is phosphorylated initially by virus-specified thymidine kinase to acyclovir monophosphate and then by cellular kinases to acyclovir triphosphate, which inhibits viral DNA polymerase. Thus, there is a marked selectivity for virus-infected cells. Acyclovir has low toxicity except for crystal deposition in renal tubules when used at high doses or when urine output is poor. No commercial ophthalmic preparation is currently available in the USA; a topical product available for treatment of genital herpes should not be used in the eye. A parenteral preparation is available for use in immunocompromised patients.

DIAGNOSTIC DYE SOLUTIONS

Sodium Fluorescein
Preparations: Solution, 2%, in single-use disposable units; as sterile paper strips; as 10% sterile solution for intravenous use in fluorescein angiography.
Dosage: 1 drop.
Comment: Used as a diagnostic agent for detection of corneal injury, in applanation tonometry, and in fitting contact lenses.

Rose Bengal
Preparation: Solution, 1%.
Dosage: 1 drop.
Comment: Used in diagnosis of keratoconjunctivitis sicca; the mucous shreds and corneal epithelial changes stain more brilliantly than with fluorescein.

TEAR REPLACEMENT & LUBRICATING AGENTS

Methylcellulose and related chemicals, polyvinyl alcohol and related chemicals, and gelatin are used in the formulation of artificial tears, ophthalmic lubricants, contact lens solutions, and gonioscopic lens solutions. These agents are particularly useful in the treatment of keratoconjunctivitis sicca. (See Chapter 7.)

To increase viscosity and prolong corneal contact time, methylcellulose is sometimes added to eye solutions (eg, pilocarpine).

OCULAR & SYSTEMIC SIDE EFFECTS OF DRUGS

F. T. Fraunfelder, MD, & S. Martha Meyer, BS

Both systemically and topically administered drugs can produce adverse ocular effects, and topical ophthalmic preparations occasionally lead to systemic effects if too much active ingredient is absorbed. Preservatives in drugs may also be associated with side effects.

Tables 28–2 to 28–4 list possible ocular and systemic side effects of some ocular and systemic medications. This is not in any way a complete listing of all drugs and their side effects. The information has been compiled from various sources. Physicians are advised to consult product labels, the references at the end of this chapter, and other appropriate sources for further information.

SYSTEMIC SIDE EFFECTS OF TIMOLOL

One example of an ocular drug with which serious side effects may occur is timolol. Timolol by topical administration is the most commonly used antiglaucoma medication in the world and has been associated with severe, even fatal, reactions. Plasma drug concentrations sufficient to cause systemic beta-adrenoceptor blocking effects can occasionally result from ocular administration. When topical ocular timolol is administered in infants, blood levels are often more than 6 times what minimum therapeutic levels would be if the drug were given orally for some other condition; these high blood levels may be present for many hours after administration. If the lacrimal system is not closed during administration, an estimated 80% of a timolol eye drop is absorbed from the nasal mucosa and passes almost directly into the vascular system. Because the drug can reach target organs before it is detoxified in the liver, the blood level following topical ophthalmic administration is proportionately higher than when the drug is given orally, as in hypertension. A genetic fault in the oxidative metabolism of beta blockers has been detected in some patients, and significantly higher levels of plasma concentrations develop in poor metabolizers.

Cardiopulmonary histories should be taken for candidates for beta-blocker glaucoma therapy. Pulmonary function studies should be considered in patients with bronchoconstrictive disease, and electrocardiograms should be ordered on selected patients with cardiac disease. Specifically, the precautions set forth in the package insert should be heeded carefully. Patients with known bronchial asthma, chronic respiratory or cardiovascular disease, or sinus bradycardia should avoid using timolol. The drug should be used with caution in patients receiving other systemic beta-blocking agents.

WAYS TO DIMINISH SYSTEMIC SIDE EFFECTS

One important principle in avoiding systemic side effects from topical ophthalmic medications is to prevent overdosing. The physician should prescribe the lowest concentration of medication that will be therapeutically effective. Only 1 drop of medication is needed at each dosage, since the volume the eye can hold is less than 1 drop.

Table 28–2. Possible adverse ocular effects of systemic drugs.

Drug	Adverse Effects	Drug	Adverse Effects
Allopurinol	Cataract	Ketamine	Nystagmus
Amiodarone	Corneal opacity	Methyldopa	Conjunctivitis
Amphetamines	Elevation of intraocular pressure	Monoamine oxidase inhibitors	Optic atrophy
Antibiotics	Conjunctivitis, keratitis		
Anticholinergics	Elevation of intraocular pressure	Morphine	Optic neuritis
Anticoagulants	Retinal hemorrhage	Nalidixic acid	Papilledema
Barbiturates	Conjunctivitis, Stevens-Johnson syndrome, ptosis, optic atrophy	Naproxen	Corneal opacity
		Oral contraceptives	Retinal occlusion, retinal hemorrhage, retinal edema, retinal vasospasm, corneal edema, nystagmus, papilledema
Busulfan	Cataract		
Cardiac glycosides	Retinal degeneration		
Chloral hydrate	Conjunctivitis		
Chlorambucil	Papilledema	Penicillamine	Extraocular muscle paralysis, ptosis, optic neuritis
Chloramphenicol	Optic atrophy, optic neuritis		
Chloroquine	Corneal opacity, retinal degeneration	Phenothiazines	Conjunctival deposits, corneal opacity, oculogyric crisis, pigmentation of lens, retinal degeneration
Chlorpropamide	Stevens-Johnson syndrome, corneal opacity, extraocular muscle paralysis		
		Phenylbutazone	Conjunctivitis, keratitis, retinal hemorrhage
Clofazimine	Conjunctival deposits, corneal opacity		
Corticosteroids	Elevation of intraocular pressure, cataract	Phenytoin	Nystagmus, extraocular muscle paralysis
Diazepam	Nystagmus	Quinacrine	Conjunctival deposits
Disulfiram	Optic neuritis	Quinine	Retinal edema, retinal vasodilation followed by vasoconstriction
Ethambutol	Optic neuritis		
Gold salts	Conjunctival deposits, corneal opacity, nystagmus, pigmentation of lens	Rifampin	Optic neuritis
		Salicylates	Nystagmus, retinal hemorrhage
		Streptomycin	Optic neuritis
Guanethidine	Ptosis	Sulfonamides	Conjunctivitis, Stevens-Johnson syndrome, retinal hemorrhage
Haloperidol	Cataract		
Hexamethonium	Retinal vasodilation	Tetracycline	Papilledema
Indomethacin	Corneal opacity	Tricyclic antidepressants	Elevation of intraocular pressure
Iodoquinol	Optic atrophy	Vitamin A	Conjunctival deposits, papilledema
Isoniazid	Optic neuritis	Vitamin D	Conjunctival deposits, corneal opacity
Isotretinoin	Conjunctivitis, corneal opacity, papilledema		

The proper method of topical administration of ophthalmic medications is as follows:

Position the patient with head tilted back toward the ceiling. Grasp the lower eyelid below the lashes and gently pull the lid away from the eye (Fig 28– 1). Instill 1 drop of medication into the inferior cul-de-sac nearest the involved area, being careful not to touch the lashes or eyelids and thus avoid contamination (Fig 28– 2). The lower eyelid should then be gently lifted to make contact with the upper lid (Fig 28– 3). Patients should position their heads so that gravity will keep the drug where medically indicated. The eyelids should be kept closed for 3 minutes or more to prevent blinking, which pumps the drug into the nose and increases systemic absorption. The patient should be shown how to obstruct the lacrimal drainage system with firm pressure over the inner corner of the closed eyelids (Fig 28– 4). Excess medication in the medial canthus should be blotted away before pressure is released or the eyelids opened. The patient receiving multiple topical medications should wait 10 minutes between doses, so that the first drug will not be washed out of the eye by the second.

NATIONAL REGISTRY OF DRUG-INDUCED OCULAR SIDE EFFECTS

The National Registry of Drug-Induced Ocular Side Effects is a clearinghouse of drug information on ocular toxicology. The principle underlying its establishment is the assumption that the suspicions of practicing clinicians regarding possible ocular toxicity of drugs can be pooled to increase the data base and decrease the lag time in recognizing adverse responses. Physicians who wish to report suspected adverse drug reactions or would like to receive references pertaining to the data in Tables 28– 2 to 28– 4 should call or write the Department of Ophthalmology, Oregon Health Sciences University, 3181 S.W. Sam Jackson Park Road, Portland, OR 97201, (503) 225-8456.

Table 28—3. Possible adverse systemic effects of topical ocular medications.

Medication	Adverse Effects
Anesthetics, topical local	
Benoxinate	Allergic reactions, anaphylactic reactions, convulsions, faintness, hypotension, syncope
Proparacaine	Same as benoxinate
Tetracaine	Same as benoxinate
Antibiotics	
Chloramphenicol	Allergic reactions; bone marrow depression, including aplastic anemia; gastrointestinal symptoms
Chlortetracycline	Photosensitivity, skin discoloration
Sulfacetamide	Photosensitivity, Stevens-Johnson syndrome
Sulfamethizole	Same as sulfacetamide
Sulfisoxazole	Same as sulfacetamide
Tetracycline	Same as chlortetracycline
Anticholinergics	
Atropine	Confusion, dermatitis, dry mouth, excitement, fever, flushed skin, hallucinations, psychosis, tachycardia, thirst
Cyclopentolate	Amnesia, ataxia, convulsions, disorientation, dysarthria, fever, hallucinations, psychosis
Homatropine	Same as atropine
Scopolamine	Same as atropine
Tropicamide	Same as cyclopentolate
Anticholinesterases, long-acting	
Demecarium	Abdominal cramps, diarrhea, fatigue, nausea, rhinorrhea, weight loss
Echothiophate	Same as demecarium
Isoflurophate	Same as demecarium
Anticholinesterases, short-acting	
Neostigmine	Abdominal cramps, depigmentation, diarrhea, nausea, vomiting
Physostigmine	Same as neostigmine
Beta-adrenoceptor blocking agent	
Timolol	Asthma, bradycardia, cardiac arrythmia, confusion, depression, dizziness, dyspnea, hallucinations, impotence, myasthenia, psychosis
Parasympathomimetics	
Carbachol	Abdominal cramps, diarrhea, hypotension, increased salivation, muscle tremors, nausea, respiratory distress, rhinorrhea, slurred speech, sweating, vomiting, weakness
Pilocarpine	Same as carbachol
Sympathomimetics	
Ephedrine	Cardiac arrhythmia, hypertension, palpitations, subarachnoid hemorrhage, tachycardia
Epinephrine	Same as ephedrine
Hydroxyamphetamine	Same as ephedrine
Phenylephrine	Same as ephedrine

Table 28—4. Possible adverse ocular effects of topical ocular medications.

Medication	Adverse Effects
Anesthetics, local	
Butacaine	Allergic reactions, corneal opacity, decreased corneal wound healing, iritis
Proparacaine	Same as butacaine
Tetracaine	Same as butacaine
Antibiotics	
Chlortetracycline	Allergic reactions, corneal discoloration
Neomycin	Allergic reactions, follicular conjunctivitis, keratitis
Tetracycline	Same as chlortetracycline
Anticholinergics	
Cyclopentolate	Angle-closure glaucoma, blurred vision, photophobia
Tropicamide	Same as cyclopentolate
Anticholinesterases, long-acting	
Demecarium	Accommodative spasm, cataract, depigmentation of lids, iris cysts, lacrimal outflow obstruction
Echothiophate	Same as demecarium
Isoflurophate	Same as demecarium
Anti-inflammatory agents	
Corticosteroids	Cataracts, corneal thinning, decreased corneal wound healing, glaucoma, infection
Antivirals	
Idoxuridine	Cicatricial pseudopemphigoid, keratitis, lacrimal outflow obstruction
Trifluridine	Same as idoxuridine
Vidarabine	Same as idoxuridine
Beta-adrenoceptor blocking agent	
Timolol	Blepharoconjunctivitis, corneal anesthesia, diplopia, dry eyes, keratitis, ptosis
Parasympathomimetic	
Pilocarpine	Accommodative spasm, cicatricial pseudopemphigoid, corneal haze (gel), myopia, retinal detachment
Preservatives	
Benzalkonium chloride	Allergic reactions, corneal opacity, keratitis
Phenylmercuric nitrate	Same as benzalkonium chloride
Thimerosal	Same as benzalkonium chloride
Sympathomimetics	
Dipivefrin	Allergic reactions, angle-closure glaucoma, follicular conjunctivitis
Epinephrine	Cicatricial pseudopemphigoid; cystoid macular edema; discoloration of cornea, conjunctiva, and soft contact lens; lacrimal outflow obstruction

Figure 28–1. With the patient's head tilted back toward the ceiling, grasp the lower eyelid below the lashes and gently pull the lid away from the eye.

Figure 28–3. While the patient is looking downward, gently lift the lower eyelid to make contact with the upper lid.

Figure 28–2. One drop of solution or a "match head" amount of ointment should be placed in the inferior cul-de-sac, without touching the bottle to the lashes or eyelids (to prevent contamination).

Figure 28–4. For 3 minutes or more, firm pressure is maintained with the forefinger or thumb over the inner corner of the closed eyelids. Any excess medication should be blotted away before pressure is released or the eye is opened.

REFERENCES

AMA Drug Evaluations, 5th ed. American Medical Association, 1983.

Dukes MNG (editor): *Meyler's Side Effects of Drugs*, 9th ed. Excerpta Medica, 1980.

Ellis PP: *Ocular Therapeutics and Pharmacology*, 7th ed. Mosby, 1985.

Fraunfelder FT: *Drug-Induced Ocular Side Effects and Drug Interactions*, 2nd ed. Lea & Febiger, 1982.

Fraunfelder FT, Roy FH (editors): *Current Ocular Therapy*, 2nd ed. Saunders, 1985.

Grant WM: *Toxicology of the Eye*, 2nd ed. Thomas, 1976.

Havener WH: *Ocular Pharmacology*, 5th ed. Mosby, 1983.

INDUSTRIAL VISUAL EVALUATION*

The following mathematical calculation of loss of visual efficiency is used for legal and industrial cases, particularly in determination of compensation for injury.†

Calculation of total visual efficiency is based on 3 factors of equal importance: percentage loss of visual acuity, percentage loss of visual field, and percentage loss of coordinated ocular movements. Percentage loss of visual acuity in one eye does not represent the individual's total disability; even a total loss of one eye would not represent a 50% disability if the remaining eye were normal. Many people lead normal lives with one eye.

For evaluation of industrial visual efficiency, therefore, 3 visual functions are measured and mathematically coordinated: (1) visual acuity, (2) visual field, and (3) ocular motility (diplopia field, binocular field).

Visual Acuity

Distance and near vision are weighted evenly.

For purposes of calculating total visual acuity loss, near visual acuity is equally as important as distance acuity.

Example: If the distance acuity is 6/24 (20/80) and the subject can read Jaeger 6—

$$\frac{40 + 50}{2} = \begin{array}{l} \text{45\% visual acuity loss, or 55\%} \\ \text{visual acuity efficiency} \end{array}$$

Visual Field

A white test object is used in 8 meridians as diagrammed on p 384. This can be done with a 3-mm object at 0.33 m, using a perimeter. A full field represents 100% function. (Illumination should be at least 120 lux.)

*Modified and reproduced, with permission, from *Arch Ind Health* 1955;**12**:439. For further explanation of the reasons behind the statistics and a legal discussion, see Spaeth EB: *Trans Am Acad Ophthalmol Otolaryngol* 1957;**61**:592.
†The method described here may differ from government standards for defining reduced vision in assessing eligibility for compensation, which vary from state to state. The State Department of Industrial Relations (or its equivalent) can be contacted for data.

AMA Method of Estimation of Percentage Visual Loss (Using Best Correcting Spectacle Lens)

Distance	
Distance Visual Acuity	% Loss
20/20 (6/6)	0
20/25 (6/7.5)	5
20/40 (6/12)	15
20/50 (6/15)	25
20/80 (6/24)	40
20/100 (6/30)	50
20/160 (6/48)	70
20/200 (6/60)	80
20/400 (6/120)	90

Near	
Jaeger Test Type	% Loss
1	0
2	0
3	10
6	50
7	60
11	85
14	95

Ocular Motility

The extent of diplopia in the various directions of gaze is best determined using a tangent screen at 1 meter. A small test light is used and diplopia plotted along the 3 meridians above the horizontal 10, 20, and 30 degrees from fixation. Diplopia fields are also plotted on the horizontal meridians and the 3 meridians below, 10, 20, 30, and 40 degrees from the straight-ahead position. Diplopia within the central 20 degrees represents 100% loss of motility efficiency of one eye, since this condition usually requires patching one eye. If diplopia is not present in the central 20 degrees, loss of ocular motility is calculated from a field diagram showing percentage loss. This value is then subtracted from 100 and expressed as "80% motility efficiency," etc.

The inferior fields are weighted heavily, since this is the position of the eyes in reading. Diplopia away from fixations in other quadrants is considered much less important.

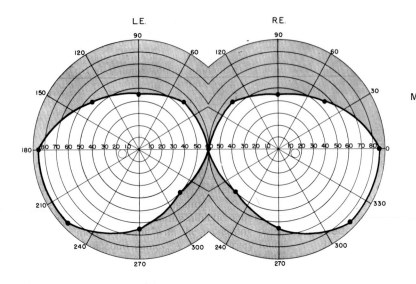

Minimum Legal Visual Field

Minimal Normal Field:

Temporally	85°
Down and temporally	85°
Down	65°
Down and nasally	50°
Nasally	60°
Up and nasally	55°
Up	45°
Up and temporally	55°
Full field	= 500°

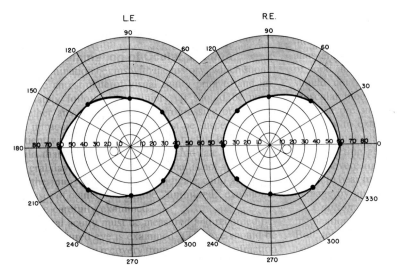

Twenty-eight Percent Loss

Moderate Loss of Field:

Temporally	60°
Down and temporally	50°
Down	40°
Down and nasally	40°
Nasally	40°
Up and nasally	40°
Up	40°
Up and temporally	50°
	360°

$$\frac{360 \times 100}{500} = \begin{array}{l}72\% \text{ field remaining, or}\\28\% \text{ field loss}\end{array}$$

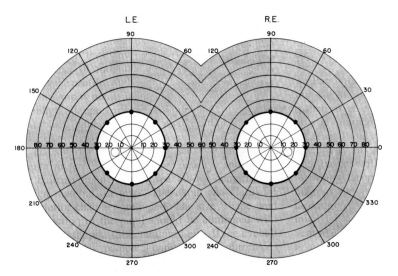

Fifty-two Percent Loss

Severe Loss of Field:

Temporally	30°
Down and temporally	30°
Down	30°
Down and nasally	30°
Nasally	30°
Up and nasally	30°
Up	30°
Up and temporally	30°
	240°

$$\frac{240 \times 100}{500} = \begin{array}{l}48\% \text{ field remaining, or}\\52\% \text{ field loss}\end{array}$$

Visual Efficiency (VE) of One Eye

The percentages of efficiency for the 3 measurements are multiplied to give the total visual efficiency.

Example: Visual acuity = 73%
Visual field = 57%
Motility = 90%

0.73 × 0.57 × 0.90 = 37% VE or 63% loss

Visual Efficiency (VE) of 2 Eyes

The 2 eyes are calculated separately; the better eye is weighted 3 times and the poorer eye once. Thus, one blind eye and one normal eye give 75% visual efficiency.

$$\frac{3 \times (\% \text{ VE better eye}) + \% \text{ VE in worse eye}}{4} = \text{binocular VE (\%)}$$

Example: RE = 90%; LE = 30%.

$$\frac{3 \times 90 + 30}{4} = 75\% \text{ binocular VE}$$

VISUAL STANDARDS FOR THE ARMED FORCES*

The visual acuity requirements outlined below apply for all branches of the services. For aircraft pilots, service academy candidates, and some other officer assignments, the requirements are much more rigid.

Standards for Disqualification

Any strabismus of 40 prism diopters or more uncorrectable by lenses to less than 40 diopters is disqualifying, as is the presence of diplopia. Any active or progressive disease of the eyes is disqualifying even though the minimal visual standards can be met.

Minimal Standards

Distance visual acuity must correct to one of the following: (1) 6/12 (20/40) in one eye and 6/20 (20/70) in the other; (2) 6/9 (20/30) in one eye and 6/30 (20/100) in the other; (3) 6/6 (20/20) in one eye and 6/120 (20/400) in the other.

Near visual acuity must correct to at least J-6 in the better eye.

VISUAL STANDARDS FOR DRIVERS' LICENSES IN THE USA

States have varying visual standards for persons applying for drivers' licenses. Failure to meet certain minimum standards may result in suspension of driv-

*Subject to change. Medical Officers for Recruitment at military hospitals or induction centers are supplied with the latest data.

ing privileges or denial of license unless a certificate is obtained from an ophthalmologist or optometrist. In recent years there has been a trend toward higher standards and more periodic visual testing, especially in persons over age 70.

EDUCATIONAL VISUAL STANDARDS IN THE USA

Twelve percent of the pupils in elementary schools have significant eye difficulty, but no more than one in 1000 requires special educational facilities because of severe visual deficiencies. Although a medical examination is mandatory for school children in all states because of assessments required by Public Law 94-142, ophthalmologic examinations are seldom included. It has therefore been found necessary to devise procedures by which it will be possible, without a highly specialized staff, to give preliminary screening tests.

The Snellen test is the single most important test. Visual acuity tests may be given by nurses, parents, or trained volunteer teachers. Visual acuity testing of preschool children is far more important than visual acuity testing of school-age children. Testing should be performed as early as possible, preferably no later than 3½– 4 years of age.

Even if a child has a significant visual handicap, it is best to try regular school. If the student cannot keep up with regular schoolwork, special "sight-saving" classes are necessary.

Education of Visually Handicapped Children

Education must be provided for partially seeing pupils at all school levels. (For educational purposes, a partially seeing child is one who has a corrected visual acuity of 6/20 [20/70] or less in the better eye.) Experience indicates that it is best to establish the first class on an elementary school level, since the earlier help is given the better will be the prospect of success. In communities in which the school population is too small to warrant the establishment of more than one class, it may be advisable to give the advantages of the special class to children above the second grade, since much less close eye work is required in the first and second grades and a great deal of material in large, clear print is available for younger children. In general, well-motivated partially sighted children have good learning potential.

Education of Blind Children

Children with poor visual acuity who are unable to take advantage of ordinary visual educational methods are entered either in special schools for the blind, where emphasis is placed upon learning by touch (Braille), or (preferably) in integrated schools where facilities are available for special training but where the child is not deprived of all contact with normal persons in the same age group.

Allen MJ: *Vision and Highway Safety*. Chilton, 1970.

Blum HL et al: *Vision Screening for Elementary Schools*. Univ of California Press, 1968.

Cameron JH, Cameron M: Visual screening of pre-school children. *Br Med J* 1978;**1**:1693.

Committee on Rating of Mental and Physical Impairment: The visual system. Chapter 7 in: *Guides to the Evaluation of Permanent Impairment*. American Medical Association, 1971.

Gardiner PA: *Vision in Children*. Appleton-Century-Crofts, 1982.

Goble JL: *Visual Disorders in the Handicapped Child*. Marcel Dekker, 1984.

Hall SM, Pugh AG, Hall DM: Vision screening in the under-5s. *Br Med J* 1982;**285**:1096.

Harrington DO: *The Visual Fields: A Textbook and Atlas of Clinical Perimetry*, 5th ed. Mosby, 1981.

Helveston EM et al: Visual function and academic performance. *Am J Ophthalmol* 1985;**99**:346.

Moller MA: The visually handicapped child. *Pediatr Clin North Am* 1983;**30**:1185.

Potts AM: *The Assessment of Visual Function*. Mosby, 1972.

Appendix II:
Practical Factors in Illumination

The physical aspects of illumination discussed below are of practical interest to the physician who may be called upon to evaluate the adequacy of light sources in factories, shops, schoolrooms, and homes. Of principal interest is light **intensity,** conventionally measured in lux. One lux is equal to 1 lumen per square meter. Lux can be measured directly with special light meters.

Proper illumination minimizes eyestrain and increases the speed and efficiency of reading. Poor lighting does not cause eye disease but increases eye fatigue. The most common error students make in adjusting their lighting arrangement is to place a desk lamp opposite them on the desk. From this position the light is reflected into the reader's eyes, causing glare. For reading, the best light source is an incandescent or fluorescent lamp coming from above that produces a diffuse light with a minimum of glare and shadows. For writing, the light source should be so adjusted that the shadow of the arm and hand on the page is eliminated.

The most common sources of light are daylight, incandescent light, and fluorescent light. Daylight is an excellent light source but quite variable, and it is difficult to control its intensity. Incandescent lamps simulate daylight and provide a steady, diffuse flow of light. Ordinary fluorescent tubes operate on an alternating current that causes flickering, but it is possible to link 2 fluorescent tubes in a couple so adjusted that when one is on the up-phase the other is on the down-phase, thus eliminating the flicker.

Illumination Factors
Affecting Visibility

A. Intensity: The amount of illumination is directly related to reading efficiency. A reader employing 80 lux reads much more slowly and less efficiently than if a 500-lux source were utilized. The following minimum intensities are recommended (assuming that all undue reflections resulting in glare have been eliminated): reading black print on white paper, 500– 650 lux; schoolrooms, 500– 650 lux at the desk and 650– 800 lux at the blackboard; passageways, halls, and closets, 80 lux; eye charts, 1350– 1700 lux; operating room illumination at the point of surgery, 5000 lux.

There is a close relationship between a person's age and the magnification and illumination required. Because they have great powers of accommodation, children can read small print in semidarkness by hold-

ing the page close to their eyes. (This does not hurt the child's eyes although it may bother the parents.) On the other hand, a 48-year-old, slightly farsighted presbyope cannot read under ordinary illumination without magnifying glasses because the power of accommodation has been lost. Using a stronger light bulb or taking the printed material into sunlight makes reading possible in such cases. The presbyope also can improve visual performance by holding printed matter farther away. ("I need longer arms.")

The basic requirement in illumination is to have enough light to see by. Once this is accomplished, the intensity of illumination and the magnification (eyeglasses) can be adjusted to increase the efficiency of visual performance.

The intensity of light on an object is inversely proportionate to the square of the distance from the light source. Therefore, if a reading lamp 0.6 m (2 feet) from the page is moved to a distance of 1.2 m (4 feet), there will be 4 times less light on the page.

B. Contrast: It is much easier to read black letters on a white page than black letters on a blue page. Eye fatigue is minimized when the surroundings are about 30– 40% darker than the object being observed. Thus, in watching a television screen it is best not to have a completely darkened room.

C. Diffuseness: Shadows and spotlight phenomena should be avoided. However, diffuseness is overdone by manufacturers of indirect lighting fixtures. Indirect "reading lamps" are usually inadequate because of the vastly decreased amount of illumination on the printed page. This can be demonstrated by observing the unwarranted amount of light cast on the ceiling by the average indirect reading lamp.

D. Age of Subject: Illumination requirements and age are closely related, as evidenced by the increased illumination required by the 45-year-old presbyope compared with a teenage daughter. Although it is not recommended, children in the 7– 16 age group can read adequately in semidarkness, whereas the same person 30 years later may be able to read the telephone book only by "taking it to the window." Conversely, many people in the 50- to 65-year range who require full correction for their presbyopia can still read fine print without glasses in sunlight.

In general, illumination should be sufficient to perform the task at hand efficiently and comfortably.

Appendix III:
Rehabilitation of the Visually Handicapped & Special Services Available to the Blind

Although no completely reliable statistics are available, the most widely used estimates place the legally blind population of the USA at 2.24 per thousand (ie, approximately 500,000). Approximately 50,000 become legally blind annually, and many others have enough visual loss to constitute a serious employment problem.

Blindness does not necessarily imply helplessness. Individual adjustment to marked visual impairment or total blindness varies with age at onset, temperament, education, economic resources, and many other factors. The older patient, for example, may accept blindness quite stoically, whereas for the younger patient the vocational or social impact of blindness is often catastrophic. Blindness is accepted more easily by persons who are born blind and by persons of any age who lose their vision gradually rather than suddenly.

The responsibility of the physician clearly does not end with the diagnosis, prevention, and treatment of ocular disorders that might result in blindness. The physician caring for the patient who is suddenly faced with actual or imminent blindness is in a position to be of great assistance. When blindness is a possibility but is not inevitable (eg, during acute ocular inflammation), optimism and reassurance are warranted. However, it is unwise to offer false hopes or to delay "breaking the news" when blindness is inevitable. If it is certain that blindness will occur, it is important to extend to the distraught patient as well as to the patient's family the warmth, understanding, encouragement, and assistance so desperately needed. The physician should be alert to the severe depressive reactions that may occur.

It is especially important to assist the patient in making the adjustment to blindness while some vision is still present. Early referral to rehabilitation agencies is essential for recently blinded adults and those with irreversible progressive visual loss. Training programs or reeducation for the many changes involved in daily living and employment are greatly simplified if the patient has the partial support provided by even limited vision.

It may be valuable to have the patient talk with a blind person who has made a satisfactory adjustment to blindness.

Many special services are available for blind persons. The aim of the rehabilitation program is to enable the patient to lead as nearly normal a life as possible. Approximately 5000 blind persons in the USA are rehabilitated and obtain paid employment each year. An additional larger number of blind homemakers are able to perform their household duties without assistance or are able to live independently of others.

The physician should work actively with both the patient and the family and with other professional people concerned with rendering services to the blind.

Rehabilitation must be individualized. Guide dogs, for example, may be extremely valuable for certain persons but totally unsatisfactory for others. The methods of sightless reading and writing must be adapted to the capabilities, needs, and preferences of each patient. Mobility training is most important; several universities* have undergraduate and postgraduate programs in mobility training for the blind.

State Services

The physician should be familiar with the many special services available to the blind. Services vary from state to state but may be illustrated by the diversified programs for the blind conducted by the State of California.†

A. Educational Services for the Blind:

1. California School for the Blind–A residential school for general education from kindergarten through the secondary grades; also provides field service, guidance, and assistance to preschool children and students in advanced courses.

2. California State Library–A repository for magazines and books in raised type (Moon and Braille), talking books and machines for use with the books, casettes and tapes, games adapted for use by the blind, and writing appliances. These materials may be secured directly from the library or by mail (postage-free).

3. Office of Special Education–Coordinates the establishment and operation of special public school programs for visually handicapped children throughout the state. This program enables blind and partially seeing students to live at home and attend school with normal children.

---

*Undergraduate level programs are at Cleveland State University in Ohio, Florida State University in Florida, and Stephen F. Austin University in Texas. Graduate programs are at Boston University, California State University (Los Angeles), Northern Colorado University, San Francisco State University, University of Arkansas, University of Wisconsin, and Western Michigan State University.

†The services referred to are those provided by public-sponsored agencies for the blind and do not include the many religious organizations, private or voluntary health and welfare agencies, sheltered workshops, and community and recreational facilities.

4. Clearinghouse Depository for Handicapped Students–Instructional aids for visually handicapped students in public or nonprofit private schools that comply with the Civil Rights Act. Also serves as a referral service on educational materials for visually handicapped students.

B. Reader Services for Blind Students: Provides reader services for blind students in high schools, junior colleges, vocational training schools, colleges, and universities.

C. Rehabilitation Services for the Blind:

1. Field rehabilitation services–Counselor-teachers provide services to the blind within their homes or in hospitals and other institutions so that individuals may learn the skills necessary to meet the demands of daily living. Counseling in adjustment to blindness is given to the visually disabled person and the family.

2. Orientation Center for the Blind (State of California Department of Rehabilitation)–Provides intensive orientation and prevocational training, including training in techniques of daily living and travel, physical conditioning, sensory training, instruction in Braille, typing, and business methods, and training in hand and machine work, homemaking, and other vocationally useful skills. Limited residence facilities are available.

3. Vocational Rehabilitation Service–Provides, for the adult blind, vocational counseling to help work out suitable employment objectives, supervised vocational training, and job placement. The following services may also be provided if needed for employment and if the applicant is unable to pay for them: medical and surgical treatment, including hospitalization; prosthetic appliances and glasses; maintenance and transportation while undergoing treatment or training; and tools or equipment needed in training, job placement, or self-employment.

4. Business enterprise program–Assists blind persons to establish and operate vending stands, snack bars, and cafeteria or other businesses they may be qualified to operate.

D. Social Welfare Programs for the Blind:

1. Supplemental Security Income (SSI)–Financial assistance paid by state and federal governments to blind persons who, because of loss or impairment of sight, are unable to provide themselves with the necessities of life.

2. Aid to Potentially Self-Supporting Blind–Financial assistance by the county and state to the adult blind who, because of loss or impairment of sight, are unable fully to provide themselves with the necessities of life but who are working on a plan for self-support.

3. Prevention of Blindness–A program designed to prevent blindness or restore vision by providing necessary medical or surgical treatment through MediCal (Medicaid in other states) and other federal, state, and local funds.

4. Counseling and support programs–County Social Service Departments provide help to visually handicapped persons through locating needed services and, when necessary, paying for in-home chore workers.

E. Provisions for Prevention of Blindness, Preventive Medicine Services Branch (California State Department of Health):

1. Prevention of blindness in newborn infants–Enforces legal requirement of (1) silver nitrate or antibiotic prophylaxis for the eyes as a preventive measure against ophthalmia neonatorum; (2) prenatal serologic test of parents for syphilis; and (3) control of excessive use of oxygen in the care of premature infants as a preventive measure against retinopathy of prematurity.

2. Control of communicable diseases apt to cause loss of vision–Requires reporting, isolation, treatment, and control of ophthalmia neonatorum, trachoma, and syphilis.

3. Aid to Physically Handicapped Children (California Children's Service)–Provides for the necessary medical care of children suffering from eye conditions leading to loss of vision if the parents or legal guardians are unable to meet these costs in whole or in part.

F. Guide Dogs for the Blind: The State Board of Guide Dogs for the Blind (California State Department of Consumer Affairs) was established for the purpose of ensuring that guide dogs are trained and that their owners also are trained to use the dogs as guides. Minimum requirements, licensing, and supervision of guide dog schools are functions of the Board.

National Services

The following organizations will provide information and send literature and catalogs upon request:

(1) American Foundation for the Blind, 15 West 16th Street, New York 10011. Provides information on almost all phases of problems of the blind; sells special watches, home appliances, etc, for the blind.

(2) American Printing House for the Blind, 1839 Frankfort Avenue, PO Box 6085, Louisville, Kentucky 40206-0085. Prints and sells Braille publications.

(3) Guide Dogs for the Blind, Inc., PO Box 1200, San Rafael, California 94915. Training of guide dogs and training of blind persons to use dogs as guides.

(4) The Hadley School for the Blind, Inc., 700 Elm Street, Winnetka, Illinois 60093. Provides free home-study courses from elementary level into college, vocational and avocational training, Braille and other useful skills. Accredited by National Home Study Council, National Accreditation Council, and North Central Association of Colleges and Schools. Affiliate member of National University Extension Association.

(5) Howe Press of Perkins School for the Blind, 175 North Beacon Street, Watertown, Massachusetts 02172. Manufactures and distributes internationally the Perkins Brailler (portable Braille typewriter) and Braille paper. Also children's stories in a special Braille

edition, games, mathematical aids, Braille maps, music, and Braille writing appliances.

(6) Library of Congress. Extensive collection of books and magazines in Braille, on disk, and on cassette available free to visually impaired US citizens. Materials and playback equipment are distributed through a system of network libraries in each state. (Consult local library for specific addresses.) Music materials only are circulated directly from the Library (Division for the Blind and Physically Handicapped, 1291 Taylor Street, NW, Washington, DC 20542).

(7) Rehabilitation Services Administration, Bureau for the Blind and Visually Handicapped, US Department of Health and Human Services, Washington, DC 20201. Conducts a nationwide program for the vocational rehabilitation of the blind; provides pamphlets and other information regarding rehabilitation services available to the blind.

(8) *Readers Digest*. Publishes *Readers Digest* in Braille and on records for the Talking Book; may be secured from the American Printing House for the Blind.

(9) Recording for the Blind, Inc., 215 East 58th Street, New York 10022. Records textbooks and educational materials free of charge for blind persons for educational, vocational, or professional use.

(10) The Seeing Eye, Inc., PO Box 375, Morristown, New Jersey 07960. First organization in USA to provide guide dogs for qualified blind persons (1929).

(11) Central Rehabilitation Section for Visually Impaired and Blinded Veterans (117A), Veterans Administration Hospital, Hines, Illinois 60141. Provides rehabilitation program lasting up to 18 weeks for veterans. Low vision and blind centers also located at Veterans Administration Hospitals in West Haven, Connecticut, and Palo Alto, California. Round trip transportation of veteran generally paid by Veterans Administration.

(12) Xavier Society for the Blind, 154 East 23rd Street, New York 10010, provides free periodical and library service in Braille, large print, and cassette or open reel tape recordings to any interested blind or partially sighted reader. Catalogs available on request.

(13) Louis Braille Foundation for Blind Musicians, Inc., 215 Park Avenue South, New York 10003. A national, nonprofit clearinghouse for professional blind musicians and composers. It transcribes and copyrights musical works; provides publicity and promotion; sponsors concerts; provides musical instruments, Braille music, and special equipment for needy musicians; sponsors the LBF Artists' Bureau; and provides scholarship aid.

American Foundation for the Blind. 1976–77 Catalog of Publications.

Carroll TJ: *Blindness*. Little, Brown, 1961.

Cholden L: *Psychiatric Aspects of Informing the Patient of Blindness*. American Academy of Ophthalmology and Otolaryngology, Instruction Section, Course No. 221, 1953.

Cholden L: *Some Psychiatric Problems in the Rehabilitation of the Blind*. Bulletin of the Menninger Clinic, Vol. 18, No. 3, May 1954.

Faye EE (editor): *Clinical Low Vision*, 2nd ed. Little, Brown, 1984.

Gloor B, Brückner R: *Rehabilitation of the Visually Disabled and the Blind at Different Ages*. University Park Press, 1980.

Hoehne CW, Cull JG, Hardy RE: *Ophthalmological Considerations in the Rehabilitation of the Blind*. Thomas, 1980.

If Blindness Occurs. The Seeing Eye, Inc.

Mallinson GG (editor): *Blindness 1977–78*. American Association of Workers for the Blind, Inc., 1978.

Sekuler R, Kline D, Dismukes K: *Aging and Human Visual Function*. Alan R. Liss, 1982.

Stetten D Jr: Coping with blindness. *N Engl J Med* 1981; **305**:458.

US Department of Health, Education and Welfare: *Support for Vision Research: Interim Report of the National Advisory Eye Council, 1976*. National Institutes of Health, DHEW Publication No. (NIH) 76-1098.

Glossary of Terms Relating to the Eye*†

Accommodation: The adjustment of the eye for seeing at different distances, accomplished by changing the shape of the lens through action of the ciliary muscle, thus focusing a clear image on the retina.

Agnosia: Inability to recognize common objects despite an intact visual apparatus.

Albinism: A hereditary deficiency of pigment in the retinal pigment epithelium, iris, and choroid.

Amaurosis fugax: Transient recurrent unilateral loss of vision.

Amblyopia: Reduced visual acuity (uncorrectable with lenses) in the absence of detectable anatomic defect in the eye or visual pathways.

Ametropia: See Refractive error.

Aniridia: Congenital absence of the iris.

Aniseikonia: A condition in which the image seen by one eye differs in size or shape from that seen by the other.

Anisometropia: Difference in refractive error of the eyes, eg, one eye hyperopic and the other myopic.

Anophthalmos: Absence of a true eyeball.

Anterior chamber: Space filled with aqueous bounded anteriorly by the cornea and posteriorly by the iris.

Aphakia: Absence of the lens.

Aqueous: Clear, watery fluid that fills the anterior and posterior chambers.

Asthenopia: Eye fatigue caused by tiring.

Astigmatism: Refractive error that prevents the light rays from coming to a single focus on the retina because of different degrees of refraction in the various meridians of the cornea.

Binocular vision: Ability of the eyes to focus on one object and to fuse the 2 images into one.

Blepharitis: Inflammation of the eyelids.

Blepharoptosis: Drooping of the eyelid.

Blepharospasm: Involuntary spasm of the lids.

Blind spot: ''Blank'' area in the visual field, corresponding to the light rays that come to a focus on the optic nerve.

Blindness: In the USA, the usual definition of blindness is corrected visual acuity of 6/60 (20/200) or less in the better eye, or a visual field of no more than 20 degrees in the better eye.

Buphthalmos: Large eyeball in infantile glaucoma.

Canal of Schlemm: A circular modified venous structure in the anterior chamber angle.

Canaliculus: Small tear drainage tube in inner aspect of upper and lower lids leading from the puncta to the common canaliculus and then to the tear sac.

Canthus: The angle at either end of the eyelid aperture; specified as outer and inner.

Cataract: A lens opacity.

Cataract extraction: Removal of a cataract, either by removal of the lens complete with its capsule (intracapsular cataract extraction), or by removal of the lens contents after opening the capsule (extracapsular cataract extraction).

Chalazion: Granulomatous inflammation of a meibomian gland.

Chemosis: Conjunctival edema.

Choroid: The vascular middle coat between the retina and sclera.

Ciliary body: Portion of the uveal tract between the iris and the choroid. It consists of ciliary processes and the ciliary muscle.

Coloboma: Congenital cleft due to the failure of some portion of the eye or ocular adnexa to complete growth.

Color blindness: Diminished ability to perceive differences in color.

Concave lens: Lens having the power to diverge rays of light; also known as diverging, reducing, negative, myopic, or minus lens, denoted by the sign (−).

Cones and rods: Two kinds of retinal receptor cells. Cones are concerned with visual acuity and color discrimination; rods, with peripheral vision under decreased illumination.

Conjunctiva: Mucous membrane that lines the posterior aspect of the eyelids and the anterior sclera.

Convergence: The process of directing the visual axes of the eyes to a near point.

*Modified and reproduced, with permission, from Publication 172 of the National Society for the Prevention of Blindness, Inc.
†See also Definitions of Strabismus, Chapter 16, and Glossary of Genetic Terms, Chapter 22.

Convex lens: Lens having power to converge rays of light and to bring them to a focus; also known as converging, magnifying, hyperopic, or plus lens, denoted by the sign (+).

Cornea: Transparent portion of the outer coat of the eyeball forming the anterior wall of the aqueous chamber.

Corneal contact lenses: Thin lenses that fit directly on the cornea under the eyelids.

Corneal graft (keratoplasty): Operation to restore vision by replacing a section of opaque cornea with transparent cornea, either involving the full thickness of the cornea (penetrating keratoplasty) or only a superficial layer (lamellar keratoplasty).

Cover test: A method of determining the presence and degree of phoria or tropia by covering one eye with an opaque object, thus eliminating fusion.

Crystalline lens: A semi-transparent biconvex structure suspended in the eyeball between the aqueous and the vitreous. Its function is to bring rays of light to a focus on the retina. Accommodation is produced by variations in the magnitude of this effect. (Now usually called simply the lens.)

Cycloplegic: A drug that temporarily puts the ciliary muscle at rest, paralyzing accommodation.

Cylindric lens: A segment of a cylinder the refractive power of which varies in different meridians.

Dacryocystitis: Infection of the lacrimal sac.

Dark adaptation: The ability to adjust to decreased illumination.

Diopter: Unit of measurement of strength of refractive power of lenses or of prisms.

Diplopia: Seeing one object as two.

"E" test: A system of testing visual acuity in illiterates, particularly preschool children.

Ectropion: Turning out of the eyelid.

Emmetropia: Absence of refractive error.

Endophthalmitis: Extensive intraocular infection.

Enophthalmos: Abnormal retrodisplacement of the eyeball.

Entropion: A turning inward of the eyelid.

Enucleation: Complete surgical removal of the eyeball.

Epiphora: Tearing.

Esophoria: A tendency of the eyes to turn inward.

Esotropia: A manifest inward deviation of the eyes.

Evisceration: Removal of the contents of the eyeball.

Exenteration: Removal of the entire contents of the orbit, including the eyeball and lids.

Exophoria: A tendency of the eyes to turn outward.

Exophthalmos: Abnormal protrusion of the eyeball.

Exotropia: A manifest outward deviation of one or both eyes.

Farsightedness: See Hyperopia.

Field of vision: The entire area that can be seen without shifting the gaze.

Floaters: Small dark particles in the vitreous.

Focus: The point to which rays are converged after passing through a lens; focal distance is the distance between the lens and the focal point.

Fornix: The junction of the palpebral and bulbar conjunctiva.

Fovea: Depression in the macula adapted for most acute vision.

Fundus: The posterior portion of the eye visible through an ophthalmoscope.

Fusion: Coordinating the images received by the 2 eyes into one image.

Glaucoma: Disease characterized by abnormally increased intraocular pressure, optic atrophy, and loss of visual field.

Gonioscopy: A technique of examining the anterior chamber angle, utilizing a corneal contact lens, magnifying device, and light source.

Hemianopia: Blindness of one-half the field of vision of one or both eyes.

Heterophoria (phoria): A tendency of the eyes to deviate.

Heterotropia: See Strabismus.

Hippus: Exaggerated spontaneous rhythmic movements of the iris.

Hordeolum, external (sty): Infection of the glands of Moll or Zeis.

Hordeolum, internal: Meibomian gland infection.

Hyperopia, hypermetropia (farsightedness): A refractive error in which the focal point of light rays from a distant object is behind the retina.

Hyperphoria: A tendency of the eyes to deviate upward.

Hypertropia: A manifest deviation of one eye in relation to the other.

Hyphema: Blood in the anterior chamber.

Hypopyon: Pus in the anterior chamber.

Hypotony: Abnormally soft eye from any cause.

Injection: Congestion of blood vessels.

Iris: Colored, circular membrane, suspended behind the cornea and immediately in front of the lens.

Ishihara color plates: A test for color vision based on the ability to trace patterns in a series of multicolored charts.

Jaeger test: A test for near vision using lines of various sizes of type.

Keratoconus: Cone-shaped deformity of the cornea.

Keratomalacia: Corneal softening, usually associated with avitaminosis A.

Keratoplasty: See Corneal graft.

Keratoprosthesis: Plastic implant surgically placed in an opaque cornea to achieve an area of optical clarity.

Lacrimal sac: The dilated area at the junction of the nasolacrimal duct and the canaliculi.

Lens: A refractive medium having one or both surfaces curved. (See also Crystalline lens.)

Leukoma: Dense corneal opacity due to any cause.

Limbus: Junction of the cornea and sclera.

Macula: Moderately dense corneal opacity due to any cause.

Macula lutea: The small avascular area of the retina surrounding the fovea.

Metamorphopsia: Wavy distortion of vision.

Microphthalmos: Abnormal smallness of the eyeball.

Miotic: A drug causing pupillary constriction.

Mydriatic: A drug causing pupillary dilatation.

Myopia (nearsightedness): A refractive error in which the focal point for light rays from a distant object is anterior to the retina.

Nearsightedness: See Myopia.

Nebula: Slight corneal opacity due to any cause.

Nystagmus: An involuntary, rapid movement of the eyeball that may be horizontal, vertical, rotatory, or mixed.

Oculist or ophthalmologist: Terms used interchangeably; a physician who is a specialist in diseases of the eye.

Ophthalmia neonatorum: Conjunctivitis in the newborn.

Ophthalmoscope: An instrument with a special illumination system for viewing the inner eye, particularly the retina and associated structures.

Optic atrophy: Optic nerve degeneration.

Optic disk: Ophthalmoscopically visible portion of the optic nerve.

Optic nerve: The nerve that carries visual impulses from the retina to the brain.

Optician: One who makes or deals in eyeglasses or other optical instruments and who fills prescriptions for glasses.

Optometrist: A nonmedical person trained in the measurement of refraction of the eye.

Orthoptist: One who gives training to those with ocular muscle imbalances.

Oscillopsia: The subjective illusion of movement of objects that occurs with some types of nystagmus.

Palpebral: Pertaining to the eyelid.

Pannus: Infiltration of the cornea with blood vessels.

Papilledema: Swelling of the optic disk.

Partially seeing child: For educational purposes, a partially seeing child is one who has a corrected visual acuity of 6/20 (20/70) or less in the better eye.

Perimeter: An instrument for measuring the field of vision.

Peripheral vision: Ability to perceive the presence, motion, or color of objects outside of the direct line of vision.

Phoria: See Heterophoria.

Photocoagulation: A method of causing artificial inflammation of the retina and choroid for treatment of certain types of retinal disorders, particularly retinal detachment.

Photophobia: Abnormal sensitivity to light.

Photopsia: Appearance of sparks or flashes within the eye due to retinal irritation.

Phthisis bulbi: Atrophy of the eyeball with blindness and decreased intraocular pressure, due to end-stage intraocular disease.

Posterior chamber: Space filled with aqueous anterior to the lens and posterior to the iris.

Presbyopia ("old sight"): Physiologically blurred near vision, commonly evident soon after age 40, due to reduction in the power of accommodation.

Pseudoisochromatic charts: Charts with colored dots of various hues and shades forming numbers, letters, or patterns, used for testing color discrimination.

Pseudophakia: Presence of an artificial intraocular lens implant following cataract extraction.

Pterygium: A triangular growth of tissue that extends from the conjunctiva over the cornea.

Ptosis: Drooping of the eyelid.

Puncta: External orifices of the upper and lower canaliculi.

Pupil: The round hole in the center of the iris that corresponds to the lens aperture in a camera.

Refraction: (1) Deviation in the course of rays of light in passing from one transparent medium into another of different density. (2) Determination of refractive errors of the eye and correction by glasses.

Refractive error (ametropia): A defect that prevents light rays from being brought to a single focus on the retina.

Refractive media: The transparent parts of the eye having refractive power.

Retina: Innermost coat of the eye, consisting of the sensory retina, which is composed of light-sensitive neural elements connecting to other neural cells, and the pigment epithelium.

Retinal detachment: A separation of the retina from the choroid.

Retinitis pigmentosa: A hereditary degeneration and atrophy of the retina.

Retinoscope: An instrument specially designed for the objective aspect of refraction.

Rods: See Cones and rods.

Sclera: The white part of the eye—a tough covering that, with the cornea, forms the external protective coat of the eye.

Scotoma: A blind or partially blind area in the visual field.

Slit lamp: A combination light and microscope for examination of the eye, principally the anterior segment.

Snellen chart: Used for testing central visual acuity. It consists of lines of letters or numbers, in graded sizes drawn to Snellen measurements.

Strabismus (heterotropia, tropia): A manifest deviation of the eyes.

Sty: See Hordeolum, external.

Sympathetic ophthalmia: Inflammation in one eye following traumatic inflammation in the fellow eye.

Synechia: Adhesion of the iris to cornea (anterior synechia) or lens (posterior synechia).

Syneresis: Degenerative process within a gel, involving a drawing together of particles of the dispersed medium, separation of the medium, and shrinkage of the gel.

Tonometer: An instrument for measuring intraocular pressure.

Trachoma: Serious infectious keratoconjunctivitis.

Tropia: See Strabismus.

Uvea (uveal tract): The iris, ciliary body, and choroid.

Uveitis: Inflammation of one or all portions of the uveal tract.

Visual acuity: Detailed central vision, as in reading.

Vitreous: Transparent, colorless mass of soft, gelatinous material filling the eyeball behind the lens.

Zonule: The numerous fine tissue strands that stretch from the ciliary processes to the lens equator (360 degrees) and hold the lens in place.

Zonulolysis: Lysis of the zonule, as with chymotrypsin, to facilitate removal of the lens in cataract surgery.

Index

Lange Medical Books are available at medical bookstores within the United States.
To order directly from the publisher, complete and mail the postage-paid card below.

BASIC SCIENCE TEXTBOOKS

1. **Correlative Neuroanatomy & Functional Neurology, 19th Ed.,** *Chusid,* A0001-6, $21.50
2. **Biochemistry: A Synopsis,** *Colby,* A0033-9, $14.00
3. **Review of Medical Physiology, 13th Ed.,** *Ganong,* A8435-8, $24.00
4. **Physiology: A Study Guide,** *Ganong,* A0032-1, $13.00
5. **Review of Medical Microbiology, 17th Ed.,** *Jawetz et al.,* A8432-5, $22.00
6. **Basic Histology, 5th Ed.,** *Junquiera et al.,* A0570-0, $24.00
7. **Basic & Clinical Pharmacology, 3rd Ed.,** *Katzung,* A0553-6, $29.50
8. **Pharmacology: A Review,** *Katzung and Trevor,* A0031-3, $14.00
9. **Harper's Review of Biochemistry, 20th Ed.,** *Martin et al.,* A0003-2, $27.50
10. **Basic & Clinical Immunology, 6th Ed.,** *Stites et al.,* A0548-6, $29.00

CLINICAL SCIENCE TEXTBOOKS

11. **Principles of Clinical Electrocardiography, 12th Ed.,** *Goldman,* A0008-1, $22.00
12. **Review of General Psychiatry,** *Goldman,* A0030-5, $27.50
13. **Electrocardiography: Essentials of Interpretation,** *Goldschlager and Goldman,* A0029-7, $16.50
14. **Basic & Clinical Endocrinology, 2nd Ed.,** *Greenspan and Forsham,* A0547-8, $27.00
15. **General Urology, 11th Ed.,** *Smith,* A0009-9, $28.00

16. **Clinical Cardiology, 4th Ed.,** *Sokolow and McIlroy,* A0023-0, $26.50
17. **General Ophthalmology, 11th Ed.,** *Vaughan and Asbury,* A3108-6, $23.50

CURRENT CLINICAL REFERENCES

18. **Current Obstetric & Gynecologic Diagnosis & Treatment, 6th Ed.,** *Pernoll and Benson,* A1412-4, $31.50
19. **Current Pediatric Diagnosis & Treatment, 9th Ed.,** *Kempe et al.,* A1414-0, $31.50
20. **Current Medical Diagnosis & Treatment 1987, 26th Ed.,** *Krupp et al.,* A1413-2, $32.50
21. **Current Emergency Diagnosis & Treatment, 2nd Ed.,** *Mills et al.,* A0027-1, $29.50
22. **Current Surgical Diagnosis & Treatment, 7th Ed.,** *Way,* A0019-8, $34.00

HANDBOOKS

23. **Handbook of Obstetrics & Gynecology, 8th Ed.,** *Benson,* A0014-9, $13.00
24. **Handbook of Poisoning, 12th Ed.,** *Dreisbach and Robertson,* A3643-2 $16.50
25. **Physician's Handbook, 21st Ed.,** *Krupp et al.,* A0002-4, $16.50
26. **Handbook of Pediatrics, 15th Ed.,** *Silver et al.,* A3635-8, $16.50

ORDER CARD

Please send the books I've circled below on 30-day approval:

1. Chusid, A0001-6, $21.50	10. Stites, A0548-6, $29.00	19. Kempe, A1414-0, $31.50
2. Colby, A0033-9, $14.00	11. Goldman, A0008-1, $22.00	20. Krupp, A1413-2, $32.50
3. Ganong, A8435-8, $24.00	12. Goldman, A0030-5, $27.50	21. Mills, A0027-1, $29.50
4. Ganong, A0032-1, $13.00	13. Goldschlager, A0029-7, $16.50	22. Way, A0019-8, $34.00
5. Jawetz, A8432-5, $22.00	14. Greenspan, A0547-8, $27.00	23. Benson, A0014-9, $13.00
6. Junquiera, A0570-0, $24.00	15. Smith, A0009-9, $28.00	24. Dreisbach, A3643-2, $16.50
7. Katzung, A0553-6, $29.50	16. Sokolow, A0023-0, $26.50	25. Krupp, A0002-4, $16.50
8. Katzung, A0031-3, $14.00	17. Vaughan, A3108-6, $23.50	26. Silver, A3635-8, $16.50
9. Martin, A0003-2, $27.50	18. Pernoll, A1412-4, $31.50	

☐ Payment enclosed. (Publisher pays postage & handling.)
  Please include your state sales tax.
☐ Bill me later.
Charge to: ☐ VISA ☐ Mastercard

Card #_____ Exp. Date_____

Signature_____

NAME_____

ADDRESS_____

CITY/STATE/ZIP_____

APPLETON & LANGE
Combining the houses of Appleton-Century-Crofts
and Lange Medical Publications.
25 Van Zant St.
E. Norwalk, CT 06855

NO POSTAGE
NECESSARY
IF MAILED
IN THE
UNITED STATES

BUSINESS REPLY MAIL
FIRST CLASS PERMIT NO. 150 E. NORWALK, CT

POSTAGE WILL BE PAID BY ADDRESSEE

APPLETON & LANGE

DEPARTMENT B.
25 VAN ZANT STREET
EAST NORWALK, CT 06855